Lecture Notes in Artificial Intelligence 9414

Subseries of Lecture Notes in Computer Science

More information about this series at http://www.springer.com/series/1244

Obdulia Pichardo Lagunas · Oscar Herrera Alcántara
Gustavo Arroyo Figueroa (Eds.)

Advances in Artificial Intelligence and Its Applications

14th Mexican International Conference
on Artificial Intelligence, MICAI 2015
Cuernavaca, Morelos, Mexico, October 25–31, 2015
Proceedings, Part II

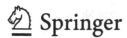

Springer

Editors
Obdulia Pichardo Lagunas
Unidad Profesional Interdisciplinaria
México, DF
Mexico

Gustavo Arroyo Figueroa
Instituto de Investigaciones Eléctricas
Cuernavaca, Morelos
Mexico

Oscar Herrera Alcántara
Universidad Autónoma Metropolitana
México, DF
Mexico

ISSN 0302-9743   ISSN 1611-3349 (electronic)
Lecture Notes in Artificial Intelligence
ISBN 978-3-319-27100-2   ISBN 978-3-319-27101-9   (eBook)
DOI 10.1007/978-3-319-27101-9

Library of Congress Control Number: 2015955367

LNCS Sublibrary: SL7 – Artificial Intelligence

Printed on acid-free paper

Springer International Publishing AG Switzerland is part of Springer Science+Business Media
(www.springer.com)

Preface

The Mexican International Conference on Artificial Intelligence (MICAI) is a yearly international conference series organized by the Mexican Society of Artificial Intelligence (SMIA) since 2000. MICAI is a major international artificial intelligence forum and the main event in the academic life of the country's growing artificial intelligence community.

MICAI conferences publish high-quality papers in all areas of artificial intelligence and its applications. The proceedings of the previous MICAI events have been published by Springer in its *Lecture Notes in Artificial Intelligence* series, vol. 1793, 2313, 2972, 3789, 4293, 4827, 5317, 5845, 6437, 6438, 7094, 7095, 7629, 7630, 8265, 8266, 8856, and 8857. Since its foundation in 2000, the conference has been growing in popularity and improving in quality.

The proceedings of MICAI 2015 are published in two volumes. The first volume, *Advances in Artificial Intelligence and Soft Computing*, contains 46 papers structured into eight sections:

- Invited Paper
- Natural Language Processing
- Logic and Multi-agent Systems
- Bioinspired Algorithms
- Neural Networks
- Evolutionary Algorithms
- Fuzzy Logic
- Machine Learning and Data Mining

The second volume, *Advances in Artificial Intelligence and Its Applications*, contains 46 papers structured into eight sections:

- Invited Papers
- Natural Language Processing Applications
- Educational Applications
- Biomedical Applications
- Image Processing and Computer Vision
- Search and Optimization
- Forecasting
- Intelligent Applications

This two-volume set will be of interest for researchers in all areas of artificial intelligence, students specializing in related topics, and the general public interested in recent developments in artificial intelligence.

The conference received for evaluation 297 submissions by 667 authors from 34 countries: Argentina, Australia, Brazil, Canada, Chile, China, Colombia, Cuba, Czech Republic, Ecuador, France, Germany, India, Iran, Israel, Italy, Japan, Kazakhstan,

Table 1. Distribution of papers by topics

Track	Submitted	Accepted	Rate
Applications	73	29	40 %
Pattern Recognition	58	15	26 %
Machine Learning	54	18	33 %
Data Mining	46	21	46 %
Natural Language Processing	41	15	37 %
Computer Vision and Image Processing	38	9	24 %
Genetic Algorithms	35	13	37 %
Expert Systems and Knowledge-Based Systems	30	6	20 %
Knowledge Representation and Management	30	12	40 %
Neural Networks	27	10	37 %
Hybrid Intelligent Systems	21	10	48 %
Planning and Scheduling	20	4	20 %
Fuzzy Logic	18	7	39 %
Robotics	18	5	28 %
Bioinformatics and Medical Applications	17	5	29 %
Multi-agent Systems and Distributed AI	14	2	14 %
Ontologies	13	5	38 %
Sentiment Analysis and Opinion Mining	12	2	17 %
Constraint Programming	10	6	60 %
Knowledge Acquisition	9	3	33 %
Intelligent Tutoring Systems	8	5	62 %
Uncertainty and Probabilistic Reasoning	8	4	50 %
Logic Programming	7	5	71 %
Intelligent Interfaces: Multimedia, Virtual Reality	5	2	40 %
Intelligent Organizations	4	–	–
Automated Theorem Proving	3	2	67 %
Spatial and Temporal Reasoning	3	2	67 %
Case-Based Reasoning	2	1	50 %
Model-Based Reasoning	2	2	100 %
Non-monotonic Reasoning	1	–	–
Philosophical and Methodological Issues of AI	1	–	–
Qualitative Reasoning	1	1	100 %

Mexico, Pakistan, Peru, Poland, Portugal, Romania, Russia, Saudi Arabia, Slovakia, Spain, Switzerland, Taiwan, Tunisia, Turkey, UK, and USA; the distribution of papers by topics is shown in Table 1. Of those submissions, 89 papers were selected for publication in these two volumes after a peer-reviewing process carried out by the international Program Committee. The acceptance rate was 29.9 %.

In addition to regular papers, the volumes contain three invited papers by the keynote speakers Alexander Gelbukh (Mexico), Gennady Osipov (Russia), and Zita Vale (Portugal).

The international Program Committee consisted of 172 experts from 27 countries: Australia, Azerbaijan, Belgium, Brazil, Canada, Colombia, Czech Republic, Denmark, Finland, France, Germany, Greece, India, Israel, Italy, Japan, Mexico, New Zealand, Poland, Russia, Singapore, Spain, Sweden, Switzerland, Turkey, UK, and USA.

MICAI 2014 was honored by the presence of renowned experts who gave excellent keynote lectures:

- Alexander Gelbukh, Instituto Politécnico Nacional, Mexico
- Gennady Osipov, Higher School of Economics, Russia
- Paolo Rosso, Universitat Politècnica de València, Spain
- Ruslan Salakhutdinov, University of Toronto, Canada
- Juan M. Torres Moreno, Université d'Avignon et des Pays de Vaucluse, France
- Zita Vale, Politécnico do Porto, Portugal

The technical program of the conference also featured tutorials presented by Roman Barták (Czech Republic), Ildar Batyrshin (Mexico), Alexander Gelbukh (Mexico), Isai Rojas González (Mexico), Luis Enrique Sucar (Mexico), Zita Vale (Portugal), and Ivan Zelinka (Czech Republic), among others. Four workshops were held jointly with the conference: the 8th Workshop on Hybrid Intelligent Systems, HIS 2015; the 8th Workshop on Intelligent Learning Environments, WILE 2015; the Second International Workshop on Recognizing Textual Entailment and Question Answering, RTE-QA 2015; and the First International Workshop on Intelligent Decision Support Systems (DSS) for Industry Application.

The authors of the following papers received the Best Paper Award based on the paper's overall quality, significance, and originality of the reported results:

First place:	"Detecting Social Spammers in Colombia 2014 Presidential Election," by Jhon Adrián Cerón-Guzmán and Elizabeth León (Colombia)
	Prize from Springer: € 400; prize from SMIA: € 400
Second place:	"Dynamic Systems Identification and Control by Means of Complex-Valued Recurrent Neural Networks," by Ieroham Baruch, Victor Arellano Quintana, and Edmundo Pérez Reynaud (Mexico)
	Prize from Springer: € 300; prize from SMIA: € 300
Third place:	"Inferring Sentiment-Based Priors in Topic Models," by Elena Tutubalina and Sergey Nikolenko (Russia)
	Prize from Springer: € 200; prize from SMIA: € 200

The authors of the following paper selected among all papers of which the first author was a full-time student, excluding the papers listed above, received the Best Student Paper Award:

First place:	"Place Recognition-Based Visual Localization Using LBP Feature and SVM," by Yongliang Qiao, Cindy Cappelle, and Yassine Ruichek (France)
	Prize from Springer: € 100; prize from SMIA: € 100

The awards included significant monetary prizes sponsored by Springer and by the Mexican Society of Artificial Intelligent (SMIA).

We want to thank everyone involved in the organization of this conference. In the first place, the authors of the papers published in this book: it is their research work that gives value to the book and to the work of the organizers. We thank the track chairs for their hard work, the Program Committee members, and the additional reviewers for their great effort spent on reviewing the submissions.

We would like to thank the Polytechnic University of Morelos (Upemor) for hosting the workshops and tutorials of MICAI 2015; in particular, we thank Dr. Mireya Gally Jordá, the rector of the university, and Dr. Yadira Toledo, the academic secretary, for their support and generosity. We also thank the Tecnológico de Monterrey Campus Cuernavaca for the hospitality and for opening its doors to the participants of MICAI 2015; we would especially like to thank Dr. Mónica Larre, the director of professional studies, for her support. We thank the INAH Delegación Morelos, Secretary of Culture of Morelos, and Secretary of Tourism of Morelos, particularly Mr. Manuel Zepeda Mata, Ministry of Promotion of the Arts, and Mr. Sergio Perea Garza, Director for Tourism, for their support in carrying out the cultural activities of MICAI 2015. We also want to thank the staff of the Electrical Research Institute (IIE) and the National Center for Research and Technology Development (CENIDET) for their support in the organization of this conference.

We gratefully acknowledge the sponsorship received from Springer for monetary prizes handed to the authors of the best papers of the conference. This generous sponsorship demonstrates Springer's strong commitment to the development of science and their sincere interest in the highest quality of the conferences published with them.

We are deeply grateful to the conference staff and to all members of the local committee headed by Gustavo Arroyo Figueroa, Yasmín Hernández, and Noé Alejandro Castro Sánchez. We acknowledge support received from the project CONACYT 240844. The entire submission, reviewing, and selection process, as well as preparation of the proceedings, was supported for free by the EasyChair system (www.easychair. org). Finally, yet importantly, we are very grateful to Springer staff for their patience and help in the preparation of this volume.

October 2015   Grigori Sidorov
                                                Sofía N. Galicia-Haro
                                             Obdulia Pichardo Lagunas
                                               Oscar Herrera Alcántara
                                             Gustavo Arroyo Figueroa

Conference Organization

MICAI 2015 was organized by the Mexican Society of Artificial Intelligence (SMIA, Sociedad Mexicana de Inteligencia Artificial) in collaboration with the Instituto de Investigaciones Eléctricas (IIE), the Centro Nacional de Investigación y Desarrollo Tecnológico (CENIDET), the Universidad Politécnica del Estado de Morelos (Upemor), the Tecnológico de Monterrey Campus Cuernavaca, the Centro de Investigación en Computación del Instituto Politécnico Nacional (CIC-IPN), the Unidad Profesional Interdisciplinaria en Ingeniería y Tecnologías Avanzadas del Instituto Politécnico Nacional (UPIITA-IPN), the Universidad Autónoma de México Azcapotzalco (UAM), and the Universidad Nacional Autónoma de México (UNAM).

The MICAI series website is www.MICAI.org. The website of the Mexican Society of Artificial Intelligence, SMIA, is www.SMIA.org.mx. Contact options and additional information can be found on these websites.

Conference Committee

General Chair

Grigori Sidorov — Instituto Politécnico Nacional, Mexico

Program Chairs

Gustavo Arroyo Figueroa — Instituto de Investigaciones Eléctricas, Mexico
Sofía N. Galicia-Haro — Universidad Autónoma Nacional de México, Mexico
Oscar Herrera Alcántara — Universidad Autónoma Metropolitana Azcapotzalco, Mexico
Obdulia Pichardo Lagunas — Instituto Politécnico Nacional, Mexico
Grigori Sidorov — Instituto Politécnico Nacional, Mexico

Workshop Chairs

Obdulia Pichardo Lagunas — Instituto Politécnico Nacional, Mexico
Noé Alejandro Castro Sánchez — Centro Nacional de Investigación y Desarrollo Tecnológico, Mexico

Tutorials Chair

Félix Castro Espinoza — Universidad Autónoma del Estado de Hidalgo, Mexico

Doctoral Consortium Chairs

Miguel Gonzalez Mendoza — Tecnológico de Monterrey CEM, Mexico
Antonio Marín Hernandez — Universidad Veracruzana, Mexico

Keynote Talks Chair

Sabino Miranda Jiménez — INFOTEC, Mexico

Publication Chair

Miguel Gonzalez Mendoza   Tecnológico de Monterrey CEM, Mexico

Financial Chair

Ildar Batyrshin   Instituto Politécnico Nacional, Mexico

Grant Chairs

Grigori Sidorov   Instituto Politécnico Nacional, Mexico
Miguel Gonzalez Mendoza   Tecnológico de Monterrey CEM, Mexico

Organizing Committee Chairs

Gustavo Arroyo Figueroa   Instituto de Investigaciones Eléctricas, Mexico
Yasmín Hernández   Instituto de Investigaciones Eléctricas, Mexico
Noé Alejandro Castro   CENIDET, Mexico
  Sánchez

Area Chairs

Natural Language Processing

Grigori Sidorov   Instituto Politécnico Nacional, Mexico

Machine Learning and Pattern Recognition

Alexander Gelbukh   Instituto Politécnico Nacional, Mexico

Data Mining

Miguel Gonzalez-Mendoza   Tecnológico de Monterrey CEM, Mexico
Félix Castro Espinoza   Universidad Autónoma del Estado de Hidalgo, Mexico

Intelligent Tutoring Systems

Alexander Gelbukh   Instituto Politécnico Nacional, Mexico

Evolutionary and Nature-Inspired Metaheuristic Algorithms

Oliver Schütze   CINVESTAV, Mexico
Jaime Mora Vargas   Tecnológico de Monterrey CEM, Mexico

Computer Vision and Image Processing

Oscar Herrera Alcántara   Universidad Autónoma Metropolitana Azcapotzalco,
  Mexico

Robotics, Planning and Scheduling

Fernando Martin   Universidad Veracruzana, Mexico
  Montes-Gonzalez

Neural Networks and Hybrid Intelligent Systems
Sergio Ledesma-Orozco   Universidad de Guanajuato, Mexico

Logic, Knowledge-Based Systems, Multi-Agent Systems and Distributed AI
Mauricio Osorio   Jose Raymundo Marcial Romero

Fuzzy Systems and Probabilistic Models in Decision Making
Ildar Batyrshin   Instituto Politécnico Nacional, Mexico

Bioinformatics and Medical Applications
Jesus A. Gonzalez   Instituto Nacional de Astrofísica, Óptica y Electrónica, Mexico
Felipe Orihuela-Espina   Instituto Nacional de Astrofísica, Óptica y Electrónica, Mexico

Program Committee

Juan C. Acosta-Guadarrama	Universidad Autónoma del Estado de México, Mexico
Teresa Alarcón	Universidad de Guadalajara, Mexico
Fernando Aldana	Universidad Veracruzana, Mexico
Jesus Angulo	Ecole des Mines de Paris, France
Marianna Apidianaki	LIMSI-CNRS, France
Alfredo Arias-Montaño	Instituto Politécnico Nacional, Mexico
Jose Arrazola	Universidad Autónoma de Puebla, Mexico
Gustavo Arroyo	Instituto de Investigaciones Eléctricas, Mexico
Victor Ayala-Ramirez	Universidad de Guanajuato, Mexico
Alexandra Balahur	European Commission Joint Research Centre, Italy
Sivaji Bandyopadhyay	Jadavpur University, India
Maria Lucia Barrón-Estrada	Instituto Tecnológico de Culiacán, Mexico
Rafael Batres Prieto	Tecnológico de Monterrey, Mexico
Ildar Batyrshin	Instituto Politécnico Nacional, Mexico
Albert Bifet	University of Waikato, New Zealand
Igor Bolshakov	Russian State University for the Humanities, Russia
Ramon F. Brena	Tecnológico de Monterrey, Mexico
Eduardo Cabal-Yepez	Universidad de Guanajuato, Mexico
Hiram Calvo	Instituto Politécnico Nacional, Mexico
Nicoletta Calzolari	Istituto di Linguistica Computazionale – CNR, Italy
Erik Cambria	Nanyang Technological University, Singapore
César Cárdenas	Tecnológico de Monterrey, Mexico
Michael Carl	Copenhagen Business School, Denmark
Heydy Castillejos	Universidad Autónoma del Estado de Hidalgo, Mexico
Oscar Castillo	Instituto Tecnológico de Tijuana, Mexico
Felix Castro Espinoza	Universidad Autónoma del Estado de Hidalgo, Mexico

Noé Alejandro Castro-Sánchez	Centro Nacional de Investigación y Desarrollo Tecnológico, Mexico
Hector Ceballos	Tecnólogico de Monterrey, Mexico
Gustavo Cerda-Villafana	Universidad de Guanajuato, Mexico
Niladri Chatterjee	Indian Institute of Technology Delhi, India
Stefania Costantini	Università degli Studi dell'Aquila, Italy
Heriberto Cuayahuitl	Heriot-Watt University, UK
Erik Cuevas	Universidad de Guadalajara, Mexico
Oscar Dalmau	Centro de Investigación en Matemáticas, Mexico
Guillermo De Ita	Universidad Autónoma de Puebla, Mexico
Maria De Marsico	University of Rome La Sapienza, Italy
Asif Ekbal	Indian Institute of Technology Patna, India
Hugo Jair Escalante	Instituto Nacional de Astrofísica, Óptica y Electrónica, Mexico
Ponciano Jorge Escamilla-Ambrosio	Instituto Nacional de Astrofísica, Óptica y Electrónica, Mexico
Vlad Estivill-Castro	Griffith University, Australia
Gibran Etcheverry	Universidad de Sonora, Mexico
Denis Filatov	Instituto Politécnico Nacional, Mexico
Juan J. Flores	Universidad Michoacana de San Nicolás de Hidalgo, Mexico
Andrea Formisano	Università di Perugia, Italy
Anilu Franco-Arcega	Instituto Nacional de Astrofísica, Óptica y Electrónica, Mexico
Claude Frasson	University of Montreal, Canada
Alfredo Gabaldon	Carnegie Mellon University, USA
Sofia N. Galicia-Haro	Universidad Nacional Autónoma de México, Mexico
Ana Gabriela Gallardo-Hernández	Universidad Nacional Autónoma de México, Mexico
Carlos Garcia-Capulin	Instituto Tecnológico Superior de Irapuato, Mexico
Ma. de Guadalupe Garcia-Hernandez	Universidad de Guanajuato, Mexico
Raúl Garduño Ramírez	Instituto de Investigaciones Electricas
Alexander Gelbukh	Instituto Politécnico Nacional, Mexico
Onofrio Gigliotta	University of Naples Federico II, Italy
Eduardo Gomez-Ramirez	Universidad La Salle, Mexico
Arturo Gonzalez	Universidad de Guanajuato, Mexico
Miguel Gonzalez-Mendoza	Tecnológico de Monterrey CEM, Mexico
Felix F. Gonzalez-Navarro	Universidad Autónoma de Baja California, Mexico
Efren Gorrostieta	Universidad Autónoma de Querétaro, Mexico
Carlos Arturo Gracios-Marin	CERN, Switzerland
Joaquin Gutierrez	Centro de Investigaciones Biológicas del Noroeste S.C., Mexico
Yasunari Harada	Waseda University, Japan
Rogelio Hasimoto	Centro de Investigación en Matemáticas, Mexico

Antonio Hernandez	Instituto Politécnico Nacional, Mexico
José Alberto Hernández Aguilar	Universidad Autónoma de Estado de Morelos, Mexico
Yasmín Hernández Pérez	Instituto de Investigaciones Eléctricas, Mexico
Oscar Herrera	Universidad Autónoma Metropolitana Azcapotzalco, Mexico
Dieter Hutter	DFKI GmbH, Germany
Pablo H. Ibarguengoytia	Instituto de Investigaciones Eléctricas, Mexico
Oscar G. Ibarra-Manzano	Universidad de Guanajuato, Mexico
Diana Inkpen	University of Ottawa, Canada
Héctor Jiménez Salazar	Universidad Autónoma Metropolitana, Mexico
Laetitia Jourdan	Inria/LIFL/CNRS, France
Pinar Karagoz	Middle East Technical University, Turkey
Ryszard Klempous	Wroclaw University of Technology, Poland
Olga Kolesnikova	Instituto Politécnico Nacional, Mexico
Konstantinos Koutroumbas	National Observatory of Athens, Greece
Vladik Kreinovich	University of Texas at El Paso, USA
Angel Kuri-Morales	Instituto Tecnológico Autónomo de México, Mexico
Mathieu Lafourcade	Le Laboratoire d'Informatique, de Robotique et de Microélectronique de Montpellier (UM2/CNRS), France
Ricardo Landa	CINVESTAV Tamaulipas, Mexico
Dario Landa-Silva	University of Nottingham, UK
Bruno Lara	Universidad Autónoma del Estado de Morelos, Mexico
Monica Larre Bolaños Cacho	Tecnológico de Monterrey Campus Cuernavaca, Mexico
Yulia Ledeneva	Universidad Autónoma del Estado de México, Mexico
Yoel Ledo Mezquita	Universidad de las Américas, Mexico
Eugene Levner	Ashkelon Academic College, Israel
Rocio Lizarraga-Morales	Universidad de Guanajuato, Mexico
Aurelio Lopez	Instituto Nacional de Astrofísica, Óptica y Electrónica, Mexico
Virgilio Lopez-Morales	Universidad Autónoma del Estado de Hidalgo, Mexico
Omar López-Ortega	Universidad Autónoma del Estado de Hidalgo, Mexico
Tanja Magoc	University of Texas at El Paso, USA
J. Raymundo Marcial-Romero	Universidad Autónoma del Estado de México, Mexico
Luis Martí	Pontifícia Universidade Católica do Rio de Janeiro, Brazil
Lourdes Martínez	Tecnológico de Monterrey CEM, Mexico
Francisco Martínez-Álvarez	Universidad Pablo de Olavide, Spain
R. Carolina Medina-Ramirez	Universidad Autónoma Metropolitana Iztapalapa, Mexico
Patricia Melin	Instituto Tecnológico de Tijuana, Mexico
Ivan Vladimir Meza Ruiz	Universidad Nacional Autónoma de México, Mexico
Efrén Mezura-Montes	Universidad Veracruzana, Mexico

Mikhail Mikhailov   University of Tampere, Finland
Sabino Miranda   INFOTEC, Mexico
Raul Monroy   Tecnológico de Monterrey CEM, Mexico
Manuel Montes-y-Gómez   Instituto Nacional de Astrofísica, Óptica y Electrónica,
                                   Mexico
Carlos Montoro   Universidad de Guanajuato, Mexico
Jaime Mora-Vargas   Tecnológico de Monterrey CEM, Mexico
Eduardo Morales   Instituto Nacional de Astrofísica, Óptica y Electrónica,
                                   Mexico
Guillermo Morales-Luna   CINVESTAV, Mexico
Masaki Murata   Tottori University, Japan
Michele Nappi   Italy
Jesús Emeterio   Society for the Promotion of Applied Computer
   Navarro-Barrientos   Science (GFaI e.V.), Germany
Juan Carlos Nieves   Umeå University, Sweden
Roger Nkambou   Université du Québec À Montréal, Canada
Leszek Nowak   Jagiellonian University, Poland
C. Alberto Ochoa-Zezatti   Universidad Autónoma de Ciudad Juárez, Mexico
Ivan Olmos   Benemérita Universidad Autónoma de Puebla, Mexico
Ekaterina Ovchinnikova   KIT, Karlsruhe and University of Heidelberg, Germany
Partha Pakray   National Institute of Technology Mizoram, India
Ivandre Paraboni   University of Sao Paulo, Brazil
Mario Pavone   University of Catania, Italy
Ted Pedersen   University of Minnesota Duluth, USA
Héctor Pérez-Urbina   Google, USA
Obdulia Pichardo   Instituto Politécnico Nacional, Mexico
David Pinto   Benemérita Universidad Autónoma de Puebla, Mexico
Volodymyr Ponomaryov   Instituto Politécnico Nacional, Mexico
Marta R. Costa-Jussà   Universitat Politècnica de Catalunya, Spain
Risto Fermin Rangel   Universidad Autónoma Metropolitana Azcapotzalco,
   Kuoppa   Mexico
Ivan Salvador Razo-Zapata   Université libre de Bruxelles, Belgium
Orion Reyes   University of Alberta Edmonton AB, Canada
Alberto Reyes Ballesteros   Instituto de Investigaciones Eléctricas, Mexico
Erik Rodner   Friedrich Schiller University of Jena, Germany
Arles Rodriguez   Universidad Nacional de Colombia, Colombia
Alejandro Rosales   Instituto Nacional de Astrofísica, Óptica y Electrónica,
                                   Mexico
Paolo Rosso   Universitat Politècnica de València, Spain
Horacio Rostro Gonzalez   Universidad de Guanajuato, Mexico
Jose Ruiz-Pinales   Universidad de Guanajuato, Mexico
Chaman Sabharwal   Missouri University of Science and Technology, USA
Luciano Sanchez   Universidad de Oviedo, Spain
Edgar Sánchez   CINVESTAV Unidad Guadalajara, Mexico
Abraham Sánchez López   Benemérita Universidad Autónoma de Puebla, Mexico
Marino Sánchez Parra   Instituto de Investigaciones Eléctricas, Mexico

Guillermo Sanchez-Diaz	Universidad Autónoma de San Luis Potosí, Mexico
Antonio-José Sánchez-Salmerón	Universitat Politècnica de València, Spain
Jose Santos	University of A Coruña, Spain
Oliver Schuetze	CINVESTAV, Mexico
Friedhelm Schwenker	Ulm University, Germany
Shahnaz Shahbazova	Azerbaijan Technical University, Azerbaijan
Oleksiy Shulika	Universidad de Guanajuato, Mexico
Patrick Siarry	Université de Paris 12, France
Grigori Sidorov	Instituto Politécnico Nacional, Mexico
Bogdan Smolka	Silesian University of Technology, Poland
Jorge Solis	Waseda University, Japan
Thamar Solorio	University of Houston, USA
Juan Humberto Sossa Azuela	Instituto Politécnico Nacional, Mexico
Efstathios Stamatatos	University of the Aegean, Greece
Josef Steinberger	University of West Bohemia, Czech Republic
Johan Suykens	Katholieke Universiteit Leuven, Belgium
Hugo Terashima	Tecnológico de Monterrey, Mexico
Leonardo Trujillo	Instituto Tecnológico de Tijuana, Mexico
Alexander Tulupyev	St. Petersburg Institute for Informatics and Automation of Russian Academy of Sciences, Russia
Fevrier Valdez	Instituto Tecnológico de Tijuana, Mexico
Edgar Vallejo	Tecnológico de Monterrey CEM, Mexico
Manuel Vilares Ferro	University of Vigo, Spain
Aline Villavicencio	Universidade Federal do Rio Grande do Sul, Brazil
Francisco Viveros Jiménez	Instituto Politécnico Nacional, Mexico
Panagiotis Vlamos	Ionian University, Greece
Piotr W. Fuglewicz	TiP Sp. z o. o., Poland
Nicolas Younan	Mississippi State University, USA
Carlos Mario Zapata Jaramillo	Universidad Nacional de Colombia, Colombia
Ramon Zatarain	Instituto Tecnológico de Culiacán, Mexico
Alisa Zhila	Independent Researcher, Russia
Reyer Zwiggelaar	Aberystwyth University, UK

Additional Reviewers

Akiko Aizawa	Brenda L. Flores-Rios
Haneen Algethami	Mercedes García Martínez
Miguel Ángel Álvarez Carmona	Marcos Angel González-Olvera
Leticia Cagnina	Braja Gopal Patra
Francisco De Asís López-Fuentes	Esteban Guerrero
Miguel Angel De La Torre Gomora	Oznur Kirmemis
Oscar H. Estrada	Pramod Kumar Sahoo

Wasakorn Laesanklang
Rodrigo Lankaites Pinheiro
Luis M. Ledesma-Carrillo
Misael Lopez Ramirez
Pascual Martínez-Gómez
Miguel Angel Medina Pérez
Gabriela Ramírez-De-La-Rosa

Claudia A. Rivera
Jorge Rodas
Salvador Ruiz-Correa
Karan Singla
Yasushi Tsubota
Pavel Vorobiev

Organizing Committee

Local Chairs

Gustavo Arroyo Figueroa	Instituto de Investigaciones Eléctricas, Mexico
Yasmín Hernández	Instituto de Investigaciones Eléctricas, Mexico
Noé Alejandro Castro Sánchez	CENIDET, Mexico

Finance Chair

Gustavo Arroyo Figueroa	Instituto de Investigaciones Eléctricas, Mexico

Sponsorships Chair

Yasmín Hernández	Instituto de Investigaciones Eléctricas, Mexico

Logistics Chair

Yasmín Hernández	Instituto de Investigaciones Eléctricas, Mexico

Registration Chair

Yasmín Hernández	Instituto de Investigaciones Eléctricas, Mexico

Design and Print Chair

Luis Arturo Domínguez Brito	Instituto de Investigaciones Eléctricas, Mexico

Promotion Chair

Noé Alejandro Castro Sánchez	CENIDET, Mexico

Website

Sara Edith Pinzon Pineda	Instituto de Investigaciones Eléctricas, Mexico

Members

Yadira Toledo Navarro	Universidad Politécnica del Estado de Morelos, Mexico
Mónica Larre Bolaños Cacho	Tecnológico de Monterrey Campus Cuernavaca, Mexico
Jose Alberto Hernández Aguilar	Universidad Autónoma del Estado de Morelos, Mexico

Contents – Part II

Educational Applications

Biomedical Applications

Image Processing and Computer Vision

Best Student Paper Award

Search and Optimization

Forecasting

Intelligent Applications

Contents – Part I

Logic and Multi-agent Systems

Bioinspired Algorithms

Neural Networks

Best Paper Award, Third Place

Evolutionary Algorithms

Fuzzy Logic

Machine Learning and Data Mining

Invited Papers

Measuring Non-compositionality of Verb-Noun Collocations Using Lexical Functions and WordNet Hypernyms

Olga Kolesnikova[1(✉)] and Alexander Gelbukh[2]

[1] Superior School of Computer Sciences,
Instituto Politécnico Nacional, Mexico City 07738, Mexico
`kolesolga@gmail.com`
[2] Centro de Investigación en Computación,
Instituto Politécnico Nacional, Mexico City 07738, Mexico
`http://www.gelbukh.com`

Abstract. In such verb-noun combinations as *draw a conclusion, lend support, take a step*, the verb acquires a meaning different from its typical meaning usually represented by the first sense in WordNet thus making a correct compositional analysis hard or even impossible. Such non-compositional word combinations are called collocations. The semantics and syntactical properties of collocations can be formalized using lexical functions, a concept of the Meaning-Text Theory. In this paper we realized two series of experiments, both with supervised learning methods on automatic detection of lexical functions in verb-noun collocations using WordNet hypernyms. In the first experimental series, we used hypernyms which correspond to the manually annotated WordNet senses of verbs and nouns in the dataset. In the second series, we used hypernyms corresponding to the typical (first) sense of the verbs. Comparing the results of both experiments we found that the performance of supervised learning on some lexical functions was better in the second case in spite of the fact that the first sense was not the sense of the verbs they have in collocations. This shows that for such lexical functions, the semantics of the verbs is closer to their typical senses and thus non-compositionality of such collocations is weaker. We propose to use the difference in lexical function detection based on the actual sense and the first sense as a simple measure of non-compositionality of verb-noun collocations.

Keywords: Lexical functions · Verb-noun collocations · Supervised learning · Non-compositionality of collocations · Wordnet hypernyms

1 Introduction

Collocation is a phrase, typically consisting of two words, which cannot be analyzed compositionally, that is, the semantics of such phrase is not obtained by adding the meaning of one word to the meaning of the other word or words. To illustrate the concept of collocation, let us consider first a compositional phrase, for example, *take a book*. The typical meaning of *take* is 'to move something or someone from one place to another', and the typical meaning of *book* is 'a written work that is published, either as

© Springer International Publishing Switzerland 2015
O. Pichardo Lagunas et al. (Eds.): MICAI 2015, Part II, LNAI 9414, pp. 3–25, 2015.
DOI: 10.1007/978-3-319-27101-9_1

printed pages inside a cover or electronically' (the definitions are taken from Macmillan Dictionary Online[1]). Applying two simple heuristics (*book* as an inanimate object and a bigger corpus frequency of *take a book* in which *book* means 'printed pages'), the meaning of *take a book* is generated correctly as 'to move a written work that is published as printed pages inside a cover from one place to another' which proves that *take a book* is compositional, that is, its semantics can be obtained directly from the semantics of its component words. Such phrases are called free word combinations.

However, in *take a step*, the same verb *take* does not have its typical meaning 'to move something or someone from one place to another', but 'to perform a particular action or series of actions' (Macmillan Dictionary Online) which differs significantly from the typical meaning. Therefore, the semantics of *take a step* cannot be interpreted as a sum of the meanings of both words, so the compositional approach fails here. Such non-compositional word combinations are termed collocations. Other examples are *draw a conclusion, lend support, make one's bed, give a presentation* – all these are verb-noun collocations, one of the syntactic types of collocations we study in this research.

Here we have to comment on what meaning of a word is viewed as its typical meaning. Commonly, it is a meaning most frequently met in texts. For example, lists of word senses in WordNet,[2] a well-known electronic dictionary accessible online [34, 35] and widely used in computational linguistics and natural language processing, are ordered by frequency, therefore, sense 1 is the most frequent meaning of a word, and it can be considered as its typical meaning. However, the issue of which meaning in the list of meanings should be considered typical is still not resolved and constitutes another research topic; in this paper, for the purpose of our work, we will adopt the interpretation of typical as most frequent.

Another example to illustrate the issue of free word combinations and collocations is the verb *have* which typically means 'to hold or maintain as a possession, privilege, or entitlement' as in the phrase *they have a new car* or in *I have my rights* (the definition taken from Merriam-Webster Dictionary Online[3]) However, in the combination *have lunch* as in *I had lunch at 3 pm today*, this verb does not mean 'possess' but 'consume', 'partake of'.

Commonly, as we have mentioned above, the most typical sense of a word is put first in the list of its senses in a dictionary, so the meaning 'to hold or maintain as a possession…' is put as sense 1 of *have*, for example, in the Merriam-Webster Dictionary Online. *Have* in its typical sense can combine with any noun denoting a physical or abstract entity; however, the meaning 'consume' is compatible only with nouns which are names of various food products, dishes, or drinks. Therefore, the first type of *have* usage is a free word combination, and the second case is a collocation or restricted lexical co-occurrence since it is limited to a much narrower category of nouns with more specific semantics.

It is very important in automatic processing of texts in natural language to determine if a given phrase is a free word combination or a collocation. In the first case of a

---

[1] Macmillan Dictionary Online, available on http://www.macmillandictionary.com/.

[2] WordNet 3.1, available on http://wordnet.princeton.edu/.

[3] Merriam-Webster Dictionary Online, available on http://www.merriam-webster.com/.

free word combination, the phrase under treatment can be submitted to a compositional analysis which outputs the meaning of the phrase as a combination of the meaning of each constituent: *have a car = have + a car =* 'to hold or maintain as a possession' + 'a vehicle that has four wheels and an engine and that is used for carrying passengers on roads' (the definitions are quoted as in the Merriam-Webster Dictionary Online); therefore *have a car* means 'to hold or maintain as a possession a vehicle that has four wheels and an engine and that is used for carrying passengers on roads'.

In the case of collocations, their compositional analysis is usually not applicable, as we mentioned previously, since their semantics is hard or impossible to derive from the meaning of their elements. The property which makes a compositional analysis so problematic is called non-compositionality; we will tackle it in more detail in the sections dedicated to this feature (Sects. 2 and 4). Here we will only mention that the degree of non-compositionality can vary among collocations: *have lunch* ('consume a midday meal'), *make one's bed* ('set one's bed in order'), *catch someone's attention* ('attract and hold someone's attention') seem to be more compositional than *big house* (meaning 'jail'), *like sauce* (meaning 'superior, dominant'), *spill the beans* (meaning 'let secret information become known'), *find one's feet* (meaning 'become more comfortable in whatever one is doing'). Therefore, it is important to determine the degree of non-compositionality of a phrase in order to choose an appropriate technique for it semantic analysis.

Collocations are 'pain in the neck' for natural language processing (NLP) [54] because of their opaque, non-motivated, and non-compositional nature. Due to this, their meaning is difficult to predict automatically, and their semantic interpretation in NLP applications is still a challenge.

An example of an NLP application which makes use of semantic analysis of utterances is machine translation. A widely used translation tool today is Google Translate so we performed some experiments with this application on August 24, 2015.

The sentences *Tom and Becky had lunch at the restaurant. Then Becky asked Tom if he had a good book to give her to read at night* were translated correctly into Spanish by Google Translate as *Tom y Becky almorzaron en el restaurante. Entonces Becky preguntó Tom si tenía un buen libro para darle a leer por la noche.* Here, the English collocation *had lunch* is correctly rendered as *almorzar*, and the free word combination *have a book* is also correctly translated as *tener un libro*. Note that *almorzar* is not a literal translation of *have lunch*; expressed literally in Spanish words it is *tener almuerzo* which is understandable to a native Spanish speaker but does not sound natural and is perceived as a 'lexical accent' of an English speaker.

Another utterance in our experiments with Google Translate was *How wonderful is to take a walk in the woods!* This sentence was translated as *¡Qué maravilloso es tomar un paseo en el bosque! Take a walk* is another English collocation translated word for word here as *tomar un paseo.* However, the correct Spanish collocation corresponding to *take a walk* is not *tomar un paseo* but *dar un paseo,* literally *give a walk. Take a walk* does not seem so difficult a collocation, nevertheless, Google Translate fails to generate its Spanish equivalent.

Although *tomar un paseo* sounds awkward, in spite of this the semantics it is supposed to transmit can be quite easily guessed and restored, so the error of generation of an unnatural phrase does not in fact prevent a Spanish speaking reader from understanding the meaning of the original English utterance. But when the semantics of collocations becomes more opaque, more non-compositional, and the distance between the meaning of a collocation as a whole and the meanings of its constituents becomes greater, its automatic translation cannot help the user to understand the meaning of the original text, moreover, it may lead to a very different interpretation.

As an example of such difficult case we took the sentence *We sat on the porch until late at night, just shooting the breeze*, borrowed from the entry for the collocation *shoot the breeze* in the Cambridge Dictionary Online.[4] *Shoot the breeze* means 'to talk with someone about unimportant things for a long time'. After receiving this example as an input, Google Translate produced the output *Nos sentamos en el porche hasta bien entrada la noche, sólo el rodaje de la brisa* which does not represent the actual meaning of the English sentence, gives a false account of the event, and does not even leave space for a guess which could lead to the original content. Google Translate generates a translation of *shoot the breeze* as *el rodaje de la brisa* failing even to produce a correct morphological analysis of this phrase, since it labels the verb *shooting* in its ing-form as a noun and interprets *shooting* as *filming* (*el rodaje* is a noun in Spanish meaning 'filming'), so in this case Google Translate was totally unable to recognize the semantics of this opaque collocation.

As we observed in our experiments with Google Translate, in spite of advanced technology and effort of many language researchers and engineers dedicated to the design and implementation of this modern tool, the issue of semantic analysis of collocations (of **any** collocation including fixed and non-compositional expressions) still remains unresolved, so there is a need of more profound and detailed studies of collocations and a search for more efficient, robust methods and techniques of their semantic analysis.

Collocations form a specific type of a broader class of word combinations called Multi-Word Expression (MWE). Beside collocations, MWEs include conjunctions like *as well as* (meaning 'including'), idioms like *kick the bucket* (meaning 'die'), phrasal verbs like *find out* (meaning 'search'), and compounds like *village community* [61]. MWEs idiosyncratic interpretations cross word boundaries and cannot be analyzed on a word-by-word level.

However, the issue of processing and correct interpretation of MWEs cannot be ignored due to the fact that collocations and other MWEs are used in texts very frequently forming a big part of the language we employ today: for example, 41 % of the WordNet entries [34, 35] are multiword expressions [54]; also, depending on a specific domain, collocations can comprise up to 85 % of vocabulary in texts [37]; consequently, their correct analysis is an important task in NLP.

Due to the non-compositional nature of collocations and other MWEs, for their correct automatic analysis and understanding we have to employ procedures different from those used for compositional analysis of phrases and utterances. Moreover, recognition and treatment of collocations may vary depending on their degree of non-compositionality. If this degree is high, we have to deal with fixed phrases better interpreted as words-with-spaces (*by and large, in short, every which way*) [54]. If the

---

[4] Cambridge Dictionary Online, http://dictionary.cambridge.org/.

degree of non-compositionality is low as, for example, in the case of 'light verb + noun' constructions (*make a decision, have a look, make an offer,* and the previous examples *take a step, draw a conclusion, lend support, make one's bed, give a presentation*), then words-with-spaces approach is not flexible enough to recognize the typical meaning of nouns and a changed semantics of verbs. On the other hand, a fully compositional technique in such a case may lead to incorrect generation of phrases like **to do a mistake* instead of *to make a mistake, *to do attention* instead of *to pay attention,* etc. [9]. Therefore, it is important to have information concerning the degree of non-compositionality of phrases to be able to decide what technique to choose for their processing.

Collocations are very useful in many important practical applications. For example, they help spotting sentiment in textual reviews. In recent works on sentiment analysis, collocations are identified using dependency tree based tree [47]; then their polarity is defined based on unsupervised sentiment flow strategy [45]. People tend to use collocations in verbal communication, i.e., while expressing opinion verbally. Such collocations are the basis of the concept-level text analysis [43, 50], which improves the accuracy of audio-visual sentiment detection by a large margin [44, 46]. Collocations are actively used in such tasks as human-computer dialog [57], information retrieval [1], database curation [52], topic identification [13], and metaphor detection [36].

The rest of the paper is organized as follows. Section 2 reviews related work on non-compositionality of collocations, Sect. 3 explains the concept of lexical functions within the theoretical framework of the Meaning-Text Theory and shows that lexical functions can be used to represent semantic classes of collocations. Section 4 presents our proposal to model non-compositionality of collocations in terms of lexical function detection using WordNet hypernyms. Section 5 describes our experiments on Spanish verb-noun collocations; Sect. 6 gives the obtained results and their discussion, while Sect. 7 outlines conclusions and future work.

2   Related Work on Non-compositionality of Collocations

The notion of non-compositionality is complex as shown in [59]; it is also disputable since there is no commonly accepted definition of this property inherent in collocations. However, it is applied widely in natural language research and engineering to distinguish collocations and other MWEs from free word combinations [19, 23, 27, 38, 42, 60].

In this paper, we use the term *non-compositionality* as negation of compositionality, the latter defined by Lyons as a phenomenon characterized by the fact that "the meaning of a composite expression is a function of the meanings of its component expressions" [25].

There have been basically two approaches in studying the non-compositional nature of collocations: the first approach, which emerged earlier and is more developed now, focuses on distinguishing non-compositional phrases from compositional ones, the second approach is more recent and is attracting a growing interest of NLP researchers: it seeks to measure the degree of non-compositionality on both coarse- and fine-grained levels. Our work is within the second approach as we are interested in identifying differences in non-compositionality of verb-noun collocations which on the surface level appear to be equal. Therefore, in this section we will pay more attention to related work belonging to the second approach.

As an example of the first approach we will mention [20], a work on detecting compositionality of verb-particle constructions (VPCs). The authors measured the degree of compositionality by semantic similarity between the VPCs and their base verbs in isolation. The semantics of both VPCs and their base verbs was represented by WordNet synsets and hypernyms; then the data was supplied to classifiers to detect two classes: compositional and non-compositional VPCs. The highest experimental result was an F-measure of 0.876.

Another work within the first approach is [7]. The authors introduced a new metric called Multiword Expression Distance (MED) to define the semantic function of n-grams and the information distance from the n-grams to their semantics. The procedure to calculate the metric takes advantage of two concepts: Kolmogorov complexity and information distance. Kolmogorov complexity of a binary string x condition to another binary string y $K_U(x|y)$ is defined as the length of the shortest (prefix-free) program for a universal Turing machine U that outputs x with input y. The concept of information distance is derived from a physical principal of von Neumann and Landauer which says that irreversibly process one bit of information costs 1KT of energy, so information distance $E(x, y)$ between two objects x and y is the energy to convert between x and y. The new metric was evaluated on detection of non-compositionality of multiword expressions in two applications: question answering and complex name entity extraction. In both applications the new metric outperformed state of the art methods.

Now we will discuss related work on measuring the non-compositionality of expressions using some specified range of values. Such work is within the second approach as we defined it previously in this section.

The authors of [26] measured the non-compositionality of verb-particle constructions (VPCs) like *eat up* by a numerical score of 0 to 10, with 10 meaning a fully compositional VPC and 0, a totally opaque one. The experiments were performed applying two strategies: a statistic one and a strategy based on Lin thesaurus [24]. Within each strategy, various techniques were implemented. The best statistic method turned out to be point-wise mutual information, and the best thesaurus-based measure was the one that took into account the number of neighbors with the same particle as in the VPC minus the equivalent number of the simplex (non-phrasal) neighbors, i.e. having the same particle as the target VPC (with a Spearman Rank-Order Correlation Coefficient of 0.490).

The research reported in [61] is dedicated to measuring the relative compositionality of verb-noun expressions with the objective to rank collocations according to such measure. Using SVM-based ranking functions, verb-noun combinations were scored from 1 to 6, where 6 corresponds to a free word combination while 1 corresponds to collocations. Each verb-noun combination was represented as a vector of two types of features: collocation-based features and context-based ones. The first type of features included frequency of the collocation in the British National Corpus, point-wise mutual information, least mutual information difference with similar collocations, distributed frequency of object (noun in a verb-noun collocation), and distributed frequency of object using the verb information. Context-based features included dissimilarity of the collocation with its constituent verb using the LSA model [4, 55], and similarity of the collocation to the verb-form of the object using the LSA model. To evaluate the results, the authors used Pearson's Rank-Order Correlation Coefficient with the human ranking. In the experiments, the correlation of obtained results reached 0.448.

We mentioned previously in this section that measuring the non-compositionality of phrases has been attracting more attention of researchers in the last years. An evidence of this interest is the organization of the ACL-HLT 2011 workshop on Distributional Semantics and Compositionality (DiSCo) with a shared task to assign a graded compositionality score to phrases in suggested corpora [6]. The golden standard was comprised by adjective-noun, subject-verb, and verb-object phrases in three languages (English, German, Italian) rated by mother-tongue speakers for semantic compositionality on a fine-grained scale between 0 and 100 (*hot dog* has a rating close to 0 since it is non-compositional, *red car* has a rating close to 100), and on a coarse-grained level as low, medium, and high compositionality. The output of the proposed systems was evaluated as an average point difference with the golden standard on the fine-grained level (a perfect score is 0) and as a ratio of the number of matches with the golden standard to the total number of phrases on a coarse-grained level (a perfect score is 1).

The first best work at the Workshop was [15]. To distinguish among various degrees of compositionality (and, therefore, of non-compositionality) on a fine-grained level, the authors used endocentricity of a word pair $w_1 w_2$. Endocentricity is based on the idea that the distribution of w_1 is likely to be similar to the distribution of $w_1 w_2$ if w_1 is the syntactic head of $w_1 w_2$. To calculate word distributions, the authors applied the COALS algorithm [53]. Their system achieved the best fine-grained score of 16.19 and a coarse-grained score of 0.356 on all three English syntactic constructions.

The second-best methodology in the shared task is presented in [51]. The authors' method implements the exemplar-based word space model. The underlying idea is to compare the cosine similarity of two vectors built for a word combination $w_1 w_2$: the first vector $V_{w_1 w_2}$ is a context vector of $w_1 w_2$ viewed as a single word, and the second vector $V_{w_1 \oplus w_2}$ is a composition of two context vectors: one built on the context of w_1 and the second, on the context of w_2. If the similarity of $V_{w_1 w_2}$ and $V_{w_1 \oplus w_2}$ is high, then $w_1 w_2$ is likely to be compositional, if this similarity is low, it is more probable that the word combination is non-compositional. This approach achieved the second best result at the DiSCo workshop: fine-grained scores of 14.62 and 15.72 for adjective noun and subject-verb, respectively, both for English. Their coarse-grained scores for the same type of expressions were 0.731 (it was the first best coarse-grained score on English adjective noun constructions) and 0.500, respectively.

In our work, we measured the non-compositionality of verb-noun collocations following the second approach: ranking collocations according to the degree of non-compositionality. However, we did not use a specific range for such measure. Nevertheless, the fundamental research question is the same: whether the non-compositional nature of collocations is equal or they differ in the degree of non-compositionality. But we go forward and expand the question by asking if the non-compositionality depends on the semantics of verb-noun collocations. By semantics we mean here the semantic classes represented as lexical functions of the Meaning-Text Theory [29, 31]. We found in this work that there is a correlation between the degree of non-compositionality and lexical functions. So, in the following section we discuss the concept of lexical function and in the subsequent section we show the correlation of the non-compositionality degree with different lexical functions.

3   Lexical Functions as a Concept of the Meaning-Text Theory

Lexical function (LF) is a formal concept proposed within the Meaning-Text Theory [29, 31] to generalize and represent both semantic and syntactic structures of a collocation. Therefore, first of all, we explain briefly the framework and fundamental ideas of the Meaning-Text Theory to better understand how multiword expressions in general and collocations in particular are considered, analyzed, and represented in this theory.

3.1   Meaning-Text Theory (MTT)

The Meaning-Text Theory (MTT) was proposed by Žolkovskij and Mel'čuk in the 1960 s in Moscow, Russia [66, 67] as a universal theory applicable to any language, and was presented in a comprehensive and detailed way on the material of the Russian language by Mel'čuk in 1974 [30]. Since this first complete presentation, MTT has been developed by a number of language researchers, mainly from Canada and Europe [17, 18, 21, 33, 63, 65], in particular, by scientists of Moscow semantic school, Russia [2, 3]. Its most recent exposition can be found in [32]. MTT international conferences have been held since 2003, see the webpage at meaningtext.net.

MTT views a natural language as a system of mappings or rules which enable its speakers to transfer meaning into text. This theory is elaborated to generalize, formalize, and represent multiple levels of such transfer, that is, the process of text synthesis or generation starting from a semantic representation of meaning a speaker intends to communicate. The semantic representation is developed using a special semantic language created for such purpose with enough power to reflect all semantic units and relations among them present in all natural languages; some relations are formalized by lexical functions – the concept we explain in the next subsection.

The focus on text generation is preferred to text understanding, which goes in the opposite direction from text to meaning, due to the fact that text production can be studied in linguistic terms only, whereas text analysis and understanding have to involve disambiguation, which beside linguistic aspects also requires extra-linguistic knowledge, commonly termed as knowledge of the world. The latter remains outside of the MTT since this theory and its formalisms are intended to stay within the purely linguistic realm.

In spite of the fact that MTT deals with text generation only, the concepts of this theory have gained wide recognition in areas other than text generation thanks to their capacity to represent in a clear and concise manner the meaning and relations of linguistic entities on the word, phrase, single utterance, and text levels. In particular, the concept of lexical function has attracted attentions of researchers working on the issue of collocations, looking for ways to generalize and represent their semantics for the purposes of automatic processing, classification, and building computer accessible systematized repositories of collocations. In this sense, determination of lexical function of a collocation is viewed as understanding of the meaning of the collocation. In the next subsection we present the concept of lexical function and illustrate it with examples.

3.2 Lexical Function

Lexical function (LF) is a tool to describe the semantic and syntactic aspects of lexical relations between words in a natural language. It is a function in the mathematical sense defined as a mapping from a word w_0 called the LF argument to a set of words $\{w_1, w_2, \ldots, w_n\}$ in which each word w_i, $1 \leq i \leq n$, has a particular (and the same) lexical relation with the argument w_0; so using mathematical notation, LF is represented as

$$LF(w_0) = \{w_i\}, 1 \leq i \leq n.$$

In the definition of lexical function given above [31], we used the simplistic term *word*. In fact, a more precise term is *lexical unit* which can be an individual word or a multiword expression (MWE). An MWE is an expression of two or more words which together form a single unit of meaning, as in *by and large, come along, bread and butter, give a try* [8]. That is, the meaning of a multiword expression is atomic rather than molecular, or composite, it does not tend to be made of the atomic meanings of the words that are constituents of the MWE.

Another comment on the definition of lexical function concerns the term *lexical relation*. Mel'čuk, defining lexical functions in [31], adds that such functions are generalizations of only lexical relations, but not the relations he calls pseudo-lexical, the latter are termed semantic by some researchers. Mel'čuk clarifies his point by the example of a part-whole or meronymy/holonymy relation saying that this relation holds between things and not between lexical units, therefore, it is not lexical.

In the documents of WordNet [34, 35], it is stated that lexical relations hold between *semantically* related word forms, and *semantic* relations hold between word meanings. In both cases there is a semantic aspect present, although to a different degree and manner, so the definitions look a bit confusing. Besides, quite often the term *lexical relation* is used in papers without any definition; supposedly in such cases it means any type of meaningful relatedness or association of lexical units; see, for example, [11, 12, 58]. In this paper, we make use of all relations, lexical and semantic, since our interest is in semantic analysis or language understanding, and within this perspective both kinds of relations covey particular meanings we seek to identify. Consequently, we apply the concept of lexical function to all lexical, pseudo-lexical, and semantic relations among words and MWEs in a lexicon and in texts, that is, on both the paradigmatic and syntagmatic levels.

We will explain this idea informally with some examples. Let us start with the hyperonymy relation. How are hypernyms detected by linguists? First, some candidate pairs of words are found by digging texts or dictionaries and observing the meaning of words in them: *cat – animal, rose – flower, chair – furniture, magazine – publication, white – color*, etc. We notice that the semantic relation between *cat* and *animal* is the same as between *rose* and *flower*, and in the other word pairs the same semantic association can be seen. Then, we try to describe, understand the meaning of such relation and define it formally, so we notice that one word in a pair represents a class of entities of which the other word of the pair is a specific instance.

At last, we need to create a name, a term, with which we can refer to this relation, and we come up with *hyperonymy*, from Greek *hupér*, 'over' and *onomas*, 'name'; so we say that *animal* a hypernym of *cat*. Moreover, we notice that this relation can be reversed and interpreted in a different but also consistent way, and propose another term, *hyponym*, formed in a similar way from the corresponding Greek words *hupó*, 'under' and *onomas*, 'name', so we say that *cat* is a hyponym of *animal*. Further on we can look for more hyponyms and hypernyms, then hyponyms of hyponyms and hypernyms of hypernyms, etc., revising all the lexicon and many texts, and in the end build a big semantic network in which lexical units would be linked by the hyperonymy/hyponymy relation. An example of such semantic network for English is WordNet [34, 35].

Earlier in this section we mentioned a very important idea which serves as a criterion for identifying relations between words; applying this criterion to the example words in the hyperonymy relation, we said that the semantic relation between *cat* and *animal* is the same as that between *rose* and *flower*, and in other similar word pairs. In other words, we look for words which are related in the same way. This equivalence of relatedness between words is a crucial feature for detecting and further defining relations.

In Table 1 we make observations of other pairs of words: the first word is a noun and the second one is the verb used with the noun in a collocation; we put the respective collocation in the third column of the table. We see here *decision* is related to *make* in the same way as *question* is related to *ask*, and the same association holds between the noun and the verb in all other pairs.

Now, what meaning is communicated by this relation? First of all, all the nouns denote actions: the actions of deciding, asking, arguing, considering, looking, analyzing, resisting, crying, proposing, and ordering. Secondly, what each corresponding verb does

Table 1. Verb-noun collocations and their elements

Noun	Verb	Collocation
Decision	*Make*	*Make a decision*
Question	*Ask*	*Ask a question*
Argument	*Develop*	*Develop an argument*
Attention	*Pay*	*Pay attention*
Look	*Take*	*Take a look*
Analysis	*Conduct*	*Conduct an analysis*
Resistance	*Put up*	*Put up resistance*
Cry	*Raise*	*Raise a cry*
Proposal	*Bring forth*	*Bring forth a proposal*
Order	*Give*	*Give an order*

is, on the one hand, verbalizing the noun, as a noun cannot express time, aspect, person, number (in the sense of the number of agents who perform this action), and all other semantic and pragmatic elements which can be conveyed by a verb, and on the other hand, the verb in each collocations has a meaning 'perform the action expressed by the respective noun'.

Beside the semantic aspect of the relation we found, all collocations have the same syntactic structure verb + noun functioning as a direct object, and, moreover, each collocation is used in utterances with similar core semantic and syntactic structure which we can represent as a semantic and syntactic pattern *Agent performs the action expressed by the noun as the direct object*. Here are some examples of sentences taken from the Corpus of Contemporary American English (COCA)[5] with 450 million words in texts dated from 1990 to 2012:

- In 1994, *Veal made the decision* to come to Arizona State.
- But *you have asked a question* that a lot of people in the country are going to ask today.
- It would be difficult for *an absolutist to develop a* moral *argument* against this behavior, since it primarily affects the person doing the dyeing.
- And apparently *he paid attention* in his military classes...
- *McClellan took a look* at Beverly Park Manor...
- Four years ago, *Luft conducted an analysis* of Iran's consumption of refined petroleum products...
- *Japanese soldiers put up* stiff *resistance* on Biak off New Guinea, but U.S. troops push closer to the island's airfields.
- Again *the ghost raised a cry* and shook his chains.
- *King Hassan brought forth a proposal* for a federalization of Morocco...
- It's easier when *the head of the VA or Department of Defense can* just *give an order* and have things happen and people obey.

Continuing to think of the meaning of the verbs in the previous examples, more fascinating facts can be brought to light. Notice how different the verbs are: *make, ask, develop, pay, take, conduct, put up, raise, bring forth, give.* If we consider them separately, without their corresponding nouns, we see a list of verbs with different and unrelated meanings, probably compiled randomly, having perhaps one aspect in common: all of them are transitive. Then if you might ask, say, a language student whether all these verbs can gain one and the same meaning and under what conditions, the probability of receiving a negative answer may be rather high and such answer will be quite logical: for example, *make* and *ask* seem to belong to different semantic fields, then, in this list two verbs, *take* and *give*, are antonyms, they have opposite meanings, so how can they be transformed into synonyms, words with similar meanings?

The language possesses a miraculous ability to 'make opposite ends meet': *take* and *give* are simply inserted in collocations *take a look* and *give an order*, and they become synonyms instead of antonyms! So what we see in the previous paragraph is a list of

---

[5] Corpus of Contemporary American English (COCA) created by Mark Davies, Brigham Young University, available on http://corpus.byu.edu/coca/.

synonyms; however, such synonyms are not of the type we are used to see in a dictionary of synonyms (moreover, *take* and *give* can be encountered in a dictionary of antonyms), but it is a synonymy acquired by verbs in collocations or under the condition of restricted lexical co-occurrence.

This new synonymy has another interesting feature. Synonymy in the traditional sense (as it is defined in WordNet [34, 35]) implies that synonymous words are interchangeable in some contexts. For example, we can interchange *big* and *large* in the utterance *We came to a large/big, high clapboard house close to the ocean* (taken from COCA). "Collocational synonymy" (as we will call it meanwhile) also allows a similar interchange: for example, *take* and *give* are collocational synonyms in *take a look* and *give an order*. We can change *take* for *give* and get a collocation with a similar meaning: *give a look* (*Tegan gave me a look and I flushed*; taken from COCA). In fact, in the Oxford Collocations Dictionary [28] such synonymous verbs are given: *a look* can be used with *have, cast, dart, give, shoot, throw* expressing the generalized semantics 'perform the action denoted by the noun'. Certainly, these synonyms differ in the manner the action is performed; however, the action realization idea is present in all of them.

Then, in spite of the fact that *take* in *take a look* can be change for any verb in the list of its synonyms from the dictionary of collocations, it cannot be substituted by *ask, conduct, put up, develop* – other verbs with the same generalized semantics 'perform the action denoted by the noun'. Notwithstanding the fact that *ask* in *ask a question* have the same meaning as *take* in *take a look*, we cannot say **ask a look* or *take a question* preserving the meaning of performing an action. **Ask a look* is awkward; *take a question* is acceptable but its meaning is not the same as that of *ask a question*; therefore, such substitutions are not possible.

Now we see that this new "collocational synonymy" is not as flexible as the traditional synonymy, it is restricted and conditioned by the nouns. *A look* in *take a look* or 'perform the action expressed by the noun *look*' can select such other verbs as *have, cast, dart, give, shoot, throw*, and *a question* in *ask a question* prefers *have, put, bombard somebody with, fire, bring up, pose, raise* [28]. We see that some verbs can be used with both nouns, but not all of them: **raise a look* is another example of an inappropriate use.

So far we have discussed a new semantic and syntactic relation found in verbal collocations, and defined it as 'Agent performs the action expressed by the noun as the direct object'. We can search more texts and collocations dictionaries and find more instances of this relation; we will see that instances of such relation are not scarce; in fact, there are a significant number of such collocations. More examples are *pursue a goal, make an error, make an announcement, make use, apply a measure, give a smile, give a hug, take a step, take a walk, take action, have lunch, deliver a lecture, lend support, commit suicide, do a favor, launch an appeal, lay a siege.*

We will also see that some verbs are more productive as they are used in many collocations with the semantics 'perform the action denoted by the noun'– such verbs have a very general meaning: *do, have, make, give, take.* Other verbs have a more narrow meaning and combine with less nouns forming collocation of the same semantic relation, they are *pursue, apply, deliver, lend, commit, launch, lay* from the collocations listed above. More study and observations can be done on the collocations of this semantic type.

As we have defined a new semantic and syntactic relation, we are in need of creating a term to refer to it. The founders of the Meaning-Text Theory who made the observations and discoveries we have just seen, proposed to use abbreviated Latin words to denote this and other types of "collocational synonymy" found in collocations. They gave the name Oper1 to the relation defined as '*Agent performs the action expressed by the noun as the direct object*'; Oper is a shortened Latin word *operari* meaning *do, carry out*, and 1 means that the word used to lexicalize the semantic role of agent of the action denoted by the verb (agent is considered the first argument of a verb) functions as the grammatical subject in a sentence, so the formalism of Oper1 also represents the syntactic structure.

3.3   Lexical Functions in Verb-Noun Collocations

As we explained previously in this section, lexical function (LF) is similar to a mathematical function and has the form $LF(w_0) = \{w_1, w_2, \ldots, w_n\}$, where w_0 is the LF argument which is the base of a collocation, and the LF value is the set $\{w_1, w_2, \ldots, w_n\}$ whose elements are words or word combinations $w_i, 0 < i \leq n$, which is/are collocate/s of a given base. In our previous work we have shown how lexical functions can be automatically detected in verb-noun collocations [22].

In the present research we consider only verb-noun collocations and, respectively, verb-noun lexical functions, so applying the above formula to this particular group of collocations we have w_0 to denote a noun (the base of a collocation) and the set $\{w_1, w_2, \ldots, w_n\}$ will now include only one element w_1 which is a verb (the collocate in a verb-noun collocation). Thus here we deal with lexical functions of the type $LF : N \rightarrow V$, where N is a set of nouns in which each noun functions as the base in a verb-noun collocation, and V is a set of all verbal collocates.

LF represents the generalized semantics of groups of verbal collocates on the one hand, and on the other hand, captures the basic syntactic and predicate-argument structure of sentences in which a collocation belonging to such group is used. Therefore, a lexical function can be viewed as a formal representation of semantic, syntactic, and governing patterns of collocations and their context. We will explain and illustrate this formalism with some of most common lexical functions found in verb-noun collocations. These LFs are used in our experiments which we describe in Sect. 5.

Oper1, from Latin *operari = do, carry out*, formalizes the action of carrying out of what is denoted by the noun (LF argument). As we indicated in the previous subsection, integers in the LF notation are used to specify the predicate-argument and syntactic structure. In Oper1, 1 means that the word used to lexicalize the semantic role of agent of the action denoted by the verb (agent is considered the first argument of a verb) functions as the grammatical subject in a sentence, so Oper1 represents the pattern *Agent performs* w_0 (w_0 is the argument of a lexical function). For example, Oper1(*decision*) = *make*, and in the sentence *The president made a decision, president* is the agent and its syntactic function is subject. Other verb-noun collocations which can be covered by Oper1 are *pursue a goal, make an error, apply a measure, give a smile, take a walk, have lunch, deliver a lecture, make an announcement, lend support, put up resistance, give an order.*

Func0, from Latin *functionare* = *to function*, represents the meaning 'happen, take place'. The noun argument w_0 of Func0 is the name of an action, activity, state, property, relation, i.e., it is such a noun whose meaning is or includes a predicate in the logical sense of the term thus presupposing arguments. Zero in Func0 means that the argument of Func0 is the agent of the verb and functions as the grammatical subject in a sentence. Therefore, Func0 represents the patterns w_0 *occurs*. For example, *snow falls, silence reigns, smell lingers, time flies*.

Each lexical function discussed above represents one simple meaning or a single semantic unit, so such functions are called simple. There are lexical functions that formalize combinations of unitary meanings; they are called complex lexical functions. Now we will consider some of them.

IncepOper1 is a combination of the semantic unit 'begin', from Latin *incipere*, and Oper1 presented above. This LF has the meaning 'begin doing something' and represents the pattern *Agent begins to do* w_0: *to open fire on ..., to acquire popularity, to sink into despair, to take an attitude, to obtain a position, begin negotiations, fall into problems*.

ContOper1 combines the meaning 'continue', from Latin *continuare*, with Oper1. It represents the pattern *Agent continues to do* w_0, for example, *maintain enthusiasm, maintain supremacy, keep one's balance*.

Caus, from Latin *causare*, represents the meaning 'cause, do something so that w_0 begin occurring'. Caus is used only in combinations with other LFs. So CausFunc0 means 'to cause the existence of w_0' and represents the pattern *Agent does something such that w_0 begins to occur*: *bring about the crisis, create a difficulty, present a difficulty, call elections, establish a system, produce an effect*. CausFunc1 represents the pattern *Non-agent argument does something such that w_0 begins to occur*, for example, *open a perspective, raise hope, open a way, cause a damage, instill a habit into somebody*.

4   Non-compositionality in Terms of Lexical Function Detection Using WordNet Hypernyms

In verb-noun collocations, the meaning of the collocate (the verb) differs from its typical meaning commonly represented in dictionaries as sense 1, while the noun is used in its typical sense. Our hypothesis is that the greater the semantic difference between the meaning of the verb in the collocation and the typical meaning of the same verb, the greater the non-compositionality degree of the verb-noun collocation is. We measure the difference between the verb meanings by the difference between two values of F-measure with which the lexical function corresponding to the verb-noun collocation is detected automatically first applying the meaning the verb has in the collocation and, second, applying the typical meaning of the verb.

Now we illustrate the above said with an example. Consider the collocation *make a decision*, it is manually annotated with Oper1. Both the verb and the noun are disambiguated with WordNet senses. In WordNet 3.1 [34, 35] *make* has sense 16 'perform or carry out', so we represent it as *make_16*, and *decision* is used in sense 1, *decision*_1. Then, we use all hypernyms of *make*_16 and *decision*_1 as features, including *make* and *decision* as zero level hypernyms. Like other positive and negative instances of Oper1, *make a decision* is represented as a vector of features, then all instances are submitted to various supervised machine learning algorithms which detect Oper1 with a certain value of F-measure denoted as F.

In another experiment we substitute the sense *make* as well as all verbs in the dataset for Oper1 have in respective collocations with their typical sense (sense 1 in WordNet), so instead of *make*_16 *decision*_1 we get *make*_1 *decision*_1, sense 1 of *make* is 'engage in' as in *make an effort, make revolution*. Then the dataset is submitted to the same algorithms, and Oper1 is detected with (probably) another value of F-measure which we denote as F^1. The difference $F - F^1$ serves as an evidence of the non-compositionality degree of the collocation. If the LF is detected better using sense 1 of the verb in a collocation, then such collocation is less non-compositional. If the LF is detected worse with sense 1, then the collocation is more non-compositional, that is, more opaque. Additionally, we interpret the difference $F - F^1$ as a degree of non-compositionality which can be applied to measure this property of collocations on a fine-grained level.

5 Experiments

For automatic detection of lexical functions, we use a dataset of Spanish verb-noun collocations[6] [10] annotated manually with lexical functions and the Spanish WordNet[7] version 2000611 [62] senses. The dataset is submitted to various supervised machine learning techniques implemented in Weka[8] 3-6-12- × 64 [64] to classify each sample in the dataset set as belonging or not to a particular LF (binary yes-no classification) using 10-fold cross validation.

Each collocation in the dataset is represented as a list of all hypernyms of the verb and all hypernyms of the noun including both verb and noun as zero level hypernyms. As explained in Sect. 4, in the first series of experiments, we detect LFs using the actual senses of the verbs. For this purpose, from the dataset of verb-noun collocations we choose only those collocations in which the verb has sense other than 1. This is because in the second series of experiments we plan to compare LF detection on the same collocations, but having substituted the actual sense of the verb by sense 1. Remember that to distinguish the results of the two series of experiments, F-measure obtained in the first experiment is denoted as F, and F-measure obtained in the second experiment is termed F^1. After obtaining the results of both experiments, we calculate the difference $F - F^1$ which is interpreted as the non-compositionality degree of the collocation.

---

[6] Spanish Verb-Noun Lexical Functions, available on http://148.204.58.221/okolesnikova/index.php?id=lex/ and http://www.gelbukh.com/lexical-functions/.

[7] Spanish WordNet: http://www.lsi.upc.edu/~nlp/web/index.php?Itemid=57&id=31&option=com_content&task=view.

[8] The University of Waikato Computer Science Department Machine Learning Group, WEKA, available on http://www.cs.waikato.ac.nz/ml/weka/downloading.html/.

Table 2. Lexical functions used in our experiments

LF	# of samples in experiments	Examples of collocations	
		Spanish	English translation
Oper1	154	*realizar un estudio*	do a study
		cometer un error	make an error
		dar un beso	give a kiss
IncepOper1	21	*iniciar un proceso*	begin a process
		tomar la palabra	take the floor
		adoptar la actitud	adopt the attitude
ContOper1	14	*seguir un curso*	follow a course
		mantener un contacto	keep in touch
		guardar silencio	keep silent
CausFunc0	80	*crear una cuenta*	create an account
		formar un grupo	form a group
		hacer ruido	make noise
CausFunc1	73	*ofrecer una posibilidad*	offer a possibility
		causar un problema	cause a problem
		crear una condición	create a condition

Table 2 presents the LFs used in our experiments. The semantics of each LF was described in Sect. 3.

6   Results and Discussion

Tables 3, 4, 5, 6 and 7 present the results of ten classifiers out of 66 classifiers implemented in Weka 3-6-12- × 64 [64] and applicable to the type of data used in our experiments. We remind the reader of the notation explained in Sect. 5: F-measure obtained in the first experiment when LFs were detected in collocations with the actual

Table 3. Experimental results for Oper1

Classifier	F	F^1	$F - F^1$
trees.SimpleCart	0.900	0.815	0.085
rules.PART	0.900	0.783	0.117
trees.LADTree	0.900	0.769	0.131
meta.END	0.900	0.832	0.068
meta.FilteredClassifier	0.900	0.832	0.068
meta.OrdinalClassClassifier	0.900	0.832	0.068
trees.J48	0.900	0.832	0.068
rules.Jrip	0.900	0.819	0.081
trees.BFTree	0.897	0.819	0.078
trees.REPTree	0.896	0.750	0.146
Average	**0.899**	**0.808**	**0.091**

Table 4. Experimental results for IncepOper1

Classifier	F	F^1	$F - F^1$
trees.Id3	0.900	0.571	0.329
rules.Prism	0.842	0.583	0.259
rules.Nnge	0.829	0.516	0.313
trees.LADTree	0.829	0.629	0.200
functions.SMO	0.821	0.571	0.250
functions.Logistic	0.810	0.435	0.375
meta.MultiClassClassifier	0.810	0.435	0.375
BayesianLogisticRegression	0.789	0.286	0.503
functions.SimpleLogistic	0.789	0.429	0.360
rules.PART	0.703	0.439	0.264
Average	**0.812**	**0.489**	**0.323**

Table 5. Experimental results for ContOper1

Classifier	F	F^1	$F - F^1$
lazy.LWL	0.857	0.880	−0.023
rules.DecisionTable	0.857	0.923	−0.066
functions.SimpleLogistic	0.857	0.923	−0.066
BayesianLogisticRegression	0.857	0.923	−0.066
rules.Ridor	0.839	0.963	−0.124
meta. AttributeSelectedClassifier	0.828	0.889	−0.061
trees.BFTree	0.828	0.889	−0.061
trees.SimpleCart	0.828	0.923	−0.095
meta.END	0.828	0.889	−0.061
meta.FilteredClassifier	0.828	0.889	−0.061
Average	**0.841**	**0.909**	**−0.068**

Table 6. Experimental results for CausFunc0

Classifier	F	F^1	$F - F^1$
trees.SimpleCart	0.756	0.532	0.224
trees.LADTree	0.744	0.744	0
meta. AttributeSelectedClassifier	0.735	0.829	−0.094
trees.BFTree	0.726	0.818	−0.092
functions.SimpleLogistic	0.714	0.812	−0.098
meta.END	0.711	0.829	−0.118
meta.FilteredClassifier	0.711	0.829	−0.118
meta.OrdinalClassClassifier	0.711	0.829	−0.118
trees.J48	0.711	0.769	−0.058
rules.Jrip	0.704	0.843	−0.139
Average	**0.722**	**0.783**	**−0.061**

Table 7. Experimental results for CausFunc1

Classifier	F	F^1	$F - F^1$
meta.RotationForest	0.771	0.855	–0.153
trees.BFTree	0.771	0.870	–0.157
trees.SimpleCart	0.771	0.859	–0.163
meta.END	0.769	0.861	–0.164
meta.FilteredClassifier	0.769	0.861	–0.193
meta.OrdinalClassClassifier	0.769	0.861	–0.167
trees.J48	0.769	0.861	–0.191
meta.LogitBoost	0.766	0.892	–0.205
trees.ADTree	0.766	0.892	–0.254
meta. AttributeSelectedClassifier	0.762	0.892	–0.145
Average	**0.768**	**0.870**	**–0.179**

sense of the verb is represented as F, and F-measure in the second experiment is represented as F^1 since in this experiment LFs were detected in the same collocations but the actual verb sense was substituted by sense 1, the typical meaning of the verb.

Then we calculated the difference $F - F^1$ and interpreted it as the non-compositionality degree of the collocation.

Now we discuss our results in terms of the average values of F, F^1, and $F - F^1$.

It can be observed in Table 3 that Oper1 is detected notably worse when the actual verb sense is substituted with sense 1, with a value of F^1 of 0.808 versus a value of F of 0.899 for the actual verb senses. Therefore, Oper1 collocations are more non-compositional, with a difference $F - F^1$ of 0.091. This fact suggests that the actual verb senses fit well the definition of Oper1, *Agent performs* w_0, where w_0 is the noun in a verb-noun collocation.

Table 4 presents the results for IncepOper1. Here the performance of classifiers in terms of average F is 0.812. However, if the actual verb sense is changed for sense 1, the performance degrades dramatically, with an F^1 of 0.644. The degree of non-compositionality $F - F^1$ is 0.323, which is higher than the non-compositionality of Oper1 collocations.

Now we discuss ContOper1 collocations in Table 5. It is interesting to note that if the actual verb senses are changed to sense 1, this improves the classifier performance: F is 0.841, but F^1 has a value of 0.909, so $F - F^1$ is –0.068. Therefore, collocations of the semantic type ContOper1 are less non-compositional and closer to free word combinations compared with Oper1 and IncepOper1.

Similar results were obtained on detection of CausFunc0 and CausFunc1 in Tables 6 and 7, respectively: the classifier performance is improved if the actual verb senses are substituted with verb sense 1. For CausFunc0, we have F of 0.722, F^1 is 0.783, and the non-compositionality degree $F - F^1$ of –0.061. For CausFunc1, F is 0.768, F^1 is 0.870, and $F - F^1$ is –0.179.

We see that verb-noun collocations represent a range of non-compositionality: from highly non-compositional IncepOper1 (0.323) and Oper1 (0.091) to less non-compositional CausFunc0 (−0.061) and ContOper1 (−0.068), and to almost compositional CausFunc1 (−0.179). It is also noteworthy that the non-compositionality degree varies across lexical functions. Moreover, our results show to what extent the meaning of the verb in a collocation is able to distinguish lexical functions, and the measure $F^n - F^m$, where n and m are the numbers of WordNet senses, can be applied to measure correlation between lexical functions and WordNet senses as well as to evaluate the quality of word sense classification and definitions.

7 Conclusions and Future Work

In this work we proposed a new measure of the non-compositionality degree of verb-noun collocations. This measure is the difference between two values of F-measure with which lexical functions of the Meaning-Text Theory [29–31], representing different semantic classes of collocations, are detected automatically by supervised machine learning techniques. The first value is obtained on a dataset in which all verbs are disambiguated using WordNet senses, and the second value is obtained on the same dataset but with actual verb senses substituted by sense 1, which is commonly the most typical sense of the verb. The intuition behind our proposal is that the greater the difference between the meaning the verb has in the collocation and the typical sense of the same verb, the higher the non-compositionality degree of the collocation is.

We found that the difference between two values of F-measure varies among lexical functions: collocations belonging to IncepOper1 and Oper1 are highly non-compositional, collocations of CausFunc0 and ContOper1 are less non-compositional, and those of CausFunc1 are almost compositional.

Our measure can be used to rank collocations according to the degree of their non-compositionality which then allows a natural language system to choose techniques most appropriate for handling each category of collocations. Also, our measure can be applied to evaluate the similarity of senses in a dictionary as well as the correlation between the semantic classes of verb-noun collocations and dictionary definitions; it can also be used to evaluate the quality and discriminative ability of dictionary word senses.

In future, we plan to perform experiments with other lexical functions not considered in the present work. Detecting collocations is useful to effectively perform many textual analysis tasks, since they can help in measuring text similarity [14, 16] and serve as features in machine learning algorithms [56]. Thus our future work will also focus on identifying and using collocations in such tasks such as personality detection [48], textual entailment [39–41], sentiment analysis [5] and emotion detection [49].

Acknowledgements. The work was done under partial support of Mexican Government: SNI and Instituto Politécnico Nacional, grants SIP 20152095 and SIP 20152100.

References

1. Alonso-Rorís, V.M., Santos Gago, J.M., Pérez Rodríguez, R., Rivas Costa, C., Gómez Carballa, M.A., Anido Rifón, L.: Information extraction in semantic, highly-structured, and semi-structured web sources. Polibits **49**, 69–75 (2014)
2. Apresjan, J.D.: Lexical Semantics. Vostochnaya Literatura, Russian Academy of Sciences, Moscow (1995). (In Russian)
3. Apresjan, J.D.: Systematic Lexicography. Oxford University Press, Oxford (2000)
4. Baldwin, T., Bannard, C., Tanaka, T., Widdows, D.: An empirical model of multiword expression decomposability. In: Proceedings of the ACL 2003 Workshop on Multiword Expressions: Analysis, Acquisition and Treatment, vol. 18, pp. 89–96. Association for Computational Linguistics (2003)
5. Agarwal, B., Poria, S., Mittal, N., Gelbukh, A., Hussain, A.: Concept-level sentiment analysis with dependency-based semantic parsing: a novel approach. Cogn. Comput. **7**(4), 1–13 (2015)
6. Biemann, C., Giesbrecht, E.: Distributional semantics and compositionality 2011: shared task description and results. In: Proceedings of the Workshop on Distributional Semantics and Compositionality, pp. 21–28. Association for Computational Linguistics (2011)
7. Bu, F., Zhu, X., Li, M.: Measuring the non-compositionality of multiword expressions. In: Proceedings of the 23rd International Conference on Computational Linguistics, pp. 116–124. Association for Computational Linguistics (2010)
8. Fazly, A., Stevenson, S.: Distinguishing subtypes of multiword expressions using linguistically motivated statistical measures. In: Grégoire, N., Evert, S., Krenn, B. (eds.) Proceedings of the ACL 2007 Workshop on a Broader Perspective on Multiword Expressions, pp. 9–16. Czech Republic, Prague (2007)
9. Fontenelle, T.: Using lexical functions to discover metaphors. In: Proceedings of the 6th EURALEX International Congress, pp. 271–278 (1994)
10. Gelbukh, A., Kolesnikova, O.: Supervised learning for semantic classification of Spanish collocations. In: Martínez-Trinidad, J.F., Carrasco-Ochoa, J.A., Kittler, J. (eds.) MCPR 2010. LNCS, vol. 6256, pp. 362–371. Springer, Heidelberg (2010)
11. Hashimoto, K., Stenetorp, P., Miwa, M., Tsuruoka, Y.: Task-Oriented Learning of Word Embeddings for Semantic Relation Classification, arXiv preprint arXiv:1503.00095 (2015)
12. Hirst, G., St-Onge, D.: Lexical chains as representations of context for the detection and correction of malapropisms. In: WordNet: An electronic Lexical Database, pp. 305–332 (1998)
13. Inkpen, D., Razavi, A.H.: Topic classification using latent Dirichlet allocation at multiple levels. Int. J. Comput. Linguist. Appl. **6**(1), 43–58
14. Jimenez, S., Gonzalez, F.A., Gelbukh, A.: Soft cardinality in semantic text processing: experience of the SemEval international competitions. Polibits **51**, 63–72 (2015)
15. Johannsen, A., Alonso, H.M., Rishøj, C., Søgaard, A.: Shared task system description: frustratingly hard compositionality prediction. In: Proceedings of the Workshop on Distributional Semantics and Compositionality, pp. 29–32. Association for Computational Linguistics (2011)
16. Huynh, D., Tran, D., Ma, W., Sharma, D.: Semantic similarity measure using relational and latent topic features. Int. J. Comput. Linguist. Appl. **5**(1), 11–25 (2014)
17. Kahane, S.: What is a natural language and how to describe it? Meaning-text approaches in contrast with generative approaches. In: Gelbukh, A. (ed.) CICLing 2001. LNCS, vol. 2004, pp. 1–17. Springer, Heidelberg (2001)

18. Kahane, S.: The meaning-text theory. Dependency Valency Int. Handb. Contemp. Res. **1**, 546–570 (2003)
19. Katz, G., Giesbrecht, E.: Automatic identification of non-compositional multi-word expressions using latent semantic analysis. In: Proceedings of the Workshop on Multiword Expressions: Identifying and Exploiting Underlying Properties, pp. 12–19. Association for Computational Linguistics (2006)
20. Kim, S.N., Baldwin, T.: Detecting compositionality of English verb-particle constructions using semantic similarity. In: Proceedings of the 7th Meeting of the Pacific Association for Computational Linguistics PACLING 2007, pp. 40–48 (2007)
21. Kittredge, R., Iordanskaja, L., Polguère, A.: Multilingual text generation and the meaning-text theory. In: Proceedings of TMI-88, Pittsburgh, PA (1988)
22. Kolesnikova, O.: Discriminative ability of WordNet senses on the task of detecting lexical functions in Spanish verb-noun collocations. Int. J. Comput. Linguist. Appl. **5**(2), 61–86 (2014)
23. Kunchukuttan, A., Damani, O.P.: A system for compound noun multiword expression extraction for Hindi. In: 6th International Conference on Natural Language Processing, pp. 20–29 (2008)
24. Lin, D.: Automatic retrieval and clustering of similar words. In: Proceedings of the 36th Annual Meeting of the Association for Computational Linguistics and 17th International Conference on Computational Linguistics, vol. 2, pp. 768–774. Association for Computational Linguistics (1998)
25. Lyons, J.: Linguistic Semantics: An Introduction. Cambridge University Press, Cambridge (1995)
26. McCarthy, D., Keller, B., Carroll, J.: Detecting a continuum of compositionality in phrasal verbs. In: Proceedings of the ACL 2003 Workshop on Multiword Expressions: Analysis, Acquisition and Treatment, vol. 18, pp. 73–80. Association for Computational Linguistics (2003)
27. McCarthy, D., Venkatapathy, S., Joshi, A.K.: Detecting compositionality of verb-object combinations using selectional preferences. In: EMNLP-CoNLL, pp. 369–379 (2007)
28. McIntosh, C., Francis, B., Poole, R. (eds.): Oxford Collocations Dictionary for Students of English. Oxford University Press, Oxford (2009)
29. Mel'čuk, I.A., Žolkovskij, A.K.: Towards a functioning 'Meaning-Text' model of language. Linguistics **8**(57), 10–47 (1970)
30. Mel'čuk, I.A.: Toward a Theory of Meaning-Text Linguistic Models. Nauka Publishers, Moscow (1974)
31. Mel'čuk, I.A.: Lexical functions: a tool for the description of lexical relations in a lexicon. In: Wanner, L. (ed.) Lexical Functions in Lexicography and Natural Language Processing, pp. 37–102. Benjamins Academic Publishers, Amsterdam, Philadelphia, PA (1996)
32. Mel'čuk, I.A.: Semantics: From Meaning to Text, vol. 3. John Benjamins Publishing Company, Amsterdam (2015)
33. Milićević, J.: A short guide to the meaning-text linguistic theory. J. Koralex **8**, 187–233 (2006)
34. Miller, G.A.: WordNet: a lexical database for English. Commun. ACM **38**(11), 39–41 (1995)
35. Miller, G.A., Leacock, C., Tengi, R., Bunker, R.T.: A semantic concordance. In: Proceedings of the Workshop on Human Language Technology Association for Computational Linguistics, pp. 303–308 (1993)
36. Mohler, M., Tomlinson, M., Rink, B.: Cross-lingual semantic generalization for the detection of metaphor. Int. J. Comput. Linguist. Appl. **6**(2), 115–136 (2015)

37. Nakagawa, H., Mori, T.: Automatic term recognition based on statistics of compound nouns and their components. Terminology **9**(2), 201–219 (2003)
38. Orliac, B., Dillinger, M.: Collocation extraction for machine translation. In: Proceedings of Machine Translation Summit IX, pp. 292–298 (2003)
39. Pakray, P., Neogi, S., Bhaskar, P., Poria, S., Bandyopadhyay, S., Gelbukh, A.: A textual entailment system using anaphora resolution. In: System Report. Recognizing Textual Entailment Track (TAC RTE). Notebook. National Institute of Standards and Technology (2011)
40. Pakray, P., Pal, S., Poria, S., Bandyopadhyay, S., Gelbukh, A.: JU_CSE_TAC: textual entailment recognition system at TAC RTE-6. In: System Report, Text Analysis Conference Recognizing Textual Entailment Track (TAC RTE). Notebook. National Institute of Standards and Technology (2010)
41. Pakray, P., Poria, S., Bandyopadhyay, S., Gelbukh, A.: Semantic textual entailment recognition using UNL. Polibits **43**, 23–27 (2011)
42. Pecina, P.: An extensive empirical study of collocation extraction methods. In: Proceedings of the ACL Student Research Workshop, pp. 13–18. Association for Computational Linguistics (2005)
43. Poria, S., Agarwal, B., Gelbukh, A., Hussain, A., Howard, N.: Dependency-based semantic parsing for concept-level text analysis. In: Gelbukh, A. (ed.) CICLing 2014, Part I. LNCS, vol. 8403, pp. 113–127. Springer, Heidelberg (2014)
44. Poria, S., Cambria, E., Gelbukh, A.: Deep convolutional neural network textual features and multiple kernel learning for utterance-level multimodal sentiment analysis. In: Proceedings of EMNLP 2015, Lisbon, pp. 2539–2544 (2015)
45. Poria, S., Cambria, E., Gelbukh, A., Bisio, F., Hussain, A.: Sentiment data flow analysis by means of dynamic linguistic patterns. IEEE Comput. Intell. Mag. **10**(4), 26–36 (2015)
46. Poria, S., Cambria, E., Howard, N., Huang, G.-B., Hussain, A.: Fusing audio, visual and textual clues for sentiment analysis from multimodal content. Neurocomputing (2015, in press). doi:10.1016/j.neucom.2015.01.095
47. Poria, S., Cambria, E., Winterstein, G., Huang, G.-B.: Sentic patterns: dependency-based rules for concept-level sentiment analysis. Knowl.-Based Syst. **69**, 45–63 (2014)
48. Poria, S., Gelbukh, A., Agarwal, B., Cambria, E., Howard, N.: Common sense knowledge based personality recognition from text. In: Castro, F., Gelbukh, A., González, M. (eds.) MICAI 2013, Part II. LNCS, vol. 8266, pp. 484–496. Springer, Heidelberg (2013)
49. Poria, S., Gelbukh, A., Das, D., Bandyopadhyay, S.: Fuzzy clustering for semi-supervised learning – case study: construction of an emotion lexicon. In: Batyrshin, I., González Mendoza, M. (eds.) MICAI 2012, Part I. LNCS, vol. 7629, pp. 73–86. Springer, Heidelberg (2013)
50. Poria, S., Gelbukh, A., Cambria, E., Hussain, A., Huang, G.-B.: EmoSenticSpace: a novel framework for affective common-sense reasoning. Knowl.-Based Syst. **69**, 108–123 (2014)
51. Reddy, S., McCarthy, D., Manandhar, S., Gella, S.: Exemplar-based word-space model for compositionality detection: shared task system description. In: Proceedings of the Workshop on Distributional Semantics and Compositionality, pp. 54–60. Association for Computational Linguistics (2011)
52. Rinaldi, F., Lithgow-Serrano, O., López-Fuentes, A., Gama-Castro, S., Balderas-Martínez, Y.I., Solano-Lira, H., Collado-Vides, J.: An approach towards semi-automated biomedical literature curation and enrichment for a major biological database. Polibits **52**, 25–31 (2015)
53. Rohde, D.L., Gonnerman, L.M., Plaut, D.C.: An improved model of semantic similarity based on lexical co-occurrence. Commun. ACM **8**, 627–633 (2006)

54. Sag, I.A., Baldwin, T., Bond, F., Copestake, A., Flickinger, D.: Multiword expressions: a pain in the neck for NLP. In: Gelbukh, A. (ed.) CICLing 2002. LNCS, vol. 2276, pp. 1–15. Springer, Heidelberg (2002)
55. Schütze, H.: Automatic word sense discrimination. Comput. Linguist. **24**(1), 97–123 (1998)
56. Sidorov, G.: Should syntactic N-grams contain names of syntactic relations? Int. J. Comput. Linguist. Appl. **5**(2), 23–46 (2014)
57. Sidorov, G., Kobozeva, I., Zimmerling, A., Chanona-Hernández, L., Kolesnikova, O.: Modelo computacional del diálogo basado en reglas aplicado a un robot guía móvil. Polibits **50**, 35–42 (2014)
58. Smadja, F.A., McKeown, K.R.: Automatically extracting and representing collocations for language generation. In: Proceedings of the 28th Annual Meeting on Association for Computational Linguistics, pp. 252–259. Association for Computational Linguistics (1990)
59. Svensson, M.H.: A very complex criterion of fixedness: non-compositionality. Phraseology Interdisc. Perspect. S. Granger **81**, 81–93 (2008)
60. Van de Cruys, T., Moirón, B.V.: Semantics-based multiword expression extraction. In: Proceedings of the Workshop on a Broader Perspective on Multiword Expressions, pp. 25–32. Association for Computational Linguistics (2007)
61. Venkatapathy, S., Joshi, A.K.: Measuring the relative compositionality of verb-noun (VN) collocations by integrating features. In: Proceedings of the Conference on Human Language Technology and Empirical Methods in Natural Language Processing, pp. 899–906. Association for Computational Linguistics (2005)
62. Vossen, P. (ed.): EuroWordNet: a Multilingual Database with Lexical Semantic Networks. Kluwer Academic Publishers, Dordrecht (1998)
63. Wanner, L. (ed.): Recent Trends in Meaning-Text Theory. John Benjamins Publishers, Amsterdam, Philadelphia (1997)
64. Witten, I.H., Frank, E., Hall, M.A.: Data mining: Practical machine learning tools and techniques. Morgan Kaufmann Publishers, MA, USA (2011)
65. Zabokrtský, Z.: Resemblances between meaning-text theory and functional generative description. In: Proceedings of Second International Conference on Meaning–Text Theory, Moscow (2005)
66. Žolkovskij, A.K., Mel'čuk, I.A.: On a possible method an instruments for semantic synthesis (of texts), in Russian. Sci. Technol. Inf. **6**, 23–28 (1965). (in Russian)
67. Žolkovskij, A.K., Mel'čuk, I.A.: On semantic synthesis (of texts), in Russian. Probl. Cybern. **19**, 177–238 (1967). (in Russian)

Fuzzy-Probabilistic Estimation of the Electric Vehicles Energy Consumption

Nuno Borges[(⊠)], João Soares, and Zita Vale

GECAD – Research Group on Intelligent Engineering and Computing for
Advanced Innovation and Development, Porto, Portugal
{ndsbs,joaps,zav}@isep.ipp.pt

Abstract. This paper presents a framework and methodology to characterize the uncertainty of the consumption in the Electric Vehicles (EVs). A Fuzzy Logic (FL) is implemented to obtain an interval of the probability that the energy consumption may take. The framework assumes the availability of Information and Communication Technology (ICT) technology and previous data records. A case study is presented using a fleet of 30 EVs considering a smart grid environment.

Keywords: Communications · Electric vehicles · Fuzzy logic · Smart grid

1 Introduction

Currently, more than 90 % of the energy used in the transportation sector is provided by oil source [1]. Oil will continue to be a major fuel for decades, but reducing this dependence on a single source is very risky because oil is a fossil source, as such, does not last forever. Other problem is the enormous quantity of CO^2 produced by the vehicles moved with fossil fuels that is prejudicial to the planet. With the increasing concern over global climate change, policy makers are promoting renewable energy sources (RESs) to reduce this problem. According to the reference [2], a partial solution to solve this problem can be mitigated by 2 measures: the first one is the use of decentralized RES, and the second is the application of next-generation plug-in vehicles, which include plug-in hybrid electric vehicles (PHEV) and electric vehicles (EVs), with vehicle-to-grid (V2G).

If we do a direct comparison, EVs convert about 59–62 % of the electrical energy from the grid to power at the wheels, the conventional gasoline vehicles only convert about 17–21 % of the energy stored in gasoline to power at the wheels [3]. In [4] it is discussed the social and technical barriers to the V2G transition, namely what policymakers need to achieve to enable a successful implementation. However, the introduction of EVs represents an unprecedented interaction between transportation and the electricity grid. The electricity grid and EVs are highly dependent due to the fact that the energy to charge the batteries comes from the grid [5]. With the increased use of the EVs the planning of the electrical infrastructures is more demanding [6], mainly due to the level of the uncertainties introduced. The impacts of the EV penetration in the grid were studied in [7] and [8].

The variability in EV's energy consumption has a high impact at the user level and the electricity system. For example, to the user this situation difficult the planning of the

© Springer International Publishing Switzerland 2015
O. Pichardo Lagunas et al. (Eds.): MICAI 2015, Part II, LNAI 9414, pp. 26–36, 2015.
DOI: 10.1007/978-3-319-27101-9_2

periods that the EV need to charge. In what regards system's impacts, daily charging of an EV would double of a typical household electricity consumption. With a significant penetration level at the distribution system, this could result in high variations in energy demand.

Due to improvements in Information and Communication Technology (ICT) big data will be available for smart grid operators [9]. Real-time records regarding EVs' location, time of charge, energy charged, charged rate and trip consumptions, could be maintained in appropriate data storage systems, e.g. a computer cloud. This data can be processed to be useful for operators in a later stage.

This paper proposes one methodology to model the uncertainties of the consumptions in the EV. The methodology presented in this paper depends on the availability of ICT technology and historical data records to obtain the probabilistic consumptions. Its ultimate goal is to be used with realistic data. EV's are very sensitive to parameters which can influence their energy consumptions, such as: driving conditions, auxiliary systems' impact (for example, electrically driven air conditioning, driver's aggressiveness and braking energy).

Recent works on the available literature use a different types of methodologies to model similar problems, for example. In [10], an EV demand model for load flow studies is developed, the model considers the EV demand has PQ buses with stochastic characteristics using Queueing Theory as a function of the charging time. The method only considers one type of vehicle in the case study and does not represent a load pattern along the day or a set of scenarios for the EV. This method has been applied in [11] to developed a probabilistic constrained load flow with the presence of EVs. The work considers the full charge and discharge power of EVs in a specific region, allowing the calculation of power flow with probabilistic constraints. However the two methods mentioned above do not consider the different types of battery capacity of the EVs. In reference [12] a Fuzzy Logic (FL) control strategy is developed for an energy management system of an EV with dual source power (battery and super capacitor). This dual source architecture is proposed in order to satisfy the EVs energy requirements, improving the EVs efficiency and the performance of the overall system. In [13] MATSim is used to obtain the arrival and departure time of each trip and the associated energy consumption for each vehicle. Based on that reference sample, a generation of different samples of driving patterns for each vehicle was made. The trip departure time and trip duration are uniformly distributed 30 min around their reference values and the trip consumption is also assumed to be uniformly distributed 1 kWh around the reference value. With these distributions is possible generate different realizations of driving patterns for each individual vehicle. However, the chosen distributions are just exemplary distributions, in practice the aggregator would need to collect data from its PEV customers to find appropriate models for their stochastic behavior. In [14], a Bootstrap technique is used to model the charging temporal uncertainties for the Plug-In Electric Vehicles (PEV). Initially, using the Bootstrap method, an input sample is generated, representing the different scenarios for the behavior of PEVs, with the various initial battery state-of-charges and arrival and departure times of the PEVs. The GA-based optimization model is used to generate 25 independent observations of the daily system peak demand and their corresponding hourly load tap charging schedules to make up the original sample, which are then used to generate a large number of Bootstrap samples in order to demonstrate the central limit theorem.

Taking into account the current literature this work proposed a framework and respective methodology to support the estimation of the fuzzy-probabilistic curves of the EVs' energy consumption. This information can be used to make an accurate planning of the journey and obtain an adequate pattern of the EV demand. This can be useful for power system operators and EVs' energy management systems in order. This methodology was tested with a realistic case study that represent one year for weekdays and weekend behavior.

This paper is organized as follows: after this introductory Sect. 2 presents the proposed framework based on FL, Sect. 3 presents the case study and finally Sect. 4 presents the conclusions.

2 Methodology

This section presents the developed framework and methodology.

2.1 Framework

Figure 1 presents the proposed framework to support the information necessary for the presented methodology and other applications beyond the scope of this paper. In this proposed framework each EV have one processing unit (CPU) with the capacity to process the information in real time, this information can be stored in a memory card

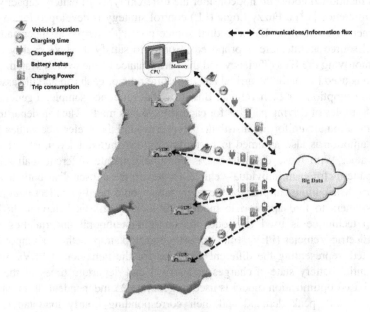

Fig. 1. Framework to support the proposed methodology

and can be transmitted for the cloud (big data), if the EV has an appropriate system with connection to the internet. Several communication technologies are considered as candidates such as WiMAX, WiFi, and power line communications are available for the smart grid system to support the information flux between the EVs and the grid using the Internet Protocol (IP) [15]. The data transmitted over the communication network can be encrypted using a secured TLS cryptographic mechanism. However, this will require an overhead resulting in larger data size to be transmitted. This system in the case of internet connection failure (e.g. driving in tunnels, parking in underground) should have an internal memory system to allow each EV to save the data temporarily. Later, with reconnection, the data can be sent to the cloud, thus preventing previous data from being lost. This implies an individual processing and storage of data with minimal computing requirements in each EV. A centralized process (cloud application) could be available to handle EVs' recorded data in a smarter way, e.g. using big data analytics. Such applications could include real-time traffic alerts, monitoring and rerouting, consumers' patterns identification, EVs' demand forecast, connected vehicles applications including accident avoidance.

The type of data available in each vehicle could be the EVs ' location, time of charge, energy charged, charged rate and trip consumptions. This might be regulated by a standard or legal requirement in the future, thus enabling a greater compatibility for the proposed framework. In order to define this standard it would be necessary to consider the types of data to be stored and transmitted, a control access to the data and the transmission mode.

Table 1 shows a very simple data scheme of the information that could be transmitted between the EVs and the cloud applications (see Fig. 1). The values depicted in the table do not consider the overhead of the encryption, the packet's header (typically 20 bytes), and the possible compression of repeated data sequences. The methodology present in this paper depends on the successful treatment and processing of data to attain the expected results.

The first parameter, Vehicle's ID, can provide one number that represent the identification of the client (EV). This ID number can be saved in class int32 format (4 bytes).

Table 1. Proposed data scheme

Data Parameters	Description of data structure		
	Type of data	*Data class*	*Size per record*
Vehicle's ID	Identification of EV	int32	4 bytes
Location	GPS location	Double	3 × 8 bytes
Battery status	Battery capacity; SOC level	int32	2 × 4 bytes
Connected to outlet	Connected (0/1); Outlet ID	Binary and int32	1 + 4 bytes
Charged energy	Charged energy; timestamp	int32 and Double	4 + 2 × 8 bytes
Charge rate	Charging power	int32	4 bytes
Trip consumptions	Energy consumption in the trip; Start and end timestamp	int32 and Double	4 + 2 × 8 bytes

The Location parameter needs to consider a 3 types of data: latitude, longitude and timestamp. The results of this is the GPS location of the EV. The type of data class is double with a size per record of 3 × 8 bytes, 8 bytes for each type of data. Other important parameter is the trip consumptions, where the types of data records are the energy consumptions in the total trip, the start and end timestamp for this trip. This parameter (energy consumption) can be saved in int32 class format (4 bytes), while the start and end timestamp can be saved in double class format (2 × 8bytes).

2.2 Fuzzy-Probabilistic Methodology

The methodology used consists in the use of Fuzzy Logic (FL) to characterize the uncertainty of the consumption data and a probabilistic distribution function.

The term FL was introduced with the 1965 proposal of fuzzy set theory by Zadeh [16], however had been studied since the 1920, as infinite-valued logic [17]. FL is a superset of conventional (Boolean) logic that has been extended to handle the concept of partial truth. The number of paper dealing, in some sense, with FL and its applications is immense, and the success in applications is evident.

The meaning of fuzzy portrays something vague, uncertain, being used to get one representation of imprecise data [18]. Fuzzy set is very convenient method for representing some form of uncertainty, because this method is a type of logic that recognizes more than simple true and false values. While variables in mathematics usually take numerical values, in FL applications, the non-numeric are often used to facilitate the expression of rules and facts. With FL, this propositions can be represented with degrees of truth. For example, the statement, today is sunny, might be 100 % true if there are no clouds, 80 % true if there are a few clouds, 50 % true if it's hazy and 0 % true if it rains all day. The FL allows an infinite range of values in the range [0, 1], which would indicate the possibility of a statement to be true (1) or false (0), assuming intermediate logical values neither completely true nor false. The process of converting the fuzzy region in a final numeric value is designated by defuzzification and resides in simply calculating the center of gravity of the end region and can be achieved by expression (1):

$$v = \frac{\int_x (x \times t(x))}{\int_x (t(x))} Z \tag{1}$$

Where:
v – defuzzification value
$t(x)$ – degree of truth in the point x

From the historical database (Big Data), we filtered the parameter of consumption that corresponded to the use of the available energy in the battery for each period of the day. When the vehicle is charging, the consumption have a null value. To apply the fuzzy logic it was necessary to make a calculation of the average energy consumption from the filtered data. For the implementation of FL we defined an upper bound value, a lower bound value and number of degrees of truth. To the results of the fuzzy function is given the value of centroid, which indicates the average value of the figure, or in other words, the point in the center of the figure which is the shortest distance for the all points of the figure. Fuzzification was applied to average and standard deviation values.

The distribution that best represents the consumption of EVs is the normal distribution [19]. The normal distribution can be obtained using (2):

$$fp(P) = \frac{1}{\sqrt{2\pi \times \sigma^2}} \times e^{\frac{-(P-\mu)^2}{2\times\sigma^2}} Z \qquad (2)$$

Where:
μ – average value of consumption;
σ – standard deviation of consumption;
P - values resulting from the fuzzy function;

With the fuzzified values previously calculated the normal distribution functions were derived. In this distribution the average value and the standard deviation are the respective FL values. As a final result is obtained the interval of probability (pessimistic and optimistic) of a given EV have one specific consumption in a period of time. This can be used to the driver make a more accurate planning of his journey and for the power system know the period of the EV need to load.

In Fig. 2 is possible to see the flowchart of the algorithm to implement the FL and the normal distribution in this specific case.

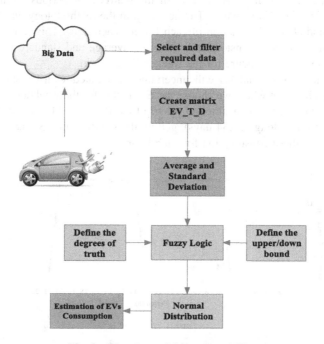

Fig. 2. Flowchart of the proposed FL

3 Numerical Example

Currently there is no enough historical data related with the operation of EVs, e.g. location, charged energy and time of charging. Hence, a scenario was generated considering a realistic study, for the city of Vila Real in Portugal, for a fleet of 30 Electric Vehicles (EV). The historical data was divided in two groups, due to the difference in behavior between weekdays and weekends. The weekdays had a total of 254 days, while the weekends and holidays corresponded to a total of 111 days. Several possibilities are taken into account. The EVs may leave earlier, breakdown can occur or the EV owner may change the charging station. The program considers possible changes in the planned route, i.e. breakdowns or failures in the EV fleet, therefore it simulates a realistic behavior. The script stores the data in Excel format, being the starting point for the FL.

To execute the FL it was necessary to prepare data and calculate the average and standard deviation of the EV's consumptions for each hour and day. To achieve this, the Excel data were loaded using MATLAB, where each excel sheet represent one day. Each sheet stored the information of the entire trip. For each EV, the information stored over a period of 24 h with a resolution of 1 h was: energy consumption, connection status ("1" in the case the EV was connected and "0" if it was not), bus connected in the grid, battery status and battery capacity. The data was properly filtered corresponding to the consumptions, i.e., for each EV and for each period of the day, the consumption of the EV's had. As a result a matrix that contained the data to be used to calculate the average and standard deviation was obtained (*EV_T_D*). The dimensions of this matrix was 30 × 24 × 254 with 30 EVs (lines of the matrix), 24 periods (columns of the matrix), and 254 days (weekdays). The next step in the methodology was to calculate the average and standard deviation of each EV for each hour. This results are in two matrices with 30 × 24 dimensions indicating the average and standard deviation of a given EV. The same procedure for the weekend's scenario.

Turning now to an analysis will uncertainty associated with consumption, considering a specific case where we choose the EV-1, this for the weekdays. Initially, we calculate the average fuel consumption per trip to a period of 24 h a day (the average value for each hour along of 254 days), getting the graph in Fig. 3 where we observe the variations of these consumption for each hour.

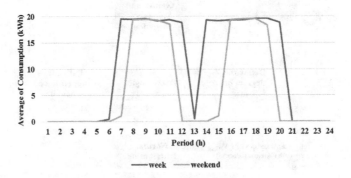

Fig. 3. Average of consumption for the EV-1

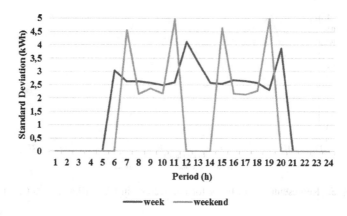

Fig. 4. Standard deviation of consumption for the EV-1

The next step is the calculation of the standard deviation of the value of consumption, as shown in Fig. 4.

After performing the calculation of the average and the standard deviation is already possible to apply the fuzzy function for the average and standard deviation values. To proceed to the implement the FL we need to define the lower bound, the upper bound, and the degrees of truth. In this study we have considered 100 degrees of truth. In order to present a better result, we considered two distinct cases, one case more pessimistic and other more optimistic. For the first case, the pessimistic, the lower bound was −10 % and the upper bound was 30 %. To the second case, the more optimistic, we utilized a value of −30 % for the lower bound and 10 % to the upper bound. The results of fuzzy method obtained in the EV-1, in the hour 7, are shown in the following Tables 2 and 3. Both tables are related with the implementation of the FL method, the first one was applied to the average value, while the second one characterizes the implementation to the standard deviation values.

The representation of the FL for the average can be seen in the Fig. 5 (Pessimistic Case) and Fig. 6 (Optimistic Case). In each figure it is possible to see the triangular fuzzy function and the centroid value for each case regarding the EV-1 in the hour 7. As it is referred in Table 2, it was obtained a fuzzy average consumption that can for

Table 2. Average Fuzzy values (kWh) for EV-1 in the hour 7

Case	Average	Lower bound	Fuzzy value	Upper bound
Pessimistic	19.52	18.15	20.17	26.22
Optimistic		13.21	18.87	20.76

Table 3. Standard deviation fuzzy values (kWh) for EV-1 in the hour 7

Case	Standard deviation	Lower bound	Fuzzy Value	Upper bound
Pessimistic	2.62	2.43	2.70	3.51
Optimistic		1.77	2.53	2.78

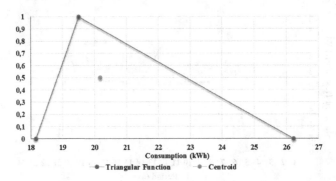

Fig. 5. Representation of fuzzy for the average in EV-1 (Pessimistic Case)

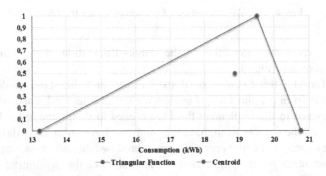

Fig. 6. Representation of fuzzy for the average in EV-1 (Optimistic Case)

the pessimistic and optimistic case, varying between 18.87 and 20.17 kWh, depending on the considered deviations.

The next stage was to implement the normal distribution with the values that were obtained with the FL (average fuzzy values and standard deviation fuzzy values) by using (2).

Figure 7 depicts the normal distributions for each case, namely the original normal distribution: Fuzzy Optimistic and Fuzzy Pessimistic. The Fuzzy Optimistic and Fuzzy Pessimistic, resulted in the calculation of the normal distribution with the fuzzy values.. The Normal Distribution, considered the original values for average and standard deviation. These values of average and standard deviation for the three cases can be seen in Table 2 and 3, respectively. The values presented regard the consumption probabilistic distribution for EV-1 in the hour 7.

With proposed fuzzy-probabilistic methodology it was possible to obtain the probabilities range that a given consumption might reach. For example, the probability of EV-1 to have a consumption higher than 20 kWh over 24 h can be verified in the Fig. 8 for the optimistic case and pessimistic case, respectively.

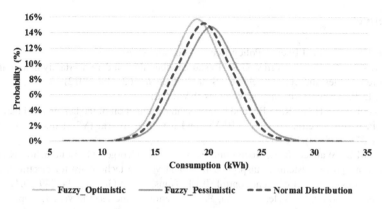

Fig. 7. Comparison with the 3 types of normal distribution

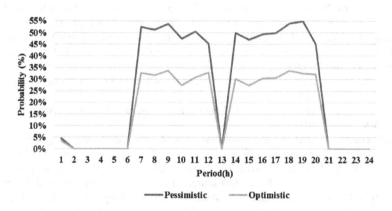

Fig. 8. Fuzzy probabilistic distribution of consumption for the EV-1

4   Conclusions

The paper presented a framework and methodology to estimate the uncertainty of the consumption of EVs. A Fuzzy Logic (FL) was implemented to estimate the probability of consumptions, but this methodology may also be applied to modulate the uncertainty of the charged energy. A case study was evaluated using a fleet of 30 Electric Vehicles (EV) and 2 different scenarios (weekdays and weekends). The methodology presented satisfactory results using low processing time that can be easily integrated with other applications. Authors aim to further develop the proposed idea as well as the data scheme necessary. This type of methodology could be used by automotive industry, network operators and electricity retailers to improve the user's experience and management of future smart grids in the presence of EVs.

References

1. IEEE-USA. National Energy Policy Recommendations (2014)
2. Saber, A.Y., Venayagamoorthy, G.K.: Resource scheduling under uncertainty in a smart grid with renewables and plug-in vehicles. Syst. J. IEEE **6**, 103–109 (2012)
3. U. S. E. P. Agency. All-Electric Vehicles (EVs) (ed)
4. Sovacool, B.K., Hirsh, R.F.: Beyond batteries: an examination of the benefits and barriers to plug-in hybrid electric vehicles (PHEVs) and a vehicle-to-grid (V2G) transition. Energy Policy **37**, 1095–1103 (2009)
5. Galus, M.D., Waraich, R.A., Noembrini, F., Steurs, K., Georges, G., Boulouchos, K., et al.: Integrating power systems, transport systems and vehicle technology for electric mobility impact assessment and efficient control. IEEE Trans. Smart Grid **3**, 934–949 (2012)
6. Morais, H., Sousa, T., Vale, Z., Faria, P.: Evaluation of the electric vehicle impact in the power demand curve in a smart grid environment. Energy Convers. Manage. **82**, 268–282 (2014)
7. Clement-Nyns, K., Haesen, E., Driesen, J.: The impact of charging plug-in hybrid electric vehicles on a residential distribution grid. IEEE Trans. Power Syst. **25**, 371–380 (2010)
8. Meliopoulos, S., Meisel, J., Cokkinides, G., Overbye, T.: Power system level impacts of plug-in hybrid vehicles. Power Systems Engineering Research Center (PSERC), Technical Report, pp. 09–12 (2009)
9. Balac, N.: "Green machine" intelligence: greening and sustaining smart grids. IEEE Intell. Syst. **28**, 0050–55 (2013)
10. Garcia-Valle, R., Vlachogiannis, J.G.: Letter to the editor: electric vehicle demand model for load flow studies (2009)
11. Vlachogiannis, J.G.: Probabilistic constrained load flow considering integration of wind power generation and electric vehicles. IEEE Trans. Power Syst. **24**, 1808–1817 (2009)
12. Silva, M.A., de Melo, H.N., Trovao, J.P., Pereirinha, P.G., Jorge, H.M.: An integrated fuzzy logic energy management for a dual-source electric vehicle. In: Industrial Electronics Society, IECON 2013-39th Annual Conference of the IEEE, pp. 4564–4569 (2013)
13. Gonzalez Vaya, M., Andersson, G.: Optimal bidding strategy of a plug-in electric vehicle aggregator in day-ahead electricity markets under uncertainty. IEEE Trans. Power Syst. **30**(5), 1–11 (2014)
14. Mehboob, N., Cañizares, C., Rosenberg, C.: Day-ahead dispatch of distribution feeders considering temporal uncertainties of PEVs. In: IEEE Power and Energy Society General Meeting, July 2015
15. Wen, M.H., Leung, K.-C., Li, V.O.: Communication-oriented smart grid framework. In: 2011 IEEE International Conference on Smart Grid Communications (SmartGridComm), pp. 61–66 (2011)
16. Zadeh, L.A.: Toward a theory of fuzzy information granulation and its centrality in human reasoning and fuzzy logic. Fuzzy Sets Syst. **90**, 111–127 (1997)
17. Pelletier, F.J.: Review of metamathematics of fuzzy logics in the bulletin of symbolic logic. JSTOR **6**(3), 342–346 (2000)
18. Harris, C.J., Moore, C.G., Brown, M.: Intelligent Control: Aspects of Fuzzy Logic and Neural Networks. World Scientific Press, 04 May 1993
19. Zhao, J., Wen, F., Dong, Z.Y., Xue, Y., Wong, K.P.: Optimal dispatch of electric vehicles and wind power using enhanced particle swarm optimization. IEEE Trans. Ind. Inform. **8**, 889–899 (2012)

Natural Language Processing Applications

Data-Driven Unsupervised Evaluation
of Automatic Text Summarization Systems

Elena Yagunova[✉], Olga Makarova, and Ekaterina Pronoza

Saint-Petersburg State University,
7/9 Universitetskaya Nab., Saint-Petersburg, Russia
{iagounova.elena,makarova.olga.e,
katpronoza}@gmail.com

Abstract. Automatic text summarization is a text compression problem with many applications in natural language processing. In this paper we focus the problem of the evaluation of text summarization system. We propose an unsupervised approach based on keywords: it does not require large amount of manual processing and can be implemented as a fully automatic procedure. We also conduct a series of experiments with naïve informants and professional experts. The results of the experiments with informants, experts and automatically extracted keywords confirm that keywords, as one of the types of text compression, can be successfully used for the evaluation of summaries quality. Our data is represented by (but not restricted to) different types of Russian news texts.

Keywords: Automatic text summarization · Evaluation of summaries · News text · Flexible summarization system · Recall · Brevity · Experiments with informants

1 Introduction

Automatic text summarization is a well-known task in natural language processing (NLP). A wide number of text summarization systems have been developed as part of various NLP applications since 1960s [2]. To build an effective text summarization system, one should be able to evaluate its performance.

In this paper we address the problem of summarization evaluation: we propose an unsupervised method for summarization evaluation which uses keywords. Our method is simple and does not require any gold standard annotation, and at the same time it enables one to build a flexible text summarization system targeting a particular audience because it takes into account differences between the judgements of different groups of informants. Our approach is data-driven in the sense that it is mostly based on the information extracted from the data, and does not require any external resources or expertise.

Large amount of manual processing is a serious problem in summarization evaluation: traditional evaluation methods usually involve experts' work. Unlike such traditional approaches, ours aims to reduce experts' processing and the method we propose is fully automatic.

O. Pichardo Lagunas et al. (Eds.): MICAI 2015, Part II, LNAI 9414, pp. 39–51, 2015.
DOI: 10.1007/978-3-319-27101-9_3

In this paper we present an approach based on keywords: it does not require large amount of manual processing and can be implemented as an automatic procedure. We also conduct a series of experiments with informants and compare our results with expert annotation. The results of the experiments with informants, experts and automatically extracted keywords confirm that keywords, as one of the types of text compression, can be successfully used for the evaluation of summaries quality.

Our data is represented by (but not restricted to) different types of Russian news texts.

2 Related Work

The approaches towards text summarization can be classified into two types: extractive and abstractive. While an extractive summary consists of the words, phrases and sentences from original text, an abstractive summary is a different text obtained from the original one by constructing semantic model of the text and then generating new text based on this model. The latter approach requires deep semantic analysis and text generation. These tasks are still unsolved, and that is why most text summarization systems use extractive methods (or combine them with abstractive methods), and ours is not an exception.

As part of the extractive method, words, phrases and other text units are extracted from the original text with their weights. Such weights can be calculated using various metrics like TF-iDF, TextRank, etc. To improve the resulting summary, some euristics can be further applied (e.g., taking into account positions of the sentences in the text, words occurring in the title, etc.).

The approaches applied for the evaluation of summarization systems can, in their turn, be classified into intrinsic and extrinsic ones [1].

Extrinsic methods evaluate the performance of the method on other tasks other than automatic text summarization. A list of questions about the content of the texts is an example of such method: if a human, after reading the summary, can answer the questions correctly, the summary is good. It is obvious that such method is costly as it requires human resources.

Intrinsic methods are based on the comparison of the original text and its summary. Thus, a traditional manual method involves the estimation by expert linguists using criteria like coherence, brevity, grammatical correctness, the complexity of perception, precision, redundancy[1]. Such traditional method is also very costly and evaluation based on this method cannot be conducted in real time.

A common intrinsic approach towards text summarization systems evaluation is represented by the ROUGE (Recall-Oriented Understudy for Gisting Evaluation) metric. There are about 20 variations of this metric, and all of them are based on the idea of using gold-standard summaries created manually by the experts. ROUGE is

---

[1] These terms (precision, etc.), well-known in NLP community, should be interpreted in a different way here: they represent metrics by which experts estimate the quality of summaries, rather than automatically calculated quality measures. For example, in [5] experts assign each summary precision and redundancy values from the rating scale.

calculated as the percentage of various text elements (lexical units, n-grams, sentences, etc.) from the gold standard occurring in the summary. Such approach has its drawbacks: it involves manual processing, and gold-standard summaries are subjective.

Another metric, called Pyramid [3], unlike previous metrics, depends on the number of important facts and topics described in the summary, and not the number of overlapping word sequences or n-grams. Such facts are called SCUs – summarization content units. SCU is a semantic unit which can be expressed in one or several words and is usually within one sentence. Its length varies because the same information can be expressed in a word, phrase or even the whole sentence. To calculate Pyramid, one should first of all manually create several summaries and annotate all the SCUs in them. These SCUs are assigned their weights, and the largest weights correspond to the SCUs occurring in all summaries. Then a pyramid is constructed: each level contains SCUs with equal weights, and SCU with the maximal weight is at the top of it. The Pyramid metric is calculated as the sum of all SCU weights in the summary divided by the sum of weights in the gold-standard summary with the same number of SCUs.

Pyramid, unlike ROUGE, is designed to evaluate summaries on the semantic level. However, this metric, although more or less objective, demands a large amount of qualified manual processing and is very costly. Moreover, experts are required not only to prepare gold-standard summaries but also to annotate every new estimated summary with SCUs.

Thus, high cost and subjectivity of the methods using gold standards has spurred the development of alternative evaluation methods. For example, there are attempts to evaluate summaries using similarity measures or search indexes (supposed that a good summary is as relevant to the query as the original document). But there are no results of the comparison of these methods with experts' summaries known to us.

In this paper we present an approach based on keywords: it does not require large amount of manual processing and can be implemented as an automatic procedure. We also conduct a series of experiments with informants and compare our results with expert annotation.

3   Our Approach

Text compression is text transformation which shortens the original text. Text can be compressed by pruning redundant text units and units which can be reconstructed using their context and by choosing short text structures.

Summary is a traditional type of text compression, while a list of keywords is an example of extreme text compression [6]. A keyword can be treated as a word which can represent the whole text together with other keywords.

In this paper our hypothesis is that we can judge the quality of one text compression method by another text compression method. Thus, by comparing a summary with the list of keywords we can see whether the most important themes from the original text are mentioned in the summary. Such idea is close to the Pyramid approach because keywords can be considered SCUs [1].

The method of text summarization systems evaluations using keywords was initially designed for news texts, namely, for estimating the quality of summaries constructed from one document. Due to the specifics of the news genre, the evaluation of the summaries coherence is not necessary.

As we have already mentioned, our approach towards summaries evaluation is based on the use of keywords. We prepare a set of top keywords for each text, depending on the level of compression. Then we calculate two metrics for each top keywords set: recall and brevity.

Recall, a standard metric in NLP, is calculated as the number of words from top keywords set occurring in the summary divided by the total number of words in the top keywords set:

$$Recall = \frac{number\_of\_top\_keywords\_in\_summary}{total\_number\_of\_the\_top\_keywords} \qquad (1)$$

Brevity, which reflects the density of important information and the absence (which is desired) of unimportant information in the summary, is calculated as the number of words from top keywords set occurring in the summary (including repetitions and synonyms) divided by the total number of words in the summary:

$$Brevity = \frac{number\_of\_top\_keywords\_in\_summary\_(repetitions, synonyms)}{total\_number\_of\_words\_in\_the\_summary} \qquad (2)$$

Both metrics range from 0 to 1. And the close they are to 1, the better the summary is. It should be noted that the brevity value does not reach 1, or else it would mean that the summary is identical with the top keywords set.

4 Data

In our experiments we use the data obtained from [5]. There are 3 types of data: news articles, their summaries constructed using 4 different text summarization systems and recall and brevity of these summaries given by the experts.

We use the news articles from Lenta.ru [7] published in autumn 2011. The articles are selected manually, and include both simple (for analysis) texts without any stylistic mistakes and text with severe stylistics and structural errors. All the texts are at least 7 sentences long, but less than 2000 symbols. We prepared 25 news articles but as the texts were to be given to the informants (to manually extract keywords – as part of the experiment), we finally selected only 12 articles to ease their task.

The 12 articles in question can be classified into the informative and emotional, simple (describing one event) and complex (describing several events) ones. Most articles are simple (9 out of 12) and informative (also 9 out of 12) which is quite typical of a news text. To illustrate the described types of news text, let us consider two examples from our data set (see Table 1).

The keywords in Table 1 are extracted automatically from the corresponding articles and the summaries are created using information content metric. The first article about bank thefts is an example of a typical news text: it is simple in the sense that it is wholly dedicated to one event, and informative (the informative side dominates the

Table 1. Examples of news articles of different types

Title	Most important keywords with their weights	Summary
In Moscow, hackers' plan of stealing money from 96 banks is thwarted	Theft (27), hackers (26), keys (23), passwords (19), software (noun) (17), banks (16), prevented (16), software (adjective) (16), storage (15), order (14), money (13), untimely update (12), malicious (11), captured (10), electronic (10)	In Moscow, the employees of the Department of Economic Security of the capital's police **prevented** the **theft** of millions of dollars of **money** from the accounts of 457 companies in 96 banks. Criminals stole electronic keys from 457 companies. Bank **keys**, user names and **passwords** of 457 customers were stolen by **hackers** using **malicious software**.
In Saint-Petersburg a FSS officer shot and killed a passerby	Shot (29), passerby (28), FSS (28), died (23), officer (23), deputy (18), in Saint-Petersburg (14), arrested (12), Saratov (12), traumatic (11), incident (10), victim (10)	**In St. Petersburg** a **FSS officer shot** a **passerby** with a **traumatic** gun. A spokesman for the Investigative Committee of St. Petersburg reported to RBC that their department does not handle this case. **Saratov** Regional Duma **deputy** from the "United Russia" Leonid Pisnoy opened fire in the city center. Around 21:45 the security forces blocked Volskaya St. Their KamAZ drove in a convoy, and the road was closed to avoid accidents when the truck was taking a turn. According to the police officers, L.Pisnoy came out of the "Volga" and rudely demanded to remove the cars from the road.

emotional one). The second article is, on the contrary, complex because it describes two different incidents: (1) shooting by a FSS officer and (2) the fire opened by a Saratov deputy in the city centre. This article is emotional rather than informative. Although it might not follow from the summary in Table 1, the author's sentiment is in fact clearly expressed in the original text: the incident with the officer is called "scandalous", the deputy is ironically called the "elect of nation", etc. The interesting point is that, as the summary was constructed using an information-oriented (and not sentiment-oriented) metric, all the emotional phrases are missing from it. We suppose that such (emotional) types of text demand an approach to summarization which takes sentiment into account, and it is confirmed by the results of our research. Unfortunately, due to space limits, we cannot give examples of other types of summaries, and neither can we go into further details about different types of news texts.

Each of the selected 12 articles is provided with 4 different quasi-summaries, each of them not larger than 1/3 of the original text. The summaries are obtained using statistical method (e.g., information content, TF-iDF), sentiment analysis-based method described in [5] and TextAnalyst [8] demo-version.

To estimate recall and brevity, 20 informants were asked to give each summary a score, and at a result of this procedure each summary was provided with 2 scores (recall and brevity) ranging from 1 (excellent) to 3 (bad).

5   Experiments. Results. Discussion

5.1   Experiment with Informants

As part of the experiments with informants each informant was given a list of 12 news articles accompanied by the following instruction: "Read the text, think about its content. Underline 10–15 words, most important for its understanding"[2].

The informants were native Russian speakers – there were no demands as to their education or occupation. They spent 30 min (on average) to fulfill the task, and the quickest answer was received in 11 min. All in all, we received 75 answers from the informants.

Then the list of keywords with their frequencies was constructed for each news text. Based on these lists, we prepared the top keywords sets which are used for summaries evaluation in our research.

The distribution of keywords frequencies is quite common in such experiments: there are usually a few keywords with top frequencies, several "plateaus" represented by keywords with lesser but not sharply decreasing frequencies, and a long "tail" of low-frequency keywords. Taking into account high level of compression (1/3 of the original text) in the summaries we decided to include into our top keywords sets all the keywords from the top until an appropriate plateau.

5.2   Preliminary Evaluation of the Summaries

We conducted a preliminary evaluation of the summaries based on the collected top keywords sets. At this stage of the research we adopted a "bag-of-words" approach,

---

[2] There initially 25 articles given to each of the informants, ant they were asked to write down the words. However, after we received the first answers, we decided to change the instruction: we asked the informants to underline the words in the text. It helped us to avoid misprints and to maintain information about the positions of the words in the text. We also reduced the number of articles to 12, because the preliminary results showed that the number of errors invariably increased with the growth of the number of articles.

ignoring any morphological or grammatical features of the words. But such an approach gave poor results on the texts where the words were often repeated in different forms. To improve the situation, we normalized each word and further analyzed the summaries on the lemma (and not on the word-) level.

To check our hypothesis that summaries can be evaluated using keywords we compare the results with the scores (recall and brevity mentioned in Sect. 3, precision and redundancy as described in [5]) previously given by the experts. We consider these pairs of scores – recall and precision, redundancy and brevity – equivalent in our case. As the experts were using different scales, we decided to assign each summary a score from 1 to 4, to reflect the best and the worst results from each of the experts scales respectively. Tables 2 and 3 present the comparison of 4 text summarization methods with the corresponding pairs of precision (P) and recall (R) scores and redundancy (R) and brevity (B) scores, contradicting scores are given in bold. Each text number is accompanied by two abbreviations which correspond to the type of the text: I (informative, intended only to inform the reader) or E (emotional, expressing strong sentiment) and S (simple, describing one event) or C (complex, describing two or more events which differ in time and/or place). Such denotation also takes place in the rest of the tables in this paper.

Table 2. Comparison of different summarization methods by precision and recall

Method	Information content		TF-iDF		Sentiment analysis		TextAnalyst	
# text	R	P	R	P	R	P	R	P
1 IS	**1**	**4**	**4**	**1**	2	2	**3**	**2**
2 IS	**1**	**4**	**4**	**3**	**3**	**2**	**2**	**1**
3 EC	3	3	4	4	2	2	1	1
4 IS	**2**	**4**	3	3	**4**	**2**	1	1
5 IS	1	1	4	4	2	2	3	3
6 EC	4	4	2	2	1	1	3	3
7 ES	4	4	3	3	1	1	2	2
8 IS	4	4	**2**	**3**	1	1	**3**	**2**
9 IS	4	4	3	3	1	1	2	2
10 IS	3	3	4	4	2	2	1	1
11 IC	4	4	2	2	1	1	3	3
12 IS	1	1	**1**	**3**	4	4	**3**	**2**
Average	2.6	3.3	3.0	2.9	2.0	1.8	2.3	1.9

The disagreement between the experts' estimates and the scores obtained using keywords occur 13 times out of 36. Full agreement takes place 7 times out of 12 (for all the four summaries). There are only 2 times when the best and the worst scores are given to the same summary (texts 1 and 2). It should also be noted that the experts agree on the texts which seem to be the hardest ones for automatic analysis (i.e., emotional and complex texts) and disagree on simple and informative texts. Another interesting point is that, according to experts' judgement, summarization method based on sentiment analysis seems to be the most successful one for emotional texts. The same tendency can be seen in Table 3, and virtually in every table further in this paper.

Table 3. Comparison of different summarization methods by brevity and redundancy

Method	Information content		TF-iDF		Sentiment analysis		TextAnalyst	
# text	B	R	B	R	B	R	B	R
1 IS	1	4	3	1	4	3	2	2
2 IS	2	2	1	1	4	4	3	3
3 EC	3	3	2	2	1	1	4	4
4 IS	2	4	1	1	4	2	3	3
5 IS	3	3	1	2	4	1	2	4
6 EC	4	4	1	1	2	2	3	3
7 ES	4	4	1	1	3	2	2	3
8 IS	1	4	3	3	2	1	4	2
9 IS	4	4	3	3	2	2	1	1
10 IS	2	4	4	2	3	3	1	1
11 IC	4	3	1	1	2	2	3	4
12 IS	2	2	1	1	3	3	4	4
Average	2.66	3.41	1.83	1.58	2.83	2.16	2.66	2.83

Experts' estimations agree with the keywords-based scores in 31 cases out of 48 when the redundancy-brevity parameter is considered. Here, again, it can be seen that disagreement mostly takes place when the text is simple and informative, and vice versa.

In general, the obtained results allows us to conclude that the method based on keywords can be applied for summarization evaluation.

5.3   Automatic Keywords Extraction

It is obvious that experiments on the extraction of keywords by the informants are still costly although not as costly as the experiments with the experts. The question is, can we make the evaluation procedure fully automatic (i.e., use automatically extracted keywords)?

There exists a wide number of metrics for extracting keywords, TF-iDF being the most well-known of them. But as one of the 4 types of summaries was created using this metric in our research, we cannot use TF-iDF for summaries evaluation. We calculate BM25 instead. It is a metric from information retrieval which is represented by a function on a bag of words and a bag of documents. It evaluates the latter based on the occurrence of the words from the query in the document. BM25 has a lot of variations and can be used for keywords extraction.

In this paper we implement one of the most well-known variations of BM25 – Okapi BM25 [4]:

$$OkapiBM25(D, q) = iDF(q) \times \frac{f(q, D) \times (k + 1)}{f(q, D) + k \times (1 - b + b \times \frac{l}{avgl})}, \quad (3)$$

where D denotes a document, q – a word, $f(q, D)$ – the frequency of the word q in the document D, l – length of the document, $avgl$ – average length of the document in the collection, k and b – arbitrary coefficients, traditionally set to 2.0 and 0.75 respectively. Inverse document frequency (iDF) is calculated as:

$$iDF(q) = \log \frac{N - n(q) + 0.5}{n(q) + 0.5}, \quad (4)$$

where N denotes the total number of documents in the collection and $n(q)$ – the number of the documents which contain the word q.

Okapi BM25 calculation requires a different collection of documents – we use the news articles from Lenta.ru published in the first half of 2012. These texts satisfy the same requirements as the texts chosen for the summaries. It should also be noted that in our research BM25 is calculated on the lemma level and not on the word level to avoid the problems which arise because of the use of different word forms in inflexional languages like Russian.

We also had to decide on the size of the automatically collected top keywords sets for summaries evaluation. We selected the same number of words as in the top keywords sets created by the informants.

Although it may seem that the scores calculated on the automatically collected keywords should be higher on the summaries evaluated automatically than on the summaries evaluated by the informants. However, the scores appear to be similar (see Tables 4 and 5). Table 4 displays recall scores and Table 4 – brevity scores.

Table 4. Comparison of different summarization evaluation methods by recall

Method	Information content		TF-iDF		Sentiment analysis		TextAnalyst	
# text	Informants	BM25	Informants	BM25	Informants	BM25	Informants	BM25
1 IS	0.73	0.73	0.47	0.6	0.6	0.53	0.4	0.33
2 IS	0.67	0.6	0.33	0.27	0.47	0.53	0.6	0.47
3 EC	0.67	0.67	0.2	0.13	**0.67**	**0.27**	0.73	0.67
4 IS	0.73	0.8	0.6	0.53	0.8	0.87	0.8	0.6
5 IS	0.6	0.6	0.47	0.27	0.6	0.6	0.53	0.47

(*Continued*)

Table 4. (*Continued*)

Method	Information content		TF-iDF		Sentiment analysis		TextAnalyst	
# text	Informants	BM25	Informants	BM25	Informants	BM25	Informants	BM25
6 EC	**0.1**	**0.33**	**0.8**	**0.27**	**0.87**	**0.53**	0.4	0.27
7 ES	0.2	0.27	**0.67**	**0.33**	**0.8**	**0.33**	0.67	0.47
8 IS	0.33	0.27	0.4	0.6	0.93	1	0.33	0.4
9 IS	0.73	0.6	0.73	0.67	1	0.8	0.73	0.6
10 IS	0.27	0.2	0.07	0.13	0.33	0.27	**0.67**	**0.27**
11 IC	0.2	0.2	0.53	0.4	0.67	0.47	0.27	0.4
12 IS	0.67	0.6	0.8	0.67	**0.67**	**0.4**	0.6	0.73
Average	0.49	0.49	0.51	0.41	0.70	0.55	0.56	0.47

Recall values which differ more than in 20 % for the same summarization method and on the same text, are given in bold. Such differences mostly take place on emotional or complex texts.

Table 5. Comparison of different summarization evaluation methods by brevity

Method	Information content		TF-iDF		Sentiment analysis		TextAnalyst	
# text	Informants	BM25	Informants	BM25	Informants	BM25	Informants	BM25
1 IS	0.25	0.23	0.21	0.23	0.15	0.15	0.24	0.2
2 IS	0.16	0.15	0.22	0.17	0.11	0.12	0.16	0.13
3 EC	0.12	0.12	0.12	0.08	**0.48**	**0.19**	0.12	0.1
4 IS	0.2	0.22	0.22	0.18	0.15	0.15	0.18	0.12
5 IS	0.12	0.11	**0.36**	**0.18**	0.09	0.08	0.12	0.1
6 EC	0.12	0.21	**0.25**	**0.09**	0.24	0.14	0.14	0.14
7 ES	0.09	0.12	**0.56**	**0.28**	**0.24**	**0.1**	0.28	0.19
8 IS	0.14	0.11	0.08	0.12	0.09	0.1	0.07	0.09
9 IS	0.14	0.12	0.18	0.16	0.16	0.13	0.18	0.15
10 IS	0.08	0.06	0.02	0.05	0.08	0.06	**0.21**	**0.08**
11 IC	0.03	0.07	0.18	0.11	0.15	0.1	0.07	0.11
12 IS	0.18	0.15	0.2	0.18	0.18	0.12	0.13	0.16
Average	0.14	0.14	0.22	0.15	0.18	0.12	0.16	0.13

As in Table 5, brevity values which differ more than in 10 % for the same summarization method and on the same text, are given in bold. And there is the same tendency as in Table 4: most differences occur when the texts are emotional or complex.

5.4   Comparison of Keywords Given by Different Groups of Informants

As we have already mentioned, there were initially no special demands to the informants. But having conducted the experiments with informants we could see that different groups of informants actually tend to extract different types of keywords. We believe that such specialty should be taken into account while developing text summarization systems with a particular target audience.

To confirm this hypothesis we divided the informants into two groups: naïve informants and experts. The latter include linguists, analysts and content managers – in other words, those who have a large amount of experience with textual data.

We compared the scores given by the naïve informants with those provided by the experts. The comparison by the two metrics: recall and brevity – is presented in Tables 6 and 7 respectively.

Table 6. Comparison of the naive informants' and by experts's scores by recall

Method	Information content		TF-iDF		Sentiment analysis		TextAnalyst	
# text	Naive	Experts	Naive	Experts	Naive	Experts	Naive	Experts
1 IS	0.73	0.8	0.47	0.53	0.6	0.53	0.4	0.4
2 IS	0.67	0.67	0.33	0.33	0.47	0.47	0.6	0.6
3 EC	0.67	0.67	0.2	0.2	0.67	0.67	0.73	0.8
4 IS	0.73	0.73	0.6	0.67	0.8	0.87	0.8	0.87
5 IS	0.6	0.67	0.47	0.53	0.6	0.67	0.53	0.6
6 EC	0.1	0.2	0.8	0.73	0.87	0.93	0.4	0.27
7 ES	0.2	0.2	0.67	0.67	0.8	0.8	0.67	0.67
8 IS	0.33	0.33	0.4	0.4	0.93	0.93	0.33	0.33
9 IS	0.73	0.73	0.73	0.73	1	1	0.73	0.73
10 IS	0.27	0.27	0.07	0.07	0.33	0.33	0.67	0.67
11 IC	0.2	0.07	0.53	0.67	0.67	0.67	0.27	0.27
12 IS	0.67	0.73	0.8	0.73	0.67	0.6	0.6	0.6
Average	0.49	0.51	0.51	0.52	0.70	0.71	0.56	0.57

Table 7. Comparison of the naive informants' and by experts's scores by brevity

Method	Information content		TF-iDF		Sentiment analysis		TextAnalyst	
# text	Naive	Experts	Naive	Experts	Naive	Experts	Naive	Experts
1 IS	0.23	0.23	0.18	0.23	0.17	0.15	0.24	0.2
2 IS	0.16	0.15	0.22	0.17	0.11	0.12	0.16	0.13
3 EC	0.12	0.12	0.12	0.08	**0.48**	**0.19**	0.11	0.1
4 IS	0.2	0.22	0.2	0.18	0.14	0.15	0.16	0.12
5 IS	0.11	0.11	**0.32**	**0.18**	0.08	0.08	0.11	0.1
6 EC	**0.07**	**0.21**	**0.27**	**0.09**	0.22	0.14	0.21	0.14

(Continued)

Table 7. (*Continued*)

Method	Information content		TF-iDF		Sentiment analysis		TextAnalyst	
# text	Naive	Experts	Naive	Experts	Naive	Experts	Naive	Experts
7 ES	0.09	0.12	**0.56**	**0.28**	**0.24**	**0.1**	0.28	0.19
8 IS	0.14	0.11	0.08	0.12	0.09	0.1	0.07	0.09
9 IS	0.14	0.12	0.18	0.16	0.16	0.13	0.18	0.15
10 IS	0.08	0.06	0.02	0.05	0.08	0.06	**0.21**	**0.08**
11 IC	0.07	0.07	0.14	0.11	0.15	0.1	0.07	0.11
12 IS	0.16	0.15	0.21	0.18	0.2	0.12	0.13	0.16
Average	0.13	0.13	0.21	0.15	0.18	0.12	0.16	0.13

It can be seen that the recall values obtained from the experts' and the naïve informants' evaluation do not differ significantly. The situation is slightly different with brevity scores (see Table 7).

Brevity values which differ more than in 10 % between experts and naïve informants are given in bold in Table 7, and the tendency is absolutely the same as in the previous tables: naïve informants and experts disagree on emotional and complex texts.

In general, we can conclude that the estimates given by the experts are similar to those given by the naïve informants but are slightly higher for recall and lower – for brevity.

It should be noted that the lists of keywords extracted by the experts are quite similar to those obtained automatically. Therefore we may conclude that involving experts into the evaluation process in the role of mere informants is not a good idea.

Thus, the described experiments allow us to confirm our hypothesis about the applicability of the keywords-based method for summaries evaluation.

6   Conclusion and Future Work

In this paper we focus on the problem of the evaluation of text summarization systems and describe experiments with informants of different groups and news texts of different types. We work with news articles in Russian but our approach is not restricted to this language. We propose an unsupervised data-driven summarization evaluation method based on the use of keywords and conduct a series of experiments with informants to prove our method. Our approach, unlike many others, does not involve large amount of manual processing. Neither does it require any gold-standard summaries which, created manually by experts, are costly and subjective. And unlike other methods, ours allows to build a flexible summarization system targeting a particular audience because it takes into account differences between (1) the different types of text the judgements and (2) different groups of informants on.

As a result of the experiments we confirm our hypothesis that keywords can be used for the evaluation of the quality of quasi-summaries of news texts. The scores of the summaries obtained automatically are similar to those given by the experts. We also show that the quality of a summary can be improved if one takes into account specific types of text: according to the results of our experiments, summarization method based on sentiment analysis achieves best scores on emotional news texts.

During our experiments with informants we also obtain some unexpected results. Namely, the scores given by the professional experts practically do not differ from those calculated on the automatically extracted keywords. We suppose that in such case, if the addressee of a text summarization system is a naïve informant, summarization method should not be evaluated by professional experts, and vice versa. In other words, an effective text summarization system should be aimed at particular tasks (and type audience: professional or not) and be trained on a particular type of texts.

As a result of this part of our research we also developed a tool for keywords extraction and summaries evaluation based on their recall and brevity values. Such tool can be used for any other experiments which involve keywords extraction.

In future we plan to improve our keywords extraction method and to experiment with other types of texts, for example, with scientific collections.

Acknowledgements. The authors acknowledge Saint-Petersburg State University for the research grant 30.38.305.2014.

References

1. Hennig, L., De Luca, E.W., Albayrak, S.: Learning summary content units with topic modeling. In: COLING 2010: Poster Volume, pp. 391–399 (2010)
2. Luhn, H.P.: The automatic creation of literature abstracts. IBM J. Res. Dev. **2**(2), 157–165 (1958)
3. Nenkova, A., Passonneau, R.: Evaluating content selection in summarization: the pyramid method. In: HLT-NAACL 2004: Main Proceedings, pp. 145–152 (2004)
4. Robertson, S.E., Walker, S., Jones, S., Hancock-Beaulieu, M., Gatford, M.: Okapi at TREC-3. In: Proceedings of the Third Text REtrieval Conference (TREC 1994) (1994)
5. Solov'ev, A.N., Antonova, A.J., Pazel'skaja, A.G.: Using sentiment-analysis for text information extraction. In: Computational Linguistics and Intelligent Technology: According to the Materials of the Annual International Conference "Dialogue" vol. 11, no. 18: B 2т. T. 1: The Main Program of the Conference, pp. 616–627. Publishing House of the Russian State Humanitarian University (2012)
6. Yagunova, E.V., Makarova, O.E., Antonov, A.Y., Solovyov, A.N.: Various compression methods in the study of understanding the text of the news. In: Understanding in Communication. Man in the Information Space, vol. 2, pp. 414–421. Publishing House of YAGPU, Yaroslavl – Moscow (2012)
7. Lenta.ru: Rambler Media Group. http://www.lenta.ru
8. TextAnalyst. http://www.analyst.ru/index.php?lang=eng&dir=content/products/&id=ta

Extractive Single-Document Summarization Based on Global-Best Harmony Search and a Greedy Local Optimizer

Martha Mendoza[1(⊠)], Carlos Cobos[1], and Elizabeth León[2]

[1] Universidad Del Cauca, Popayán, Colombia
{mmendoza, ccobos}@unicauca.edu.co
[2] Universidad Nacional de Colombia, Bogotá D.C., Colombia
eleonguz@unal.edu.co

Abstract. Due to the great amount of documents available on the Web, end users need to be able to access information in summary form – keeping the most important information in the document. The methods employed for automatic text summarization generally allocate a score to each sentence in the document, taking into account certain features. The most relevant sentences are then selected, according to the score obtained for each sentence. In this paper, the extractive single document summarization task is treated as a binary optimization problem and, based on the Global-best Harmony Search metaheuristic and a greedy local search procedure, a new algorithm called ESDS-GHS-GLO is proposed. This algorithm optimizes an objective function, which is a lineal normalized combination of the position of the sentence in the document, sentence length, and coverage of the selected sentences in the summary. The proposed method was compared with the state of the art methods MA-SingleDocSum, DE, FEOM, UnifiedRank, NetSum, QCS, CRF, SVM, and Manifold Ranking, using ROUGE measures on the DUC2001 and DUC2002 datasets. The results showed that ESDS-GHS-GLO outperforms most of the state-of-the-art methods except MA-SingleDocSum. ESDS-GHS-GLO obtains promissory results using a fitness function less complex than MA-SingleDocSum, therefore requiring less execution time.

Keywords: Single-document summarization · Memetic algorithms · Global-best harmony search · Greedy search

1 Introduction

Today, automatic text summarization constitutes a key service for a range of application types, including internet, library, scientific, and business uses [1]. The vast quantities of information stored in digital text documents need summaries in order to help users find the required information with the least time and effort possible. For many years, the automatic generation of summaries has attempted to create summaries that closely approximate those generated by humans [1, 2], but until now, this research area is still unresolved.

Different taxonomies for summaries exist [1, 2] based on the way the summary is generated, the target audience of the summary, the number of documents to be

© Springer International Publishing Switzerland 2015
O. Pichardo Lagunas et al. (Eds.): MICAI 2015, Part II, LNAI 9414, pp. 52–66, 2015.
DOI: 10.1007/978-3-319-27101-9_4

summarized, and so on. According to how it is generated, the summary can be either extractive or abstractive [1, 2]. Extractive summaries are formed from the reuse of portions of the original text. Abstractive summaries [3] on the other hand are rather more complex, requiring linguistic analysis tools to construct new sentences from those previously extracted. Taking account of the target audience, summaries may be [1, 2] generic, query-based, user-focused or topic-focused. Generic summaries do not depend on the audience for whom the summary is intended. Query-based summaries respond to a query made by the user. User-focused ones generate summaries to tailor the interests of a particular user, while topic-focused summaries emphasize those summaries on specific topics of documents. Depending on the number of documents processed, summaries [1, 2] can be either single document or multiple document. As regards the language of the document, they may be monolingual or multilingual, and regarding document genre may be scientific article, news, blogs, and so on. The summarization algorithm (method) proposed in this paper is extractive, for a single document, and for any type of document, although the evaluation was performed on a set of news.

Automatic summarization is an area that has explored different methods for the automatic generation of single document summaries, such as (1) statistical and prob-abilistic approaches, which use information such as the frequency of occurrence of a term in a text, the position of the sentences in the document, and the presence of keywords or words from the document title in the sentences [4]; (2) Machine learning approaches, including Bayes' Theorem [5, 6], Hidden Markov Models [7, 8], Neural networks [9], Conditional Random Fields [10], Probabilistic Support Vector Machine (PSVM) and Naïve Bayes [11]; (3) Text connectivity approaches [12, 13], including lexical chains [14] and rhetorical structure theory [15]; (4) Graph-based approaches [16, 17], which represent sentences in the vertices of the graph and the similarity between the text units by means of the edges, then an iterative process is carried out and the summary with sentences from the first vertices is obtained; (5) Algebraic approaches using Latent Semantic Analysis [18] based on Singular Value Decomposition [19–21] or Non-negative Matrix Factorization [22]; (6) Metaheuristic approaches that seek to optimize an objective function to find the sentences that will be part of the summary. These works include genetic algorithms, [23–28], particle swarm optimization (PSO) [29], Harmony Search [30], and Differential Evolution (DE) algorithm [31, 32]; and (7) Fuzzy approaches that combine fuzzy set theory with swarm intelligence (binary PSO) [33] or with clustering and evolutionary algorithms in a new fuzzy evolutionary optimization model (FEOM) [34] for document summarization.

Algebraic, clustering, probabilistic, metaheuristic and fuzzy approaches are language independent and unsupervised, two key aspects on which more emphasis is being placed in the most recent research. Research based on a memetic algorithm (combination of metaheuristics) for single document summarization [35] has recently shown good results, making this a promising area. Therefore, in this paper, a new memetic algorithm for the automatic generation of extractive and generic single document summaries is proposed.

The new memetic algorithm is based on Global-best Harmony Search (GHS) bearing in mind that "No Free Lunch theorems for optimization state that no one algorithm is better than any other when performances are averaged over the whole set of possible problems. However, it has been recently suggested that algorithms might show performance differences when a set of real-world problems is under study" [36] and that GHS [37] is showing promissory results in a great variety of real problems (continuos, discrete, and binary problems) [38]. The memetic algorithm also includes a greedy search as local search operator. The new algorithm, ESDS-GHS-GLO optimizes an objective function expressed by the lineal and normalized combination of three factors: position of the sentences selected in the candidate summary; length of sentences selected in the candidate summary; and coverage of the candidate summary, i.e. cosine similarity between all candidate sentences in the summary and a global representation of the document.

The rest of the paper is organized as follows: Sect. 2 introduces document representation and characteristics of the objective function proposed in the algorithm. Section 3 describes the proposed algorithm; while the results of evaluation using data sets, along with a comparison and analysis with other state-of-the-art methods, are presented in Sect. 4; finally, Sect. 5 presents conclusions and future work.

2 Problem Statement and Its Mathematical Formulation

The representation of a document is made based on the vector space model proposed by Salton [39]. Thus, a document is represented by the sentences that compose it, i.e. $D = \{S_1, S_2, ..., S_n\}$, where S_i corresponds to the i-th sentence of the document and n is the total number of sentences in the document. Likewise, a sentence is represented by the set $S_i = \{t_{i,1}, t_{i,2}, ..., t_{i,j}, ..., t_{i,o}\}$, where $t_{i,j}$ is the j-th term of the sentence S_i and o is the total number of terms in the sentence. Thus, the vector representation of a sentence of the document is a vector containing the weights of the terms, as shown in Eq. (1)

$$S_i = \{w_{i,1}, w_{i,2}, ..., w_{i,k}, ..., w_{i,m}\} \tag{1}$$

where m is the number of distinct terms in the document collection and $w_{i,k}$ is the weight of the k-th term in sentence S_i.

The component $w_{i,k}$ is calculated using the Okapi BM25 formula [39] (see Eq. (2))

$$w_{i,k} = \frac{(k_1 + 1) \times f_{i,k}}{k_1 \times \left((1 - B) + B \times \left(\frac{L_i}{L_{AVG}}\right)\right) + f_{i,k}} \times log\left(\frac{n}{n_k}\right) \tag{2}$$

where $f_{i,k}$ represents the frequency of the k-th term in sentence S_i, L_i is the length of sentence S_i, L_{AVG} is the average of all sentences in the document, n_k denotes the number of sentences in which the k-th term appears, and n is the number of sentences in the document collection. k_1 and B are two tuning parameters equal to 2 and 0.75 respectively.

Thus the aim of generating a summary of a single document is to obtain a subset of D with the sentences that contain the main information of the document. To do this, characteristics are used whose purpose is to evaluate the subset of sentences to determine the extent to which they cover the most relevant information of the document. One of these characteristics (coverage) is based on measures of similarity between sentences. The similarity between two sentences S_i and S_j, according to the vector representation described, is measured in the same way as the cosine similarity [39], which relates to the angle of the vectors S_i and S_j.

In the proposed algorithm, the objective function is in charge of guiding the search for the best summaries based on sentence characteristics. In this paper, an objective function based on the lineal normalized combination of sentence position, sentence length, and coverage of the selected sentences is proposed [40, 41].

Position Factor. According to previous studies, the relevant information in a document, regardless of its domain [42], tends to be found in certain sections such as titles, headings, the leading sentences of paragraphs, the opening paragraphs, etc. In this research, the position factor (PF) is calculated using Eq. (3)

$$PF_s = \frac{APF_s - \min_{\forall Summary} PF}{\max_{\forall Summary} PF - \min_{\forall Summary} PF}$$

$$APF_s = \sum_{\forall S_i \in Summary} \frac{PositionRanking(S_i)}{O} \tag{3}$$

where APF_s is the average sentence position in the summary S, O is the number of sentences in the summary S, $\max_{\forall summary} PF$ is the average of the maximum O values obtained from the position rankings of all sentences in the document (i.e. the average top maximum O position rankings of all sentences), $\min_{\forall summary} PF$ is the average of the minimum O values obtained from the position rankings of all sentences in the document, and PF_s is the position factor of the sentences of the summary S. $PositionRanking(S_i)$ is the position ranking of sentence S_i calculated by Eq. (4)

$$PositionRanking(S_i) = \frac{2 - 2 * \left(\frac{i-1}{n-1}\right)}{n} \tag{4}$$

where i is the position of the sentence in order of occurrence in the document, and n is the total number of sentences in the document. This formula is based on that used in the linear-rank selection method in genetic algorithms. The best ranking receives a value of $2/n$ and the lowest ranking is close to zero but not zero.

PF_s is close to one (1) when sentences in the summary are the first sentences in the document and PF_s is close to zero (0) when sentences in the summary are the last in the document. The *max* and *min* components in PF_s allow the normalization of the factor between zero and one (Min-Max normalization commonly used in data mining and other areas).

Length Factor. Some studies have concluded that the shortest sentences of a document ought to be less likely to appear in the document summary [6]. Equation (5) shows the calculation of length factor for the sentences of a summary:

$$LF_s = \frac{ALF_s - \min_{\forall Summary} LF}{\max_{\forall Summary} LF - \min_{\forall Summary} LF}$$

$$ALF_s = \sum_{\forall S_i \in Summary} \frac{Length(S_i)}{O} \tag{5}$$

where ALF_s is the average sentence length in the summary S, $Length(S_i)$ is the length (in words) of sentence S_i, O is the number of sentences in the summary S, $max_{\forall summary}$ LF is the average of the maximum O values obtained from the lengths of all sentences in the document (i.e. the average top maximum O lengths of all sentences), $min_{\forall summary}$ LF is the average of the minimum O values obtained from the lengths of all sentences in the document, and LF_s is the length factor of the sentences of the summary S. LF_s is close to one (1) when sentences in the summary are the largest sentences in the document and LF_s is close to zero (0) when sentences in the summary are the shortest in the document. The *min* and *max* components in LF_s allow the normalization of the factor between zero and one.

Coverage Factor. A summary ought to contain the main aspects of the documents with the least loss of information. The sentences selected should therefore cover the largest amount of information contained within the set of sentences in the document. As such, coverage factor is calculated taking into account the cosine similarity between the text of the candidate summary and all sentences of the document, as shown in Eq. (6).

$$CF_s = sim_{cos}(R, D) \tag{6}$$

where R represents the text with all the candidate summary sentences; D represents all the sentences of the document collection (in this case, it is the centroid of the document). This factor therefore takes values between zero and one, but bearing in mind that length summary is just a portion θ of the entire document, the real range of this factor is between θ-ε and $\theta + \varepsilon$, where θ-$\varepsilon > 0$ and $\theta + \varepsilon \ll 1$. NB: in order to compare this factor with position and length factors, all values for candidate summaries in the iterative process should be normalized based on a Min-Max strategy using current solution values in the optimization algorithm.

Thus the objective function to be maximized is defined as the linear normalized combination of sentence position (PF$_s$), sentence length (LF$_s$), and coverage (CF$_s$) factors (see Eq. (7)). Alfa (α), Beta (β), and Gamma (γ) coefficients are introduced, which gives flexibility to the objective function allowing more or less weight to be given to each factor. The sum of these coefficients should be equal to one, i.e. $\alpha + \beta + \gamma = 1$. Equation (8) includes a restriction to maximize the information included in the summary by selecting sentences containing relevant information but few words.

$$\text{Maximize } f(x) = \alpha * PF_s + \beta * LF_s + \gamma * CF_s \tag{7}$$

$$\text{subject to } \sum_{i=1}^{r} l_i x_i \leq L \tag{8}$$

where x_i indicates one if the sentence S_i is selected and zero otherwise; l_i is the length of the sentence S_i (measured in words) and L is the maximum number of words allowed in the generated summary.

3 The Proposed Memetic Algorithm

Global-best Harmony Search (GHS) is a stochastic optimization algorithm proposed in 2008 by Mahamed G.H. Omran and Mehrdad Mahdavi [37], which hybridizes the original Harmony Search (HS) with the concept of swarm intelligence proposed in PSO (Particle Swarm Optimization) [37], in which a swarm of individuals (called particles) fly through the search space. Each particle represents a candidate solution to the optimization problem. The position of a particle is influenced by the best position visited by itself (own experience) and the position of the best particles in the swarm (swarm experience). GHS modifies the pitch adjustment step in the original HS in such a way that the newly-produced harmony can mimic the best one in the harmony memory. This allows GHS to work efficiently in continuous and discrete problems. GHS is generally better than the original HS when applied to problems of high dimensionality and when noise is present [37].

In Fig. 1, the general outline of ESDS-GHS-GLO, the proposed memetic algorithm for automatically generating extractive summaries based on Global-best Harmony Search [37] and greedy search, is shown.

Harmony Memory Initialization (HM.Initialize). The initial population is composed of p agents, generated randomly, taking into account the constraint of the maximum number of words allowed in the summary (the number of sentences in the agent is controlled by means of Eq. (8)). Each agent represents the presence of the sentence in the summary with a one, absence with a zero. The most common strategy for initializing the population ($t = 0$) is to randomly generate each agent. In order that all the sentences in the document have the same probability of being part of the agent, a random number between one and n (number of sentences in the document) is defined, the gene corresponding to this value is chosen and a value of one is given, so that this sentence will become part of the summary in the current agent. Thus, the c-th agent of the initial population is created as shown in Eq. (9):

$$X_c(0) = \left[x_{c,1}(0), x_{c,2}(0), \ldots, x_{c,n}(0)\right], x_{c,s}(0) = a_s \qquad (9)$$

where a_s is a random value in $\{0,1\}$, $c = 1,2, \ldots, p$ and $s = 1,2, \ldots ,n.$, p is the population size and n is the number of sentences.

Evaluation (HM.Evaluate) and Optimization (HM.Optimize) of the Initial Population. After generating the initial population randomly, the fitness value of each agent is calculated using Eqs. (7) and (8). A percentage op of the population is then optimized using greedy local search, which is explained further on. Finally, the fitness is recalculated and the resulting population is ordered (**HM.Sort**) from highest to lowest based on this new fitness value. Bearing in mind that Coverage Factor needs a special normalization process based on values registered for agents in current harmony memory, minimum (min) and maximum (max) values are calculated and used to normalize values in all agents of the memory. Every time these values change, the coverage factor is recalculated and the fitness function is thus also recalculated in an incremental and efficient way.

Improvisation of a New Harmony. A new harmony is created empty, then using the original rules of the Global-best Harmony Search algorithm (memory consideration, pitch adjustment using Particle Swarm Optimization (PSO) concept, and random selection) some sentences are selected in order to be part of the new improvised version (harmony). The fitness value of this new harmony is calculated (**newHarmony. Evaluate**), and if the min or max values of coverage change, the fitness value is updated for all agents in the harmony memory. Later, the optimization (**newHarmony. Optimize**) of the new harmony occurs, only with an *op* probability (see the Greedy local optimizer section below). Finally, in order to avoid a premature convergence or loss of diversity, the algorithm ensures that only different solutions (new harmonies) will be included in the harmony memory; therefore, if newHarmony exists in the harmony memory the process is repeated.

L: maximum allowed agent length; *hms*: harmony memory size; *hmcr*: harmony memory consideration rate; *parmin*: minimum pitch adjustment rate; *parmax*: maximum pitch adjustment rate; *nofe*: current number of objective function evaluations; *mnofe*: maximum number of objective function evaluations.

```
HM.Initialize();        // Random initialization of Harmony Memory (hms agents), each meme represents
                        // the absence or presence of the sentence in the summary. Each agent must meet
                        // the length restriction (total words <= L)
HM.Evaluate();          // Calculate min-max values of coverage and Calculate fitness for all agents in HM.
HM.Optimize();          // Only a percentage of agents in HM is optimized.
HM.Sort()               // Sort based on fitness value. Best solution is HM[0]. Worst solution is HM[hms]
While nofe < mnofe do
    currentPar = parmin+(parmax-parmin)*(nofe/mnofe); // From original Global-best Harmony Search
    Do
        newHarmony.Length = 0; // New Harmony is created empty (no sentence is selected)
        While (newHarmony.Length <= L)                  // Total words <= L
            If (U(0,1) < hmcr)                          // Memory consideration rule
                i = rand(hms)                           // Select a random position in HM
                If (U(0,1) < currentPar)                 // Pitch adjustment rule
                    i=0;                                // Position of best solution in HM
                End If
                dimension = rand(HM[i].selectedSentences)  // Select the number of an active meme
            Else                                        // Random selection rule
                dimension = rand(n);                    // Randomly select a dimension from all possibilities
            End if
            If (newHarmony[dimension] = 1) continue while;  // Ignore this dimension if it was
                                                            // previously selected
            newHarmony[dimension] = 1;                   //Active this sentence (dimension)
            newHarmony.Length += SentenceLength[dimension];
        End While
        newHarmony.Evaluate();      // Calculate fitness for new Harmony, if the min-max values of
                                    // coverage change then update fitness for all agents in HM.
        newHarmony.Optimize();      // Tries to optimize the newHarmony.
        If (nofe >= mnofe) exit while;
    While (HM.Exists(newHarmony) )
    If (newHarmony.Fitness > HM[HMS].Fitness)
        HM[hms] = newHarmony;       // Replace the worst solution in HM by newHarmony.
        HM.Sort();
    End if
End While;
Return (HM[0]); // The agent with best fitness in HM is returned;
```

Fig. 1. Scheme of the ESDS-GHS-GLO memetic algorithm

Replacement. If the new harmony has a better fitness than the worst harmony in harmony memory, the new harmony replaces the worst harmony. The harmony memory is sorted in order to define the best and the worst harmony. It should be noted that to improve the performance of the algorithm, the sorting process can be avoided and only the best and worst harmonies in memory are calculated.

Stopping Criterion. The running of the memetic algorithm terminates when the stop condition is met. The stop condition was established earlier as a maximum number of evaluations of the objective function (*mnofe* parameter). Finally, the best founded solution (harmony) is returned, i.e. the first solution in the sorted harmony memory.

3.1 Greedy Local Optimizer

Regarding local search, ESDS-GHS-GLO uses a Greedy approach [43]. Taking into account the optimization probability (*op*), an agent is optimized a maximum number of times (*maxnumop*), adding and removing a sentence from the summary, and controlling the number of sentences in the agent by means of Eq. (8). If the fitness value of the new agent improves on the previous agent, the replacement is made. Otherwise, the previous agent is retained. A movement is then made again in the neighborhood, repeating the previous steps (Fig. 2 summarizes the greedy search used).

Lss: a list of sentences sorted by a reduced version of the fitness function equal to $f_i = \alpha \times \left(\frac{RankingPosition_i}{MaxRanking}\right) + \beta \times \left(\frac{Length_i}{MaxLength}\right) + \gamma \times SimCos(S_i, \overline{D})$.
op: optimization probability; *maxnumop*: maximum number of optimizations; *OriginalAgent*: original agent (agent to optimize);

If (U(0,1) > op) Then Return;   // Do not optimize
For *i*=1 ... *Maxnumop* do
   CurrentAgent = Copy (*OriginalAgent*);
   Add_sentence (*CurrentAgent*);   // A sentence with the highest value of the reduced fitness of
                                     // the list *Lss* that is not part of the current agent is activated.
   Delete_sentence (*CurrentAgent*);   // A sentence with the lowest value of similarity of
                                       // the list *Lss* is turned off in the current agent.
   Length_restriction (*CurrentAgent*); // The restriction of the summary length is executed.
   Evaluate (*CurrentAgent*);   // Calculate fitness for current agent. If max-min values of
                                       // coverage factor change, update fitness for all agents in HM
   If (Fitness(*CurrentAgent*) > Fitness(*OriginalAgent*)) Then *OriginalAgent* = *CurrentAgent*;
End For

Fig. 2. Procedure of greedy local optimization

The neighborhood is generated based on a scheme of elitism in which the sentence denoted as a one (i.e. included in the candidate summary) is selected from a list sorted according to the similarity of the sentence to the document centroid; and the sentence denoted as a zero (being thus removed from the candidate summary) contains least similarity to the document centroid. This means the coverage factor is the criterion used to include or remove a sentence from the candidate summary.

4 Experiment and Evaluation

To evaluate the ESDS-GHS-GLO algorithm, Document Understanding Conference (DUC) datasets for the years 2001 and 2002 were used. These collections are a product of research by the National Institute of Standards and Technology and are available online at http://www-nlpir.nist.gov. The DUC2001 collection comprises 309 documents; and DUC2002 comprises 567 documents. In these collections, the summary generated should be less than 100 words and have several reference summaries for each document.

Pre-processing of the documents involves linguistic techniques such as segmentation of sentences or words [39], removal of stop words, removal of capital letters and punctuation marks, stemming and indexing [39]. This process is carried out before starting to run the algorithm for the automatic generation of summaries.

The segmentation process was done using an open source segmentation tool called "splitta" (available at http://code.google.com/p/splitta). Stop word removal was carried out based on the list built for the SMART information retrieval system (ftp://cs.cornell.edu/pub/smart/english.stop). The Porter algorithm was used for the stemming process. Finally, Lucene (http://lucene.apache.org) was used to facilitate the entire indexing and searching in information retrieval tasks.

Evaluation of the quality of the summaries generated was performed using metrics provided by the assessment tool ROUGE (Recall-Oriented Understudy for Gisting Evaluation) [44] version 1.5.5 (available on internet), which has been widely handled (official metric) by DUC in evaluating automatic summaries. Because the proposed algorithm is not deterministic, the algorithm was run thirty (30) times over each document to obtain the average of each ROUGE measure.

Comparison of the proposed algorithm was made against MA-SingleDocSum [35] and DE [31] (metaheuristic approach), FEOM (fuzzy evolutionary approach) [21], UnifiedRank (graph-based approach) [17], NetSum (machine learning approach based on neural nets) [9], CRF (machine learning approach based on Conditional Random Fields) [10], QCS (machine learning approach based on Hidden Markov Model) [7], SVM (algebraic approach) [20], and Manifold Ranking (probabilistic approach using greedy algorithm) [17].

4.1 Parameter Tuning

Parameter tuning was carried out based on the Meta Evolutionary Algorithm (Meta-EA) [45], using a version of harmony search [46]. The configuration of parameters for the ESDS-GHS-GLO algorithm is as follows: Harmony memory size $hms = 10$, harmony memory consideration rate $hmcr = 0.85$, minimum pitch adjustment rate $parmin = 0.01$, maximum pitch adjustment rate $parmax = 0.99$, optimization probability $op = 0.25$, maximum number of optimizations $maxnumop = 5$ (maximum number of times an agent is optimized), maximum length of summary to evolve $mlse = 110$ (during the evolutionary process), maximum number of objective function evaluations $mnofe = 1600$, $\alpha = 0.50$, $\beta = 0.30$, and $\gamma = 0.20$. The algorithm was implemented on a PC Intel Core I7 3.0 GHz CPU with 12 GB of RAM in Windows 8.1.

As regards the objective function, the process of tuning the weights of the ESDS-GHS-GLO objective function was divided into two stages. In the first, a subset of all documents (DUC2001 and DUC2002) was selected as a training set. Using a Meta-EA approach based on HS the best weights for all factors were defined. In the second stage, the best weights obtained were used over all documents in order to obtain the results shown in the next section.

4.2   Results

Table 1 presents the results obtained in ROUGE-1 and ROUGE-2 measures, for ESDS-GHS-GLO and other state-of-the-art methods on the DUC2001 and DUC2002 data sets. The best solution is represented in bold type. The number in the right part of each ROUGE value in the table shows the ranking of each method. As shown in this table, MA-SingleDocSum improves upon the other methods in all ROUGE-2 measures for DUC2001 and DUC2002, and ESDS-GHS-GLO obtains second place. DE obtains best ROUGE-1 results on DUC2001 and UnifiedRank obtains best ROUGE-1 results on DUC2002.

Table 1. ROUGE values for each method on DUC2001 and DUC2002.

Method	DUC2001		DUC2002	
	ROUGE-1	ROUGE-2	ROUGE-1	ROUGE-2
MA-SingleDocSum	0.44862 7	**0.20142** 1	0.48280 2	**0.22840** 1
ESDS-GHS-GLO	0.45402 5	0.19565 2	0.47896 3	0.22138 2
DE	**0.47856** 1	0.18528 4	0.46694 4	0.12368 6
FEOM	0.47728 2	0.18549 3	0.46575 5	0.12490 5
UnifiedRank	0.45377 6	0.17646 7	**0.48487** 1	0.21462 3
NetSum	0.46427 3	0.17697 6	0.44963 6	0.11167 7
QSC	0.44852 8	0.18523 5	0.44865 7	0.18766 4
CRF	0.45512 4	0.17327 8	0.44006 8	0.10924 8
SVM	0.44628 9	0.17018 9	0.43235 9	0.10867 9
Manifold Ranking	0.43359 10	0.16635 10	0.42325 10	0.10677 10

Because the results do not identify which method gets the best results on both data sets, a unified ranking of all methods is presented, taking into account the position each method occupies for each measure. Table 2 shows the unified ranking. The resultant rank in this table (last column) was computed according to Eq. (10)

$$Rank(method) = \sum_{r=1}^{10} \frac{(11 - r + 1) \times R_r}{10} \qquad (10)$$

where R_r denotes the number of times the method appears in the r-th rank. The denominator 10 corresponds to the total number of compared methods. High values of Rank are desired.

Table 2. The resultant rank of the methods.

Methods	$R_r =$										Rank
	1	2	3	4	5	6	7	8	9	10	
MA-SingleDocSum	2	1	0	0	0	0	1	0	0	0	3.3
ESDS-GHS-GLO	0	2	1	0	1	0	0	0	0	0	3.2
DE	1	0	0	2	0	1	0	0	0	0	2.9
FEOM	0	1	1	0	2	0	0	0	0	0	2.9
UnifiedRank	1	0	1	0	0	1	1	0	0	0	2.7
NetSum	0	0	1	0	0	2	1	0	0	0	2.2
QSC	0	0	0	1	1	0	1	1	0	0	2.0
CRF	0	0	0	1	0	0	0	3	0	0	1.6
SVM	0	0	0	0	0	0	0	0	4	0	0.8
Manifold Ranking	0	0	0	0	0	0	0	0	0	4	0

Considering the results of Table 2 the following can be observed:

- The MA-SingleDocSum algorithm takes first place in the ranking (the highest value of the column Rank in the Table 2), focusing optimization on sentences position, sentences length, similarity of the sentence with the document title, cohesion and coverage of the summary. The fitness function uses five factors, and those factors are not normalized, so the weight of each factor is not in fact so meaningful.
- The ESDS-GHS-GLO method takes second place in the ranking, but MA-SingleDocSum used more execution time and uses a more complex fitness function. ESDS-GHS-GLO outperforms other methods based on metaheuristic approach (DE proposal), fuzzy evolutionary approach (FEOM), graph-based approach (UnifiedRank), machine learning approach (NetSum, QCS, and CRF), algebraic approach (SVM), and probabilistic approach using greedy algorithm (Manifold Ranking).
- The metaheuristic approach outperforms all remaining methods (machine learning, algebraic reduction, and probabilistic methods). Machine learning approach (using neural nets, conditional random fields, and hidden markov models) outperforms the algebraic and probabilistic methods. Finally, the algebraic reduction approach outperforms the probabilistic approach.

The experimental results indicate that optimization that combines global search based on population (Global-best Harmony Search) with a heuristic local search for some of the agents (greedy search) - as is the case with the ESDS-GHS-GLO memetic algorithm - is a promising area of research for the problem of generating extractive summaries for a single document. This approach is similar to previous research where a genetic algorithm was combined with guided local search, but it now features an easier and more meaningful fitness function.

5   Conclusions and Future Work

This paper proposes a new memetic algorithm for automatically generating extractives summaries from a single document - ESDS-GHS-GLO, based on Global-best Harmony Search and greedy search. For this problem, the agent is represented using many "zeros" and very few "ones" (sentences selected for the summary) but can also be implemented as a list featuring only the selected sentences. Using the Global-best Harmony Search algorithm, the design process of the algorithm is easier, because the designer does not have to worry about the selection, crossover, mutation and replacement tasks common in genetic algorithms.

The ESDS-GHS-GLO method proposed was evaluated by means of ROUGE-1 and ROUGE-2 measures on DUC2001 and DUC2002 datasets. Metaheuristic methods (including the proposed ESDS-GHS-GLO) surpass all methods in the state of the art over all measures. The best solutions are achieved by MA-SingleDocSum, ESDS-GHS-GLO, and DE. Therefore, regarding results obtained in the task of automatically generating summaries using memetic algorithms, the use of these in this type of problem is promising, but it is necessary to continue to conduct research in order to achieve better results than those obtained in this paper.

Considering possible future work, it is necessary to carry out experiments on other data sets, and to include other characteristics in the objective function that allow the selection of sentences relevant to the content of the documents and obtain a summary that is closer to the reference summaries built by humans; likewise to evaluate the use of other similarity measures such as soft cosine measure [47]; furthermore local search algorithms should also be explored, taking into account the characteristics specific to the automatic generation of summaries.

Acknowledgments. The work in this paper was supported by the University of Cauca and the National University of Colombia. We are especially grateful to Colin McLachlan for suggestions relating to English text.

References

1. Nenkova, A., McKeown, K.: A survey of text summarization techniques. In: Aggarwal, C. C., Zhai, C. (eds.) Mining Text Data, pp. 43–76. Springer, New York (2012)
2. Lloret, E., Palomar, M.: Text summarisation in progress: a literature review. Artif. Intell. Rev. **37**(1), 1–41 (2012)
3. Miranda, S., Gelbukh, A., Sidorov, G.: Generación de resúmenes por medio de síntesis de grafos conceptuales. Revista Signos. Estudios de Lingüística **47**(86) (2014)
4. Edmundson, H.P.: New methods in automatic extracting. J. ACM **16**(2), 264–285 (1969)
5. Aone, C., et al., Trainable, scalable summarization using robust NLP and Machine Learning. In: Mani, I., Maybury, M.T. (eds.) Advances in Automatic Text Summarization, pp. 71–80 (1999)
6. Kupiec, J., Pedersen, J., Chen. F.: A trainable document summarizer. In: Proceedings of the 18th Annual International ACM SIGIR Conference on Research and Development in Information Retrieval. ACM, Seattle, Washington, USA (1995)

7. Dunlavy, D.M., et al.: QCS: a system for querying, clustering and summarizing documents. Inf. Process. Manage. **43**(6), 1588–1605 (2007)
8. Conroy, J., O'leary, D.: Text summarization via hidden Markov models. In: Proceedings of the 24th Annual International ACM SIGIR Conference on Research and Development in Information Retrieval. ACM, New Orleans, Louisiana, USA (2001)
9. Svore, K., Vanderwende, L., Burges, C.: Enhancing single-document summarization by combining RankNet and third-party sources. In: Proceedings of the EMNLP-CoNLL (2007)
10. Shen, D., et al.: Document summarization using conditional random fields. In: Proceedings of the 20th International Joint Conference on Artificial Intelligence. Morgan Kaufmann Publishers Inc., Hyderabad, India (2007)
11. Wong, K.-F., Wu, M., Li, W.: Extractive summarization using supervised and semi-supervised learning. In: Proceedings of the 22nd International Conference on Computational Linguistics. Association for Computational Linguistics, Manchester, UK (2008)
12. Marcu, D.: Improving summarization through rhetorical parsing tuning. In: Proceedings of the Sixth Workshop on Very Large Corpora, Montreal, Canada (1998)
13. Ono, K., Sumita, K., Miike, S.: Abstract generation based on rhetorical structure extraction. In: Proceedings of the 15th Conference on Computational Linguistics. Association for Computational Linguistics, Kyoto, Japan (1994)
14. Barzilay, R., Elhadad, M.: Using lexical chains for text summarization. In: Proceedings of the ACL/EACL 1997 Workshop on Intelligent Scalable Text Summarization, Madrid, Spain (1997)
15. Louis, A., Joshi, A., Nenkova, A.: Discourse indicators for content selection in summarization. In: Proceedings of the 11th Annual Meeting of the Special Interest Group on Discourse and Dialogue, pp. 147–156. Association for Computational Linguistics, Tokyo, Japan (2010)
16. Mihalcea, R., Tarau, P.: Text-rank: bringing order into texts. In: Proceeding of the Conference on Empirical Methods in Natural Language Processing, Barcelona, Spain (2004)
17. Wan, X.: Towards a unified approach to simultaneous single-document and multi-document summarizations. In: Proceeding of the 23rd International Conference on Computational Linguistics (Coling 2010), Beijing (2010)
18. Gong, Y.: Generic text summarization using relevance measure and latent semantic analysis. In: Proceedings of the 24th Annual International ACM SIGIR Conference on Research and Development in Information Retrieval (2001)
19. Steinberger, J., Jezek, K.: Using latent semantic analysis in text summarization and summary evaluation. In: Proceedings of the 7th International Conference ISIM (2004)
20. Yeh, J.-Y., et al.: Text summarization using a trainable summarizer and latent semantic analysis. Inf. Process. Manage. **41**(1), 75–95 (2005)
21. Steinberger, J., Ježek, K.: Sentence compression for the LSA-based summarizer, pp. 141–148 (2006)
22. Lee, J.-H., et al.: Automatic generic document summarization based on non-negative matrix factorization. Inf. Process. Manage. **45**(1), 20–34 (2009)
23. Dehkordi, P.-K., Kumarci, F., Khosravi, H.: Text summarization based on genetic programming. In: Proceedings of the International Journal of Computing and ICT Research (2009)
24. Qazvinian, V., Sharif, L., Halavati, R.: Summarising text with a genetic algorithm-based sentence extraction. Int. J. Knowl. Manage. Stud. (IJKMS) **4**(4), 426–444 (2008)
25. García-Hernández, R.A., Ledeneva, Y.: Single extractive text summarization based on a genetic algorithm. In: Carrasco-Ochoa, J.A., Martínez-Trinidad, J.F., Rodríguez, J.S., Baja, G.S. (eds.) MCPR 2012. LNCS, vol. 7914, pp. 374–383. Springer, Heidelberg (2013)

26. Litvak, M., Last, M., Friedman, M.: A new approach to improving multilingual summarization using a genetic algorithm. In: Proceedings of the 48th Annual Meeting of the Association for Computational Linguistics. Association for Computational Linguistics, Uppsala, Sweden (2010)

27. Fattah, M.A., Ren, F.: GA, MR, FFNN, PNN and GMM based models for automatic text summarization. Comput. Speech Lang. **23**(1), 126–144 (2009)

28. Meena, Y.K., Gopalani, D.: Evolutionary algorithms for extractive automatic text summarization. Procedia Comput. Sci. **48**, 244–249 (2015)

29. Binwahlan, M.S., Salim, N., Suanmali, L.: Swarm diversity based text summarization. In: Leung, C.S., Lee, M., Chan, J.H. (eds.) ICONIP 2009, Part II. LNCS, vol. 5864, pp. 216–225. Springer, Heidelberg (2009)

30. Shareghi, E., Hassanabadi, L.S.: Text summarization with harmony search algorithm-based sentence extraction. In: Proceedings of the 5th International Conference on Soft Computing as Transdisciplinary Science and Technology. Cergy-Pontoise, France (2008)

31. Aliguliyev, R.M.: A new sentence similarity measure and sentence based extractive technique for automatic text summarization. Expert Syst. Appl. **36**(4), 7764–7772 (2009)

32. Abuobieda, A., Salim, N., Kumar, Y.J., Osman, A.H.: An improved evolutionary algorithm for extractive text summarization. In: Selamat, A., Nguyen, N.T., Haron, H. (eds.) ACIIDS 2013, Part II. LNCS, vol. 7803, pp. 78–89. Springer, Heidelberg (2013)

33. Binwahlan, M.S., Salim, N., Suanmali, L.: Fuzzy swarm diversity hybrid model for text summarization. Inf. Process. Manage. **46**, 571–588 (2010)

34. Song, W., et al.: Fuzzy evolutionary optimization modeling and its applications to unsupervised categorization and extractive summarization. Expert Syst. Appl. **38**(8), 9112–9121 (2011)

35. Mendoza, M., et al.: Extractive single-document summarization based on genetic operators and guided local search. Expert Syst. Appl. **41**(9), 4158–4169 (2014)

36. Garcia-Martinez, C., Rodriguez, F.J., Lozano, M.: Analysing the significance of no free lunch theorems on the set of real-world binary problems. In: 2011 11th International Conference on Intelligent Systems Design and Applications (ISDA) (2011)

37. Omran, M.G.H., Mahdavi, M.: Global-best harmony search. Appl. Math. Comput. **198**(2), 643–656 (2008)

38. Geem, Z.W.: Music-Inspired Harmony Search Algorithm: Theory and Applications. Studies in Computational Intelligence, vol. 191, 206. Springer Publishing Company, Incorporated, Rockville, Maryland (2009)

39. Manning, C., Raghavan, P., Schütze, H.: Introduction to Information Retrieval. Cambridge University Press, Cambridge (2008)

40. Hachey, B., Murray, G., Reitter, D.: The Embra System at DUC 2005: query-oriented multi-document summarization with a very large latent semantic space. In: Proceedings of the Document Understanding Conference (DUC), Vancouver, Canada (2005)

41. Alguliev, R.M., et al.: MCMR: Maximum coverage and minimum redundant text summarization model. Expert Syst. Appl. **38**, 14514–14522 (2011)

42. Lin, C.-Y., Hovy, E.: Identifying topics by position. In: Proceedings of the Fifth Conference on Applied Natural Language Processing, San Francisco, CA, USA (1997)

43. Ochoa, G., Verel, S., Tomassini, M.: First-improvement vs. best-improvement local optima networks of NK landscapes. In: Schaefer, R., Cotta, C., Kołodziej, J., Rudolph, G. (eds.) PPSN XI. LNCS, vol. 6238, pp. 104–113. Springer, Heidelberg (2010)

44. Lin, C.-Y.: Rouge: a package for automatic evaluation of summaries. In: Proceedings of the ACL-04 Workshop on Text Summarization Branches Out, Barcelona, Spain (2004)

45. Eiben, A.E., Smit, S.K.: Evolutionary algorithm parameters and methods to tune them. In: Monfroy, E., Hamadi, Y., Saubion, F. (eds.) Autonomous Search, pp. 15–36. Springer, Berlin (2012)
46. Cobos, C., Estupiñán, D., Pérez, J.: GHS + LEM: global-best Harmony Search using learnable evolution models. Appl. Math. Comput. **218**(6), 2558–2578 (2011)
47. Sidorov, G., et al.: Soft similarity and soft cosine measure: similarity of features in vector space model. Computación y Sistemas **18**(3) (2014)

SVD-LDA: Topic Modeling for Full-Text Recommender Systems

Sergey Nikolenko[1,2,3]([✉])

[1] Steklov Institute of Mathematics at St. Petersburg, St. Petersburg, Russia
`sergey@logic.pdmi.ras.ru`
[2] Laboratory for Internet Studies, National Research University –
Higher School of Economics, St. Petersburg, Russia
[3] Kazan (Volga Region) Federal University, Kazan, Russia

Abstract. In recommender systems, matrix decompositions, in particular singular value decomposition (SVD), represent users and items as vectors of features and allow for additional terms in the decomposition to account for other available information. In text mining, topic modeling, in particular latent Dirichlet allocation (LDA), are designed to extract topical content of a large corpus of documents. In this work, we present a unified SVD-LDA model that aims to improve SVD-based recommendations for items with textual content with topic modeling of this content. We develop a training algorithm for SVD-LDA based on a first order approximation to Gibbs sampling and show significant improvements in recommendation quality.

1 Introduction

Modern recommender systems deal with items of very different nature, including images, videos, tagged items, goods and services, and texts; many of these items have some kind of meaningful content that can be used to improve recommendations. Therefore, one natural direction of research in recommender systems would be to mine the content of the items being recommended. This is especially relevant for the cold start problem: to recommend new content with no history of preferences it would be very useful to make first recommendations to users who prefer this kind of content. In practice, such models usually represent a modification of some classical collaborative filtering model, usually based either on similarity between users or items [1,2] or on matrix decompositions. Over the last decade, collaborative filtering, starting from the Netflix Prize Challenge and beyond, have been dominated by various matrix decomposition techniques, mainly singular value decomposition (SVD) and nonnegative matrix factorization (NMF) [3,4]. On the other hand, again over the last decade, topic modeling, starting from probabilistic latent semantic analysis [5] and continuing with its Bayesian version, latent Dirichlet allocation [6], has become the method of choice for understanding large text corpora. Topic modeling is basically a dimensionality reduction technique, in many aspects very similar to an SVD decomposition,

O. Pichardo Lagunas et al. (Eds.): MICAI 2015, Part II, LNAI 9414, pp. 67–79, 2015.
DOI: 10.1007/978-3-319-27101-9_5

where the word-document matrix is decomposed into the "product" of word-topic and topic-document matrices.

In this work, we combine the SVD and LDA decompositions into a single unified model that optimizes a joint likelihood function and thus infers topics that are especially useful for improving recommendations. We provide an inference algorithm based on Gibbs sampling. However, it turns out that straightforward Gibbs sampling would have prohibitive computational costs, as each iteration of Gibbs sampling would require iterating over all ratings in the recommender dataset. Therefore, we develop an approximate sampling scheme based on a first order approximation to Gibbs sampling. The resulting algorithm has the same complexity as the original LDA Gibbs sampling and provides both meaningful topics and improved recommendations. We also add user metadata (demographic features), showing that the resulting topic factors are meaningful and provide a snapshot of the corresponding demographic group's tastes.

The paper is organized as follows. In Sect. 2, we remind the basic facts about latent Dirichlet allocation and briefly survey relevant extensions; Sect. 3 does the same for singular value decomposition as applied to recommender systems. In Sect. 4, we introduce the novel SVD-LDA model, show the inference for Gibbs sampling in this model, and approximate it to make the sampling tractable. Section 5 shows practical evaluation on a large dataset of full-text recommended items, and Sect. 6 concludes the paper.

2   LDA and sLDA

2.1   Latent Dirichlet Allocation

We begin with the basic latent Dirichlet allocation (LDA) model that we extend in the next section. The graphical model of LDA [6,7] is shown on Fig. 1a. We assume that a corpus of D documents contains T topics expressed by W different words. Each document $d \in D$ is modeled as a discrete distribution $\theta^{(d)}$ on the set of topics: $p(z_w = j) = \theta^{(d)}$, where z is a discrete variable that defines the topic of each word $w \in d$. Each topic, in turn, corresponds to a multinomial distribution on words: $p(w \mid z_w = k) = \phi_w^{(k)}$. The model also introduces prior Dirichlet distributions with parameters α for the topic vectors θ, $\theta \sim \mathrm{Dir}(\alpha)$, and β for the word distributions ϕ, $\phi \sim \mathrm{Dir}(\beta)$. A document is generated word by word: for each word, we (1) sample the topic index k from distribution $\theta^{(d)}$; (2) sample the word w from distribution $\phi_w^{(k)}$. Inference in LDA is usually done via either variational approximations or Gibbs sampling; we use the latter since it is easy to generalize to further extensions. In the basic LDA model, Gibbs sampling reduces to the so-called *collapsed Gibbs sampling*, where θ and ϕ variables are integrated out, and z_w are iteratively resampled according to the following distribution:

$$p(z_w = t \mid \boldsymbol{z}_{-w}, \boldsymbol{w}, \alpha, \beta) \propto \frac{n_{-w,t}^{(d)} + \alpha}{\sum_{t' \in T}\left(n_{-w,t'}^{(d)} + \alpha\right)} \frac{n_{-w,t}^{(w)} + \beta}{\sum_{w' \in W}\left(n_{-w,t}^{(w')} + \beta\right)}, \text{ where } n_{-w,t}^{(d)} \text{ is the}$$

number of words in document d chosen with topic t and $n_{-w,t}^{(w)}$ is the number of times word w has been generated from topic t apart from the current value z_w;

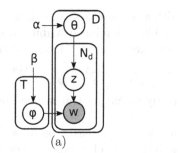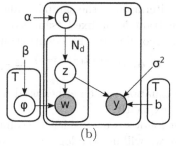

(a)   (b)

Fig. 1. The (a) LDA and (b) sLDA graphical models.

both counters depend on the other variables z_{-w}. Samples are then used to esti-
mate model variables: $\theta_{d,t} = \dfrac{n_{-w,t}^{(d)}+\alpha}{\sum_{t' \in T}\left(n_{-w,t'}^{(d)}+\alpha\right)}$, $\phi_{w,t} = \dfrac{n_{-w,t}^{(w)}+\beta}{\sum_{w' \in W}\left(n_{-w,t}^{(w')}+\beta\right)}$, where
$\phi_{w,t}$ denotes the probability to draw word w in topic t and $\theta_{d,t}$ is the probability
to draw topic t for a word in document d.

After it was introduced in [6], the basic LDA model has been subject to many
extensions, each presenting either a variational or a Gibbs sampling algorithm
for a model that builds upon LDA to incorporate some additional information or
additional presumed dependencies. In this work, we will further extend a specific
extension of LDA named Supervised LDA.

2.2   Supervised LDA

The SVD-LDA model we present in Sect. 4 is, in a way, an extension of the
Supervised LDA (sLDA) model [8]. In fact, in [8] the authors give recommender
systems as an example, albeit more in the context of sentiment analysis: the
authors predict the rating a user gives a movie based on the text of this user's
review. The sLDA graphical model is shown on Fig. 1b. Each document is now
augmented with a response variable y; in sLDA, y is drawn from a normal distribution centered around a linear combination of the document's topical distribution ($\bar{z}$, average z variables in this document) with some unknown parameters
b, a that are also to be trained when learning the model: $y \sim \mathcal{N}(y \mid b^\top \bar{z}+a, \sigma^2)$.

The original work [8] presents an inference algorithm for sLDA based on
variational approximations, but in this work we operate with Gibbs sampling
which will be easier to extend to SVD-LDA later. Thus, we show an sLDA
Gibbs sampling scheme. It differs from the original LDA in that the model
likelihood gets another factor corresponding to the y variable: $p(y_d \mid z, b, \sigma^2) =$
$\exp\left(-\frac{1}{2}\left(y_d - b^\top \bar{z} - a\right)^2\right)$, and the total likelihood is now

$$p(z \mid w, y, b, \alpha, \beta, \sigma^2) \propto \prod_d \frac{B(n_d + \alpha)}{B(\alpha)} \prod_t \frac{B(n_t + \beta)}{B(\beta)} \prod_d e^{-\frac{1}{2}\left(y_d - b^\top \bar{z}_d - a\right)^2}.$$

On each iteration of the sampling algorithm, we now first sample $\boldsymbol{z}$ for fixed $\boldsymbol{b}$ and then train $\boldsymbol{b}$ for fixed (sampled) $\boldsymbol{z}$. The sampling distribution of each z variable, according to the equation above, are $p(z_w = t \mid \boldsymbol{z}_{-w}, \boldsymbol{w}, \alpha, \beta) \propto$
$$q(z_w, t, \boldsymbol{z}_{-w}, \boldsymbol{w}, \alpha, \beta) e^{-\frac{1}{2}(y_d - \boldsymbol{b}^\top \bar{\boldsymbol{z}} - a)^2} = \frac{n^{(d)}_{-w,t} + \alpha}{\sum_{t'} \left(n^{(d)}_{-w,t'} + \alpha\right)} \frac{n^{(w)}_{-w,t} + \beta}{\sum_{w'} \left(n^{(w')}_{-w,t} + \beta\right)} e^{-\frac{1}{2}(y_d - \boldsymbol{b}^\top \bar{\boldsymbol{z}} - a)^2}.$$
The latter equation can be either used directly or further transformed by separating $\boldsymbol{z}_{-w}$ explicitly.

In what follows, we consider a recommender system based on likes and dislikes, where we will use the logistic sigmoid $\sigma(x) = 1/(1 + \exp(-x))$ of a linear function to model the probability of a "like": $p = \sigma\left(\boldsymbol{b}^\top \bar{\boldsymbol{z}} + a\right)$. In this version of sLDA, the graphical model remains the same, only conditional probabilities change. The total likelihood is now $p(\boldsymbol{z} \mid \boldsymbol{w}, \boldsymbol{y}, \boldsymbol{b}, \alpha, \beta, \sigma^2) \propto$

$$\prod_d \frac{B(\boldsymbol{n}_d + \alpha)}{B(\alpha)} \prod_t \frac{B(\boldsymbol{n}_t + \beta)}{B(\beta)} \prod_d \prod_{x \in X_d} \sigma\left(\boldsymbol{b}^\top \bar{\boldsymbol{z}}_d + a\right)^{y_x} \left(1 - \sigma\left(\boldsymbol{b}^\top \bar{\boldsymbol{z}}_d + a\right)\right)^{1-y_x},$$

where X_d is the set of experiments (ratings) for document d, and y_x is the binary result of one such experiment. The sampling procedure also remains the same, except that now we train logistic regression with respect to $\boldsymbol{b}$, a for fixed $\boldsymbol{z}$ instead of linear regression, and the sampling probabilities for each z variable are now $p(z_w = t \mid \boldsymbol{z}_{-w}, \boldsymbol{w}, \alpha, \beta) \propto$

$$q(z_w, t, \boldsymbol{z}_{-w}, \boldsymbol{w}, \alpha, \beta) \prod_{x \in X_d} \left[\sigma\left(\boldsymbol{b}^\top \bar{\boldsymbol{z}}_d + a\right)\right]^{y_x} \left[1 - \sigma\left(\boldsymbol{b}^\top \bar{\boldsymbol{z}}_d + a\right)\right]^{1-y_x}$$
$$= \frac{n^{(d)}_{-w,t} + \alpha}{\sum_{t' \in T} \left(n^{(d)}_{-w,t'} + \alpha\right)} \frac{n^{(w)}_{-w,t} + \beta}{\sum_{w' \in W} \left(n^{(w')}_{-w,t} + \beta\right)} e^{s_d \log p_d + (|X_d| - s_d) \log(1 - p_d)},$$

where s_d is the number of successful experiments among X_d, and $p_d = \frac{1}{1 + e^{-\boldsymbol{b}^\top \bar{\boldsymbol{z}}_d - a}}$.

3   SVD in Recommender Systems

3.1   Basic SVD Model in Collaborative Filtering

Recommender systems usually rely on collaborative filtering which can be expressed with the "like like like" maxim: users are similar if they like similar items (movies, musical compositions, web pages etc.), objects are similar if similar users have liked them, and similar users will keep liking similar items in the future. Collaborative filtering is usually based either on nearest neighbors [1,9] or, more importantly for this work, on matrix decompositions. Matrix decompositions, such as SVD, are used to extract from the data and estimate latent factors that influence the rating a user assigns to an item. In collaborative filtering based on singular value decomposition (SVD), the rating is represented as a sum of baseline predictors for both user and item and the scalar product of user features and item features: $\hat{r}_{i,a} = \mu + b_i + b_a + q_a^\top p_i$, where μ is a general mean, b_i and b_a are the user and item baseline predictors respectively, p_i and q_a are the user and item feature vectors. In case of a linear scale of ratings $\hat{r}_{i,a}$ can be used directly as an estimate of $r_{i,a}$ with Gaussian noise. However, in our case we have binary ratings, likes and dislikes, so we adopt the logistic SVD model where the probability of a like is modeled as $p(\text{like}_{i,a}) = \sigma(\hat{r}_{i,a})$ for the logistic sigmoid $\sigma(x) = 1/(1+e^{-x})$. Such models can be trained with stochastic gradient descent (SGD) or alternating least squares (ALS). Thus, the rating matrix that has many unknown components (ratings to be predicted) undergoes a low-rank approximation: an $N \times M$ matrix for N users and M items is decomposed into a product of $N \times F$ and $F \times M$ matrices, where F is the number of features which is usually several orders of magnitude smaller than both N and M. There are many different variations of this model; see, e.g., [3] and other works.

3.2   Cold Start, Additional Information, and Content

A key issue of all recommender systems is the cold start problem: how do we recommend content to a new user with no history of rated items and how do we recommend a new item that has no history of being rated by users? Basic collaborative filtering works very well for users and items with sufficient statistics already accumulated, and if we have no additional information except for the matrix of ratings, there is little we can do to cope with cold start; lists of top rated items are usually recommended to new users.

However, real life recommender systems almost always have some additional information about their users and/or items. Such information is often well structured; for instance, a movie may come with its genre, director, release date etc. Structured additional information, where there is a closed and relatively small list of possible values (e.g., movie genres), and they are known for items in the dataset, can be directly incorporated in the SVD model: $\hat{r}_{i,a} = \mu + b_i + b_a + q_a^\top p_i + r_a^\top s_i$, where r_a represents the additional information about the items, and s_i are feature vectors (or perhaps one-dimensional predictors) for the additional information in question; s_i can be trained individually for each user, but this often leads to overfitting, so s_i are often shared among users in a cluster. The clustering can be based either on the ratings themselves or on additional information about the users, such as, for instance, demographic information from the user profile (age, gender, country etc.). In the latter case, the resulting features can be used for cold start recommendations: a new user who has filled out his/her profile can have recommendations that are suitable for his/her demographic group. Note that the training algorithms do not change at all, we simply introduce new additive terms in the model, so both partial derivatives are still easy to compute for SGD and the model still reduces to linear or logistic regression with respect to user or item features in case of ALS.

The situation becomes more complicated, however, when the additional information also has to be trained. In this work, we concentrate on the case when the items being recommended have textual content (in the dataset below they will be web pages), and the additional information that we want to use represents topical content of the items extracted with a topic model as discussed in Sect. 2. One could, of course, first train the LDA model separately and then use the topic distributions θ_a for each document a as additional information, adding new features l_i for each user or cluster of users and each topic: $\hat{r}_{i,a} = \mu + b_i + b_a + q_a^\top p_i + \theta_a^\top l_i$. This approach was formalized and further developed in the fLDA model [10], which is an extension of regression-based latent factor models (RLFM) [11]. We will develop a new unified model that trains LDA topics in such a way as to improve SVD recommendations, similar to how sLDA extracts topics that are relevant for its response variable.

4   SVD-LDA

In this section, we present the new SVD-LDA model that combines logistic SVD for modeling the probability of a like with additional terms based on LDA topics that are trained together with SVD. In Sect. 4.1, we begin with a Gibbs sampling scheme that proves to be too computationally intensive, so in Sect. 4.2 we present an approximation which makes it tractable but still useful.

4.1   SVD-LDA: Exact Sampling

In the SVD-LDA model, for recommendations we use an SVD model with additional predictors corresponding to how much a certain user or group of user likes the topics trained in the LDA model; since our dataset is binary (like-dislike), we use a logistic version of the SVD model:

$$p(\text{success}_{i,a}) = \sigma\left(\hat{r}_{i,a}\right) = \sigma\left(\mu + b_i + b_a + q_a^\top p_i + \theta_a^\top l_i\right),$$

where p_i may be absent in case of cold start, and l_i may be shared among groups (clusters) of users. The total likelihood of the dataset with ratings comprised of triples $D = \{(i, a, r)\}$ (user i rated item a as $r \in \{-1, 1\}$) is a product of the likelihood of each rating (assuming, as usual, that they are independent): $p(D \mid \mu, b_i, b_a, p_i, q_a, l_i, \theta_a) = \prod_D \sigma\left(\hat{r}_{i,a}\right)^{[r=1]} \left(1 - \sigma\left(\hat{r}_{i,a}\right)\right)^{[r=-1]}$, and the logarithm is

$$\ln p(D \mid \mu, b_i, b_a, p_i, q_a, l_i, \theta_a) = \sum_D \ln\left([r = -1] - \sigma\left(\hat{r}_{i,a}\right)\right),$$

where $[r = -1] = 1$ if $r = -1$ and $[r = -1] = 0$ otherwise, and θ_a is the vector of topics trained for document a in the LDA model, $\theta_a = \frac{1}{N_a}\sum_{w \in a} z_w$, where N_a is the length of document a. Sampling probabilities for each z variable now look like
$$p(z_w = t \mid \mathbf{z}_{-w}, \mathbf{w}, \alpha, \beta) \propto q(z_w, t, \mathbf{z}_{-w}, \mathbf{w}, \alpha, \beta)p(D \mid \mu, b_i, b_a, p_i, q_a, l_i, \theta_a^{w \to t})$$

$$= \frac{n_{-w,t}^{(d)} + \alpha}{\sum_{t' \in T}\left(n_{-w,t'}^{(d)} + \alpha\right)} \frac{n_{-w,t}^{(w)} + \beta}{\sum_{w' \in W}\left(n_{-w,t}^{(w')} + \beta\right)} p(D \mid \mu, b_i, b_a, p_i, q_a, l_i, \theta_a^{w \to t})$$

$$= \frac{n_{-w,t}^{(d)} + \alpha}{\sum_{t' \in T}\left(n_{-w,t'}^{(d)} + \alpha\right)} \frac{n_{-w,t}^{(w)} + \beta}{\sum_{w' \in W}\left(n_{-w,t}^{(w')} + \beta\right)} e^{\sum_D \ln\left([r=-1] - \sigma\left(\hat{r}_{i,a}^{\text{SVD}} + l_i^\top \theta_a^{w \to t}\right)\right)},$$

where $\hat{r}_{i,a}^{\text{SVD}} = \mu + b_i + b_a + q_a^\top p_i$, and $\theta_a^{w\to t}$ is the vector of topics for document a where topic t is substituted in place of z_w. We see that in the formula above, to compute the sampling distribution for a single z_w variable one has to take a sum over all ratings all users have provided for this document, and due to the presence of the sigmoid function one cannot cancel out terms and reduce the sum to updating counts. It is possible to store precomputed values of $\hat{r}_{i,a}^{\text{SVD}}$ in memory, but it does not help because the z_w variables change during sampling, and when they do all values of $\sigma(\hat{r}_{i,a}^{\text{SVD}} + l_i^\top \theta_a^{w\to t})$ also have to be recomputed for each rating from the database. We have developed an implementation of this sampling algorithm; as expected, it works well on toy examples but cannot run in any reasonable time on a real-world sized dataset.

4.2   SVD-LDA: First Order Approximation

To make the model feasible, we had to develop a simplified SVD-LDA training algorithm that could run reasonably fast on large datasets. For the purposes of this simplification, we used a first order approximation to the value of the log likelihood, decomposing it into a Taylor series at the point where log likelihood is zero. Such an approximation will be very bad far from zero, but note that this is the logarithm of a value proportional to a multinomial probability: large negative values will all be sufficiently close to zero after exponentiation as to not matter, and large positive values will all yield a dominating advantage over alternatives. The only values where we need the approximation to be relatively precise are exactly the values around zero, where there are several alternative topics with comparable and significant probabilities. To construct the approximation, we differentiate $\ln p(D \mid \mu, b_i, b_a, p_i, q_a, l_i, \theta_a)$ with respect to θ_a; it is convenient to use the fact that $\sigma'(x) = \sigma(x)(1 - \sigma(x))$, which means that $\frac{\partial \ln \sigma(x)}{\partial x} = 1 - \sigma(x)$, $\frac{\partial \ln(1 - \sigma(x))}{\partial x} = -\sigma(x)$, so

$$\frac{\partial \ln p(D \mid l_i, \theta_a, \dots)}{\partial \theta_a} = \sum_D \left[[r = 1] \left(1 - \sigma(\hat{r}_{i,a}^{\text{SVD}} + \theta_a^\top l_i) \right) l_i \right.$$

$$\left. - [r = -1] \sigma(\hat{r}_{i,a}^{\text{SVD}} + \theta_a^\top l_i) l_i \right] = \sum_D \left[[r = 1] - \sigma(\hat{r}_{i,a}^{\text{SVD}} + \theta_a^\top l_i) \right] l_i.$$

We denote $s_a = \sum_D \left([r = 1] - \sigma \left(\hat{r}_{i,a}^{\text{SVD}} + \theta_a^\top l_i \right) \right) l_i$. We can now precompute s_a (it is a vector over topics) for each document right after SVD is trained (this requires additional memory of the same size as to hold the θ matrix) and then use it on the LDA sampling step as follows:

$$p(z_w = t \mid \boldsymbol{z}_{-w}, \boldsymbol{w}, \alpha, \beta) \propto q(z_w, t, \boldsymbol{z}_{-w}, \boldsymbol{w}, \alpha, \beta) p(D \mid \mu, b_i, b_a, p_i, q_a, l_i, \theta_a^{w\to t})$$

$$\approx \frac{n_{-w,t}^{(d)} + \alpha}{\sum_{t' \in T} \left(n_{-w,t'}^{(d)} + \alpha \right)} \frac{n_{-w,t}^{(w)} + \beta}{\sum_{w' \in W} \left(n_{-w,t}^{(w')} + \beta \right)} e^{s_a \theta_a^{w\to t}},$$

and the latter is proportional to simply $\dfrac{n^{(d)}_{-w,t}+\alpha}{\sum_{t'\in T}\left(n^{(d)}_{-w,t'}+\alpha\right)}\dfrac{n^{(w)}_{-w,t}+\beta}{\sum_{w'\in W}\left(n^{(w')}_{-w,t}+\beta\right)}e^{s_t}$
because $s_a\theta^{w\to t}_a = s_a\theta_a - s_w z_w + s_t z_t$, and the first two terms do not depend on t which is being sampled. Thus, the first order approximation yields a very simple modification of LDA sampling that incurs relatively small computational overhead as compared to the sampling itself. In Sect. 5, we will see that this approximation does indeed work.

4.3   Variations of SVD-LDA

We have outlined a general approximate sampling scheme; however, several different variations are possible depending on which predictors are shared in the basic SVD model, $p(\text{success}_{i,a}) = \sigma\left(\hat{r}_{i,a}\right)$. In general, it hardly makes sense to train a separate set of l_i features for every user, as each user will be represented by far too many independent variables, which will lead to heavy overfitting. We used two variations:

(1) share $l_i = l$ among all users; in this case, we simply want to find out which topics are better received by the user base in general;
(2) share $l_i = l_c$ among certain clusters of users, preferably inferred from some external information; in our experiments below, we used demographic information (age and gender) to divide the users into 20 approximately equal clusters; in this case, we can infer topics that are better or worse received by specific demographic groups of users.

Both variations can be used for cold start with respect to users; for cold start recommendations, we simply substitute $p_i = 0$ in the prediction formula above.

5   Evaluation

5.1   Dataset

For our experimental evaluation, we have used a dataset provided by the recommender system *Surfingbird*[1]; this system recommends web pages that will hopefully be of interest to users (it is similar to *StumbleUpon*), so most items available for recommendation (except pictures and videos) come with full text (usually in Russian) that has already been parsed by *Surfingbird*. The dataset contains 515K users and 1364K items (web pages). We split it into a training set with 29M ratings (users rate items with likes and dislikes) containing ratings provided by the users from December 2011 through April 2014, and a test set with 1.7M ratings which entered the system in May 2014. Note that the dataset is imbalanced, there are about 8 times more likes than dislikes, so the values of all ranking metrics like AUC are close to 1 by default, and small changes are even more important than usually in recommender systems.

---

[1] http://surfingbird.ru.

For the experiments, we have developed an implementation of the SVD-LDA training algorithm with Gibbs sampling in the C++ programming language. In particular, we have implemented the basic LDA training, supervised LDA, SVD-LDA with exact sampling as shown in Sect. 4.1 (impractical on this scale), SVD-LDA with approximate sampling as in Sect. 4.2, and a natural extension of the algorithm where SVD has both base predictors and LDA topic predictors for demographic user clusters.

5.2 RMSE Improves with LDA Training

In the first series of experiments, we used RMSE (root mean squared error) to support that approximate inference in the SVD-LDA model does indeed work and does make LDA topics gradually more relevant to improving prediction quality in the SVD model. As we have seen in Sect. 4 on each iteration of LDA training the SVD-LDA model training algorithm learns an SVD model with predictors corresponding to current document-topic distributions θ_a. Figure 2 shows a sample graph of how final RMSE (on the test set) after SVD training declines as LDA iterations progress. The graph indicates that better LDA topics do indeed help SVD train better, significantly increasing its predictive power.

5.3 SVD-LDA Recommends Better Than SVD

The second series of experiments uses results of SVD-LDA training to further provide content recommendations to the users, in particular to recommend new web pages and/or make recommendations to new users ("cold start"). We have trained the following models on the training set: (1) SVD model without additional predictors; (2) SVD-LDA model with additional topic predictors; (3) SVD-LDA-DEM model with additional topic predictors for each demographic cluster.

To evaluate the results, we use ranking evaluation metrics: recommendations are represented as an ordered list (the order of recommendations is all that matters for the user), and the perfect ranking would be to have all "likes" in front of the list followed by all "dislikes". We used the following metrics:

- NDCG – Normalized Discounted Commulative Gain [12];
- AUC – Area Under (ROC) Curve, which is in the binary case equivalent to the share of correctly ranked pairs of items [13, 14];
- Top-N metrics that show the share of "likes" in the top N recommendations, including Top-1 under the name of WTA (winner takes all) and Top-10 traditionally called MAP (mean average precision).

In the experiments, we varied the number of topics in SVD-LDA training, the number of features in the SVD model, and the regularization coefficient λ used for SVD training. Table 1 shows the best results we obtained for each model. It is clear that SVD-LDA outperforms SVD on all counts, while SVD-LDA-DEM provides an additional improvement over SVD-LDA. Note that in an imbalanced dataset, even small changes in the ranking metrics convert to significant improvements in recommendation quality.

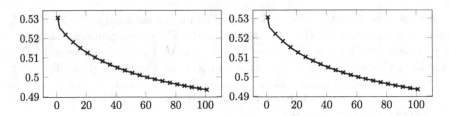

Fig. 2. RMSE at the end of each SVD-LDA training step as it changes through LDA iterations. Left: SVDLDA, 50 topics; right: SVDLDA with demographic user clusters, 200 topics.

Table 1. Ranking metrics on the test set. Only the best results w.r.t. λ and the number of features are shown.

Model	Topics	Features	λ	NDCG	AUC	MAP	WTA	Top3	Top5
SVD		5	0.1	0.9814	0.8794	0.9406	0.9440	0.9434	0.9424
SVD		10	0.15	0.9815	0.8801	0.9405	0.9448	0.9434	0.9425
SVD		15	0.2	0.9815	0.8802	0.9405	0.9453	0.9435	0.9426
SVD		20	0.2	0.9816	0.8803	0.9406	0.9453	0.9437	0.9427
SVD-LDA	50	5	0.025	0.9829	0.8893	0.9418	0.9499	0.9466	0.9445
SVD-LDA	100	10	0.025	0.9829	0.8893	0.9418	0.9500	0.9465	0.9445
SVD-LDA	200	15	0.01	0.9830	0.8895	0.9417	0.9524	0.9470	0.9446
SVD-LDA-DEM	50	10	0.01	**0.9840**	0.8901	**0.9428**	**0.9531**	**0.9481**	**0.9456**
SVD-LDA-DEM	100	5	0.01	**0.9840**	**0.8904**	**0.9428**	0.9528	0.9480	**0.9456**
SVD-LDA-DEM	200	10	0.01	**0.9840**	0.8898	**0.9428**	0.9524	**0.9481**	**0.9456**

It is interesting to note that our results, both in these experiments and in terms of RMSE shown in Sect. 5.2, do not depend much on the number of LDA topics; results from 50 through 200 topics are very similar, although the topics themselves do not deteriorate in quality, and inspection shows that LDA models with more topics do indeed uncover new meaningful distinctions in the content of web pages. This suggests that in reality, while there may be plenty of different topics in recommended items (our dataset is a collection of general interest web pages, so topics are very distinctive), not many topics do indeed have a distinctive effect on the recommendations, and it may suffice to use a small number of topics, e.g., 50 or 100, for similar systems in the future. This is important because LDA training with Gibbs sampling is computationally intensive, and it scales linearly with the number of topics.

5.4 Predictors for Demographic Clusters

One more demonstration of the of our approach comes from inspecting the predictors trained in the SVD-LDA-DEM model. Table 2 shows some of the best and worst topics for a selection of demographic groups characterized by gender and age (we have removed topics consisting of common words that are hard to interpret and topics that are good or bad uniformly across all demographic

Table 2. Topic predictors for some demographic groups (transl. from Russian).

l_{ct}	Topic	l_{ct}	Topic
Male, age ≤ 15		Female, age ≤ 15	
0.016	Movie song music album cinema musical	0.015	Girl star model wedding session singer
0.016	Car auto model engine company driver	0.011	Online free dog animal video cat
0.015	Bird forest animal height rock beach	0.010	Butter dish meat salt egg taste
0.013	Planet space Sun star gas satellite	0.009	Facebook social blog post vkontakte video
...		...	
0.004	Law political Putin deputy society	−0.002	Olympic games Sochi winner medal gold
0.001	Hair skin color shade mask make-up	−0.003	Wall room design style furniture
Male, age 25-29		Female, age 25-29	
0.014	Facebook social blog post vkontakte video	0.024	Music head buy read girl favorite
0.011	Xbox console company playstation world	0.023	Butter dish meat salt egg taste
0.010	Company user google mobile client phone	0.021	Movie song music album cinema musical
...		...	
0.000	Olympic games Sochi winner medal gold	0.006	Airplane tank war machine vessel flight
−0.002	Problem business reply plan company client	0.005	Exhibition museum art curated message

groups in order to emphasize the differences). Topics are characterized by a list of their top words; note that the values of predictors are incomparable across different groups because they can be redistributed with individual baseline predictors b_i (one can add and subtract a constant from all b_i and l_i inside a cluster, and predictions will not change). While sociological conclusions based on this data would not be sufficiently justified, we do believe that these results match sociological expectations, perhaps even stereotypes, very well.

6   Conclusion

In this work, we have presented a probabilistic model that unifies SVD as it is used in recommender systems and LDA for topic modeling into a single SVD-LDA model that attempts to train LDA topics that are useful for further recommendations. We have evaluated the resulting model on a real life full-text recommender system dataset, showing that both RMSE in SVD training and final ranking metrics improve significantly with the new model and that resulting topic predictors do indeed make sense in the context of demographic user clusters. As for further work, recent advances in pLSA regularization [15,16] suggest that it may be an interesting idea to develop regularizers that would lead to supervised pLSA and ultimately an SVD-pLSA model similar to SVD-LDA developed in this work. Another idea for further study might be to extend the SVD-LDA model to matrix decomposition techniques other than LDA (for the content of recommended items) and/or SVD (for the recommender system itself). This would let one process datasets with one-sided recommendations (e.g., with only likes and no dislikes) by switching from SVD to NMF [4] and process items with non-textual context with LDA variations for images [17], music [18], and other content.

Acknowledgements. This work was supported by the Samsung Research Center grant "Recommendation Systems based on Probabilistic Graphical Models", the Government of the Russian Federation grant 14.Z50.31.0030, and the Russian Foundation for Basic Research grant no. 15-29-01173.

References

1. Resnick, P., Iacovou, N., Sushak, M., Bergstrom, P., Riedl, J.T.: Grouplens: an open architecture for collaborative filtering of netnews. In: 1994 ACM Conference on Computer Supported Collaborative Work Conference, pp. 175–186, Chapel Hill, NC, Association of Computing Machinery (1994)
2. Said, A., Jain, B.J., Albayrak, S.: Analyzing weighting schemes in collaborative filtering: cold start, post cold start and power users. In: Proceedings of the 27th Annual ACM Symposium on Applied Computing, SAC 2012, pp. 2035–2040, New York (2012)
3. Koren, Y., Bell, R.M.: Advances in collaborative filtering. In: Ricci, F., Rokach, L., Shapira, B., Kantor, P.B. (eds.) Recommender Systems Handbook, pp. 145–186. Springer, US (2011)
4. Hu, Y., Koren, Y., Volinsky, C.: Collaborative filtering for implicit feedback datasets. In: Proceedings of the 8th IEEE International Conference on Data Mining, pp. 263–272, Pisa, Italy. IEEE Computer Society (2008)
5. Hoffmann, T.: Unsupervised learning by probabilistic latent semantic analysis. Mach. Learn. **42**, 177–196 (2001)
6. Blei, D.M., Ng, A.Y., Jordan, M.I.: Latent Dirichlet allocation. J. Mach. Learn. Res. **3**, 993–1022 (2003)
7. Griffiths, T., Steyvers, M.: Finding scientific topics. Proc. Nat. Acad. Sci. **101**(Suppl. 1), 5228–5335 (2004)
8. Blei, D.M., McAuliffe, J.D.: Supervised topic models. In: Advances in Neural Information Processing Systems, vol. 22 (2007)
9. Linden, G., Smith, B., York, J.: Amazon.com recommendations: item-to-item collaborative filtering. IEEE Internet Computing **7**(1), 76–80 (2003)
10. Agarwal, D., Chen, B.C.: fLDA: matrix factorization through latent Dirichlet allocation. In: Proceedings of the 3rd WSDM, pp. 91–100, New York. ACM (2010)

11. Agarwal, D., Chen, B.C.: Regression-based latent factor models. In: Proceedings of the 15th KDD, pp. 19–28 New York. ACM (2009)
12. Jarvelin, K., Kekalainen, J.: Cumulated gain-based evaluation of IR techniques. ACM Trans. Inf. Syst. **20**, 422–446 (2002)
13. Fawcett, T.: An introduction to ROC analysis. Pattern Recogn. Lett. **27**, 861–874 (2006)
14. Ling, C.X., Huang, J., Zhang, H.: AUC: a statistically consistent and more discriminating measure than accuracy. In: Proceedings of the International Joint Conference on Artificial Intelligence 2003, pp. 519–526 (2003)
15. Potapenko, A., Vorontsov, K.: Robust PLSA performs better than LDA. In: Serdyukov, P., Braslavski, P., Kuznetsov, S.O., Kamps, J., Rüger, S., Agichtein, E., Segalovich, I., Yilmaz, E. (eds.) ECIR 2013. LNCS, vol. 7814, pp. 784–787. Springer, Heidelberg (2013)
16. Vorontsov, K.: Additive regularization for topic models of text collections. Doklady Mathematics **89**, 301–304 (2014)
17. Cao, L., Fei-Fei, L.: Spatially coherent latent topic model for concurrent segmentation and classification of objects and scenes. In: IEEE 11th International Conference on Computer Vision, ICCV 2007, pp. 1–8 (2007)
18. Hu, D., Saul, L.K.: A probabilistic topic model for unsupervised learning of musical key-profiles. In: Hirata, K., Tzanetakis, G., Yoshii, K. (eds.) ISMIR, International Society for Music Information Retrieval, pp. 441–446 (2009)

Movies Recommendation Based on Opinion Mining in Twitter

Marcelo G. Armentano[1(✉)], Silvia Schiaffino[1], Ingrid Christensen[1], and Francisco Boato[2]

[1] ISISTAN (CONICET/UNICEN), Campus Universitario, Tandil, Argentina
{marcelo.armentano,silvia.schiaffino,
ingrid.christensen}@isistan.unicen.edu.ar
[2] Fac. de Ciencias Exactas, UNICEN, Campus Universitario, Tandil, Argentina
francisco.boato@gmail.com

Abstract. A traditional way for movie recommendation in a real scenario is by word of mouth. People ask their friends or relatives their opinion about a movie and then make their own judgment about whether to go to see the movie. In this article, we take this paradigm to evaluate Twitter as a source of information for movie recommendation. We built a balanced dataset consisting of 3036 tweets expressing opinions regarding movies. Then, we evaluated different tokenization strategies, pre-processing techniques and algorithms to build classification models that are able to determine the sentiment (opinion + polarity) expressed in the short texts published in Twitter. Finally, the best classifier is used to extract the main sentiment of Twitter users regarding a target movie in order to help users to decide to see the movie or not, obtaining promising results.

1 Introduction

Opinion Mining (OM) refers to the area where the opinions, emotions, attitudes and perceptions of people towards institutions, other people, events and attributes of each of these are analyzed. In particular, Sentiment Analysis can be defined as the task, within the area of Opinion Mining, which seeks to determine the polarity (positive, neutral or negative) of a sentence or text, or to make texts classification based on their polarity [6]. Opinion Mining is an area that is receiving every day more attention from many companies interested in the subjective opinions emitted by users in relation to a particular product or service.

Twitter[1] is a social networking and microblogging service that allows users to write and read messages up to 140 characters, called *tweets*. Twitter has had a great worldwide impact in the last years: in February 2015, Twitter was the second largest social network after Facebook, with 488 million registered users and 288 million active users (users who accessed their account in the last month), publishing a total of 500 million Tweets per day.

---

[1] https://twitter.com.

O. Pichardo Lagunas et al. (Eds.): MICAI 2015, Part II, LNAI 9414, pp. 80–91, 2015.
DOI: 10.1007/978-3-319-27101-9_6

The massive and globalized use of Twitter has generated a source of extremely large, constantly updated, and mostly public information accessible to all users. Users of Twitter, among other things, express their opinions about a variety of issues (politics, technology, books, films, religion, food). The common aspect shared by all these opinions is the subjectivity, since users express their own thinking or feeling about someone or something with a text shorter than 140 characters. By applying Opinion Mining techniques on data collected from Twitter we might be able to know the general feeling of users in relation to a variety of topics. These opinions can be very useful for large companies, but may also be useful to private individuals, for example to know the general opinion of users in relation to a product or service, to decide whether to purchase that product or service or not.

Particularly, a common situation we face is that of deciding whether or not to watch a particular film. The traditional mechanism we use is to ask several friends or acquaintances what they think about the film, thus forming our own opinion and finally deciding whether to watch or not the film. Thanks to the potential of Twitter, users can instantly know the opinion of many people in relation to an issue, in our case a particular movie. This information can be vital for recommender systems, which can take advantage of opinions for making recommendations [4, 12].

In this article we focus on micro-blogging social websites that are characterized by the publication of short texts. Short texts are usually informal and do not follow a defined semantics. Particularly, we focus on the analysis of microblogs to help users to take the decision about watching a movie or not, searching and evaluating the tweets related to it. Then, from the main sentiment of the tweets collected, the system presents a recommendation to the user. We evaluate different pre-processing techniques to improve the quality of the information contained in short texts. Then, we evaluate different classification models capable of extracting the polarity of the sentiment expressed by users in short texts. Finally, we use the model which performed best in the offline experiments to make recommendations to users regarding the general sentiment on Twitter about particular movies used as queries.

The remaining of the article is organized as follows. Section 2 describes the different steps we use to build classification models for opinion mining. Section 3 presents the different experiments we carried out combining different strategies for the different steps involved in the classification model. We also present in this section, results regarding recommendations to watch or not particular movies used as query. Then, in Sect. 4 we discuss some related works. Finally, in Sect. 5 we present our conclusions and outline some future works.

2   Classification Models for Opinion Mining

Figure 1 shows the pipeline with the different steps and strategies we evaluated in this article. In this section, we first describe the tokenization alternatives that we evaluated (subsect. 2.1). Then, we describe the pre-processing tasks we selected and applied to tweets (subsect. 2.2). Finally, we mention different classification techniques we can consider (subsect. 2.3).

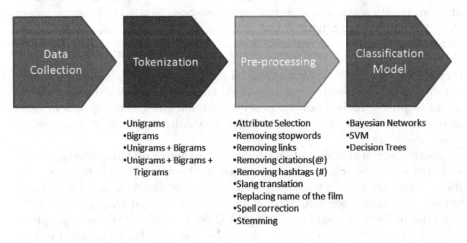

Fig. 1. Pipeline for tweets processing

2.1 Tokenization

The first step after data collection (See Sect. 3.1) is the tokenization of the tweets. Tokenization refers to transforming the raw text in a sequence of tokens or attributes. The standard tokenization strategy for English and many other languages, consists in splitting the raw text at the blanks (whitespaces). However, this simple strategy not always performs well. For example, the word "Los Ángeles" has a completely different meaning that the words "Los" and "Ángeles" independently. To face this problem, a common strategy used is to consider tuples of N words as tokens, which are known as n-grams. In computational linguistics an n-gram is a contiguous sequence of n items from a given sequence of text or speech. In the case of this article, the items we consider are words, so a unigram (n-gram of size 1) will be a word, a bigram (n-gram of size 2) a sequence of two words that appeared one after the other in a tweet, a trigram a sequence of three words, and so on.

2.2 Pre-processing

Data pre-processing is a fundamental task in the process of Knowledge Discovery. When working with short texts, data pre-processing is even more relevant since data tend to be more inconsistent and noisy. Firstly, tweets collected form online social networks are unstructured texts written by people and might contain misspellings and slang language. Another aspect that influences the poor quality of the data is the limit of characters allowed in each message (no more than 140 in the case of tweets). Since users should limit the idea they want to communicate to 140 characters, they frequently use abbreviations and unconventional language called *Internet slang*.

The preprocessing techniques evaluated in this study are:

- Removing stopwords
- Removing links to other websites
- Removing references to other users in Twitter (words starting with @)
- Removing hashtags (words starting with #)
- Translating slang to conventional language
- Replacing the name of the film by a custom tag [FILM]
- Spelling correction
- Stemming
- Attribute selection

To remove links and references to other users we used regular expressions.

Spelling correction was performed following the approach presented in [13]. The spelling correction algorithm is based primarily on the elimination of repeated letters (a typical practice used in internet and sms to emphasize an idea) and is divided into 2 steps. The first step is to remove letters that are repeated more than 2 times (leaving only 2 letters), since in the English language the triple repetition of a letter is not allowed. The second step is to eliminate duplication of letters that are not commonly repeated, allowing only the following duplications of letters "ss", "ee", "tt", "ff", "ll", "mm" and "oo".

Slang is detected and translated using the "No Slang" online dictionary[2].

For removing stopwords we tested three different stopwords lists. The first, taken from [9], only considers the most used articles in English ("a", "an" y "the"). According to [5] the most common stopwords in English are "a", "about", "an", "are", "as", "at", "be", "by", "for", "from", "how", "in", "is", "of", "on", "or", "that", "the", "these", "this", "to", "was", "what", "when", "where", "who", "will", and "with". Finally, we consider a most complete list of stopwords extracted from the ranks.nl[3] website.

The stemming step reduces words to its morphological root. We used the Lovins and Iterated Lovins algorithms [7] for this filter.

Regarding attribute selection, we used Information Gain to reduce the number of attributes in the dataset. We evaluated two strategies: keeping all words with information gain greater than 0, and keeping the N words with greater information gain.

2.3   Classification Models

According to [2], *classification* is defined as "the process of finding a model (or function) that describes and distinguishes data classes or concepts, for the purpose of being able to use the model to predict the class of objects whose class

---

[2] http://www.noslang.com.

[3] http://www.ranks.nl/resources/stopwords.html.

label is unknown. The derived model is based on the analysis of a set of training data (i.e., data objects whose class label is known)".

Several previous studies [9–11] concluded that two algorithms that performed well for short and noisy texts are Bayesian Networks and Support Vector Machine (SVM). In this article we also included decision trees, because of their easy configuration and straightforward interpretation of results.

3   Experimental Results

In this section we first describe the dataset we used in our experiments (subsect. 3.1). In subsect. 3.2 we show the result for different tokenization strategies, and in subsect. 3.3 we analyze the impact of different pre-processing alternatives. Finally, subsect. 3.4 present a experimental study on movie recommendation with different classifiers for ten movies in theaters.

3.1   Data Collection

To perform the experiments, it is necessary to have a dataset for training and validating the classification models. With this aim we crawled the Twitter network in search for tweets with a reference to a movie and an opining about it. We used a set of queries containing different movies currently in theaters at the moment of the experiment, in combination with a set of keywords expressing positive feelings (such as advice, applaud, encourage, recommend, suggest), negative fillings (such as annoying, waste, awful, horrible), neutral feelings (such as feel, presume, conclude, think) and mixed feelings (but, though, except, however, otherwise).

After combining the results for each query, the tweets collected were manually annotated by the authors of the paper. Tweets for which there was a dissagreement in the assigned label, duplicate tweets, and irrelevant tweets were discarded. The resulting dataset consisted of 755 negative tweets, 615 neutral tweets, 1040 positive tweets and 626 "mixed" tweets.

We performed a set of experiments with this dataset in order to find the most effective pre-processing tasks for building classification algorithms. We selected and compared three classification algorithms: decision trees, bayesian networks and support vector machines.

3.2   Tokenization Strategies

In this first set of experiments, we tested how filtering stopwords and stemming affected the accuracy of the classification algorithms for different tokenization options.

Unigrams. We first considered different pre-processing tasks for unigrams, that is, tokens consisting in only one word. We configured three different variables for these experiments: maximum number of attributes to be considered, filtering

Table 1. Best classification results for unigrams

Stemming	Stopwords list	Algorithm	Attr. Selection	Acc
NO	NO	SVM	InfoGain	75.43
NO	WebDM	SVM	InfoGain	75.23
NO	Senti	SVM	InfoGain	75.20
Lovins	Senti	SVM	InfoGain	75.13

(a) Accuracy

Stemming	Stopwords list	Algorithm	Attr. Selection	K
NO	No	SVM	InfoGain	66.81
NO	WebDM	SVM	InfoGain	66.52
NO	Senti	SVM	InfoGain	66.49
Lovins	Senti	SVM	InfoGain	66.40

(b) Kappa

Stemming	Stopwords list	Algorithm	Attr. Selection	AUC
Lovins	Senti	SVM	InfoGain	87.78
Lovins	NO	SVM	InfoGain	87.77
IterativeLovins	NO	SVM	InfoGain	87.57
IterativeLovins	Senti	SVM	InfoGain	87.45

(c) ROC area

stopwords and applying a stemming algorithm. We also applied an attribute selection strategy, keeping only those terms whose information gain was greater than 0. The total number of attributes after applying the attribute selection strategy varied from 156 (when applying a stemming algorithm and filtering stopwords) to 195 (without applying stemming and without filtering stopwords).

Table 1 shows the best four configurations for the tokenizers using unigrams.

We can observe that SVM algorithms give better classification results (ACC = 75.43 %, K = 66.81 % and AUC = 87.78 %). In all cases, not applying any stemming algorithm and not filtering stopwords lead to better or similar results. This suggests that we can omit applying these pre-processing tasks without affecting the classification results.

n-Grams. In this section, we analyze the results when evaluating the classifiers performance when tokenizing the tweets using n-grams with n varying from 1 to 3. As before, we considered applying different stemming algorithms and using a different set of stopwords list. We also applied an attribute selection strategy based on information gain. Table 2 shows the results obtained.

Results showed us that a better performance is obtained when adding n-grams to the vocabulary to consider them as attributes for classification. Consistent with the results from the previous subsection, the best results where

Table 2. Best classification results for n-grams

Min-gram	Max-gram	Stemming	Stopwords	Algorithm	Acc	K	AUC
1	2	NO	NO	SVM	77.37	69.39	88.96
1	2	Lovins	NO	SVM	77.31	69.31	88.87
1	3	Lovins	NO	SVM	76.78	68.58	88.76
1	3	NO	NO	SVM	76.15	67.71	88.52

obtained with support vector machine classifiers, considering both uni-grams and bi-grams, without using stemming and without filtering stopwords.

3.3 Pre-processing Strategies

The experiments performed in Sect. 3.2 were focused on analysing different configurations for the tokenizer to be applied to tweets. In this section, we evaluate how different pre-processing strategies affect the performance of the classifier for predicting the sentiment polarity of short texts. For all experiments in this section, we built support vector machines classifiers since these models proved to perform better in the experiments shown above.

We first considered the application of all pre-processing strategies but one. For each configuration, we tested four different configurations of the tokenizer (using uni-grams, bi-grams, tri-grams, and combinations of them) with attribute selection based on information gain. Results shown than using only uni-grams lead to worse results than using n-grams. The configuration for 1-2 n-grams got better accuracy than 1-3 ngrams (76.91 % vs 76.71 %). The application of a stemming algorithm did not lead to significatively better classification results. Table 3 shows the results for these set of experiments.

Table 3. Best classification results when applying all pre-processing techniques but one

n-gram	Stemm	Lower	Link	User	Hash	Film	Spell	Slang	Acc(%)	K(%)	AUC(%)
1-2	Lovins	x	x	x	x	x	-	x	77.37	69.41	88.98
1-2	Lovins	x	x	x	x	-	x	x	77.37	69.41	88.98
1-2	Lovins	x	x	x	-	x	x	x	77.37	69.41	88.98
1-2	Lovins	x	x	-	x	x	x	x	77.37	69.41	88.98
1-2	Lovins	x	-	x	x	x	x	x	77.37	69.41	88.98
1-2	Lovins	-	x	x	x	x	x	x	77.37	69.41	88.98
1-2	Lovins	x	x	x	x	x	x	x	77.37	69.41	88.98
1-2	NO	x	x	x	x	x	x	x	77.37	69.41	88.98
1-2	NO	x	x	x	x	-	x	x	77.08	69.00	88.82
1-2	NO	x	x	x	-	x	x	x	77.08	69.00	88.82

Table 4. Best classification results for different combinations of pre-processing techniques

n-gram	Stemm	Lower	Link	User	Hash	Film	Spell	Slang	Acc(%)	K(%)	AUC(%)
1-2	Lovins	x	x	-	-	x	x	x	77.57	69.67	88.89
1-2	NO	-	x	x	-	x	x	-	77.57	69.66	89.11
1-2	NO	-	-	-	-	-	-	-	77.57	69.66	89.11
1-2	Lovins	-	x	x	-	x	-	-	77.47	69.54	88.90
1-2	Lovins	-	-	-	-	-	-	-	77.47	69.54	88.90
1-2	NO	x	x	x	x	x	-	-	77.40	69.44	88.96
1-2	NO	x	x	x	-	x	-	-	77.34	69.35	88.95
1-2	NO	-	-	-	x	x	x	x	77.34	69.35	88.95

The only task that seems to affect the classification results is the translation of slang to natural language (Acc=77.37 % vs. Acc=76.81 %). For the remaining configurations, by setting the same configuration of the tokenizer we got the same results when ommiting only one pre-processing strategy.

Next, we tried to improve the classification performance by applying different combinations of the pre-processing strategies. As shown in Table 4, results are not significatively different from those presented in Table 3. Accuracy varied from 75.26 % in the worst case (using uni-grams) to 77.57 % in the best case (using combination of uni-grams and bi-grams).

3.4 Movies Recommendation

In the previous sections, we performed a set of experiments using a dataset created specially for evaluating different tokenization and preprocessing strategies for tweets and different classification algorithms. We kept this dataset balanced with respect to different categories (negative, neutral, possitive, mixed) and removed not relevant tweets to build different classifiers. In this section, we evaluate the performance of those classifiers for movies recommendation: given the title of a new movie, we aim to recommend to the user to see it or not based on the opinion for that movie collected from Twitter. We evaluate the performance of different classifiers for ten movies in theaters. Although it is not a requirement, it is better to select movies in theaters since Twitter is a real-time micro-blogging system in which it is easier to collect massive tweets only for movies that are on everyone's lips in a given moment.

For each selected movie, we search for tweets using the movie name (in English) and filtering conversations. We collect a dataset of 150 tweets for each movie, which was automatically annotated using the different classifiers built as described in the previous sections. The category assigned by the classifiers for each tweet was revised by the authors of this article in order to be able to compute the accuracy of each classifier.

Table 5 show the average accuracy for the ten testing movies using different classifiers. Results obtained varied from 62.57 % to 65.52 %. The classifiers that

Table 5. Performance for movies recommendation

Classifier	accuracy (%)
Uni-gram and bi-gram / Loving stemmer / Attribute selection (threshold) / All pre-processing	65.52
Uni-gram and bi-gram / Loving stemmer / Attribute selection (threshold)	65.46
Uni-gram / Attribute selection (threshold) / All pre-processing	64.61
Uni-gram / Attribute selection (threshold)	64.47
Uni-gram / Attribute selection (430 attributes)	63.66
Uni-gram / Attribute selection (threshold) / Pre-processing without slang filter	63.59
Uni-gram / Loving stemmer / Attribute selection (threshold) / Pre-processing	63.44
Uni-gram and bi-gram/ Attribute selection (threshold)	63.10
Uni-gram and bi-gram/ Attribute selection (threshold) / All pre-processing	62.57

obtained best accuracy used uni-grams and bi-grams, with Lovins stemming and selecting attributes based on a threshold information gain. Particularly, the classifier built using all the pre-processing tasks obtained 65.52 % accuracy, while the dataset built using no pre-processing tasks obtained 65.46 % accuracy. We also compute the weighted average and recall for each class and we verify that the best classifiers (according to those metrics) were the same models mentioned above.

An important conclusion for this experiment is that the pre-processing techniques do not significantly affect the performance of the classifiers.

Figure 2 shows a screenshot of the recommendation for a particular movie ("The secret life of Walter Mitty"). Since the main sentiment on Twitter regarding the provided movie is positive, the system recommends the user to watch the movie.

4   Related Work

Regarding sentiment analysis in social networks, some works have addressed this problem in Twitter [1,3,9]. In [1] the authors extract the polarity (positive or negative) of any tweet. Several tasks were carried out for pre-processing the training dataset. Tweets containing emoticons expressing both polarities were eliminated. Emoticons contained in the tweet were removed. To build the vector of attributes different alternatives were considered: only unigrams, only bigrams, unigrams + bigrams and POS. For the selection of attributes different mechanisms were considered: frequency of occurrence of an attribute, Mutual Information between each attribute and each class, and χ^2. The authors used the

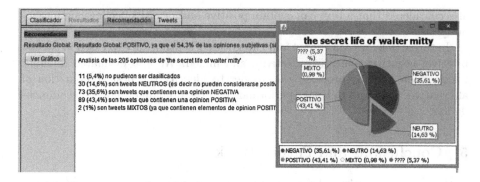

Fig. 2. Screenshot of a particular movie recommendation

accuracy measure to evaluate the performance of 4 supervised algorithms: Naive Bayes, SVM, MaxEnt NLP, and MaxEnt Stanford classifier. The best accuracy was obtained using Naive Bayes (with feature selection based on the calculation of the Mutual Information) on the unigrams dataset.

In [9] the authors continue with the analysis of sentiment of Tweets, trying to extract their polarity. The main difference lies in the fact that the authors seek to improve the performance of a ternary classification (positive, negative or neutral). The pre-processing tasks carried out were: removal of links, of references to other Twitter users, of Twitter special words (e.g. "RT"), of stop-words and emoticons. To tokenize the dataset, the POS representing the words were extracted and different alternatives were used: only unigrams, only bi-grams, and only tri-grams. Classification models based on different algorithms (Naive Bayes, SVM and Conditional Random Fields or CRF) are built. The best accuracy is achieved using bi-grams.

In [3], along with a ternary classification of Tweets sentiment, an analysis of the appearance (or target) to whom it is addressed is performed. This allows to differentiate in a tweet different feelings towards different aspects or entities. Furthermore, an analysis of the context of the tweet is performed, incorporating feelings of re-tweets or responses or other tweets posted by the same user, and thus improving the original classification. Some of the pre-processing tasks that were performed are the extraction of POS and stemming. The authors also normalized tweets, which corrects certain misspellings.

In the above-mentioned projects, when the polarity of an opinion is mentioned only two approaches are considered: positive vs negative or positive vs. negative vs. neutral. However, some works consider also "mixed" sentiments [8]. In [15] various classifiers are tested (SVM with the best performance) to evaluate the polarity of sentences, first it is determined whether the sentence is neutral (objective) or polar (subjective). In case of polar, the authors proceed to determine whether the polarity is positive, negative, double (when the sentence contains positive and negative polarity) or neutral (when it is a subjective sentence that is neither positive nor negative, e.g. speculation). In [13,14], it is also considered that a text can contain positive and negative feelings simultaneously.

In this article, we considered four categories of sentiments expressed in tweets: positive, negative, neutral (objective), and mixed. We also evaluated different tokenization and pre-processing strategies to identify the best combination of alternatives that lead to better performance in the domain of movies recommendation.

5   Conclusions and Future Work

In this article we evaluated different tokenization strategies, pre-processing techniques and algorithms to build classification models that are able to determine the opinion and polarity expressed in the short texts published in Twitter. We then used the best classifier to extract the main sentiment of Twitter users regarding a set of target movies in order to help users to decide to see the movie or not.

Regarding the desired configuration for a classification model for opinion mining, we discovered that the models based on SVM obtain better performance than those based on Bayesian Networks and Decision Trees. Also, the most effective models are those that employ a feature selection method (such as Information Gain). We also observed that the models that considered uni-grams and bi-grams together behaved better than those that only considered uni-grams. Those considering only bi-grams or tri-grams obtained the worst results. Finally, we did not observe significant differences as regards pre-processing tasks. In summary, we can say that to build a good classification model in the context of this work, depends mainly on the technique used to tokenize tweets and the technique used to classify them.

Although in this work we considered tweets in the movies domain, we consider that our findings can be extended or adapted to other application domains.

Acknowledgements. This study was partially supported by research projects PICT-2011-0366 and PICT-2014-2750

References

1. Go, A., Bhayani, R., Huang, L.: Twitter sentiment classification using distant supervision. Technical report, Stanford University (2009). https://cs.stanford.edu/people/alecmgo/papers/TwitterDistantSupervision09.pdf
2. Han, J., Kamber, M., Pei, J. (eds.): Data Mining: Concepts and Techniques. Morgan Kaufmann, San Francisco (2006)
3. Jiang, L., Yu, M., Zhou, M., Zhao, T.: Target-dependent twitter sentiment classification. In: Proceedings of the 49th Annual Meeting of the Association for Computational Linguistics: Human Language Technologies (2011)

4. Li, X., Wang, H., Yan, X.: Accurate recommendation based on opinion mining. In: Sun, H., Yang, C.-Y., Lin, C.-W., Pan, J.-S., Snasel, V., Abraham, A. (eds.) Genetic and Evolutionary Computing. Advances in Intelligent Systems and Computing, vol. 329, pp. 399–408. Springer, Heidelberg (2015)

5. Liu, B.: Web Data Mining: Exploring Hyperlinks, Contents, and Usage Data. Data-Centric Systems and Applications. Springer, Heidelberg (2011)

6. Liu, B.: Sentiment Analysis: Mining Opinions, Sentiments, and Emotions. Cambridge University Press, Cambridge (2015)

7. Lovins, J.B.: Development of a stemming algorithm. Mech. Trans. Comput. Linguist. **11**, 22–31 (1968)

8. Ounis, I., MacDonald, C., Soboroff, I.: On the trec blog track. In: Proceedings of the International Conference on Weblogs and Social Media (ICWSM) (2008)

9. Pak, A., Paroubek, P.: Twitter as a corpus for sentiment analysis and opinion mining. In: Proceedings of the Seventh Conference on International Language Resources and Evaluation, pp. 1320–1326 (2010)

10. Pang, B., Lee, L: A sentimental education: sentiment analysis using subjectivity. In: Proceedings of ACL, pp. 271–278 (2004)

11. Read, J.: Using emoticons to reduce dependency in machine learning techniques for sentiment classification. In: Proceedings of the ACL Student Research Workshop, ACLstudent 2005, pp. 43–48, Stroudsburg, Association for Computational Linguistics (2005)

12. Stavrianou, A., Brun, C.: Expert recommendations based on opinion mining of user-generated product reviews. Comput. Intell. **31**(1), 165–183 (2015)

13. Thellwall, M., Buckley, K., Paltaglou, G., Cai, D., Kappas, A.: Sentiment strength detection in short informal text. J. Am. Soc. Inf. Sci. Technol. **61**(12), 2544–2558 (2010)

14. Thelwall, M., Buckley, K., Paltaglou, G.: Sentiment strength detection for the social web. J. Am. Soc. Inf. Sci. Technol. **63**(1), 163–173 (2012)

15. Wilson, T., Wiebe, J., Hoffmann, P.: Recognizing contextual polarity: an exploration of features for phrase-level sentiment analysis. Comput. Linguist. **35**(3), 399–433 (2009)

Inferring Sentiment-Based Priors
in Topic Models

Elena Tutubalina[1] and Sergey Nikolenko[1,2,3]([⊠])

[1] Kazan (Volga Region) Federal University, Kazan, Russia
tlenusik@gmail.com
[2] Steklov Institute of Mathematics, St. Petersburg, Russia
[3] Laboratory for Internet Studies, National Research University-Higher
School of Economics, St. Petersburg, Russia
sergey@logic.pdmi.ras.ru

Abstract. Over the recent years, several topic models have appeared
that are specifically tailored for sentiment analysis, including the Joint
Sentiment/Topic model, Aspect and Sentiment Unification Model, and
User-Sentiment Topic Model. Most of these models incorporate sentiment knowledge in the β priors; however, these priors are usually set
from a dictionary and completely rely on previous domain knowledge to
identify positive and negative words. In this work, we show a new approach to automatically infer sentiment-based β priors in topic models for
sentiment analysis and opinion mining; the approach is based on the EM
algorithm. We show that this method leads to significant improvements
for sentiment analysis in known topic models and also can be used to
update sentiment dictionaries with new positive and negative words.

1 Introduction

Sentiment analysis and opinion mining is one of the oldest and most comprehen-
sively studied fields of natural language processing. Modern sentiment analysis
often emphasizes the problem of extracting opinions and evaluations regarding
certain goods and services from user-generated texts such as online reviews, e.g.,
movie reviews, item reviews in online stores and aggregators, hotel and trip
reviews and so on.

An important direction of study in this regard is *aspect-based sentiment
analysis*. The idea is that one review can touch upon many different aspects of a
product; e.g., a laptop review can touch upon design, performance, and usability,
and in all these aspects, sentiments would be expressed differently, sometimes
ambiguously; e.g., "heavy" would be a positive word for a desktop case (less
vibration), negative for a laptop (more to carry), and a neutral style marker for
music (e.g., heavy metal). Hence, it is desirable to separate the aspects and learn
different sentiment characteristics for different aspects. This idea, again, has a
long history; comprehensive surveys of both aspect-based sentiment analysis and
the entire field in general can be found in [1,2].

© Springer International Publishing Switzerland 2015
O. Pichardo Lagunas et al. (Eds.): MICAI 2015, Part II, LNAI 9414, pp. 92–104, 2015.
DOI: 10.1007/978-3-319-27101-9_7

In the last years, aspect-based sentiment analysis has been tighly linked with topic modeling. Topic modeling is a field of probabilistic modeling that infers the topical structure of a text corpus in an unsupervised way. In essence, a topic model decomposes the sparse word-document matrix into a product of dense word-topic and topic-document matrices; this idea was first fleshed out in probabilistic latent semantic analysis (pLSA) [3], and now the topic model of choice is latent Dirichlet allocation (LDA), which is a Bayesian version of pLSA [4,5]. In opinion mining, the idea is to try and get different aspects of a review into different topics; topic models are usually extended with sentiment labels and separate word-topic distributions for each such label; we survey these models in Sect. 2.3.

Existing topic models for aspect-based sentiment analysis almost invariably assume a predefined dictionary of sentiment words, usually incorporating this information into the β priors for the word-topic distributions in the LDA model. However, in many cases such dictionaries may be unavailable, e.g., when, as above, different words have different sentiments for different aspects, or in languages where detailed word sentiment dictionaries are unavailable. In this work, we propose a modification of several recently developed LDA extensions for sentiment analysis that allows for automatic updates of sentiment labels for individual words in a semi-supervised fashion, starting from a small seed dictionary. This modification works as an expectation-maximization generalization of the topic models, learning word-topic priors β on E-steps and doing regular inference based on Gibbs sampling on M-steps. We evaluate the proposed EM scheme with three different topic models on several large-scale real world datasets, showing substantial improvements in sentiment analysis quality and showing that new interesting sentiment words may be uncovered with this approach.

The paper is organized as follows. In Sect. 2, we remind the main definitions and notation of latent Dirichlet allocation, present a brief overview of the most important LDA extensions, and concentrate on LDA extensions related to aspect-based sentiment analysis; in particular, we show Gibbs sampling formulas for all considered models. In Sect. 3, we present our main contribution: an automatic inference technique for sentiment-related β priors in several LDA extensions related to sentiment based on the EM algorithm; we extend all previously surveyed models with this modification. Section 4 presents a comprehensive experimental evaluation of the proposed models on real life sentiment datasets, including sample new sentiment words found with our approach. Section 5 concludes the paper.

2   Latent Dirichlet Allocation

2.1   Notation and the Basic LDA Model

We begin by recalling the basic latent Dirichlet allocation (LDA) model that we build upon in this work. The graphical model of LDA [4,5] is shown on Fig. 1a. We assume that a corpus of D documents contains T topics expressed by W different words. Each document $d \in D$ is modeled as a discrete distribution $\theta^{(d)}$ on the set of topics: $p(z_w = t) = \theta_{td}$, where z is a discrete variable that defines the topic of each word $w \in d$. Each topic, in turn, corresponds to a multinomial distribution on words: $p(w \mid z_j = t) = \phi_{wt}$ (note that w denotes words in the vocabulary and j denotes individual instances of these words: many different j may correspond to the same w). The model also introduces prior Dirichlet distributions with parameters α for the topic vectors θ, $\theta \sim \mathrm{Dir}(\alpha)$, and β for the word distributions ϕ, $\phi \sim \mathrm{Dir}(\beta)$ (we assume the Dirichlet priors are symmetric, as they usually are). A document is generated word by word: for each word, we (1) sample the topic index t from distribution θ_d, $t \sim \mathrm{Mult}(\theta_d)$; (2) sample the word w from distribution ϕ_t, $w \sim \mathrm{Mult}(\phi_t)$.

There are two main approaches to Bayesian inference in LDA: variational approximations and Gibbs sampling; the latter is usually easier to generalize to further extensions, and it has been used in all extensions we use in this work.

We begin with some common notation: we denote by $n_{w,t,d}$ the number of words w generated with topic t in document d; partial sums over such variables are denoted by asterisks, e.g., $n_{*,t,d} = \sum_w n_{w,t,d}$ is the number of all words generated with topic t in document d, $n_{w,*,*} = \sum_{t,d} n_{w,t,d}$ is the total number of times word w occurs in the corpus and so on; we denote by $\neg j$ a partial sum over "all instances except j", e.g., $n_{w,t,d}^{\neg j}$ is the number of times word w was generated by topic t in document d except position j (which may or may not contain w).

In the basic LDA model, Gibbs sampling reduces to the so-called *collapsed Gibbs sampling*, where θ and ϕ variables are integrated out, and z_j are iteratively resampled according to the following distribution:

$$p(z_j = t \mid \boldsymbol{z}_{-j}, \boldsymbol{w}, \alpha, \beta) \propto \frac{n_{*,t,d}^{\neg j} + \alpha}{n_{*,*,d}^{\neg j} + T\alpha} \cdot \frac{n_{w,t,*}^{\neg j} + \alpha}{n_{*,t,*}^{\neg j} + W\beta},$$

where $\boldsymbol{z}_{-j}$ denotes the set of all z values except z_j. Samples are then used to estimate model variables: $\theta_{td} = \frac{n_{w,t,d} + \alpha}{n_{w,*,d} + T\alpha}$, $\phi_{wt} = \frac{n_{w,t,*} + \beta}{n_{*,t,*} + W\beta}$.

2.2   LDA Extensions

The basic LDA model has been used in numerous applications including studies that survey scientific literature [5] and attempt to mine how topics change in time [6–8]. After it was introduced in [4], the basic LDA model has been subject to many extensions, each presenting either a variational or a Gibbs sampling algorithm for a model that builds upon LDA to incorporate some additional information or additional presumed dependencies.

One large class of extensions deals with imposing new structure on the set of topics that are independent and uncorrelated in the base LDA model. *Correlated topic models* (CTM) avoid this unrealistic assumption, admitting that some topics are closer to each other and share words with each other; CTMs use logistic normal distribution instead of Dirichlet to model correlations between topics [9]. *Markov topic models* use Markov random fields to model interactions between topics in different parts of the dataset, connecting a number of different hyperparameters β_i in

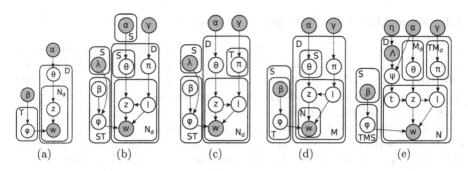

Fig. 1. LDA and its sentiment-related extensions: (a) the basic LDA model; (b) JST; (c) Reverse-JST; (d) ASUM; (e) USTM.

a Markov random field that can model a wide class of prior constraints [10]. *Syntactic topic models* introduce syntactic constraints inside a document that replace the bag-of-words model with syntactic parse trees [11]. *Relational topic models* construct a hierarchical model that reflects the structure of a document network as a graph [12], while *Spatial LDA* extends the LDA approach to image recognition by imposing spatial structure on "visual words" [13].

Another class of extensions takes into account additional information that may be available together with the documents and may reveal additional insights into the topical structure. For instance, the *Topics over Time* model applies when documents have timestamps of their creation (e.g., news articles or blog posts); it represents the time when topics arise in continuous time with a beta distribution [14]. *Dynamic topic models* represent the temporal evolution of topics through the evolution of their hyperparameters α and β, either with a state-based discrete model [15] or with a Brownian motion in continuous time [16]. Online topic detection with a temporal component (based on tensor factorization) has been applied to topic mining in continuous streams [17]. *DiscLDA* assumes that each document is assigned with a categorical label and attempts to utilize LDA for mining topic classes related to this classification problem [18]. The *Author-Topic model* incorporates information about the author of a document, assuming that texts from the same author will be more likely to concentrate on the same topics and will be more likely to share common words [19,20]. Yet other extensions improve upon the bag-of-words assumption, modeling correlations between words and individual sentences [21].

Finally, a lot of work has been done on nonparametric LDA variants based on Dirichlet processes, where the number of topics is not predefined but is also sampled automatically in the generative process. We do not go into the details here; see, e.g., [22–25] and references therein.

In this work, we build upon a specific class of LDA extensions devoted to sentiment analysis.

2.3   Topic Models for Sentiment Analysis

Topic models in sentiment analysis fall into the area of aspect-based sentiment analysis. Usually, traditional aspect-based approaches extract phrases that contain words from predefined and usually manually constructed lexicons or words that have been shown by trained classifiers to predict a sentiment polarity. These works usually distinguish *affective* words that express feelings ("happy", "disappointed") and *evaluative* words that express sentiment about a specific thing or aspect ("perfect", "awful"); these words come from a known dictionary, and the model is supposed to combine the sentiments of individual words into a total estimate of the entire text and individual evaluations of specific aspects. Recently, several topic models, i.e., several LDA extensions have been proposed and successfully used for sentiment analysis; in this section, we introduce the topic models for sentiment analysis that we will extend below.

In [26] authors proposed sentiment modifications of LDA, called Joint Sentiment-Topic (JST) and Reverse Joint Sentiment-Topic (Reverse-JST) models. The basic assumption was that in the JST model, topics depend on sentiments from a document's sentiment distribution π_d and words are generated conditional on sentiment-topic pairs, while in the Reverse-JST model sentiments are generated conditional on the document's topic distribution θ_d. In [26], a domain-independent sentiment lexicon MPQA [27] was used to incorporate prior knowledge into the models as the word prior sentiment polarity.

The JST graphical model is shown on Fig. 1(b). Formally speaking, for S different possible sentiment labels (usually S is small, e.g., for $S = 3$ we have "positive", "neutral", and "negative" labels) it extends the ϕ word-topic distributions, generating separate distributions ϕ_{lt} for each sentiment label $l \in \{1, \ldots, S\}$ (with a corresponding Dirichlet prior λ) and a multinomial distribution on sentiment labels π_d (with a corresponding Dirichlet prior γ) for each document $d \in D$. Each document now has S separate topic distributions for each sentiment label, and the generative process operates as follows: for each word position j, (1) sample a sentiment label $l_j \sim \text{Mult}(\pi_d)$; (2) sample a topic $z_j \sim \text{Mult}(\theta_{d,l_j})$; (3) sample a word $w \sim \text{Mult}(\phi_{l_j,z_j})$. The work [26] derives Gibbs sampling distributions for JST by marginalizing out π_d; denoting by $n_{w,k,t,d}$ the number of words w generated with topic t and sentiment label k in document d and extending the notation accordingly, a Gibbs sampling step can be written as

$$p(z_j = t, l_j = k \mid \nu) \propto \frac{n_{*,k,t,d}^{\neg j} + \alpha_{tk}}{n_{*,k,*,d}^{\neg j} + \sum_t \alpha_{tk}} \cdot \frac{n_{w,k,t,*}^{\neg j} + \beta_{kw}}{n_{*,k,t,*}^{\neg j} + \sum_w \beta_{kw}} \cdot \frac{n_{*,k,*,d}^{\neg j} + \gamma}{n_{*,*,*,d}^{\neg j} + S\gamma},$$

where α_{tk} is the Dirichlet prior for topic t with sentiment label k, and $\nu = (z_{-j}, w, \alpha, \beta, \gamma, \lambda)$ is the set of all other variables and model hyperparameters.

The Reverse-JST graphical model is shown on Fig. 1(c). In JST, topics were generated conditional on sentiment labels drawn from π_d; in Reverse-JST, it works in the opposite direction: for each word w, first we draw a topic label $z_j \sim \text{Mult}(\theta_d)$ and then draw a sentiment label k conditional on the topic and a word conditional on both topic and sentiment label. Again, inference is a modification of Gibbs sampling:

$$p(z_j = t, l_j = k \mid \nu) \propto \frac{n^{-j}_{*,*,t,d} + \alpha_t}{n^{-j}_{*,*,*,d} + \sum_t \alpha_t} \cdot \frac{n^{-j}_{w,k,t,*} + \beta}{n^{-j}_{*,k,t,*} + W\beta} \cdot \frac{n^{-j}_{*,k,t,d} + \gamma}{n^{-j}_{*,*,t,d} + S\gamma},$$

and in the sentiment estimation step Reverse-JST evaluates document sentiment as $p(k \mid d) = \sum_z p(k \mid z, d)p(z \mid d)$.

The work [28] presents the aspect and sentiment unification model (ASUM); it is indended to analyze user reviews of goods and services and incorporates both aspect-based analysis and sentiment, e.g., which specific characteristics of a good the review has been positive and negative about. In spirit the model is similar to JST, but it breaks a review down into sentences, assuming that all words in a single sentence are generated from the same topic (aspect), i.e., a single sentence is assumed to speak about only one aspect of the item under review. In the basic model with this assumption, Sentence LDA (SLDA), for each review d with topic distribution θ_d, for each sentence in d we: (1) draw the topic (aspect) for sentence s, $z_s \sim \text{Mult}(\theta_d)$, (2) generate words $w \sim \text{Mult}(\phi_{z_s})$. The ASUM model extends Sentence LDA with sentiment labels; similar to JST, there is a separate distribution ϕ_{st} for each sentiment label s and topic t. The generative process works as follows: for each sentence s in a document d, (1) choose its sentiment label $l_s \sim \text{Mult}(\pi_d)$, (2) choose topic $t_s \sim \text{Mult}(\theta_{dl_s})$ conditional on the sentiment label l_s, (3) generate words $w \sim \text{Mult}(\phi_{l_s t_s})$. ASUM's graphical model is shown on Fig. 1(d). Inference is done, again, with Gibbs sampling; denoting by $s_{k,t,d}$ the number of sentences (rather than words) assigned with topic t and sentiment label t in document d and extending notation with asterisks and $\neg$, we get the following Gibbs sampling distribution:

$$p(z_j = t, l_j = k \mid \nu) \propto \frac{s^{-j}_{k,t,d} + \alpha_t}{s^{-j}_{k,*,d} + \sum_t \alpha_t} \cdot \frac{s^{-j}_{k,*,d} + \gamma_k}{s^{-j}_{*,*,d} + \sum_{k'} \gamma_{k'}} \times$$

$$\times \frac{\Gamma\left(n^{-j}_{*,k,t,*} + \sum_w \beta_{kw}\right)}{\Gamma\left(n^{-j}_{*,k,t,*} + \sum_w \beta_{kw} + W_{*,j}\right)} \prod_w \frac{\Gamma\left(n^{-j}_{w,k,t,*} + \beta_{kw} + W_{w,j}\right)}{\Gamma\left(n^{-j}_{w,k,t,*} + \beta_{kw}\right)},$$

where $W_{w,j}$ is the number of words w in sentence j, and $\nu = (l_{-j}, z_{-j}, w, \gamma, \alpha, \beta)$ is the set of all other variables and model hyperparameters.

Both JST and ASUM make use of a predefined set of sentiment words to set asymmetric β priors for the models. The model assigns the lexicon's sentiment words their sentiment in the initialization step. The models were evaluated on datasets about electronic devices and restaurants in the classification task, and the corresponding papers have shown substantial improvements over supervised classifiers and other generative models; in particular, ASUM was shown to improve over JST.

Another take on the same problem deals with very recently developed User-aware Sentiment Topic Models (USTM) [29]; USTM incorporates user meta-data tags (e.g., location, gender, or age) together with topics and sentiment. In this model, each document is assigned with an observed tag or a combinations of tags, topics are generated conditioned on the document's tags, sentiment labels are generated conditioned on the (document, tag, topic) triples, and words are conditioned on the latent topics, sentiments and tags. Formally, a tag distribution ψ_d is generated for every document (with a Dirichlet prior η), for each position j a tag $a_j \sim \text{Mult}(\psi_d)$ is drawn from ψ_d, and distributions of topics, sentiments, and words are conditional on the tag a_j. The USTM graphical model is shown on Fig. 1(e). Denoting by $n_{w,k,t,m,d}$ the number of words w generated with topic t, sentiment label k, and metadata tag m in document d and extending the notation accordingly, a Gibbs sampling step can be written as

$$p(z_j = t, l_j = k, a_j = m \mid \nu) \propto$$

$$\frac{n^{-j}_{*,*,t,m,d} + \alpha}{n^{-j}_{*,*,*,m,d} + TM_d\alpha} \cdot \frac{n^{-j}_{w,*,t,m,*} + \beta}{n^{-j}_{*,*,t,m,*} + W\beta} \cdot \frac{n^{-j}_{w,k,t,m,*} + \beta_{wk}}{n^{-j}_{*,k,t,m,*} + \sum_w \beta_{wk}} \cdot \frac{n^{-j}_{*,k,t,m,d} + \gamma}{n^{-j}_{*,*,t,m,d} + S\gamma},$$

where M_d is the number of tags in document d.

We also note a nonparametric hierarchical extension of ASUM called HASM [30] and nonparametric extensions of USTM models, USTM-DP(W) and USTM-DP(S) [29]. In these extensions, the number of topics and (in case of USTM) the number of topics associated with different metadata attributes is not defined in advance but rather inferred with the help of Dirichlet processes; we do not consider nonparametric topic models further in this paper but note them as a possible direction for further work.

3 Learning Sentiment Priors β with the EM Algorithm

All of the models surveyed in Sect. 2.3 assume that we have prior sentiment information from an external vocabulary: (1) in JST and Reverse-JST, word-sentiment priors λ are drawn from an external dictionary and incorporated into β priors; $\beta_{kw} = \beta$ if word w can have sentiment label k and $\beta_{kw} = 0$ otherwise; (2) in ASUM, prior sentiment information is also encoded in the β prior, making β_{kw} asymmetric similar to JST; (3) in USTM, again, Dirichlet priors β_{kw} are asymmetric, and prior sentiment information is fixed in the priors. In other words, sentiment priors β basically contain predefined dictionaries of sentiment words.

However, this information is often incomplete; for instance, the Russian language which we would ultimately like to process does not have an accessible good sentiment vocabulary, certainly not one usable for reviews of specific goods or services (hotels, cars, movies). Therefore, it would be interesting to extend topic models for sentiment analysis to train sentiment for new words automatically. We can assume access to a small seed vocabulary with predefined sentiment, but the goal is to extend it to new words and learn their sentiment from the model.

Our modification of the models above learns the priors β_{kw} for every word and every sentiment. We treat β_{kw} as latent variables in the general model and train them with an expectation-maximization (EM) scheme. The high-level algorithm is shown below.

Algorithm 1. GENERALEMSCHEME

1: **while** inference has not converged **do**
2:     **for** N steps **do**   ▷ M-step
3:         run one Gibbs sampling update step
4:     update β_{kw} priors   ▷ E-step

This scheme works for every LDA extension considered above. At the E-step, we obviously should update $\beta_{kw} \propto n_{w,k,*,*}$, but the normalization coefficient is in our hands: Dirichlet parameters do not have to sum up to 1, and their sum affects the variance of the Dirichlet distribution. Here, it makes sense to start with relatively large variance at the stage where we are unsure of the sentiments and then gradually refine the β_{kw} estimates. Hence, in the algorithm we use a simulated annealing approach, $\beta_{kw} = \frac{1}{\tau} n_{w,k,*,*}$, where τ is a regularization coefficient (temperature) that should start large (large variance) and then decrease (smaller variance).

Thus, the final algorithm is as follows. Start with some initial approximation of the sentiments β_s^w (obtained from a small seed dictionary and maybe some simpler learning method used for initialization and then smoothed). Then, iteratively,

(1) at the E-step of iteration i, update β_{kw} as $\beta_{kw} = \frac{1}{\tau(i)} n_{w,k,*,*}$ with, e.g., $\tau(i) = \max(1, 200/i)$;
(2) at the M-step, perform several iterations of Gibbs sampling for the corresponding model with fixed values of β_{kw}.

In this work, we have extended the JST, Reverse-JST, ASUM, and USTM models in this way; in the next section, we show the results of our experiments.

4   Experimental Results

To evaluate the document sentiment prediction, we used two different corpora: the Amazon review dataset[1] and a dataset of hotel and car reviews adopted from [29], further called *Hotels+Cars*. As pre-processing we removed stopwords, converted word tokens to lowercase, applied stemming for all words with the NLTK library (http://www.nltk.org), added neighboring negations to tokens, and split both dataset into train and test parts.

Statistics of the Amazon's corpora are presented in Table 1. If the average rating score is greater than 3, we mark this review with positive sentiment; if the average rating is ≤ 3, the review is marked with negative sentiment. For the experiments, we adopted the publicly available sentiment lexicon MPQA [27] which is often used in real world sentiment analysis problems as the seed dataset of sentiment words.

Similar to recent works, we use domain-independent knowledge about sentiment polarity of words to set the sentiment priors for the reviews' words in

---

[1] Available at https://snap.stanford.edu/data/web-Amazon.html.

the corpus. In our experiments, we divided sentiment priors into three different values: neutral, positive, and negative. We first set the β priors for all words in the corpus to $\beta_{kw} = 0.01$; then, if a word is contained in the seed sentiment dictionary, we set the sentiment priors for a positive word to $\beta_{*w} = (1, 0.1, 0.01)$ (1 for positive, 0.1 for neutral, and 0.01 for negative); for a negative word, to $\beta_{*w} = (0.01, 0.1, 1)$.

Table 1. Summary statistics for Amazon datasets.

Product domain	#reviews with overall rating r				
	$r = 1$	$r = 2$	$r = 3$	$r = 4$	$r = 5$
Electronics	1410	701	811	2013	5066
Baby products	1180	723	864	1821	5413
Home tools	1230	553	814	1789	5615
Cars	848	354	600	1370	4836
Music	832	494	763	1983	5927
Phones	1998	984	1140	2186	3693
Shoes	517	432	786	1772	6494
Software	2787	890	978	1686	3660
Watches	810	527	778	2116	5769

For all models, posterior inference was done with 1000 Gibbs iterations with hyperparameters $\alpha = 50/K$, $\gamma = 0.01 * \text{AvgLen}/S$, where AvgLen is the average review length in words, S is the total number of sentiment labels, and $K = 5$ topics (aspects). In our experiments, a document d is classified as positive if its probability of positive label $p(l_{\text{pos}} \mid d)$ is higher than its probabilities of negative and neutral classes $p(l_{\text{neg}} \mid d)$ and $p(l_{\text{neu}} \mid d)$, and vice versa. The probabilities $p(l \mid d)$ were calculated based on the topic-sentiment-word distribution ϕ [29].

Tables 2 and 3 present classification results on the Amazon datasets and the Hotels + Cars dataset; models with our EM-based modifications are marked with "+EM". The results clearly show that JST + EM, Reverse-JST + EM, and USTM + EM give a substantial improvement over the original models with sentiment priors based on a predefined sentiment lexicon. ASUM + EM shows a less significant improvement, only slightly better than original ASUM, improving in 7 datasets out of 11. A possible explanation for ASUM's results is that we learn sentiment priors for every word and every sentiment, while ASUM presupposes that all words in a sentence are generated from the same sentiment. Therefore, many non-lexicon neutral words that co-occur with positive or negative adjectives in a sentence are updated with positive and negative labels. JST + EM, Reverse-JST + EM, and USTM + EM have had more significant improvements since all words are conditioned on the latent sentiments.

Table 2. Sentiment prediction quality with different topic models, Amazon reviews dataset.

Domain	JSTs		Reverse-JSTs		ASUMs	
	JST	JST + EM	Rev.-JST	R.-JST + EM	ASUM	ASUM + EM
Electronics	0.6003	**0.6398**	0.5784	**0.5934**	0.6082	**0.6198**
Cars	**0.6872**	0.6418	**0.6429**	0.5717	0.475	**0.504**
Home tools	0.5609	**0.6054**	0.5859	**0.6118**	0.4955	**0.4975**
Baby domains	0.5714	**0.6178**	0.5709	**0.6169**	0.5606	**0.5791**
Music	0.6363	**0.6948**	0.6028	**0.6513**	0.444	**0.5204**
Phones	0.5314	**0.5344**	0.5629	**0.5869**	0.536	**0.5415**
Shoes	0.6923	**0.7672**	**0.6373**	0.6149	**0.592**	0.5680
Software	0.5289	**0.5329**	0.5254	**0.5559**	**0.5445**	0.5435
Watches	0.6930	**0.7305**	0.62	**0.6438**	**0.644**	0.61

Table 3. Sentiment prediction quality with different topic models, Hotels+Cars reviews dataset.

Domain	JSTs		Reverse-JSTs		ASUMs		USTMs	
	JST	JST + EM	R.-JST	R.-JST + EM	ASUM	ASUM + EM	USTM	USTM + EM
Hotels	0.3881	0.41	0.3881	0.4250	0.5045	0.5714	0.5514	**0.5959**
Cars	0.4465	0.4485	0.3746	0.4021	0.5854	0.5721	0.6645	**0.7902**

Table 4. Topic examples with sentiment words discovered by JST and JST modification based on the EM algorithm.

Cars				Hotels				Software			
JST		JST + EM		JST		JST + EM		JST		JST + EM	
neu	pos	neu	pos	neu	pos	pos	pos	neg	pos	neg	pos
work	price	batteri	**fit**	room	stay	room	**great**	donat	**learn**	**problem**	program
great	part	**power**	buy	bed	hotel	hotel	**nice**	rent	program	**tri**	**learn**
good	**fit**	unit	*qualiti*	night	**nice**	**great**	*full*	**dead**	softwar	review	book
plug	amazon	*charg*	bought	stay	**good**	bed	*realli*	**treat**	languag	day	*read*
price	order	*gener*	item	door	room	room	experi	tax	word	**free**	**good**
gaug	ship	*run*	made	shower	night	*decor*	**expens**	**sad**	**good**	*final*	tool
littl	plug	day	**nice**	water	clean	bit	*big*	**battl**	quot	*issu*	*understand*
easi	purchas	**back**	*receiv*	open	price	size	bar	**blah**	*teach*	call	*teach*
connect	*replac*	**long**	**sound**	sleep	**great**	**modern**	breakfast	**complic**	video	*anoth*	*anyone*

As for mining new sentiment words, Table 4 shows the words extracted by the models for several datasets. Seed sentiment words from the MPQA dictionary are marked in bold, new sentiment words discovered by the models, in italics. Manual examination of different topics has confirmed that models with the proposed EM-based modification have extracted more verb expressions (e.g., *neg_work, replace, return, fit, wet*) and domain-specific product characteristics (e.g., *waterproof, quality, stainless, cool, fast*); these resulting expressions can be used to augment aspect-specific sentiment dictionaries and can ultimately be more helpful in business applications than sentiment words extracted by the original models.

5   Conclusion

In this work, we have presented a novel extension for several topic models for sentiment analysis; we have shown how to automatically update sentiment priors for individual words with a combination of the EM algorithm and standard Gibbs sampling. Our extensive experimental evaluation has proven that this idea leads to significant improvements in most considered cases and often uncovers new interesting sentiment words. One natural direction for further study would be to try to construct a unified algorithm for the entire model that would join topic inference with inference over β priors in the same step; such an algorithm might achieve better local maxima in the likelihood and might converge to these maxima faster. Another direction is to extend this idea to nonparametric topic models so that the number of topics could also be learned in the process. Finally, we also intend to study in more detail the process of learning sentiment priors for individual words and try to refine it further to be able to learn high-quality sentiment labels in a semi-supervised fashion (with a small seed dataset which is further extended by topic modeling with the EM modifications we propose). In general, we believe that this work is only the beginning of a large-scale effort that will let us bring sentiment analysis to languages and domains where extensive sentiment dictionaries are yet unavailable.

Acknowledgements. This work was supported by the Russian Science Foundation grant no. 15-11-10019.

References

1. Liu, B.: Sentiment Analysis and Opinion Mining. Synthesis Lectures on Human Language Technologies, vol. 5. Morgan & Claypool Publishers, San Rafael (2012)
2. Pang, B., Lee, L.: Opinion mining and sentiment analysis. Found. Trends Inf. Retrieval **2**, 1–135 (2008)
3. Hoffmann, T.: Unsupervised learning by probabilistic latent semantic analysis. Mach. Learning **42**, 177–196 (2001)
4. Blei, D.M., Ng, A.Y., Jordan, M.I.: Latent Dirichlet allocation. J. Mach. Learning Res. **3**, 993–1022 (2003)
5. Griffiths, T., Steyvers, M.: Finding scientific topics. Proc. Nat. Acad. Sci. U.S.A. **101**(Suppl. 1), 5228–5335 (2004)
6. Wu, Q., Zhang, C., Hong, Q., Chen, L.: Topic evolution based on LDA and HMM and its application in stem cell research. J. Inf. Sci. **40**(5), 611–620 (2014)
7. Wu, Q., Zhang, C., An, X.: Topic segmentation model based on ATNLDA and co-occurrence theory and its application in stem cell field. J. Inf. Sci. **39**, 319–332 (2013)

8. He, Q., Chen, B., Pei, J., Qiu, B., Mitra, P., Giles, L.: Detecting topic evolution in scientific literature: how can citations help? In: Proceedings of the 18th ACM Conference on Information and Knowledge Management, CIKM 2009, pp. 957–966. ACM, New York (2009)

9. Blei, D.M., Lafferty, J.D.: Correlated topic models. In: Advances in Neural Information Processing Systems, vol. 18 (2006)

10. Li, S.Z.: Markov Random Field Modeling in Image Analysis. Advances in Pattern Recognition. Springer, Heidelberg (2009)

11. Boyd-Graber, J.L., Blei, D.M.: Syntactic topic models. In: Koller, D., Schuurmans, D., Bengio, Y., Bottou, L. (eds.) Advances in Neural Information Processing Systems, pp. 185–192. Curran Associates, Inc., Red Hook (2008)

12. Chang, J., Blei, D.M.: Hierarchical relational models for document networks. Ann. Appl. Stat. **4**, 124–150 (2010)

13. Wang, X., Grimson, E.: Spatial latent Dirichlet allocation. In: Advances in Neural Information Processing Systems, vol. 20 (2007)

14. Wang, X., McCallum, A.: Topics over time: a non-Markov continuous-time model of topical trends. In: Proceedings of the 12th ACM SIGKDD International Conference on Knowledge Discovery and Data Mining, pp. 424–433. ACM, New York (2006)

15. Blei, D.M., Lafferty, J.D.: Dynamic topic models. In: Proceedings of the 23rd International Conference on Machine Learning, pp. 113–120. ACM, New York (2006)

16. Wang, C., Blei, D.M., Heckerman, D.: Continuous time dynamic topic models. In: Proceedings of the 24th Conference on Uncertainty in Artificial Intelligence (2008)

17. Guo, X., Xiang, Y., Chen, Q., Huang, Z., Hao, Y.: LDA-based online topic detection using tensor factorization. J. Inf. Sci. **39**, 459–469 (2013)

18. Lacoste-Julien, S., Sha, F., Jordan, M.I.: DiscLDA: discriminative learning for dimensionality reduction and classification. In: Advances in Neural Information Processing Systems, vol. 20 (2008)

19. Rosen-Zvi, M., Griffiths, T., Steyvers, M., Smyth, P.: The author-topic model for authors and documents. In: Proceedings of the 20th Conference on Uncertainty in Artificial Intelligence, pp. 487–494. AUAI Press, Arlington (2004)

20. Rosen-Zvi, M., Chemudugunta, C., Griffiths, T., Smyth, P., Steyvers, M.: Learning author-topic models from text corpora. ACM Trans. Inf. Syst. **28**, 1–38 (2010)

21. Bagheri, A., Saraee, M., de Jong, F.: ADM-LDA: an aspect detection model based on topic modelling using the structure of review sentences. J. Inf. Sci. **40**, 621–636 (2014)

22. Blei, D.M., Jordan, M.I., Griffiths, T.L., Tennenbaum, J.B.: Hierarchical topic models and the nested chinese restaurant process. In: Advances in Neural Information Processing Systems, vol. 13 (2004)

23. Teh, Y.W., Jordan, M.I., Beal, M.J., Blei, D.M.: Hierarchical Dirichlet processes. J. Am. Stat. Assoc. **101**, 1566–1581 (2004)

24. Williamson, S., Wang, C., Heller, K.A., Blei, D.M.: The IBP compound Dirichlet process and its application to focused topic modeling. In: Proceedings of the 27th International Conference on Machine Learning, pp. 1151–1158 (2010)

25. Chen, X., Zhou, M., Carin, L.: The contextual focused topic model. In: Proceedings of the 18th ACM SIGKDD International Conference on Knowledge Discovery and Data Mining, pp. 96–104. ACM, New York (2012)

26. Lin, C., He, Y., Everson, R., Ruger, S.: Weakly supervised joint sentiment-topic detection from text. IEEE Trans. Knowl. Data Eng. **24**, 1134–1145 (2012)

27. Turney, P., Littman, M.: Measuring praise and criticism: inference of semantic orientation from association. ACM Trans. Inf. Syst. **21**(4), 315–346 (2003)

28. Jo, Y., Oh, A.H.: Aspect and sentiment unification model for online review analysis. In: Proceedings of the Fourth ACM International Conference on Web Search and Data Mining, WSDM 2011, pp. 815–824. ACM, New York (2011)
29. Yang, Z., Kotov, A., Mohan, A., Lu, S.: Parametric and non-parametric user-aware sentiment topic models. In: Proceedings of the 38th ACM SIGIR (2015)
30. Kim, S., Zhang, J., Chen, Z., Oh, A.H., Liu, S.: A hierarchical aspect-sentiment model for online reviews. In: Proceedings of the Twenty-Seventh AAAI Conference on Artificial Intelligence, 14–18 July 2013, Bellevue, Washington, USA (2013)

Analysis of Negation Cues for Semantic Orientation Classification of Reviews in Spanish

Sofía N. Galicia-Haro[1]([✉]), Alonso Palomino-Garibay[1],
Jonathan Gallegos-Acosta[2], and Alexander Gelbukh[3]

[1] Faculty of Sciences, UNAM, Mexico City, Mexico
sngh@fciencias.unam.mx, alonsop@ciencias.unam.mx
[2] Postgraduate Program in Computer Science and Engineering, UNAM,
Mexico City, Mexico
j_gallegos_a@uxmcc2.iimas.unam.mx
[3] Centro de Investigación En Computación, Instituto Politécnico Nacional,
Mexico City, Mexico
http://www.gelbukh.com

Abstract. We study the effect of negation cues on semantic orientation prediction. State-of-the-art approaches to semantic orientation derivation are based on automatic classification. We analyze the use of negation cues as features for both supervised and unsupervised methods. We apply such methods on a collection of washing-machine reviews in Spanish. We compare the results of the two approaches and discuss the performance of each negation cue. We found that simple features performed similarly to using more resources.

Keywords: Semantic orientation · Opinion reviews · Linguistic features · Supervised methods · Unsupervised methods

1 Introduction

The huge amount of customer reviews of products and services, freely accessible on the Web, has allowed turning such opinions into valuable resources for decision-making. In particular, people interested in such products can make purchases based on other customers' information. Due the high volume of these resources, manual processing of this information is difficult; much time and effort is required to choose and compare opinions about target products of customer interest. Furthermore, in the review texts could be sentences that express positive and negative judgments about product features, making more difficult to use them.

Opinion Mining or Sentiment Analysis techniques have been tried to classify opinions automatically; they are based on what an author express in a review. This subfield combines Natural Language Processing (NLP) and Text Mining methods, and currently it comprises a large number of tasks, some more developed than others. For example, Pang and Lee [1] considered opinion identification, sentiment polarity, and summary of the opinion orientation; Liu [2] took account of sentiment analysis in comparison sentences, spam detection, recognition of opinions that do not evaluate and

© Springer International Publishing Switzerland 2015
O. Pichardo Lagunas et al. (Eds.): MICAI 2015, Part II, LNAI 9414, pp. 105–120, 2015.
DOI: 10.1007/978-3-319-27101-9_8

detection of fake opinions. There are many aspects that are still open and are considered a challenge, such as the treatment of negation, analysis at aspect level, the treatment of irony and sarcasm, etc. [3].

One of the main tasks of Opinion Mining is the semantic orientation of the opinions in an entire document, in sentences or as restricted to some features. The result of this approach is polarity opinion classification into positive or negative opinions. The main approaches to solve this problem correspond to the broader classification of machine learning methods: supervised and unsupervised methods. Although this problem has been studied extensively, polarity classification remains a challenge for natural language processing.

Pang and Lee [1] explained that accuracy of sentiment classification could be influenced by the domain of the items to which it is applied. One reason is that the same phrase can indicate different sentiments in different domains; for example, 'go read the book' most likely indicates a positive sentiment for book reviews but a negative sentiment for movie reviews.

In this work, we have worked with a set of reviews on washing machines in the Spanish language. In the case of such basic products of modern life, classification of reviews is a challenge because the authors of these opinions primarily use colloquial language, including anecdotal passages, and do not pay attention to necessary punctuation. Therefore, we decided to use simple tools and the complete collection to compare results in such conditions with more elaborated works.

Negation is a very common linguistic construction that affects polarity and, therefore, needs to be taken into consideration in sentiment analysis [4]. However, negation is a complex phenomenon with peculiarities in each language. Negation is marked at different levels, for example at words as in 'nobody' and prefix 'un-'; at syntactic structure as in *no vendrá nadie* 'no one will come'; for negative sense as in *¿Voy a ser yo quien lo haga todo?* 'Will I be the one to do it all?'; for colloquial language as in *naranjas* 'no', etc. Researchers have been considering negation cues mainly at lexical and syntactical levels, but we argue that a deep analysis on the effect of each cue on the semantic orientation classification of review texts that could yield more effective cues is needed. An automated approach using negation cues should be centered on ones that could be quantified on each orientation. In this work, we chose the following negative cues, *ninguno* 'none', *no* 'no', *nunca* 'never', *jamás* 'ever' and *nada* 'at all', to analyze their effect on the semantic orientation classification for the washing machine reviews and their causes.

We first developed a simple baseline approach proposing some adapted linguistic features for unsupervised and supervised methods where negation cues were not included. Then, we analyzed the addition of negation features in both methods. Finally, we analyzed the usefulness of each negation compound in semantic orientation classification.

This paper is organized as follows. In Sect. 2, the related work is presented; then, the corpus and linguistic knowledge considered are described. Section 4 provides a description of the machine learning methods applied: unsupervised and supervised. In Sect. 5, we give the results of our experiments and discuss them. Finally, we present our conclusions.

2   Related Work

Since sentiment analysis has been assumed as an NLP challenge, one of the most studied tasks in this area is the polarity classification of an entire document as positive or negative (semantic orientation). As established by [1], most of the work on polarity classification has been carried out in product review texts. The authors emphasized that, in this context, positive and negative opinions are often evaluative (e.g. *to like*, *to dislike*), but there are other problems in interpreting them. Among such problems, they mentioned that the task of defining whether a piece of factual information is good or bad is still not the same as classifying it in one of several classes and that the distinction between subjective and objective information can be subtle.

From the beginning, different works have considered modifiers, for example, adjectives. The work of [5] to predict the semantic orientation of adjectives considered a clustering algorithm that divided adjectives in groups of different orientations. The algorithm was based on the correlation between linguistic features and semantic orientation. For example, adjectives joined by the conjunction *and* correspond to adjectives of the same orientation as *fair and legitimate*, in opposition to *quiet but lazy*.

The main approaches that have been proposed since then to solve the polarity classification correspond to the broad classification of machine learning methods: unsupervised and supervised. Among the former ones, [6] is an important work where the semantic orientation of the text bigrams was defined for product reviews in English. This orientation was used to compute the sentence and the entire opinion of semantic orientation for a corpus of 410 opinions from the *Epinions* site. In the supervised approach, the work [7] analyzed the results of three methods, Naive Bayes, MaxEnt, and Support Vector Machines (SVM), which were used to classify the polarity of movie reviews. They included different linguistic features for each method; in general, they considered single words, sequences of two words, parts of speech, and word position.

Recent trends in opinion mining and sentiment analysis focus on the use of deep neural networks, such as Convolutional Neural Network [8]. Bag-of-concepts-based approach is also gaining attention in sentiment analysis context [9–11]. These approaches focus on extracting multiword expressions from texts and from their features. Concept-level features enhance the performance of audio-visual sentiment analysis [12, 13] and emotion detection [14, 15].

As to work done to classify semantic orientation in Spanish texts, the work of [16] used the MuchoCine [17] movie reviews corpus, for an experimental study of the combination of supervised and unsupervised algorithms in a parallel English-Spanish corpus. They used diverse tools: a translator from Spanish to English and Senti-WordNet.[1] In [18] researchers proposed an unsupervised algorithm based on dependency syntax analysis to determine the semantic orientation of texts, assigning a value for the semantic orientation of some syntactic constructions. In [17] the authors

---

[1] http://sentiwordnet.isti.cnr.it/, lexical resource for opinion mining that assigns three sentiment scores: positivity, negativity and objectivity.

compiled a corpus of almost 4,000 movie reviews, and they applied the unsupervised approach of [6] to a review set of 200 positives and 200 negatives.

For the baseline method in this work, we followed the work of [6] for the unsupervised method, and we used SVM as a supervised method according to [19]. In this study, they showed that SVM outperformed most published results on sentiment analysis datasets.

For the English language, there has been interest in negation for semantic orientation. In [7], the authors attempted to model the contextual effect of negation, for example, 'good' and 'not very good' as indicating opposite sentiment orientations. In the work of [20], a supervised polarity classifier was trained with a set of negation features derived from a list of cue words and a small window around them in the text. In [21], the authors presented a classifier that treated negation from a compositional point of view by first calculating the polarity of terms independently and then applying inference rules to arrive at a combined polarity score. They also included content-word negation.

Linguistic patterns-based approaches have been found to be useful in ensemble with supervised approaches [22, 23]. Linguistic patterns are used to detect explicit and implicit negation in sentences. Negation detection has been found very important for product review analysis and for Twitter sentiment analysis [24, 25].

As for work done to include negation in semantic orientation classification in Spanish texts, [18] considered negation among the syntactic structures extracted as features from the SFU Spanish Review Corpus[2] for an unsupervised dependency parsing based method. In [26] the authors applied an unsupervised approach to the MuchoCine movie reviews corpus where three semantic resources were used to assign the semantic orientation of the terms in the texts: SentiWordNet, a one-domain lexicon and a general-purpose lexicon. Domain lexicons contain words in the specific domain used to state opinions (e.g. positive or negative) and sentiment scores. Their compilation usually relies on manual effort that is time consuming, and their domain coverage needs to be continuously improved. More recent work has focused, for example, on estimation of the frequency with which a word is used with a sense related to an emotion (joy, anger, fear, sadness, surprise and disgust) [27].

Our work differs from the above-mentioned studies in several aspects; we used very simple and similar linguistic features for the unsupervised and supervised methods, we analyzed the effect of each linguistic feature in the supervised method and we considered all reviews, including spam.

3 Corpus and Linguistic Knowledge

3.1 Review Texts Corpus

In this work, we used the corpus compiled in [28]. The collection was retrieved automatically from the website *ciao.es*; it contains 2,800 reviews on washing machines. The average size per file in tokens is 345. The total number of tokens in the collection

---

[2] http://www.sfu.ca/~mtaboada/research/SFU_Review_Corpus.html.

is 845,280. The collection was annotated with lemma and part of speech information using FreeLing [29], an open source library for NLP tasks.

From the review text corpus, we extracted a significant subset of different opinions: 2,598 reviews. Each review has a score assigned by the authors of the texts, which, considering a balanced scale, correspond to very poor (one star), poor (two stars), average (three stars), good (four stars) and very good (5 stars).

We did not delete the reviews that were clearly advertisements for maintenance business (i.e. spam) since texts such as these advertisements and reviews paid by manufacturers appear in any collection of product reviews. We did not consider spelling correction in any form because of the diversity of errors and the kind of grammatical and orthographic rules that reviewer authors violate, but FreeLing gave the correct tag in some spelling mistakes. We did not consider any kind of normalization.

The characteristics of the collection in terms of the number of opinions by score are shown in Table 1. As we can observe, and as might be expected for opinions on appliances whose use is so widespread, favorable opinions are higher in a ratio of 7:1 between positive and negative opinions.

Table 1. Corpus of washing machines reviews

Polarity	# Reviews	Stars
Very good	1,190	5
Good	838	4
Average	239	3
Poor	127	2
Very poor	204	1

In the machine-learning field, the problem of class imbalance in the number of training examples for each class has been addressed. The solutions to this problem have been classified by [30] as follows:

- Algorithmic modification: This approach is aimed to adapt machine-learning methods to be more sensitive to the problems of imbalanced datasets, for example, [31].
- Assignment of different weights to training examples, introducing different costs to positive and negative instances: This approach gives higher costs for misclassification of the majority class with respect to the minority class during the classifier training, for example, [32].
- Data sampling includes low-sampling, oversampling and hybrid methods. The low sampling deletes instances of most frequent classes while oversampling creates new instances of the less frequent class. Hybrid methods combine the above methods, for instance, [33].

The machine-learning tool used in this work for supervised learning does automatic assignment of different weights, and, for the unsupervised method, we carried out the evaluation of the classifiers' performance using specific metrics in order to take into account the class distribution. However, according to the results obtained by [34], for a similar collection in terms of the imbalance ratio, the authors did not obtain improvements with different balancing techniques. In the work of [35], they concluded that classification algorithms are more sensitive to noise than to imbalance, but as imbalance increases in severity, it plays a larger role in the performance of classifiers and sampling techniques. They also showed that the most robust classifiers tested over imbalanced and noisy data were Bayesian classifiers and SVMs. In [36], the authors found that precision decreased from 85.8 for the unbalanced corpus to 81.6 for the balanced one using the SVM classifier.

3.2   Linguistic Knowledge

Many opinion mining systems are lexicon-based or based on solutions that do not take into account the relations between words because more complex tools are required, such as a parser that could assign the correct syntactic structures of the complete texts and normalization to obtain the correct structures, for example [18].

If the inclusion of word bigram features, i.e. sequences of two words, gave consistent gains on sentiment analysis tasks, as according to [19], we considered that they could be applied as features to unsupervised and supervised methods. So, in this paper, we considered the following morpho-syntactic bigrams as features for both the unsupervised and supervised methods:

1. Noun-adjective
2. Verb-adverb
3. Adverb-adjective
4. Adjective-adverb

We wrote a program that, from the entire collection of reviews, extracted all two-word sequences whose grammatical categories met the above rules. Their distribution is shown in Table 2. For the noun-adjective bigram, our program verified the gender and number agreement to prove their syntactic association. Applying this pattern, it should be possible to obtain properties (*lavadora silenciosa* 'silent washing machine'), and the properties are product attributes that describe aspects of the product. The verb-adverb bigram should attempt to obtain attributes of washing machine functions, like *centrifuga bastante* 'spin enough', i.e. it can catch verb modifications.

We considered the adverb-adjective sequence since adjectives and adverbs modify or describe other words and their syntactic association has special meanings. When an adverb joins an adjective, its semantic function is quantifying or qualifying [37], the

Table 2. Bigrams distribution in the collection

	# Bigrams	# Opinions
Adjective-adverb	504	401
Adverb-adjective	7,484	2,024
Noun-adjective	21,144	2,598
Verb-adverb	27,900	2,006

most frequent case when an adverb has the quantifying role. We also considered the adjective-adverb bigram; though in Spanish adverb-adjective is the most common form, we found that the reverse order is present in some reviews in our collection (*super bien* 'super good', *barato siempre* 'always cheap').

3.3   Negation

Negation is present in all human languages, and it is used to reverse the polarity of the part of statements that is otherwise affirmative by default, as stated by [38]. The authors highlighted that a negated statement often carries positive implicit meaning, but to determine the positive part from the negative part is rather difficult. For example, *all vegetarians do not eat meat* means that vegetarians do not eat meat and the universal quantifier 'all' has scope over the negation. However, *all that glitters is not gold* means that it is not the case that all that glitters is gold; the negation has scope over 'all', i.e. out of all things that glitter, some are gold and some are not.

In [4], the authors described the methods for negation modeling in a chronological sequence, and they divided them into representations that did not contain any explicit knowledge of polar expressions and representations that did contain such knowledge. An example of the former is the bag-of-words representation. They concluded that, despite the lack of linguistic plausibility, supervised polarity classifiers using bag-of-words (in particular, if training and testing are done on the same domain) offer fairly good performance.

An example of methods that contain explicit knowledge of polar expressions is the model implemented by [15] where negation is encoded in features and combined with supervised machine learning. They used a lexicon of over 8,000 subjectivity cues and a dependency parser to extract the features, negation features, shifter features and polarity modification features. They also created a corpus for the experiments adding contextual polarity judgments to the subjective expressions.

Negation in Spanish was divided by [39] into total and partial negation, and the effect of partial negation was analyzed on syntagms, on adjacent to syntagms and on negation words. Among this last, she mentioned the indefinite pronouns *nadie* 'no one', *ninguno* 'none', *nada* 'lit. nothing' and the adverbs *nunca* 'never', *jamás* 'ever' and *nada* 'at all'. In [40] the author clarified that, as an adjective, the normal position of *ninguno* is before a noun; the alternation between before and after a noun is only possible in cases when the sequence is placed after the verb. He indicated that *nunca* and *jamás* have an identical function. He also analyzed negation words according their position before and after the verb; in a preverbal position, negative words in Spanish will never be accompanied by a negation adverb.

Following these criteria in this work, we handled negation at the shallow level of morpho-syntactic sequences. The negated forms were obtained by searching specific patterns formed with sequences of POS categories. We defined the following patterns:

1. $ninguno_{LEMMA\_DET}$-noun
2. $nada_{PRONOUN}$-adjective
3. $[jamás_{ADVERB} \mid nunca_{ADVERB} \mid no_{ADVERB}]$-verb

4. no$_{\text{ADVERB}}$-verb$_{\text{AUX\_PAST PARTICIPLE}}$
5. no$_{\text{ADVERB}}$-pronoun-verb

Table 3. Cue frequencies in the collection

Cue	POS	Freq	%	Cue	POS	Freq	%
no	Noun	52	0.4	ninguno	Pronoun	55	0.5
no	Adverb	9,388	83.7	nada	Noun	4	0.035
nunca	Noun	5	0.04	nada	Pronoun	786	7.0
nunca	Adverb	348	3.1	nada	Adverb	125	1.1
ninguno	Determinant	427	3.8	jamás	Adverb	20	0.17

Statistical analysis of the selected negation cues for the washing machine corpus is shown in Table 3. Note that the cue no$_{\text{ADVERB}}$ constitutes 83.7 % of all the selected cues in the collection.

4 Methods for Semantic Orientation Classification

4.1 Unsupervised Method

The work with unsupervised methods, i.e. methods that do not have examples previously annotated with the classification to learn, is based on the counting of positive and negative terms, determining automatically if the term is positive or negative. Turney [6] determined the semantic orientation of an opinion by an algorithm that first extracted bigrams where one of the words was a modifier. Then it took each bigram to search the Web using the AltaVista NEAR operator to find how many documents have that bigram near of a positive term (*excellent*) and a negative term (*poor*). The score for the two sets was done by Pointwise Mutual Information (PMI). The difference score for the two sets was used to determine the score for the semantic orientation (SO). This results in the degree to which each (bigram, term) is positive or negative. Considering the number of results (hits) obtained from the Web search, the calculation of the semantic orientation of a phrase was made as follows:

$$SO(\text{phrase}) = \log_2 \frac{\text{hits(phrase NEAR excellent) hits(poor)}}{\text{hits(phrase NEAR poor) hits(excellent)}}.$$

When a phrase of the review appeared more often with 'excellent', then the semantic orientation was positive. It was negative when the phrase appeared more often with 'poor'. The semantic orientation of each bigram was used to determine the semantic orientation of complete sentences and of the entire opinion.

We wrote a program that used Google Search to retrieve the hits for the association of each bigram with the words *excelente* 'excellent' and *mala* 'bad$_{\text{FEMENINE}}$' by means of the AROUND operator set to 10 words. The form of the query was "word$_1$ word$_2$" AROUND (10) "*excelente*". The hits returned by this search corresponded to the pages that contained the bigram with the corresponding adjective around 10 words. When Google suggested proving the "results without quotes" because no results were obtained, the number of hits was set to zero. The semantic orientation value was calculated by adding the SO of each bigram in the review. When this value was bigger than zero, the review classification was set positive; otherwise, it was negative.

Traditionally, the accuracy rate has been the most commonly used empirical measure of evaluation criteria of classification performance, as well as of F1, precision and recall [41]. However, in the framework of imbalanced datasets, accuracy is no longer a proper measure [30] since it does not distinguish between the numbers of correctly classified examples of different classes. In imbalanced domains, the evaluation of the classifiers' performance must be carried out using specific metrics in order to take into account the class distribution. The authors proposed to obtain the following four metrics to measure the classification performance of both positive and negative classes independently:

Measure	Formula	Percentage of
True positive	$TP_{rate} = \dfrac{TP}{TP+FN}$	Positive instances correctly classified
True negative	$TN_{rate} = \dfrac{TN}{FP+TN}$	Negative instances correctly classified
False positive	$FP_{rate} = \dfrac{FP}{FP+TN}$	Negative instances misclassified
False negative	$FN_{rate} = \dfrac{FN}{TP+FN}$	Positive instances misclassified

The results obtained with the unsupervised learning method are shown in Table 4 using the features described in Sect. 3.2. The percentages obtained for true positives and true negatives were included in columns 3 and 4. Many works neglected the user scores in the middle; we decided, in addition to neglecting them (row 3), to obtain the results considering them positive (row 2) and also negative (row 1).

Table 4. Results of the unsupervised method for the base line

Classes	Metric	Value	True positives	True negatives
Negative: 1–3 stars	F1score	0.6632		
Positive: 4–5 stars	Recall$_E$	0.8606	86.8 %	26.5 %
	Precision	0.5394		
Negative: 1–2 stars	F1score	0.6759		
Positive: 3–5 stars	Recall	0.8554	82.21 %	32.44 %
	Precision	0.5587		
Negative: 1–2 stars	F1score	0.6786		
Positive: 4–5 stars	Recall	0.8606	86.8 %	32.44 %
	Precision	0.5602		

In the work [17], they applied the unsupervised method of [6] to a collection of 200 positive reviews (user scores 4 and 5) and 200 negative reviews (user scores 1 and 2) of the MuchoCine corpus. They obtained 35.5 % for the true negatives and 91.5 % for the true positives. The results that could be compared were those of the last line where reviews with three stars were neglected; the differences were −3.06 % for the true negatives and −4.7 % for the true positives. These lower values could be associated with the quantity of the reviews that we considered, more than 2,000 and the spam (user score 4–5).

4.2   Supervised Method

Since many studies consider SVM as the best semantic orientation classifier, we also decided to use SVM. We confirmed that SVM obtained better results than Naïve Bayes for our baseline did. However, future work may consider analyzing other classifiers.

The SVM training was carried out using the *scikit-learn*[3] tool, an open source machine learning library for the Python programming language that incorporated LibSVM supporting *C*-SVC [42] (two-class and multi-class). We used the multiclass classification and linear kernel that obtained the best results among polynomial and the Radius Basis Function (rbf). The collection was trained with 70 % of the opinions, and 30 % were used for testing. For this supervised method, we wrote a program to extract not the words but the lemmas of the bigrams described in Sect. 3.2; this allowed us to group several bigrams in a single feature. For example, *prenda vaquera* 'denim clothing' and *prendas vaqueras* 'denim clothings' and *lavadora nueva* 'new washing machine' and *lavadoras nuevas* 'new washing machines' were grouped in single bigrams.

Table 5 shows the results of the SVM method; note that introducing the adverb-adjective bigram decreased the measures of the previous results.

Table 5. SVM results for the base line

Features	Metric	Value
Noun-adjective	F1score	0.8419
	Recall	0.8287
	Precision	0.8556
Noun-adjective	F1score	0.9287
Verb-adverb	Recall	0.9266
	Precision	0.9309
Noun-adjective	F1score	0.9258
Verb-adverb	Recall	0.9230
Adverb-adjective	Precision	0.9286
Noun-adjective		
Verb-adverb	F1score	0.9339
Adverb-adjective	Recall	0.9312
Adjective-adverb	Precision	0.9366

---

[3] http://scikit-learn.org/stable/.

5   Results and Discussion

In this section, we present the overall results for the semantic orientation classification when the negation cues derived in bigram features were included in both unsupervised and supervised methods.

5.1   Unsupervised Method

Results including bigrams of negation for the unsupervised method are shown in Table 6. The comparison of true negatives is discussed in Sect. 5.3. Regarding the recognition of true positives, our results changed to −0.2 %, 3.69 % and 0 % when features of negation were included for diverse orientation assignment of the reviews with a user score of three. The increased value corresponded to the case when reviews with a user score of three were considered with positive orientation.

Table 6. Results of the unsupervised method when negation bigrams were included

Classes	Metric	Value	True positives	True negatives
Negative: 1–3 stars	F1score	0.6762		
Positive: 4–5 stars	Recall$_E$	0.8681	86.6 %	30 %
	Precision$_E$	0.5539		
Negative: 1–2 stars	F1score	0.6887		
Positive: 3–5 stars	Recall	0.8590	85.9 %	36.5 %
	Precision	0.5748		
Negative: 1–2 stars	F1score	0.6935		
Positive: 4–5 stars	Recall	0.8681	86.8 %	36.5 %
	Precision	0.5774		

5.2   Supervised Method

Results including bigrams of negation for the supervised method are shown in Table 7. The first column shows the four patterns that correspond to the baseline. The second column shows, in each row, the measure values obtained for each one of the patterns for negation.

Making a comparison with the last line of the base line results (see Table 5) for each row in the measured values obtained in Table 7, we note that the only pattern that did not increase the results is the one corresponding to no$_{\text{ADVERB}}$-verb$_{\text{AUX\_PAST PARTICIPLE}}$ in the first row.

The range of enhancements went from 0.41 % to 1.85 %. Two patterns have overtaken the 1 %: nunca$_{\text{ADVERB}}$–verb and nada$_{\text{PRONOUN}}$–adjective. nunca$_{\text{ADVERB}}$–verb appeared in 77 positive reviews and 17 negative reviews, nada$_{\text{PRONOUN}}$–adjective appeared in 401 positive reviews and 90 negative reviews.

5.3   Discussion

We compared the results of both approaches to the corresponding baseline. The results for the unsupervised method with all bigrams of negation are shown in Table 6. Although there is no a real base for direct comparison with other works, we found that these results are similar to those of [26]. They used two term lists, SentiWordNet and the dependency parser of [29] to calculate the semantic orientation of 2,625 reviews of the MuchoCine corpus. The lists corresponded to Spanish words indicating opinion; one list was domain independent with 2,509 positive terms and 5,626 negatives, and a second list included terms of the movie review's domain of the first one.

Table 7. SVM results when negation bigrams were included

Features		Metric	Values
Noun-Adjective	+ no_{ADVERB}-$verb_{AUX\_PAST\ PARTICIPLE}$	F1 score	0.9315
		Recall	0.9289
		Precision	0.9342
+	+ $ninguno_{LEMMA\_DET}$ -noun	F1 score	0.9406
		Recall	0.9382
		Precision	0.9431
Verb-Adverb	+ $jamás_{ADVERB}$-verb	F1 score	0.9380
		Recall	0.9359
		Precision	0.9401
+	+ $nunca_{ADVERB}$ -verb	F1 score	0.9524
		Recall	0.9510
		Precision	0.9537
Adverb-Adjective	+ no_{ADVERB} -verb	F1 score	0.9407
		Recall	0.9382
		Precision	0.9432
+	+ $nada_{PRONOUN}$ -adjective	F1 score	0.9501
		Recall	0.9487
		Precision	0.9515
Adjective-Adverb	+ no_{ADVERB}-pronoun-verb	F1 score	0.9395
		Recall	0.9370
		Precision	0.9420

Their results showed an increase in ranges of 1.69 %, 1.4 % and 1.54 % in the F1 measure when negation features were considered using SentiWordNet, the domain independent list and the domain list respectively. Our results indicated increases of 1.3 %, 1.28 %, and 1.49 % when features of negation were included for diverse orientation assignment to the reviews with a user score of three. These results were obtained without a domain lexicon or semantic resource. Regarding recognition of true negatives, our results increased by 3.5 %, 4.06 %, and 4.06 % when features of negation were included for diverse orientation assignment of the reviews with a user score of three.

The work developed in [18] considered the negators *no*, *nunca* and *sin* 'without' for treatment of negation in an unsupervised method. They applied a set of syntactic heuristic rules to identify the scope of a negation term and a shift method to modify the semantic orientation of affected tokens, giving diverse values according to the specific negator. The results of their negation approach on a collection of 400 reviews of diverse products increased the negative accuracy from 0.455 to 0.745 and diminished the positive accuracy by 12 %. The authors concluded that, in a general domain, their syntactic approach works better than machine learning approaches, but the same is not always true for a specific field, where semantic dictionaries are affected by a low recall.

Regarding the supervised method, our results for all bigrams of negation that increased the base line values are shown in Table 8. The improvement in relation to the last row of the results for the base line was 1.09 % for the F1 measure, less than the best value obtained for one of the two best patterns.

SVM has been considered one of the best classification methods for NLP in general and for opinion mining in particular. We did not contrast the final SVM results with other works since they did binary classification instead of multiclass classification. Regarding multiclass classification, the confusion matrix for the results in Table 8 showed that the worst result values were those for the reviews with a user score of three. In this experiment, 25 % of reviews were misclassified as reviews with user scores of four or five. For class 5, there were no misclassified reviews, and, for class 4, 5 % were classified with a user score of five. There were more misclassified reviews for classes 1 and 2, 16 % and 18 % respectively. Most of the misclassified reviews were assigned to classes 4 and 5.

Table 8. Results for all bigrams of negation in the SVM

Features		Metric	Value
	+		
Noun-Adjective	ninguno$_{\text{LEMMA\_DET}}$ -noun		
Verb-Adverb	jamás$_{\text{ADVERB}}$-verb	F1score	0.9448
Adverb-Adjective	nunca$_{\text{ADVERB}}$-verb		
Adjective-Adverb	no$_{\text{ADVERB}}$-verb	Recall	0.9429
	nada$_{\text{PRONOUN}}$ -adjective		
	no$_{\text{ADVERB}}$-pronoun-verb	Precision	0.9467

6   Conclusions

In this paper, we presented an analysis of the effect of negation cues on semantic orientation prediction. The sources were opinion reviews in Spanish. We presented the results when bigrams based on such negative cues were applied on supervised and unsupervised methods. We analyzed the appropriateness of each such kind of bigram.

We contrasted our results with other works, and we found that similar results were obtained when using semantic resources, but since negation is complex, proper treatment of certain syntactic structures could be enhanced with a longer range of the negative accuracy results.

Detection of negation is useful for many text analytics tasks, e.g., personality recognition [43] or recognizing textual entailment [44], among many others. Our future work will focus on the use of these features for such NLP tasks.

Acknowledgments. The fourth author recognizes the support of the Instituto Politécnico Nacional, grants SIP 20152095 and SIP 20152100.

References

1. Pang, B., Lee, L.: Opinion mining and sentiment analysis. Found. Trends Inf. Retrieval **2**(1–2), 1–135 (2008)
2. Liu, B.: Sentiment analysis and subjectivity. Handb. Nat. Lang. Process. **2**, 627–666 (2010)
3. Liu, B.: Sentiment Analysis and Opinion Mining. Synthesis Lectures on Human Language Technologies. Morgan & Claypool Publishers, San Rafael (2012)
4. Wiegand, M., Balahur, A., Roth, B., Klakow, D., Montoyo, A.: A survey on the role of negation in sentiment analysis. In: Proceedings of the Workshop on Negation and Speculation in Natural Language Processing, pp. 60–68 (2010)
5. Hatzivassiloglou, V., McKeown, K.R.: Predicting the semantic orientation of adjectives. In: Proceedings of the Eighth Conference of the European Chapter of the Association for Computational Linguistics, EACL 1997, pp. 174–181 (1997)
6. Turney, P.D.: Thumbs up or thumbs down? Semantic orientation applied to unsupervised classification of reviews. In: Proceedings of the 40th Annual Meeting of the Association for Computational Linguistics, pp. 417–424 (2002)
7. Pang, B., Lee, L., Vaithyanathan, S.: Thumbs up? Sentiment classification using machine learning techniques. In: Proceedings of EMNLP, pp. 79–86 (2002)
8. Poria, S., Cambria, E., Gelbukh, A.: Deep convolutional neural network textual features and multiple kernel learning for utterance-level multimodal sentiment analysis. In: Proceedings of EMNLP 2015, Lisbon, pp. 2539–2544 (2015)
9. Poria, S., Gelbukh, A., Hussain, A., Howard, N., Das, D., Bandyopadhyay, S.: Enhanced SenticNet with affective labels for concept-based opinion mining. IEEE Intell. Syst. **28**(2), 31–38 (2013)
10. Agarwal, B., Poria, S., Mittal, N., Gelbukh, A., Hussain, A.: Concept-level sentiment analysis with dependency-based semantic parsing: a novel approach. Cogn. Comput. **7**(4), 487–499 (2015)
11. Cambria, E., Fu, J., Bisio, F., Poria, S.: AffectiveSpace 2: enabling affective intuition for concept-level sentiment analysis. In: Proceedings of Twenty-Ninth AAAI Conference on Artificial Intelligence, pp. 508–514 (2015)
12. Poria, S., Cambria, E., Hussain, A., Huang, G.-B.: Towards an intelligent framework for multimodal affective data analysis. Neural Netw. **63**, 104–116 (2015)
13. Poria, S., Cambria, E., Howard, N., Huang, G.-B., Hussain, A.: Fusing audio, visual and textual clues for sentiment analysis from multimodal content. Neurocomputing (2015, in press). doi:10.1016/j.neucom.2015.01.095

14. Cambria, E., Poria, S., Bisio, F., Bajpai, R., Chaturvedi, I.: The CLSA model: a novel framework for concept-level sentiment analysis. In: Gelbukh, A. (ed.). LNCS, vol. 9042, pp. 3–22. Springer, Heidelberg (2015)

15. Poria, S., Gelbukh, A., Cambria, E., Hussain, A., Huang, G.-B.: EmoSenticSpace: a novel framework for affective common-sense reasoning. Knowl.-Based Syst. **69**, 108–123 (2014)

16. Martín-Valdivia, M.T., Martínez-Cámara, E., Perea-Ortega, J.M., Ureña López, L.A.: Sentiment polarity detection in Spanish reviews combining supervised and unsupervised approaches. Expert Syst. Appl. **40**, 3934–3942 (2013)

17. Cruz Mata, F., Troyano Jiménez, J.A., de Salamanca Ros, F.E., Rodríguez, F.J.O.: Clasificación de documentos basada en la opinión: experimentos con un corpus de críticas de cine en español. Procesamiento del lenguaje natural **41**, 73–80 (2008)

18. Vilares, D., Alonso, M.A., Gómez-Rodríguez, C.: A syntactic approach for opinion mining on Spanish reviews. Nat. Lang. Eng. **1**(1), 1–26 (2013)

19. Wang, S., Manning, C.D.: Baselines and bigrams: simple, good sentiment and topic classification. In: Proceedings of the 50th Annual Meeting of the Association for Computational Linguistics: Short Papers, vol. 2, pp. 90–94 (2012)

20. Wilson, T.,, Wiebe, J., Hoffmann, P.: Recognizing contextual polarity in phrase-level sentiment analysis. In: Proceedings of Human Language Technology Conference and Conference on Empirical Methods in Natural Language Processing, pp. 347–354 (2005)

21. Choi, Y., Cardie, C.: Learning with compositional semantics as structural inference for subsentential sentiment analysis. In: Proceedings of the Conference on Empirical Methods in Natural Language Processing, pp. 793–801 (2008)

22. Poria, S., Cambria, E., Winterstein, G., Huang, G.-B.: Sentic patterns: dependency-based rules for concept-level sentiment analysis. Knowl.-Based Syst. **69**, 45–63 (2014)

23. Poria, S., Cambria, E., Gelbukh, A., Bisio, F., Hussain, A.: Sentiment data flow analysis by means of dynamic linguistic patterns. IEEE Comput. Intell. Mag. **10**(4), 26–36 (2015)

24. Chikersal, P., Poria, S., Cambria, E.: SeNTU: sentiment analysis of tweets by combining a rule-based classifier with supervised learning. In: Proceedings of the International Workshop on Semantic Evaluation, SemEval 2015, pp. 647–651 (2015)

25. Chikersal, P., Poria, S., Cambria, E., Gelbukh, A., Siong, C.E.: Modelling public sentiment in Twitter: using linguistic patterns to enhance supervised learning. In: Gelbukh, A. (ed.). LNCS, vol. 9042, pp. 49–65. Springer, Heidelberg (2015)

26. Jiménez Zafra, S.M., Cámara, E.M., Valdivia, M.T.M., González, M.D.M.: Tratamiento de la negación en el análisis de opiniones en español. Procesamiento del Lenguaje Natural **54**, 37–44 (2015)

27. Díaz-Rangel, I., Sidorov, G., Suárez-Guerra, S.: Creación y evaluación de un diccionario marcado con emociones y ponderado para el español. Onomazein **29**, 31–46 (2014)

28. Galicia-Haro, S.N., Gelbukh, A.: Extraction of semantic relations from opinion reviews in Spanish. In: Gelbukh, A., Espinoza, F.C., Galicia-Haro, S.N. (eds.) MICAI 2014, Part I. LNCS, vol. 8856, pp. 175–190. Springer, Heidelberg (2014)

29. Padró, L., Stanilovsky, E.: Freeling 3.0: towards wider multilinguality. In: Proceedings of the Language Resources and Evaluation Conference (LREC 2012), Istanbul, Turkey, pp. 2473–2479. ELRA (2012)

30. López, V., Fernández, A., García, S., Palade, V., Herrera, F.: An insight into classification with imbalanced data: empirical results and current trends on using data intrinsic characteristics. Inf. Sci. **250**, 113–141 (2013)

31. Sun, Y., Kamel, M.S., Wong, A.K.C., Wang, Y.: Cost-sensitive boosting for classification of imbalanced data. Pattern Recogn. **40**(12), 3358–3378 (2007)

32. Pazzani, M., Merz, C., Murphy, P., Ali, K., Hume, T., Brunk, C.: Reducing misclassification costs. In: Proceedings of the Eleventh International Conference on Machine Learning, pp. 217–225 (1994)

33. Tang, Y., Zhang, Y.-Q., Chawla, N.V., Krasser, S.: Svms modeling for highly imbalanced classification. IEEE Trans. Syst. Man Cybern. B Cybern. **39**(1), 281–288 (2009)

34. Akbani, R., Kwek, S.S., Japkowicz, N.: Applying support vector machines to imbalanced datasets. In: Boulicaut, J.-F., Esposito, F., Giannotti, F., Pedreschi, D. (eds.) ECML 2004. LNCS (LNAI), vol. 3201, pp. 39–50. Springer, Heidelberg (2004)

35. Seiffert, C., Khoshgoftaar, T.M., Van Hulse, J., Folleco, A.: An empirical study of the classification performance of learners on imbalanced and noisy software quality data. Inf. Sci. **259**, 571–595 (2014)

36. Sidorov, G., Miranda-Jiménez, S., Viveros-Jiménez, F., Gelbukh, A., Castro-Sánchez, N., Velásquez, F., Díaz-Rangel, I., Suárez-Guerra, S., Treviño, A., Gordon, J.: Empirical study of machine learning based approach for opinion mining in Tweets. In: Batyrshin, I., González Mendoza, M. (eds.) MICAI 2012, Part I. LNCS, vol. 7629, pp. 1–14. Springer, Heidelberg (2013)

37. Spitzová, E.: Sintaxis de la lengua española. Masarykova Univerzita, Brno (1994)

38. Blanco, E., Moldovan, D.: Semantic representation of negation using focus detection. In: Proceedings of the 49th Annual Meeting of the Association for Computational Linguistics: Human Language Technologies (ACL-HLT 2011), pp. 581–589 (2011)

39. Sanz Alonso, B.: La negación en español. In: Actuales tendencias en la enseñanza del español como lengua extranjera II: actas del VI Congreso Internacional de ASELE. pp. 379–384 (1996)

40. Bergareche, B.C.: Negación doble y negación simple en español moderno. Revista de filología románica (9), 63–102 (1992)

41. Manning, C.D., Raghavan, P., Schuetze, H.: Information Retrieval. Cambridge University Press, Cambridge (2008)

42. Chang, C.-C., Lin, C.-J.: Libsvm: a library for support vector machines. ACM Trans. Intell. Syst. Technol. (TIST) **2**(3), 27 (2011)

43. Poria, S., Gelbukh, A., Agarwal, B., Cambria, E., Howard, N.: Common sense knowledge based personality recognition from text. In: Castro, F., Gelbukh, A., González, M. (eds.) MICAI 2013, Part II. LNCS, vol. 8266, pp. 484–496. Springer, Heidelberg (2013)

44. Pakray, P., Poria, S., Bandyopadhyay, S., Gelbukh, A.: Semantic textual entailment recognition using UNL. Polibits **43**, 23–27 (2011)

Detecting Social Spammers in Colombia 2014 Presidential Election

Jhon Adrián Cerón-Guzmán[(⊠)] and Elizabeth León

MIDAS Research Group, Department of Industrial and Systems Engineering,
Universidad Nacional de Colombia, Bogotá D.C., Colombia
{jacerong,eleonguz}@unal.edu.co

Abstract. The large amount of user-generated content has turned social media into an appealing source of information for understanding social behavior. Around elections time, Twitter data have been used to measure public opinion on issues such as predicting outcomes, voting intention or political alignment. However, the effect of proliferation of new forms of spam on social media in this type of measurements has not been completely recognized and tackled in research. In this paper, we focus on detecting malicious accounts on Twitter, which aim to spread spam in an electoral process (e.g., disseminate rumors, misinform, or artificially inflate support for a candidate). To achieve this, a dataset of 149 K users referring to Colombia 2014 presidential election was collected, and 1.7 million tweets and 341 K URLs were crawled from their timeline. To distinguish malicious accounts from non-spammer ones in the dataset, several machine learning techniques were implemented on a labeled collection of users, semi-automatically classified into spammer and non-spammer. Experimental results reveal that with ten tweets, the proposed strategy detects 93 % of spammers and 92 % of non-spammers. Results also highlight the importance of noise removal when measurements of public opinion are conducted using Twitter data, with approximately 22 % of accounts in the dataset classified as spammers.

Keywords: Social spammers · Spammer detection · Twitter · Politics · Presidential election · Colombia

1 Introduction

Social media has turned into a rich source of information about individuals, society and, potentially, the world in general [18]. Thus, the impressive amount of user-generated content on a diversity of issues and topics, has brought new research opportunities for understanding social behavior. Among them, the one related to public opinion has caught the attention of current research. Data collected from social media are nowadays used to measure public opinion in regards with important events such as political elections. Around elections time, a significant number of research works have used Twitter data to predict election outcomes, based on opinions or possible voting intentions expressed by users [15].

© Springer International Publishing Switzerland 2015
O. Pichardo Lagunas et al. (Eds.): MICAI 2015, Part II, LNAI 9414, pp. 121–141, 2015.
DOI: 10.1007/978-3-319-27101-9_9

In the same way that social media provides an appealing source of information, it could, however, contain noise, useless, and irrelevant information. For instance, new forms of spam have been spread to manipulate social media discourse with rumors, misinformation, political astroturf, slander, or simply noisy messages [14]. Here, two known cases are described. The first one is related to fake followers (also known as bots) used to create the appearance of wide support for politicians, as indeed has been denounced by mass media [28]. The second one, a more complex case, has to do with the use of bots with the intention of discrediting one candidate, while the image of another is indirectly benefited [14].

With this in mind, removing spam, propaganda and, in general terms, any form of noise in tweets becomes a major issue, in order to achieve reliable measurements of public opinion. However, few papers in the literature, on the line of work discussed, have adopted such measures [15].

The research presented in this paper focuses on the spammer detection problem on Twitter. In particular, we have focused on detecting malicious accounts which aim to spread spam in a political context. Colombia 2014 presidential election was proposed as a case study in order to gain insights into how much those unwanted entities populate the Twitter ecosystem, and how they could potentially affect measurements of public opinion conducted using data collected from Twitter. To that end, a dataset of 513.324 tweets dealing with the election, and the 149.831 users have posted them, was crawled from Twitter. Next, a three-part strategy was designed to create a ground truth set of users labeled as spammers and non-spammers. Then, a spammer detection system was implemented following machine learning approaches: semi-supervised and supervised learning. With a spammer detection rate of 93 %, it was found that approximately 22 % of users in the dataset are spammers, who generated 15.67 % of tweets crawled. In this paper, it is referred as spammers to computer algorithms designed to spread any form of unwanted content and, in general, to intentionally harm the experience on Twitter. The spammer and malicious user terms are used interchangeably, while the social term is used to reference the social media context. In contrast, the non-spammer and legitimate user terms are used to reference users who generate original, intelligent, or human-like contents.

The remainder of this paper is organized as follows. Section 2 surveys related work on exploiting social media for measuring public opinion and the spammer detection problem on Twitter. Next, a brief background on Colombia 2014 presidential election is discussed in Sect. 3. The methodology for collecting data and creating a labeled collection of users is described in Sect. 4. Section 5 describes the proposed detection system and evaluates its performance. In Sect. 6, results are obtained by applying the proposed system on the collected data. Finally, conclusions are drawn in Sect. 7.

2   Related Work

The impressive amount of user-generated content on social media platforms has generated a growing interest from different fields of knowledge, among them, computer science and social sciences [18]. Predicting electoral outcomes and conduct measurements of public opinion on a diversity of issues, are cases for which researchers have used data harvested from social media for understanding social behavior, and capture large-scale trends. In [26], O'Connor et al. reported a high correlation between public opinion measured from polls and sentiments measured from tweets, stating the potential of social media as a substitute and supplement for traditional polling. In [33], Tumasjan et al. found that Twitter is a platform for political deliberation, stating that the mere number of tweets reflects voting preferences. In general, several works have reported a relative success in exploiting social media for purposes of predicting, forecasting, and measuring [18]. However, social media poses problems regarding the quality and credibility of the data. In this regard, Metaxas et al. [23] warned: "spammers and propagandists write programs that create lots of fake accounts and use them to tweet intensively, amplifying their message, and polluting the data for any observer." Those problems, therefore, need to be tackled in order to achieve reliable measurements of public opinion. Nevertheless, Gayo-Avello [15] reported that most of researches have assumed that all tweets are trustworthy, while few papers have recognized the problem, and accordingly adopted measures for denoising in Twitter data.

The spammer detection problem on Twitter has been widely studied in the literature. Mainly, there have been proposed several detection models using machine learning techniques to classify users into two classes: spammer and non-spammer. In [6], Benevenuto et al. proposed a set of features, grouped into content-based features and behavior-based features, to support an automatic classification of Twitter users. In [9], a new user class was aggregated: cyborg, a mix between spammers and non-spammers. To conduct the classification, they designed a four-component system to detect patterns in posting behaviors, identify spam content in tweets, and capture spammer-like behaviors. Instead, other works [5,41] have focused on studying evasion tactics and designing new and more robust features for achieving a high detection rate of spammers, while a negligible fraction of non-spammers are misclassified. In this research, the features used for distinguishing malicious accounts from legitimate ones have been widely used in the literature by their proven highly effectiveness. While most of works have followed a supervised learning approach, in this paper, in addition to a supervised classification, an approximation of solution is implemented under a semi-supervised setting. In [24], Miller et al. posed the spammer detection as an anomaly detection problem. They used clustering techniques to predict a class for a given Twitter account, treating outliers as spammers. In spite of all those efforts, the spammer detection problem on Twitter is still an open challenge [32].

3   Background on the Colombian Election

In race for the presidency of 2014–2018, five candidates competed for the most important Colombia political office, including the incumbent President Juan Manuel Santos. Óscar Iván Zuluaga, Marta Lucía Ramírez, Clara López, and

Enrique Peñolosa were the other candidates. The former was supported by the grand center-right coalition called "Unidad Nacional", composed by the political parties "Partido de la U", "Cambio Radical", and "Partido Liberal Colombiano". Óscar Iván Zuluaga was the candidate for the "Centro Democrático" right-wing party, founded by the former president of Colombia Álvaro Uribe. Marta Lucía Ramírez, also a right-wing alternative, was chosen as the "Partido Conservador Colombiano" candidate. The main opposition party, "Polo Democrático Alternativo", supported the left-wing candidacy of Clara López. Enrique Peñalosa was the "Partido Alianza Verde" candidate.

The presidential election was held under a two-round voting system. In the first round, held on May 25, 2014, no candidate received an absolute voting majority, and for that, a run-off took place 21 days later between Óscar Iván Zuluaga and Juan Manuel Santos, who were the highest-polling candidates with 29.25 % and 25.69 % support from voters, respectively. In the run-off election, Santos was re-elected President with 50.95 % support. Table 1 shows important events of Colombia 2014 presidential election. Regarding to presidential debates, those where all contenders participated and national television broadcasted them are cited.

Table 1. Schedule of important events of the presidential election

Date	Event
May 6, 2014	A person hired by the Zuluaga campaign was captured and accused of illegally obtaining classified information [12]
May 8, 2014	Accusation against the Santos campaign for the presidency in 2010, for allegedly received funds from drug trafficking activities [10]
May 17, 2014	A video revealed publicly shows that Zuluaga met with the person captured and accused of spying [11]
May 22, 2014	First presidential debate
May 25, 2014	Election day
Jun 5, 2014	Second presidential debate
Jun 9, 2014	Third presidential debate
Jun 15, 2014	Run-off election day

4   Data Collection and Ground Truth Creation

The main contribution of this paper is to detect spammer accounts on Twitter. To address the problem, Colombia 2014 presidential election was proposed as a case study in order to gain insights into how much these unwanted entities populate the Twitter ecosystem, and how they could potentially affect measurements of public opinion conducted using data collected from this social media platform. In this section a Twitter dataset collected during the presidential election is described. Additionally, the strategy designed to create a labeled collection of spammers and non-spammers is discussed.

4.1 Dataset

During the course of the presidential election, in a two-month period between April 30, 2014, and June 24, 2014, a dataset of 513.324 tweets and 149.831 users was collected from Twitter's Search API [37]. To conduct the study relying on users referring to the aforementioned political context, a set of criterias was defined to filter tweets unrelated to the topic of interest. Thus, only tweets containing at least one keyword or hashtag related to the presidential election (i.e., *elecciones, presidenciales, #Elecciones2014, #ColombiaElige, #Elecciones-Colombia, #ColombiaDecide*), and full name or user mention that identifies a given candidate, were collected. Under this approach, a dataset for each candidate was created (even for *blank vote*). Note that one same tweet could be in two or more datasets according to candidates mentioned in it. Table 2 shows the amount of collected data in terms of users and tweets per candidate, and the query terms related to each. It may be noted that a larger amount of data were collected for the candidates Santos and Zuluaga, as well for blank vote, because they were the contestants in the run-off election. Figure 1 shows the daily activity of data collection, divided in periods comprising the first round election and the run-off election; Fig. 2 shows the daily tweet mention distribution per candidate. As can be seen in Fig. 1, local maximums were produced one day after the presidential debates, and during and after the election days, being the global maximum the run-off election day with over 93 K tweets; Fig. 2 could explain the challenging first-round election, in terms of user mention, where the protagonists were Juan Manuel Santos and Óscar Iván Zuluaga, and likewise how Santos took advantage in race for Colombia presidency in the run-off election.

Table 2. Summary of the collected data on the electoral process

Candidate	Collection period	Query terms	Tweets	Users
Santos	Apr 30–Jun 24, 2014	"Juan Manuel Santos", @JuanManSantos	332.575	117.783
Zuluaga	Apr 30–Jun 24, 2014	"Oscar Ivan Zuluaga", @OIZuluaga	202.405	81.979
Ramírez	Apr 30–May 29, 2014	"Marta Lucia Ramirez", @mluciaramirez	9.273	6.198
López	Apr 30–May 29, 2014	"Clara Lopez", @ClaraLopezObre, @ClaraPresidenta	13.711	9.457
Peñalosa	Apr 30–May 29, 2014	"Enrique Penalosa", @EnriquePenalosa	12.072	7.391
Blank vote	Apr 30–Jun 24, 2014	"Voto Blanco", Blanco	39.203	27.148

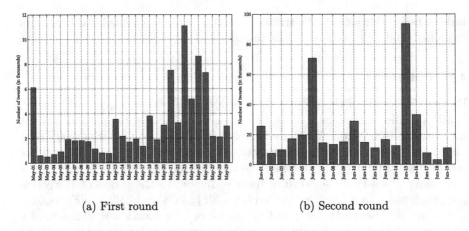

(a) First round   (b) Second round

Fig. 1. Daily number of tweets collected

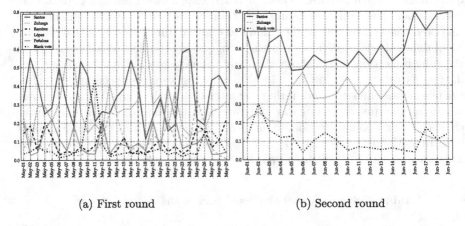

(a) First round   (b) Second round

Fig. 2. Fraction of tweets mentioning each presidential candidate. Vertical dotted lines in this figure (and in Fig. 5) represent the events highlighted in Table 1.

Because of not enough data were collected per user,[1] up to 40 most recent tweets were crawled from its timeline. From 149.831 users initially, in a second stage of data collection, conducted between February 19, 2015 and March 26, 2015, a dataset of 134.625 users and 1.765.225 tweets was collected using the public timeline API [36], since 4.805 users set their profile as private, 8.462 users changed their @username, and 1.939 were suspended by Twitter. For the work presented in hereafter was used the dataset created in this second stage.

---

[1] Average number is 1 tweet.

4.2   Ground Truth

For the purpose of this research, a collection of Twitter accounts labeled as either spammer or non-spammer, was needed to support the ability of the detection system to distinguish malicious accounts from legitimate ones. To this end, a random sample of 49.358 users was drawn from the dataset, and a three-part strategy was designed to label it in a semi-automatic way. As result of this strategy, a set of 3.455 users was created, including 2.660 spammers and 795 non-spammers.[2]

Detecting Harmful Links. The first part of the strategy consisted in automatically identify spam using five URL blacklists. From the 1.765.225 tweets in the dataset, 341.352 URLs were extracted and resolved of obfuscation using a web crawler developed to follow chain of redirects until reach target pages. The web crawler was able to resolve HTTP status code, META tags and Javascript used for redirects.

While the second data collection proccess ran, URLs in tweets were extracted and their target pages, whole chain of redirects, and tweet ids containing them, were saved in a database. Then, a batch script was developed to check the URLs crawled against the following blacklists: Google Safe Browsing, PhishTank, SURBL, Spamhaus, and URIBL [1–4,16]. The first one enables to check URLs against Google's constantly updated lists of suspected phishing and malware pages. Phishtank is a crowding service in which phishing sites are submitted, verified, and tracked in a semi-automatic way. The last three provide constantly updated lists of domain names that have appeared in unsolicited emails. Due to slow detection rate of these services [17], the blacklist detection process was performed multiple times and until April 20, 2015. If an URL was marked as harmful by two blacklists, no more checks were needed.

As result of this process, 3.302 URLs were detected as malicious links. However, during a manual revision of those URLs, it was found that only 12 of them, shared in 34 tweets, corresponded to true positives; therefore the 7 users tweeting them were labeled as spammers. To explain this high false positive rate, it is important to note that 2.576 URLs, from 9 unique domains, possibly were erroneously marked because spammers abuse of them (e.g., URL shortener services, such as *bit.ly*), or DNSBL services mark domains as spam when they appeared in unsolicited messages and not because they hosted malicious or harmful content, e.g., like happened with 873 URLs from four major news media. In this regard, the scientific community is encouraged to define a clear spam policy when URL blacklists are used, like it was done in [17] where a URL whitelist was created to minimize false positive rate.

Additional to the 7 spammer accounts resulting of this process, 86 accounts were labeled as malicious because URLs shared by them were detected by Twitter's anti-spam filter, and in a further revision of their profile, enough evidence

---

[2] The labeled collection will be available at http://www.midas.unal.edu.co/data

was found to label them as such. Of those accounts, 56 users belonged to a political astroturf campaign intended to artificially inflate support for the Zuluaga campaign.

Suspended Accounts. The first part of the strategy detected spam if an URL shared in a tweet was marked by blacklists. However, spam is not limited to posting harmful links, but rather, in a broader meaning, to any unsolicited, repeated actions that negatively impact other users [35]. This includes aggressive following behavior, posting unsolicited mentions and duplicate tweets, abusing of trending topics to grab attention, and share links unrelated to tweet content [38]. Based on Twitter's algorithm for suspending accounts that fall into some of prohibited behaviors, the second part of the strategy labeled as spammers to the suspended accounts identified in the second stage of data collection. Of the 49.358 Twitter accounts, 674 were suspended, while 1.939 were found in the population of 149.831 users.

By labeling in this way, an assumption was made that the suspended accounts were manipulated to spam purposes, and they were not legitimate accounts, e.g., belonging to real people. Although any false positive can be resolved by user requesting to be unsuspended [34], a further process was conducted to verify that suspensions were caused by prohibited behaviors. Thus, a random sample of 100 accounts was drawn from the 674 suspended, and their *timeline* was reconstructed from all tweets collected in the first stage of data collection. Considering tweet content, shared URLs, tweeting sources, numbers of followers and friends, longevity of account, and number of tweets posted, suspended accounts were manually investigated.

Of the 100 accounts under analysis, 89 of these were accordingly labeled as spammers, while for the remaining ones not enough evidence, because few tweets were collected. It is important to highlight that, in contrasts to results in [31], no harmful links were found in 356 tweets from the timeline reconstructed of the suspended accounts sample. However, 30 accounts were suspended because, in addition to automation behavior, their tweeting source pointed to a same spam URL. From these results, it is possible to conclude that the majority of accounts manually investigated were presumably well suspended, although more evidence is necessary to label the entire sample as spammers. In this way, all suspended accounts were used as spammers in the labeled collection of users.

We acknowledge that the strategy here discussed might not be potentially useful, because few tweets were collected per user in the first stage of data collection and Twitter already have identified what characterize those accounts. However, a hypothesis is made in the direction that some (additional) knowledge could be extracted from Twitter's anti-spam algorithm, and this would be acquired by the proposed detection system.

Manual Labeling. A common strategy used in the literature to create a ground truth set is manually label a sample of users [6,9,40]. Taking into account this, the third part of the strategy consisted in draw a random sample of 1.245 users from the 49.358 Twitter accounts, and label them as either spammer or non-spammer, based on their profile data and up to 100 most recent tweets from timeline from each user.

To conduct the manual labeling, a set of criterias was defined to classify users in the sample. In this way, every user was analyzed taking into consideration its tweet content, shared URLs, tweeting sources, numbers of followers and friends, and number of statuses posted. So, an user was labeled as spammer if not evidence exists of original, intelligent, or human-like contents; URLs posted are spam or unrelated to tweet content; it abuses of trending topics to grab attention, or its tweet content is unrelated to hashtags; posting duplicate content; and automation predominates account's behavior, like tweeting from automated sources or automatic statuses from news sites or blogs. This set of criterias was motivated by the work in [9]. Otherwise, an user was classified as non-spammer. From the set of 1.245 users, 599 were classified as spammers, while 117 were not labeled because doubt predominated to assign a class or few tweets had been posted by them, so they were excluded from the labeled collection.

While the manual labeling process was conducted, duplicate tweets were found over multiple accounts,[3] including 29 users that were not in the sample. In particular, 243 of those accounts were grouped into two political astroturf campaigns. The first one consisted of 150 spammers accounts used during the election to artificially inflate support for the Santos campaign. Likewise, the second one was intended to create the appearance of wide support for the Zuluaga campaign. Although this second campaign shared the same goal that the aforementioned one in the harmful links detection, they differ each due to tweet content and because the activity of the first one is based on mainly retweets, while the another one post some tweets with human-like contents.

From this third part of the strategy, a labeled collection of 1.128 users was obtained, including 628 spammers and 500 non-spammers, plus 295 verified accounts in the dataset of 149.831 users that were used as non-spammer instances.

5   Detecting Social Spammers

In this section, the proposed system for detecting spammers on Twitter is discussed. Firstly, a set of features is defined to support the discriminative power among spammer instances from non-spammer ones. Secondly, a first approximation of the detection system is implemented following a semi-supervised approach, where in addition to the ground truth set, the system infers a classification function on the entire data space, including unlabeled data. Lastly, a supervised approach is followed to implement a second approximation of the detection system. Here, it is also discussed the least number of tweets used for spammer detection, and the importance of the attributes to achieve this goal.

---

[3] Using Twitter's search page: https://twitter.com/search-home

5.1 Features

Unlike legitimate accounts, spammer ones presumably are designed to infiltrate social media without being detected by security systems like spam filters and mimic human behavior to gain confidence of real people, in order to obtain benefits for which they were made. These can be of kind commercial (e.g. advertising), harmful (e.g. malware or phishing), or even political (e.g. artificially inflate support for a candidate) [14]. That is why it would be expected that spammers differ from non-spammers on what they post, like shared URLs, user mentions, hashtags, and content originality; on their behavior, like devices used, tweeting frequency, etc.

Based on these assumptions, here a set of features is proposed to support the ability of the detection system to distinguish malicious accounts from legitimate ones; these are grouped into three categories. The features were collected from different works in the literature, and most of them have been widely used for detecting spammers on Twitter.

User-Based Features. The first category of features is based on account's information that an user provides, summarizes its lifetime on Twitter, or describes its friendship network. These features are extracted from the tweet's metadata, and comprise a list of 9 attributes presented in Table 3. First two attributes have value of 1 when the condition is satisfied.

Content-Based Features. These features are computed from tweet content, and are defined to discriminate content that spammers usually post from original, intelligent, or human-like contents. To determine what is the least amount of data required to successfully distinguish spammer from non-spammer instances, the attributes of this category (as seen in Table 3) are computed from 5, 10, 20, and 40 most recent tweets from each user. In particular, the following text preprocessing technique was applied to normalize tweet content and compute the *average of tweet content similarity* feature: remove URLs, user mentions, hashtags, emoji unicode,[4] and HTML symbols; replace time patterns with a standard text (e.g. "HORA"); normalize character repetition (based on grammatical rules of spanish language, e.g. "holaaa" → "hola"); replace emoticons with textual portrayals; normalize and replace laughs (e.g. "jajaja" → "RISA"); unification of punctuation marks [39]; replace numeric patterns with a standard text; detection of negation [25]; whitespace-based tokenization, and remove stop words. Once tweets are normalized, they are represented as vectors using the TF-IDF weighting scheme [21], and the cosine similarity is applied between them. Final value of the aforementionated feature is the average of similarity between set of unique pairs of tweets.

---

[4] http://apps.timwhitlock.info/emoji/tables/unicode

Table 3. List of features

Category	Feature
User	User has profile description
User	Account is verified
User	Age of the user account, in days (AGE)
User	Number of followings ($NFing$)
User	Number of followers ($NFers$)
User	Reputation ($\frac{NFers}{NFing+NFers}$)
User	Number of tweets
User	fofo rate ($NFers/NFing$)
User	Following rate ($NFing/AGE$)
Content	User mention (@) ratio
Content	Unique user mention (@) ratio [20]
Content	URL ratio
Content	Hashtag (#) ratio
Content	Average of tweet content similarity [20]
Behavior	Retweet rate
Behavior	Reply rate
Behavior	Mean of inter-tweeting delay
Behavior	Standard deviation of inter-tweeting delay [5]
Behavior	Average of tweets per day
Behavior	Average of tweets per week
Behavior	Number of tweets from manual devices [9]
Behavior	Number of tweets from automated devices [9]
Behavior	Distribution of tweets in each of the 8–3 h periods within a day [22]

Behavior-Based Features. The last category of features is proposed to capture the behavior that characterizes each user. Like content-based features, the attributes of this category (as seen in Table 3) are computed from 5, 10, 20, and 40 most recent tweets from each user.

To count number of tweets posted from manual and automated devices, 773 different sources found in the 20 most recent tweets collection, were manually classified. Thus, if a device requires human participation, it was classified as manual. Otherwise, the device was classified as automated.

5.2 Semi-Supervised Detection

The first approximation for social spammer detection on Twitter was posed as a semi-supervised task. Semi-supervised learning is halfway between supervised and unsupervised learning, where in addition to unlabeled data, the algorithm is provided with some supervision information [8]. Inspired by this approach, a two-stage study was conducted. In the first stage, a clustering algorithm was applied, and using labeled samples in the ground truth, a class was assigned to each cluster. Here, it was assumed that if points are in the same cluster, they are like to be of the same class [8]. In the second stage, a non-generalizing machine learning technique was used to predict a class for a given Twitter account, based on the clustered data space.

Clustering. To conduct the clustering analysis, a dataset of 46.074 users from the sample of 49.358 users was created from their 20 most recent tweets, including 1.350 samples (658 spammers, and 692 non-spammers) in the ground truth, since for 3.080 users were not collected enough tweets, and 204 (101 spammers, and 103 non-spammers) were excluded to test the prediction system (to be discussed later).

The CHAMELEON algorithm [19] and the set of features proposed were used to find groups of users with similar characteristics, which could be clustered instances of the spammer and non-spammer classes. CHAMELEON is a clustering algorithm that finds clusters of diverse shapes, densities, and sizes, modeling data items in a sparse graph, where several subclusters are found using a graph-partioning algorithm, and then, repeatedly combining subclusters using an agglomerative hierarchical technique. As a result of the analysis, a 12-way clustering solution was found, using the 1.350 samples labeled like clue about what is the cluster tendency towards a class. However, in a further statistical analysis conducted per feature, and a manual labeling of samples randomly drawn from each cluster, 7 clusters were discovered like the best candidates to potentially contain spammer and non-spammer instances, including 4 clusters that sum 2.046 samples with spammer-like behaviors, and the remaining ones of 17.211 samples with non-spammer's behaviors. Table 4 shows the clustering validation. External measures, *Entropy* and *Purity* [30] were computed using 837 users labeled within the 7 clusters, plus 354 users manually classified (108 spammers, and 246 non-spammers) of random samples drawn from each cluster. Overall *Entropy* and *Purity* for the cluster solution are 0.153 and 0.975, respectively. *Samples labeled* column shows percentage of instances per class that a cluster contains of the 1.191 users labeled, while I_1 is an internal measure computed using the Euclidean distance.

Predicting. Using the collection of 19.257 users labeled (the clustered data space), and the set of features discussed, a non-generalizing machine learning technique was implemented to predict a class for a given Twitter account. Here, it was investigated the feasibility of applying an inductive method inferred on the (partial) data space, instead of one that only takes into account labeled points. The k-Nearest Neighbors (k-NN) algorithm was chosen to classify unseen data points because, in addition to it has been commonly used in previous researches on spammer detection, this one possibly best matches with the CHAMELEON algorithm, where a k-nearest neighbor graph is used to cluster the dataset.

Table 4. Clustering validation results

Cluster	Tendency	Size	Samples labeled		I_1	Entropy	Purity
			Spammer	Non-spammer			
1	Spammer	45	11.48 %	0.00 %	0.01	0.0	1.0
2	Spammer	224	26.79 %	0.00 %	0.01	0.08	0.99
3	Spammer	756	20.41 %	0.29 %	0.75	0.1	0.99
4	Spammer	1.021	37.5 %	0.29 %	0.42	0.06	0.99
5	Non-spammer	1.665	0.5 %	33.24 %	0.28	0.13	0.98
6	Non-spammer	5.161	1.28 %	25.3 %	0.21	0.31	0.95
7	Non-spammer	10.385	2.04 %	40.88 %	0.33	0.3	0.95

The Scikit-learn [27] implementation of the k-NN algorithm was used to classify Twitter accounts into two classes: spammer and non-spammer. Firstly, the number of neighbors (i.e., the k parameter) was searched using cross validation with 5-folds on the clustered data space. Secondly, unseen data points were classified based on the class the majority of the 7 closest samples for each one on the aforementioned space. Table 5 shows the result obtained by applying the semi-supervised system on the test dataset of 204 users (101 spammers, and 103 non-spammers). This result indicates that the system correctly identifies 86.14 % of spammers (true positive rate), at a cost of misclassifying 11.65 % of non-spammers (false positive rate).

Table 5. Confusion matrix for the semi-supervised detection

		Predicted	
		Spammer	Non-spammer
Actual	Spammer	87	14
	Non-spammer	12	91

Manually examining the users being classified by mistake, it was observed that for non-spammers misclassified as spammers, synchronization of their activity on other social media platforms (such as YouTube[5] and Instagram[6]), which it generates a high number of tweets from automated devices, and posting a significant number of their tweets to trending topics or with several mentions, correspond to typical behaviors of spammers [5]. Regarding to false negative ones (spammers misclassified as non-spammers), some of them are legitimate accounts hijacked by spammers to spread spam without permission of their owners, while others are occasional spammers and a large number of tweets (e.g., 100) are required to make a correct classification.

---

[5] https://www.youtube.com/
[6] https://instagram.com/

5.3   Supervised Detection

The common strategy to tackle the spammer detection problem on Twitter is based on a supervised setting. In this one, a machine learning algorithm infers a classification model from a labeled collection, and then the extracted knowledge is applied to classify an unseen user as either spammer or non-spammer. Following this approach, here a spammer detection system is proposed. Firstly, it is discussed the classification algorithm selection between a range of machine learning techniques widely used in the literature. Secondly, it is determined the least amount of information (i.e., number of tweets) required to the proposed system detects a large number of spammers in early stages, at a cost of misclassifying a small number of non-spammers. Lastly, the importance of the features is presented.

Selecting the Classification Technique. To conduct the selection, three machine learning techniques were implemented on the ground truth set, and then the performances of them were compared using the standard information retrieval metrics of recall, precision, and F1-score. In this stage, the features were computed from 20 most recent tweets from each user. Thus, a set of 1.554 users was created (759 spammers, and 795 non-spammers), since for the remaining ones in the ground truth not enough tweets were collected. This dataset was randomly partitioned into sets of training and test. The first one (consisting of 66 % of samples) was used to optimize the hyperparameters for each technique using 5-fold cross validation. The second one was used to perform an independent test for each classification algorithm, and accordingly to select the best among them.

The Scikit-learn implementations of the Support Vector Machines (SVM), Random Forest (RF), and Gaussian Naive Bayes (NB) were used to train the algorithms and conduct the evaluation for each. In particular, two flavors of the SVM technique were implemented. In the first one, based on the LIBLINEAR library [13], only the complexity parameter was optimized, since the 'linear' kernel is fixed. In the second one, based on the LIBSVM library [7], both the kernel and the complexity parameters were optimized. Figure 3 shows the performance for each algorithm on the test dataset. To select between SVM with 'radius basis function' kernel and RF, who achieve the highest performance, the following tiebreaker rule was applied: for each spammer correctly classified, 1 point was added, while for each non-spammer misclassified as spammer, 1.5 points were subtracted. Thus, the RF was selected as the best classification technique, and therefore the system implementation was based on it.

Number of Tweets Required for Detecting Spammers. A critical limitation of previous works [29] is related to the number of tweets required to detect spammers, before than these achieve the purpose for which they were designed, i.e., to spread viruses and malwares, and a large amount of Twitter accounts may be harmed. In this stage, the goal is to determine the least number of tweets

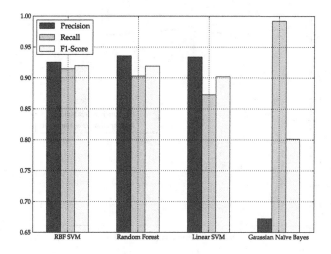

Fig. 3. Performance comparison of the classification techniques

required to detect a large number of spammers, at a cost of misclassifying a small number of non-spammers. Here, an assumption is made that a small number of tweets could reduce the delay between spammer account creation and its detection.

Figure 4 shows the numbers of tweets used for detecting spammers and true positive and false positive rates for each.[7] This result was obtained by implementing the RF algorithm on the ground truth set, and computing the features from 5, 10, 20, and 40 most recent tweets from each user in it. The experimental setup described in the previous section was also applied here. Of this result, it is determined that 10 tweets is the least amount of information required for achieving a balance between detecting a large number of spammers, at a cost of misclassifying a relatively small number of non-spammers, with true positive and false positive rates of 93.02 % and 7.78 %, respectively. Table 6 shows the performance of the detection system using 10 tweets on the test dataset. In order to improve the performance of the RF algorithm, the standard boosting

Table 6. Confusion matrix for the supervised detection using 10 tweets

		Predicted	
		Spammer	Non-spammer
Actual	Spammer	253	19
	Non-spammer	21	249

---

[7] Note that when no tweets are used to detect spammers, only the user-based features are computed to make classification.

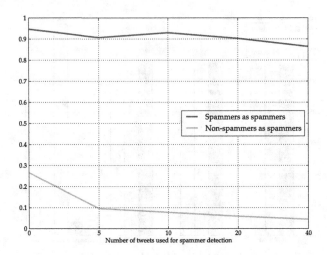

Fig. 4. Number of tweets required for detecting spammer

and bagging techniques [30] were applied to build ensemble classifiers. However, no significant improvement was obtained.

In a further manual revision of the users misclassified as spammers, it was observed that the following reasons could cause the unwanted performance: several tweets are generated from automated devices, because users have granted permissions to third parties apps for automatic tweeting; time interval between tweet posting is short, what could seem to a regular timing pattern; a significant number of tweets are posted with several mentions and URLs. Regarding to spammers misclassified as non-spammers, randomness on the inter-tweet time interval and posting tweets from manual devices (mainly from Twitter's web interface), cause spammers acquire non-spammer's characteristics.

Importance of the Features. The detection ability of the proposed system depends on the relative power of its features in discriminating between spammer instances and the non-spammer ones. Thus, to identify which features are the most important at time of discriminating each user class, the effectiveness of each of the 30 features was evaluated. In every test, only one feature was used to implement the Random Forest algorithm, under the experimental setup described above, and then evaluate its performance. Table 7 shows the top 10 features, sorted by following the tiebreaker rule described in the classification technique selection. Surprisingly, the *url ratio* is not among the most important features, as it has been reported in [6,9,20], which would indicate that spammers have evolved their tactics, and possibly redefined their objectives. However, devices used for tweeting are still highly discriminative features [9]. This is because spammers are more enticed by automated devices, due to the cheap and practical, instead of interact with devices that require human participation, e.g., when logging into Twitter's web interface. The other features correspond to the

Table 7. Ranking of the detection performance using only one feature

Category	Feature	TPR (%)	FPR (%)
Content	User mention (@) ratio	68.02	17.41
User	Age of the user account	77.57	26.67
Behavior	Number of tweets from manual devices	41.91	8.15
Behavior	Number of tweets from automated devices	41.91	8.15
Behavior	Retweet rate	81.99	35.19
User	fofo rate	69.12	30.74
Content	Unique user mention (@) ratio	68.02	31.85
Behavior	Distribution of tweets between 3 and 5 am	36.03	13.33
Behavior	Mean of inter-tweeting delay	69.12	35.56
User	Number of followers	70.96	38.52

results in the literature [6,9,20], among them, short lifetime that characterizes spammer accounts.

6   Discussion

So far, it has been discussed that social media has turned into an appealing source of information, due to the large amount of user-generated content on a diversity of issues and topics [18]. However, new forms of spam have been spread to manipulate social media discourse with rumors, misinformation, political astroturf, slander, or just noisy messages [14]. Because of this, it is imperative to distinguish noise, useless, and irrelevant information from valuable data. To this end, it has been proposed two approaches of solution to the spammer detection problem on Twitter, based on machine learning approaches: semi-supervised and supervised learning. In the first approach, it was investigated the feasibility of applying an inductive method inferred on the entire data space, including unlabeled data. Although the performance of the semi-supervised detection is good, even outperforming to other works in the literature [6] (in terms of accuracy), it is not better that the performance of the supervised detection, the second approach. In this one, an achievement of this research was to obtain an overall accuracy of 93 %, using 10 tweets and only one Twitter API method.[8] Instead, other works have required a larger amount of data (e.g. 40 tweets [5,41], and up to 100 tweets [9]), and several API methods (e.g., to compute features such as *bi-directional links* [41], and *unsolicited mentions* [5]), to achieve an overall accuracy ranging from 96 % [9] to 98 % [5].

Moreover, to quantify the importance of adopting measures to filter noise in Twitter data, the proposed detection system was applied on the dataset of

---

[8] *GET statuses/user_timeline*: https://dev.twitter.com/rest/reference/get/statuses/user_timeline

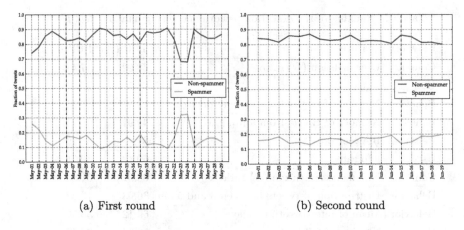

(a) First round   (b) Second round

Fig. 5. Daily fraction of tweets generated by each user class

513.324 tweets dealing with Colombia 2014 presidential election, and the 149.831 users that have posted them. As result, 22.01 % of users in the aforementioned dataset were classified as spammers, who generated 15.67 % of tweets. Figure 5 shows the daily fraction of tweets generated by each user class during the course of the presidential election; as can be seen, the fraction of tweets generated by spammers remained above 10 %, achieving a maximum peak of 32 % one day before of the election day. These findings prove that spammers could significantly affect measurements of public opinion conducted using data harvested from Twitter, and thus, for example, it can be stated that the mere number of tweets is not a reliable source of voting preferences, as it was reported in [33]. In this way, with relatively high fractions of spammers and tweets generated by them, it is emphasized the importance of adopting measures to distinguish noise, useless, and irrelevant information from valuable data, in order to achieve reliable measurements of public opinion.

7   Conclusions and Future Work

In this paper, the spammer detection problem on Twitter has been studied. In particular, the study was focused on users tweeting about Colombia 2014 presidential election, in order to gain insights into how spammers could potentially affect measurements of public opinion conducted using Twitter data. To this end, a spammer detection system based on machine learning techniques was implemented on a labeled collection of users, semi-automatically classified as spammers and non-spammers. Using few resources for the detection task, in terms of number of tweets and Twitter API methods, the proposed system achieves a high detection rate of spammers and its overall accuracy is competitive to the state-of-the-art. The results also highlight the importance of adopting measures to filter noise in data harvested from Twitter, in order to achieve reliable measurements of public opinion.

As future work, it is planned to continue researching the feasibility of using data collected from Twitter to conduct measurements of public opinion, and likewise the design of features that make the detection system more robust. Firstly, it is posed to analyze user sentiments in the collected dataset, to determine the extent of correlation between text sentiments and the Colombia 2014 presidential election outcomes. Secondly, it is planned to design new features that lead to increase the spammer detection rate, while keeping a lower false positive rate, using no more resources that those used in this work.

Acknowledgments. This work has been partially supported by COLCIENCIAS and the Vicerrectoría de Investigación of the Universidad Nacional de Colombia. We sincerely thank Arles Rodríguez and Róbinson Alvarado for their valuable comments and suggestions.

References

1. PhishTank - Join the fight against phishing. https://www.phishtank.com/. Accessed 7 March 2015
2. SURBL. http://www.surbl.org/. Accessed 7 March 2015
3. The Spamhaus project. http://www.spamhaus.org/. Accessed 7 March 2015
4. URIBL.COM - Realtime URI Blacklist. http://uribl.com/. Accessed 7 March 2015
5. Amleshwaram, A.A., Reddy, N., Yadav, S., Gu, G., Yang, C.: Cats: characterizing automation of twitter spammers. In: 2013 IEEE Fifth International Conference on Communication Systems and Networks (COMSNETS) (2013)
6. Benevenuto, F., Magno, G., Rodrigues, T., Almeida, V.: Detecting spammers on twitter. In: Collaboration, Electronic Messaging, Anti-Abuse and Spam Conference (CEAS) (2010)
7. Chang, C.C., Lin, C.J.: LIBSVM: a library for support vector machines. IEEE Trans. Intell. Syst. Technol. **2**, 1–27 (2011)
8. Chapelle, O., Schlkopf, B., Zien, A.: Semi-Supervised Learning, 1st edn. The MIT Press, Cambrdige (2010)
9. Chu, Z., Gianvecchio, S., Wang, H., Jajodia, S.: Detecting automation of twitter accounts: are you a human, bot, or cyborg? IEEE Trans. Dependable Secur. Comput. **9**(6), 811–824 (2012)
10. ElEspectador.com: Uribe dice que J.J. Rendón entregó US\$2 millones a campaña de Santos en 2010. http://www.elespectador.com/noticias/politica/uribe-dice-jj-rendon-entrego-us2-millones-campana-de-sa-articulo-491135. Accessed 23 May 2015
11. ElTiempo.com: 'Hacker' dijo a Zuluaga que tenía acceso a información de inteligencia. http://www.eltiempo.com/politica/justicia/hacker-dijo-a-zuluaga-que-tenia-acceso-a-informacion-de-inteligencia/14002995. Accessed 23 May 2015
12. ElTiempo.com: Óscar Iván Zuluaga reconoce que hacker capturado trabaja en su campaña. http://www.eltiempo.com/archivo/documento/CMS-13943188. Accessed 23 May 2015
13. Fan, R.E., Chang, K.W., Hsieh, C.J., Wang, X.R., Lin, C.J.: LIBLINEAR: a library for large linear classification. J. Mach. Learning Res. **9**, 1871–1874 (2008)
14. Ferrara, E., Varol, O., Davis, C., Menczer, F., Flammini, A.: The rise of social bots. CoRR abs/1407.5225 (2014). http://arxiv.org/abs/1407.5225

15. Gayo-Avello, D.: A meta-analysis of state-of-the-art electoral prediction from twitter data. Soc. Sci. Comput. Rev. **31**(6), 649–679 (2013)
16. Google: Safe Browsing API. https://developers.google.com/safe-browsing/. Accessed 7 March 2015
17. Grier, C., Thomas, K., Paxson, V., Zhang, M.: @Spam: the underground on 140 characters or less. In: Proceedings of the 17th ACM Conference on Computer and Communications Security, CCS 2010, pp. 27–37. ACM, New York (2010). http://doi.acm.org/10.1145/1866307.1866311
18. Harald, S., Daniel, G.A., Panagiotis, T.M., Eni, M., Markus, S., Peter, G.: The power of prediction with social media. Internet Res. **23**(5), 528–543 (2013). http://dx.doi.org/10.1108/IntR-06-2013-0115
19. Karypis, G., Han, E.H.S., Kumar, V.: Chameleon: hierarchical clustering using dynamic modeling. Computer **32**(8), 68–75 (1999). http://dx.doi.org/10.1109/2.781637
20. Lee, K., Eoff, B.D., Caverlee, J.: Seven months with the devils: a long-term study of content polluters on twitter. In: AAAI International Conference on Weblogs and Social Media (ICWSM) (2011)
21. Manning, C.D., Raghavan, P., Schütze, H.: Scoring, term weighting and the vector space model. In: An Introduction to Information Retrieval. Cambridge University Press, New York (2008)
22. McCord, M., Chuah, M.: Spam detection on twitter using traditional classifiers. In: Calero, J.M.A., Yang, L.T., Mármol, F.G., García Villalba, L.J., Li, A.X., Wang, Y. (eds.) ATC 2011. LNCS, vol. 6906, pp. 175–186. Springer, Heidelberg (2011)
23. Metaxas, P., Mustafaraj, E., Gayo-Avello, D.: How (not) to predict elections. In: 2011 IEEE Third International Conference on Privacy, Security, Risk and Trust (PASSAT) and 2011 IEEE Third Inernational Conference on Social Computing (SocialCom), pp. 165–171, October 2011
24. Miller, Z., Dickinson, B., Deitrick, W., Hu, W., Wang, A.H.: Twitter spammer detection using data stream clustering. Inf. Sci. **260**, 64–73 (2014)
25. Mohammad, S., Kiritchenko, S., Zhu, X.: Nrc-canada: building the state-of-the-art in sentiment analysis of tweets. In: Proceedings of the Seventh International Workshop on Semantic Evaluation Exercises (SemEval-2013), Atlanta, Georgia, USA, June 2013
26. O'Connor, B., Balasubramanyan, R., Routledge, B., Smith, N.: From tweets to polls: linking text sentiment to public opinion time series. In: International AAAI Conference on Weblogs and Social Media (2010)
27. Pedregosa, F., Varoquaux, G., Gramfort, A., Michel, V., Thirion, B., Grisel, O., Blondel, M., Prettenhofer, P., Weiss, R., Dubourg, V., Vanderplas, J., Passos, A., Cournapeau, D., Brucher, M., Perrot, M., Duchesnay, E.: Scikit-learn: machine learning in python. J. Mach. Learning Res. **12**, 2825–2830 (2011)
28. Samuelsohn, D.: Pols have a #fakefollower problem. http://www.politico.com/story/2014/06/twitter-politicians-107672.html. Accessed 12 June 2015
29. Song, J., Lee, S., Kim, J.: Spam filtering in twitter using sender-receiver relationship. In: Sommer, R., Balzarotti, D., Maier, G. (eds.) RAID 2011. LNCS, vol. 6961, pp. 301–317. Springer, Heidelberg (2011)
30. Tan, P.N., Steinbach, M., Kumar, V.: Cluster analysis: basic concepts and algorithms. In: Introduction to Data Mining. Addison-Wesley Longman Publishing Co., Inc., Boston (2005)

31. Thomas, K., Grier, C., Song, D., Paxson, V.: Suspended accounts in retrospect: an analysis of twitter spam. In: Proceedings of the 2011 ACM SIGCOMM Conference on Internet Measurement Conference, IMC 2011, pp. 243–258. ACM, New York (2011). http://doi.acm.org/10.1145/2068816.2068840

32. Tiku, N., Newton, C.: Twitter CEO: we suck at dealing with abuse. http://www.theverge.com/2015/2/4/7982099/twitter-ceo-sent-memo-taking-personal-responsibility-for-the. Accessed 13 June 2015

33. Tumasjan, A., Sprenger, T., Sandner, P., Welpe, I.: Predicting elections with twitter: what 140 characters reveal about political sentiment. In: International AAAI Conference on Weblogs and Social Media (2010)

34. Twitter: My account is suspended. https://support.twitter.com/articles/15790. Accessed 17 March 2015

35. Twitter: Reporting spam on Twitter. https://support.twitter.com/articles/64986-reporting-spam-on-twitter. Accessed 16 March 2015

36. Twitter: REST APIs. https://dev.twitter.com/rest/public. Accessed 6 March 2015

37. Twitter: The search API. https://dev.twitter.com/rest/public/search. Accessed 6 March 2015

38. Twitter: The Twitter Rules. https://support.twitter.com/articles/18311-the-twitter-rules. Accessed 16 March 2015

39. Vilares, D., Alonso, M.A., Gómez-Rodríguez, C.: On the usefulness of lexical and syntactic processing in polarity classification of twitter messages. J. Assoc. Inf. Sci. Technol. **66**, 1799–1816 (2014)

40. Wang, A.H.: Don't follow me - spam detection in twitter. In: Katsikas, S.K., Samarati, P. (eds.) SECRYPT, pp. 142–151. SciTePress (2010). http://dblp.uni-trier.de/db/conf/secrypt/secrypt2010.html#Wang10

41. Yang, C., Harkreader, R.C., Gu, G.: Die free or live hard? Empirical evaluation and new design for fighting evolving twitter spammers. In: Sommer, R., Balzarotti, D., Maier, G. (eds.) RAID 2011. LNCS, vol. 6961, pp. 318–337. Springer, Heidelberg (2011)

NLP Methodology as Guidance and Verification of the Data Mining of Survey ENSANUT 2012

Víctor Manuel Corza Vargas[1]([⊠]), Christopher R. Stephens[2,3],
Gerardo Eugenio Sierra Martínez[4], and Azucena Montes Rendón[4]

[1] Posgrado en Ciencia e Ingeniería de la Computación,
UNAM, Mexico D.F., Mexico
victorcorza@comunidad.unam.mx
[2] C3 – Centro de Ciencias de la Complejidad,
UNAM, Mexico D.F., Mexico
Stephens@nucleares.unam.mx
[3] Instituto de Ciencias Nucleares, UNAM, Mexico D.F., Mexico
[4] Instituto de Ingeniería, UNAM, Mexico D.F., Mexico
{GSierraM, AMontesR}@iingen.unam.mx

Abstract. Data Mining represents the cutting edge when we think about extracting information; however it always implicates a considerable spent provided that it needs "structured data". Following this idea, text mining appears in the horizon, as a little spent, reliable alternative. It is able to provide meaningful expert information without the availability of plenty of resources, all we need is a fair big (real big) corpus of text in order to conduct a research on almost every topic. By themselves, both approaches provide valuable information at the end, nevertheless what would happen if both processes were linked in a way that one approach's results could be verify by the result of a second process? With this idea on mind we are relaying on one hypothesis this is possible to generate a bound between both mining process and using them back and forth to verify one another. Hence, we describe thoroughly both methodologies making a special emphasis on mentioning those phases which have a propensity to establish a strong bound between them. We found that bound in the fact that once a Natural Language Processing has been performed on the chosen corpora what we got as an output is a list of meaningful nouns which can be used as features that will guide in a reliable way a data mining process.

Keywords: Text mining · Data mining · Naïve Bayes · Classifier · Feature detection · Diabetes · Obesity

1   Introduction

Data mining and text mining are both important tools for generating knowledge from data bases. Although, in both cases they have the same goal – knowledge generation – they differ radically in the types of data considered. Data mining traditionally works with relational data bases, where the data is considered to be "structured". Text mining,

© Springer International Publishing Switzerland 2015
O. Pichardo Lagunas et al. (Eds.): MICAI 2015, Part II, LNAI 9414, pp. 142–152, 2015.
DOI: 10.1007/978-3-319-27101-9_10

on the other hand, works with natural language, which is considered to be "unstructured". However, in reality, the structure that exists in natural language – lexical, syntactical, semantic etc. – is much more complex than the simple structures that exist in relational data bases. What is more, because of the complexity of natural language, text mining often reduces this complexity by transforming text data into structured data bases [3], where, once in the appropriate format, standard data mining tools can be used.

One may ask which of the two approaches offers better information at the end? Provided that Data Mining works with already transformed information, one might imagine that the information mined from a database is more predictive than that extracted from a large corpus of text. Text Mining should aim not only to extract information and then convert it immediately into a structured spreadsheet but also look for any meaningful information in the text data obtained by natural language processing before this is done.

Given that information in a relational database and in texts might just represent two sets of complementary information for the same problem it is natural to ask how the two can be combined or used in a complementary form for knowledge generation. In this article we will combine data from texts and from a relational database with the objective of showing how the two together can offer advantages in the process of knowledge generation. In particular, we will show how text mining can be used to improve the data mining process in a public health application where domain specific knowledge is important in developing a predictive model. Specifically, we will show how text mining can be used to incorporate "expert" knowledge in the feature selection component of the model generation process using it to construct a Naive Bayes classifier. Although, we consider only one specific problem we believe that it points the way to other possible ways in which text mining and standard data mining may be fruitfully combined to obtain knowledge that is not so readily available in only one information set.

The article is organized as follows: Sect. 2 describes the corpus of data used for each process (NLP and Data Mining); Sect. 3 provides methodological details about the NLP pipeline; Sect. 4 presents the model and results of applying a naïve Bayes classifier to the prediction of patients with both obesity and type 2 diabetes, and, finally, Sect. 5 is devoted to our conclusions.

2   Data

The area of application we chose is that of obesity and type 2 diabetes mellitus given their importance in public health and the depth of domain specific knowledge required to understand them given that they represent highly complex, multi-factorial diseases. Given this context, both the data mining and text mining will be framed by those two keywords. For the data mining part we chose a specialized data base: the National Health Survey 2012 (ENSANUT 2012[1]) a recompilation of data about the health status

---

[1] http://ensanut.insp.mx/.

of Mexican population based on extensive health questionnaires and physical measurements. For the text mining component we used the esTenTen11 (European, Freeling, Lempos) corpus available in the Sketch Engine [7] web page[2]. This is a general purpose corpus in Spanish with around 2,500,000,000 tokens. We chose not to use a specialized health corpus due to the lack of scientific or expert papers written in Spanish.

3 NLP Pipeline

The text mining component will be used to guide the feature selection process for a naïve Bayes classifier, applying a NLP methodology for information extraction. The esTenTen11 corpora represents the input of this pipeline, while the output consist of one list of meaningful nouns, classified by a category lemma and intentionality (positive or negative). This section explains all the phases of the NLP pipeline.

3.1 Text Annotation

For the purpose of carrying out the other phases in the pipeline it is necessary to prepare the corpus by adding important annotations which, among other things, facilitate the identification of lemmas related to the keywords, take part in the definition of regular expressions for dividing the corpus and, finally, identify the nouns to build the list we use for the feature selection. The annotations we use are: tokenization, lemmatization, POS-tagging and NER, we use the Stanford Core NLP tools[3] to add those annotations (Fig. 1).

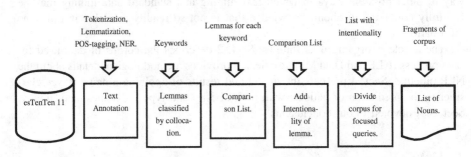

Fig. 1. Natural language processing pipeline.

3.2 Lemma Classification by Collocation

This phase carries out the extraction of those lemmas that occur in the close neighborhood of the keyword provided. It also counts the frequency for each word and

---

[2] http://www.sketchengine.co.uk.

[3] http://nlp.stanford.edu/software/corenlp.shtml [4–6].

finally classifies lemmas into groups based on their collocational behavior. To do this, we use the Sketch engine's word sketch[4] feature. There are five different collocations that word sketch assigns words to: object_of, subject_of, n_modifier, modifies and y_o. It is very important to mention that the collocational group "y_o" implicitly holds information on comorbidities, the most important relationship being between diabetes and obesity themselves, the two illnesses under consideration.

3.3   Merging Lists of Lemmas and Adding Intentionality

During this phase the two lists of lemmas obtained in the previous step (one list for each keyword) are combined and classified manually. Lemmas included in both lists appear as one record, while non-matching lemmas are discarded. Finally, we add one extra field to the combined list to aggregate the intentionality (Positive or Negative) of each lemma, this process is aiming to reflect/emphasize the interpretational character of the Text Mining process.

3.4   Corpus Division for Focused Queries

This phase performs a small document clustering by the application of several regular expressions which browse the corpus to find fragments that match with the lemma and collocation specified on each entry of the combined list. Once those fragments are located a subcorpus is created including only those matching fragments. It is then stored in a file system which specifies the lemma, the collocation and the keyword that that subcorpus is based on. It is important to mention that this phase takes advantage of the annotated corpora obtained in the first phase of this methodology where regular expressions are applied to it.

Table 1 describes the valid regular expressions for the top five lemmas of the collocational group "object_of". These regular expressions are obtained from paragraphs in which the lemma and the keyword are together or there are at the most two words between them.

Table 1. Regular expressions generated by the first five lemmas of the collocational group "object of".

Lemma	Regular expression
padecer	"<padec[a-z]+><[a-zA-Z0-9]+>([<a-zA-Z0-9>]+){0,2}<(diabetes|obesidad)>"
desarrollar	"<desarr[a-z]+><[a-zA-Z0-9]+>([<a-zA-Z0-9>]+){0,2}<(diabetes|obesidad)>"
sufrir	"<sufr[a-z]+><[a-zA-Z0-9]+>([<a-zA-Z0-9>]+){0,2}<(diabetes|obesidad)>"
prevenir	"<prev[i.e.][a-z]+><[a-zA-Z0-9]+>([<a-zA-Z0-9 >]+){0,2}<(diabetes|obesidad)>"
diagnosticar	"<diagnos[a-z]+><[a-zA-Z0-9]+>([<a-zA-Z0-9>]+){0,2}<(diabetes|obesidad)>"

---

[4] http://www.sketchengine.co.uk/ [7].

3.5   Feature Extraction

This phase extracts a list of nouns and their frequencies from the fragments obtained in the previous step. Again we are using the annotated text from phase 1, so that we can filter out everything different to a noun. The program to achieve this is coded in java[5] along with the Stanford NLP core [4–6].

Provided that we are using two keywords, the output of this phase is a pair of noun lists, one for each lemma. In order to carry out an experiment we chose the lemma "prevenir" with a positive classification against the lemma "sufrir", which is negative, both lemmas included in the "object_of" collocational group. As soon as we obtained both lists, we ordered them by frequency and then manually combined them into one list by matching those nouns that appear in both lists. Once the combinations were done, we could use those nouns as features to be considered in the data mining process.

4   Model and Results

The data base we used for this experiment is a national survey on health and nutrition carried out by INEGI[6], ENSANUT 2012[7], it was applied to around 85,000 respondents. The information is divided into two main groups: health and nutrition. The tables hold information on morbidities, eating habits, anthropometry and physical activity, among others. These tables are often found divided into three age groups: children, teenagers and adults. Our experiment focuses on adults given that this is the age group where diabetes and obesity are most frequent. (Need to mention how many are in the set to be modeled and how many in the class).

To carry out the data mining process on this database, we followed the process shown below with five distinct phases (Fig. 2).

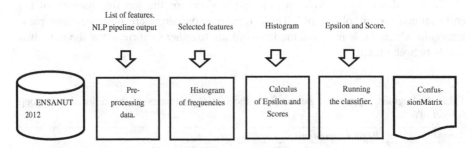

Fig. 2. Phases of the data mining process

---

[5] http://www.oracle.com/technetwork/es/java/javase/downloads/index.html.

[6] http://www.inegi.org.mx/.

[7] http://ensanut.insp.mx/.

4.1   Pre-processing Data Using the Selected Features

The objective of this phase was to explicitly establish several bounds between the two approaches, make the necessary modification to fit them and finally define the size of the sample. The input of this step is the list of nouns extracted by the NLP pipeline, Table 2 shows that list divided into positively and negatively connotated features.

Table 2. Features extracted from NLP pipeline, for the lemmas sufrir and padecer.

Negative features	#	Positive features
Sobrepeso	8	Ejercicio
Azúcar	9	Dieta
Mala alimentación	10	Hipertensión
Hipertensión	11	Madre
Herencia		
Mujer/Hombre (Género)		
Embarazo		

These features were matched with the fields that appear in the database ENSANUT 2012. In the Tables 3 and 4 we show the result of this search.

Table 3. Matching negative features with the data fields in ENSANUT

#	Negative Features	Match with	Justification
1	SobrePeso	Obesidad (Calculated Field)	Body Mass Index (BMI) used to determine if a person is obese (BMI > 30) or just overweight (25 < BMI < 30).
2	Azúcar	Alimento	Different kinds of food were classified through alimentary groups, one of them was Azúcares y Grasas.
3	Mala Alimentación	Alimento	7 coarse grained groups were added, each represents one alimentary group, at least 2 represent groups of junk food diet.
4	Hipertensión	A401 (Presión alta o hipertensión)	Full Matching
5	Herencia Diabetes	A701a y A701b	Full Matching
6	Herencia Hipertensión	A703a y A703b	Full Matching
7	Género	sexo	Full Matching
8	Embarazo	A303	Full Matching

Table 4. Matching positive features with the data fields in ENSANUT

#	Positive Features	Match with	Justification
1	Ejercicio		Fields regarding exercise were discarded.
2	Hipertensión	A401 (Presión alta o hipertensión)	Full Matching
3	Dieta	Alimento	7 coarse grain groups were added, each represents one alimentary group, at least 4 represent groups of a good diet.
4	Herencia Madre	Diabetes: A701a	Full Matching

The second bound is the selection of the class for the classifier. In phase 3.2 of the NLP pipeline we found that the collocational group "y_o" implicitly stores comorbidity information, i.e., illnesses linked to the ailment of diabetes and obesity. As expected, obesity and diabetes are strongly related given that the number of occurrences of one word linked to the other through these two conjunctions (and/or) is the most frequent. As a consequence we decided to select both illnesses as the class for the classifier.

Finally, to determine the size of the sample we defined the quantity of available records after the Diabetes and Obesity fields were joined. Table 5 describes the results. In the same fashion Table 6 describes the size of the class, i.e. those respondents who have been diagnosed with both diabetes and obesity.

Table 5. Size of the sample

Table – column 1	Table - column 2	Size	Represents
Salud_Adultos -A301 (Diabetes)	Salud_Adultos -Obesidad	36608	N

Table 6. Size of the class

Classification	Size	Represents
Class	1555	NC
No Class	35053	NC'

With these counts we calculate the class probability, P(C), it is 0.042.

4.2   Frequency Histograms

This phase represents the first step in verifying the accuracy of the features selected by the NLP process. However it is just the first step before we can decide whether the features selected are predictive or not. The histogram shows the number of occurrences of a certain feature value. The importance of this step is that we define NX for each variable and we are then ready to calculate NXC by joining the sets NC and NX. In Table 7, the fifth column "NX" shows the frequencies of the selected features.

4.3   Epsilon and Scores

This is the second verification step. It is based on the correlation between the class and every feature chosen by the NLP pipeline, this correlation will be measured by epsilon, a binomial test that measures the statistical significance of the feature X for the class relative to the null hypothesis P(C), the equation is described as follows:

$$\varepsilon = \frac{NX(P(C|X) - P(C))}{\sqrt{NX\ P(C)(1 - P(C))}} \tag{1}$$

P(C) in the numerator represents the expected value (Class priori probability), P(C|X) is the value obtained (Likelihood), both are to be multiplied by the number of occurrences of a certain feature value.

Denominator represents the standard deviation of a binomial distribution. This will work as a reference framework that will make it possible to decide whether a feature is biased or not.

Thus, this phase determines how predictive the chosen features will be for the classifier. Table 7 describes the 18 most predictive drivers. The list is ordered in ascendant order considering the absolute value of Epsilon.

These results prove that the features selected by text mining are predictive, given that the corresponding epsilon values are high. The highest epsilon is 35.98 and

Table 7. Epsilon and Scores

Description	ValCol1	ValCol2	Histogram NX	NXC	EPSILON	Score
¿Presión alta o Hipertensión?	Sí		6101	826	35,9843	1,26103
¿Diabetes durante alguno de sus embarazos?	Sí		170	89	31,1003	3,20724
¿Diabetes durante alguno de sus embarazos?	nunca embarazada		66	33	18,4303	3,11415
¿Presión alta o Hipertensión?	No		30507	729	-16,092	-0,5943
¿Madre sufrió diabetes?1Si, 2No, 3NS/NR	Sí		7864	591	14,3678	0,60560
¿Padre sufrió diabetes? 1Si, 2No, 3NS/NR	Sí		5202	350	8,87091	0,48759
¿Madre sufrió diabetes?1Si, 2No, 3NS/NR	No		26745	867	-8,15751	-0,28083
Género del entrevistado	hombre		15160	472	-6,92478	0,32160
Género del entrevistado	Mujer		21448	1083	5,821 868	0,18094
¿Padre sufrió diabetes? 1Si, 2No, 3NS/NR	No		28484	1069	-4,14008	-0,12931
¿Padre sufrió Hipertensión? 1Si, 2No, 3NS/NR	Sí		5280	281	3,87058	0,23887
¿Madre sufrió Hipertensión? 1Si, 2No, 3NS/NR	Sí		10084	502	3,63723	0,16700
CoarseGrainAzucar	0<Azúcar_al_dia <1		452	32	2,98539	0,56803
¿Madre sufrió Hipertensión? 1Si, 2No, 3NS/NR	No		24056	933	-2,83979	-0,09499
¿Padre sufrió Hipertensión? 1Si, 2No, 3NS/NR	No		27713	1088	-2,65588	-0,08247
Café sin azucar	café:-café sin azúcar	1 vez al dia	555	36	2,61520	0,47124
Café sin azucar	café:-café sin azúcar	0veces por semana	1879	58	-2,49532	-0,31599
¿Padre sufrió Hipertensión? 1Si, 2No, 3NS/NR	ns/nr		2801	145	2,43797	0,21281

corresponds to the feature "hipertensión". This means that it is one of the variables more correlated with suffering diabetes and obesity. Another important feature correlation is "Diabetes durante el embarazo" which has an epsilon of 31.10.

In the same fashion the score associated with the Naïve Bayes classifier is also calculated in this step, the equation used for that objective is the following:

$$s = \log\left[\frac{P(C|X)}{P(\bar{C}|X)}\right] \tag{2}$$

This equation considers all possible Xi that are included in the set of features; therefore this could be better expressed like follows:

$$s = \sum_1^n \log\left[\frac{P(Xi|C)}{P(Xi|\bar{C})}\right] \tag{3}$$

It is important to mention that the conditional probability changes due to the application of the naïve Bayes theorem:

$$P(c|x) = \frac{P(X|C)P(C)}{P(X)} \tag{4}$$

The summation of those scores characterizes each individual and at the end those with a positive summation are considered classified as part of the class.

4.4 Testing the Classifier

In order to complete the data mining process, considering that the naïve Bayes algorithm is a supervised learning method, we divided the population into a training set, which holds a 70 % of the sample, and a test set with the remaining 30 %. The Naïve Bayes classifier is built on the training set. The performance of the classifier on the training set is given below in terms of the corresponding confusion matrix (Table 8).

Table 8. Confusion matrix describing the performance of the classifier in the training set.

		Prediction Outcome		
		p	n	total
Actual Value	p'	True Positive 886	False Negative 5674	P'
	n'	False Positive 201	True Negative 18862	N'
	total	P	N	

4.5   Confusion Matrix of the Test Set

Finally to conclude the experiment we test the constructed classifier on the test set. In this case the size of the sample is the left 30 %, the results are described below through the confusion matrix (Table 9).

Table 9. Confusion matrix describing the performance of the classifier in the test set.

			Prediction Outcome		
		p	n	total
	p'	True Positive 386	False Negative 2620	P'
Actual Value				
	n'	False Positive 82	True Negative 7897	N'
	total	P	N	

5   Conclusion

We have shown in this paper how NLP techniques can be used to extract expert information that can then be used to guide the feature selection process for a classifier associated with a more standard data mining approach.

We can conclude that although both text mining and data mining methodologies by themselves can yield valuable information; their combination can be even more beneficial. By combining both approaches a very predictive Naïve Bayes classifier was obtained for predicting patients with both obesity and diabetes. This means that the features selected by the Text Mining process were predictive, i.e. the information extracted from the corpora was reliable, and at the same time it verified the data mining process, so the text mining model was verified by the results of the classifier.

We have stablish one route from Text Mining to Data Mining, nonetheless, this does not discard the possibility of doing the process in the opposite order, let us assume we perform a Data Mining process with the objective of finding not evident correlations between the class and the wide options of features, those hidden relations could open fields of study to enrich the experts knowledge.

Acknowledgments. VMCV is grateful to CONACYT (Consejo Nacional de Ciencia y Tecnología) for support, to Dr. César Cruz, for his support and advice during the planning phase of the NLP methodology and to various classmates for useful discussions. CRS is grateful for financial support from PAPIIT project IN113414. This work was partially funded by the C3 – Centro de Ciencias de la Complejidad.

References

1. Hand, D.J., Mannila, H., Smyth, P.: Principles of Data Mining, pp. 211–234. The MIT Press, Cambridge (2001)
2. Orallo, J.H., Quintana, M.J.R., Ramírez, C.F.: Introducción a la minería de datos, pp. 257–278. Universidad Politécnica de Valencia, Pearson, Prentice Hall, Madrid (2004)
3. Weiss, S.M., Indurkhya, N., Zhang, T., Damerau, F.J.: Text Mining, Predictive Methods for Analyzing Unstructured Information, pp. 47-82–85-101. Springer, United States of America (2010)
4. Manning, C.D., Surdeanu, M., Bauer, J., Finkel, J., Bethard, S.J., McClosky, D.: The Stanford CoreNLP natural language processing toolkit. In: Proceedings of 52nd Annual Meeting of the Association for Computational Linguistics: System Demonstrations, pp. 55–60 (2014)
5. Toutanova, K., Manning, C.D.: Enriching the knowledge sources used in a maximum entropy part-of-speech tagger. In: Proceedings of the Joint SIGDAT Conference on Empirical Methods in Natural Language Processing and Very Large Corpora (EMNLP/VLC-2000), pp. 63–70 (2000)
6. Toutanova, K., Klein, D., Manning, C.D., Singer, Y.: Feature-rich part-of-speech tagging with a cyclic dependency network. In: Proceedings of HLT-NAACL 2003, pp. 252–259 (2003)
7. Kilgarriff, A., et al.: The sketch engine: ten years on. Lexicography **1**, 1–30 (2014)
8. Orallo, J.H., Quintana, J.R., Ferri, C.: Introducción a la Minería de Datos, pp. 260–271. Pearson Prentice Hall, Englewood Cliffs (2004)

Educational Applications

A Comparative Framework to Evaluate Recommender Systems in Technology Enhanced Learning: a Case Study

Matteo Lombardi[✉] and Alessandro Marani

School of Information and Communication Technology, Griffith University,
170 Kessels Road, Nathan, QLD 4111, Australia
{matteo.lombardi,alessandro.marani}@griffithuni.edu.au

Abstract. When proposing a novel recommender system, one difficult part is its evaluation. Especially in Technology Enhanced Learning (TEL), this phase is critical because those systems influence students or educators in educational tasks. Our research aims to propose a framework for conducting comparative experiments of different recommender systems in a same educational context. The framework is expected to provide the accuracy of subject systems within a single experiment, depicting the benefits of a novel system against others. We also present an application of such framework for a comparative experiment of popular systems in TEL like Google, Slideshare, Youtube, MERLOT, Connexions and ARIADNE. Our results show that the proposed framework has been effective in comparing the accuracy of those systems, with a clear picture of their performance compared one another. Moreover, the results of the experiment can be used as a benchmark when evaluating novel recommender systems in TEL.

Keywords: Recommender systems · Technology Enhanced Learning · Comparative evaluation · Evaluation experiment · Accuracy performance evaluation

1 Introduction

Recommender systems are widely studied and developed in literature to assist users in the retrieval of relevant goods and services. Those systems use different approaches to perform the recommendation, mostly content-based filtering, collaborative filtering, knowledge-based filtering and their hybridisations [29]. Such approaches are currently applied for the recommendation of items in several areas including education with Technology Enhanced Learning (TEL) systems [7].

Indeed, many resources available on the Web may represent a potential educational content, therefore educators consider Internet as a place where they can search for materials [15]. However, searching for educational resources is a more complex task than for other goods/services, even for recommender systems that meet more challenges to perform proper suggestions. The recommendation of

O. Pichardo Lagunas et al. (Eds.): MICAI 2015, Part II, LNAI 9414, pp. 155–170, 2015.
DOI: 10.1007/978-3-319-27101-9_11

educational resources is more complex for (i) the many aspects involved in the selection of a resource, and (ii) the low amount of educational data available compared to other areas [29]. In addition, users' interests and preferences alone are not enough for a proper recommendation of educational content, because the recommended resources shall meet users' educational context as well as users' characteristics [3].

In general, the evaluation of recommender systems is a critical step when proposing a novel recommendation algorithm, because of (i) the many properties that should be evaluated (e.g. accuracy, robustness, scalability), (ii) the datasets and (iii) the number of users that such evaluations may require [23]. When evaluating a recommender system, three experimental settings are expected: offline experiment, user studies and online experiment [23]. According to Shani and Gunawardana (2011), the former is towards the calibration of the recommendation algorithm and process, or even for comparing the performances of different algorithms. For such phase, a number of existing real datasets or synthetic datasets may be used. The second experiment is towards the analysis of the system behavior with a set of test users. For this experiment, the test users interact with the system performing a set of tasks. In such scenario, the researchers record some quantitative data about the system, the users and the interaction system-user in order to have a first understanding of the system performances and influence on users. Finally, online experiment is for the evaluation of the system in real applications, where it is mainly measured how much the recommendations proposed by the system actually influence the users, as well as other properties. When evaluating recommender systems in TEL, the same three experiments are expected [7].

As the next section reports, there are many contributions about recommender systems in TEL, but there is not a comparison of their performance in similar educational contexts, which makes a comprehensive understanding of their effectiveness difficult. Even if those systems perform well on recommending educational resources considering some specific aspects, it is worth to see whether or not their overall performance is better than current practices. What we find in this study is that generic IR systems such as Slideshare, Google and Youtube are very popular among users of TEL systems and they do not perform bad either (see Sect. 6). Therefore, it is important to prove that the performance of novel systems are at least the same even if their recommendations are more appropriate for some educational aspects (e.g. educational profile of users). Hence, it would be more interesting to see different recommendation systems compared in a same framework or evaluation setting. In this way, the resulting performance of a novel system can be compared against a set of systems that are quite popular, providing a more clear evidence of the effective progress in the field of recommender systems in TEL. Indeed, in TEL we can find different ways to recommend educational resources [7], thus, for a more effective and expressive evaluation, it is important to use the same experimental setting. In this regard, we suggest a comparative framework which consists of a set of information that depicts the educational context on which to conduct the comparison of recommender systems in TEL.

Finally, we present an application of our framework for organising a comparative experiment. The objective of such experiment is the evaluation of the accuracy performance of Information Retrieval (IR) systems practically used by users of TEL systems, namely students and educators. The results here reported can be a first starting point for measuring the performance of novel TEL recommender systems. During this contribution we explore the accuracy performance of Google, Youtube and Slideshare, which are very popular among educators and students [4], although they are generic search engines, not focused only on educational resources. In addition to them, we evaluate Connexions[1], MERLOT[2] and ARIADNE[3] which are the most popular Learning Object repositories in literature and practical life of students and educators [4,14,25].

2   Background

As said in the introduction, the retrieval of educational resources is a complex task mostly because of the many aspects that are involved in the recommendation process. The literature proposes the Learning Object for the description of educational characteristics of digital content through metadata [26]. Such information is helpful for recommender systems to find a match between the user query and metadata of digital resources. Learning Objects are available on the Web in Learning Object Repositories such as MERLOT, Connexions and ARIADNE. Those systems differently gather and manage Learning Objects that they host. In particular, MERLOT does not actually store the materials that it offers, but it only records the link to the website of the resource and the metadata, as stated on its website[4]. Moreover, it is particularly appreciated for the peer review of its materials. MERLOT currently refers to 40.000 resources.

In opposite to MERLOT, Connexions stores the materials, presently over 26.000 Learning Objects according to the information reported on its website[5]. Differently, ARIADNE [10] is a federated repository based on GLOBE[6], a network of Learning Objects coming from different repositories [19]. So, ARIADNE actually uses Learning Objects available in other repositories but stored with the IEEE LOM standard[7], which presently is the most popular standard of the metadata of Learning Object [19].

The main contribution of Learning Object Repositories is that the user can search for Learning Objects typing a phrase containing the keywords, then the Learning Object Repository will present all the available resources matching with the query, similarly to Google. The search engines of Learning Object Repositories

---

[1] https://cnx.org

[2] http://www.merlot.org

[3] http://www.ariadne-eu.org

[4] http://info.merlot.org/merlothelp/index.htm#merlot_collection.htm   accessed   on 12/05/2015.

[5] http://cnx.org/ contents accessed on 12/05/2015.

[6] http://globe-info.org/

[7] IEEE 1484.12.1-2002, IEEE standard for learning object metadata.

are more appropriate for recommender systems in TEL, but they can access to a more limited number of resources than Google, Youtube or other big IR systems.

Currently, interesting systems based on Learning Object are proposed with the aim to produce proper recommendations for students and educators [7,29], some of them also based on user profiling [12,13,22]. Although we have those systems, users still mostly rely on generic search engines. In this situation, we believe that a comparative evaluation against generic IR systems represents a stronger evidence of the effectiveness of novel systems. In this regard, a comparative experiment based on a same benchmark provides the research community, industries and end users with a valid motivation to change their attitude towards novel systems and practices.

Table 1. A review of some recommender systems in TEL focused on the evaluation experiments.

System	Online evaluation	Offline evaluation	Comparative evaluation	Accuracy measures	Predictive accuracy
[18] (2007)		x			x
[16] (2008)	x (50 students)				x
[25] (2010)		x			x
[30] (2011)	x (10 students)				x
[2] (2011)		x		x	x
[5] (2012)	x (Java course)				x
[21] (2013)		x		x	
[31] (2013)	x (24 students)			x	
[9] (2014)		x		x	
[1] (2014)		x		x	x
[22] (2015)		x			x

In literature, we found some surveys of recommender systems in TEL [7,17,29] where it is depicted a very good overview of those systems and their approaches. Unfortunately, a comparative evaluation of the resulting performance of such systems is difficult to conduct because of the different experimental settings conducted in those studies. However, the performance of those systems (e.g. accuracy) can still be compared if they are evaluated in the same experiment. To the best of our knowledge, no works either conduct a comparative evaluation of accuracy performance or propose a comparative framework of recommender systems in TEL. In this regard, Table 1 reports some recommender systems in TEL and their experimental settings. As we can see, none of them has conducted a comparative evaluation with other systems, neither with current practices of their end users. In addition, the performance analysis is mostly based on predictive accuracy measures, that however cannot be used for big IR systems for the absence of ratings of their items from the educational point of view. Therefore, in this work we adopt Top-N accuracy measures of recommender systems [8], which are largely used also for the evaluation of generic search engines [11,28].

3   The Proposed Comparative Framework

The framework proposed in this contribution consists of a set of features used for conducting a comparative experiment of accuracy performance of recommender systems in TEL. In practice, our framework expresses the keywords for describing some educational features that the retrieved resources are expected to meet. The framework must be as generic as possible in order to make the comparison possible for most of the systems; the more the framework is generic, the more IR systems can be evaluated with it. Moreover, the framework must be based on information that is user independent. As result, the framework proposed in this contribution consists of:

1. Concept Name (CN)
2. Course Title (CT)
3. Difficulty (D)
4. Education Level (E)
5. Prerequisite Knowledge (PK)

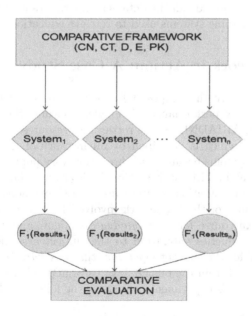

Fig. 1. Structure of a comparative experiment based on the proposed comparative framework.

Those elements represent a piece of information that is essential when searching for educational resources and independent of user characteristics [12,24]. Moreover, the order as they are here presented is important too. In fact, the framework submits 5 queries to the subject systems, where in each query is added one of those elements following that order (e.g. Query1 has only CN, then Query2 has CN and CT, and so forth). With this approach we expect to provide a more wide evaluation of the systems with different queries of increasing depth. So, we can have a spectrum of the systems' performance for the different specificity of the queries.

Figure 1 shows the structure of a comparative experiment using the proposed framework. As we can see, an instance of the framework is used to query different systems. Then, it is possible to compare the results using well-known accuracy measures of recommender systems. The framework is proposed with accuracy measures, instead of predictive accuracy or other measures, because it is not easy to find educational datasets for recommender systems in TEL, even more with ratings from users [3,29]. Being the goal of the comparative experiment the analysis of accuracy performance of subject systems, *Precision (P)* and relative *Recall (R)* [23] have been used as accuracy measures. For an expressive comparative experiment, we suggest to combine P and R in one score using the F_1 score that is, in essence, the harmonic mean of P and R [8,23]. The formula of the F_1 score is the following:

$$F_1 = \frac{2PR}{P+R} \tag{1}$$

In the next section we provide all the details about the framework and its application for comparing some systems used to retrieve educational material.

4   The Framework in Action: A Case Study

In this section we apply the proposed framework to conduct a comparative experiment of accuracy performance of Google, Youtube, Slideshare, Connexions, MERLOT and ARIADNE for the retrieval of resources appropriate for an educational context, which is described by an instance of the framework. We have selected those systems because they are either very popular among users of recommender systems in TEL, such as Google, Youtube, Slideshare and MERLOT [4], or with high attention in literature, like Connexions and ARIADNE [6,14,20]. The instance of the framework involved for this evaluation is about a *Java Programming* course for *Undergraduate* students and *Beginners* as difficulty level. All the queries submitted to the subject systems are about the retrieval of material for the concept *Operators* that has *Variables* as prerequisite in such course (derived from the official Java tutorial[8]). Therefore, the instance of the framework for this experiment consists of the following data:

---

[8] https://docs.oracle.com/javase/tutorial/java/index.html

1. Concept Name: Operators
2. Course Title: Java Programming
3. Difficulty: Beginners
4. Education Level: Undergraduate
5. Prerequisite Knowledge: Variables

From this set of information, we query each subject system five times, each time increasing the depth of the query adding a piece of information of the framework. So, we start with a query formed by only *Operators*, then the second query consists of *Operators* and *Java Programming*, and so on. The last query contains all the elements of the framework. The set of queries used for this comparative experiment is reported in Table 2.

In order to reduce every possible bias due to the automated user profiling that most of the analysed systems perform, we have decided to (i) completely delete the cache, history, cookies and any other browsing data of the browser before to perform each query, and (ii) execute the queries browsing in private (incognito). The browser used in this experiment is Internet Explorer.

Table 2. Set of queries used to evaluate the performance of the test systems.

Query #	Query	Contextual Information
1	Operators	CN
2	Operators Java programming	CN, CT
3	Operators Java programming beginners	CN, CT, D
4	Operators Java programming beginners undergraduate	CN, CT, D, E
5	Operators Java programming beginners undergraduate variables	CN, CT, D, E, PK

Specifically for this experiment, the same authors (with expertise in teaching Java Programming courses for Undergraduate) decided the relevance of the retrieved items, because of their expertise in Java Programming and their impartiality in evaluating the subject systems (the authors are not linked in any way to any of the analysed systems), as performed in other literature for the evaluation of big IR systems [28].

In addition, only the items displayed in the first page of the results are considered, given the fact that just few users go to the second page or beyond when browsing the results of large IR systems [27]. Given that all the test systems present at least ten results for each page, P and R are calculated according to the relevance of the first ten results (top-10 accuracy measure). As said, the relevance of a retrieved document is established by the same authors with a binary value (1 if relevant, 0 otherwise). A retrieved item is considered relevant when (i) it covers all the concept *Operators* and not just a part of it, even if it covers also other topics, and (ii) it complies with all the features of the educational context as described by the framework.

For the computation of the F_1 scores, the set of relevant items of each subject system consists of the union of relevant resources retrieved by the individual system during the execution of the five queries. In the following section, we present the subject systems that are evaluated in our experiment, with a particular focus on how they perform the recommendations.

4.1   Brief Overview of Subject Systems

As said earlier, during the comparative experiment presented in this paper, Google, Youtube, Slideshare, Connexions, MERLOT and ARIADNE are evaluated. With more focus on the data used for their recommendation processes and the structure of such processes, companies like Google Inc. (owner of Google search engine and Youtube platform) and LinkedIn (which is behind Slideshare) do not use only the keywords in the string query to perform their recommendations. Information about the user is deducted even if the person is not logged in, via an automated user profiling.

For example, as stated in the privacy policy of Google Inc.[9], Google can depict a user profile through the previous queries, visited web pages, Youtube videos watched in the past, the location of the user via the IP address, the device of the user and even the movements of the mouse pointer. This is applied not only for the Google search engine, but also for Youtube. Hence, recommendations are personalised using such user data collected in background of user's activities on the web.

According to the privacy policy of Slideshare[10], also this system collects information about the chronology of visualised content and queries performed by the user. In addition, if the user is logged in the system, Slideshare can deduct different data in several ways. For instance, the sex of users can be acquired analysing their name, and the users' qualifications are used to deduct age, fields of interest and range of income.

Those three subject systems mostly use generic user profiles to personalise the query results, but they do not build or use an educational profile of users. Although those systems are not focused in education, the experimental setting here proposed can still be applied. For the proposed experimentation, educational features of the retrieved items are not required for comparing the relevance of the results, but the comparative framework itself is used for querying the subject systems and then evaluate the relevance of their results; an approach valid also for Google, Slideshare and Youtube. In this manner, the comparative evaluation can show the performance of the subject systems in retrieving educational resources for the same context as described by the instance of the comparative framework.

---

[9] http://www.google.com/intl/en/policies/privacy/
[10] https://www.linkedin.com/legal/privacy-policy

5   Performance Analysis

In this section we present and discuss the performance of the subject systems involved in the comparative experiment presented in this contribution. Along the next subsections, we report the results and discussions for each analysed system.

5.1   Google

The chart of the performance of Google search engine is shown in Fig. 2. Google has retrieved 8 relevant items after the five queries. As we can see, there is an increment of Precision and Recall until the second query, reaching the best values which are 0.3 and 0.375 respectively. The performance remains steady with query number three, but it presents a drop when the query is expanded with *Education Level*. Adding the *Prerequisite Knowledge* to the query, Precision and Recall rise again to their maximum value. Overall, Google has a F_1 score which is always just over 0.3 throughout the experiment, except for query Q1 and Q4. It is not an excellent performance, but we have to consider that Google dataset is the entire web, not only educational resources, so it is acceptable that it does not have the best performance.

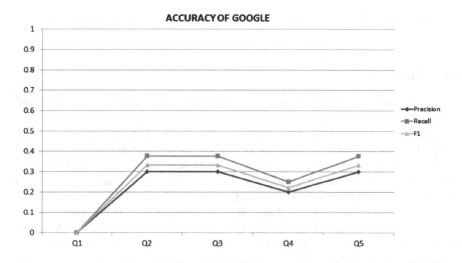

Fig. 2. Results of accuracy performance of Google using the framework.

5.2   Slideshare

Throughout the experiment, Slideshare retrieved 5 relevant resources. Figure 3 shows that Precision and Recall of Slideshare have an increasing trend until the fourth query reaching the maximum value of 0.4 for Precision and 0.8 for

Recall. The same performance is recorded for the last query. So, in opposite to Google, Slideshare benefits of the *Education Level* element and, overall, it performs better than Google. However, we expected still better results because Slideshare is more focused in education than Google.

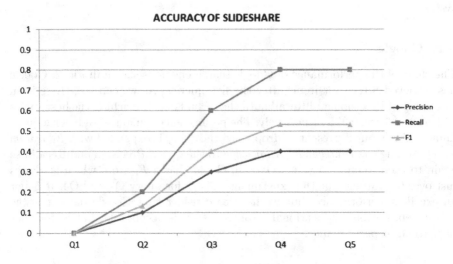

Fig. 3. Results of accuracy performance of Slideshare using the framework.

5.3 Youtube

The third system involved in this experimentation is Youtube, with 6 relevant items retrieved over the entire experiment, and Fig. 4 reports its accuracy performance. We can say that Youtube has a steady trend during the experiment except for the first and the last queries where it is registered a relevant drop of the accuracy. In particular, the first query produces a F_1 score of 0, because the retrieved items were not sufficient to cover the entire concept, but just a part of it. From the second to the fourth query, there is the best performance of Youtube, with Precision $= 0.2$ and Recall just over 0.3. Then, with the last query, Precision falls to 0.1 and Recall to less than 0.2. We can say that Youtube did not perform well against the other systems analysed so far. The main problem of such a low performance of Youtube is due to the granularity of its items, which might be too much fine for educational purposes according to the results of this experiment. In fact, although *Operators* is not a wide concept, most of the retrieved items are short videos which explain only a portion of it.

5.4 Connexions

Throughout the entire experiment Connexions has retrieved 2 relevant items and the accuracy performance is shown in Fig. 5. For this system, we can see that

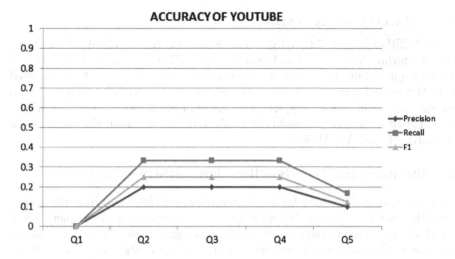

Fig. 4. Results of accuracy performance of Youtube using the framework.

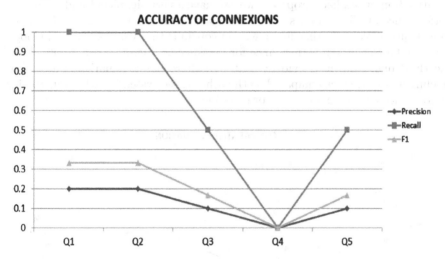

Fig. 5. Results of accuracy performance of Connexions using the framework.

the best values for precision and recall are achieved straight away with the first two queries, namely Recall $= 1$ and Precision $= 0.2$, because the only two relevant items are both retrieved in these two first queries. After that, the trend starts to fall until 0 when, in query Q4, the *Education Level* is added. A significant increment is recorded for the fifth query. The main problem of this system is the low availability of relevant material. In fact, the highest recorded value of recall is 1 because the two relevant items have been retrieved right away in the first two queries. However, it is interesting to note that it is the unique system in this experiment that reached its maximum accuracy in the first query.

5.5   MERLOT and ARIADNE

Both MERLOT and ARIADNE had issues in the retrieval of Learning
Objects during this experiment. In particular, MERLOT retrieved items only for
the first query, but none of them were relevant. No results have been reported
from the second query to the last one. Similarly, ARIADNE was not able to
retrieve any resource for any query, and, in addition, it mostly retrieved broken
links. For these reasons, we could not produce the charts about the performance
of MERLOT and ARIADNE.

6   Summarising the Results: Comparative Analysis

During our analysis we have been able to retrieve relevant items from the majority of the tested IR systems, but with different performance for each query. From
the charts presented in the previous section, we can see that Slideshare achieved
the best results in terms of precision and recall, especially when nearly all the
elements of the framework were in the query. With the application of the comparative framework here proposed, we can have a very significant and expressive
performance of all the four systems of this experiment, as Fig. 6 clearly shows.
In fact, just looking on that figure we can conclude that Connexions and Google
have the best accuracy performance for low-specific queries (Q1 and Q2). From
the third query on, it is evident that Slideshare has a remarkable and over-
whelming performance compared to the other three systems, with an increasing
performance as the queries are more specific.

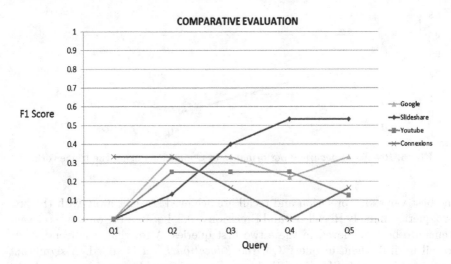

Fig. 6. Comparative evaluation of Google, Slideshare, Youtube and Connexions based
on F_1 scores resulting from the application of an instance of the comparative framework.

In conclusion of this experiment, we have shown the benefit of the proposed
framework for comparing recommender systems in TEL. Such approach is simple

but very effective in properly conducting comparative experiments and producing comparable results. Moreover, the results found in this experiment can be a benchmark for comparative evaluation of novel systems in TEL. Indeed, new recommender systems in TEL are expected to have an overall accuracy performance higher than 0.53 in terms of F_1 score. That value is the highest F_1 score observed in this experiment, achieved by Slideshare with the fourth and fifth query (refer to Fig. 6). Finally, the comparative framework can also help to understand what educational information enhance the accuracy performance of a novel system.

6.1 Limitations of the Experiment

The analysis presented in this contribution has been performed on several IR systems with the most possible attention to avoid any bias or other condition that could invalidate the experiment, but it is limited to only one domain. However, this limitation does not weak this experiment, because Java programming courses are taught in several universities around the world in Undergraduate classes, so the instance of the framework used in this experiment is a very popular scenario in the real world. Furthermore, it is highly probable that an educator or student could use the discussed IR systems to look for educational resources about the topic included in our analysis. More important, in this paper we have been able to show how it is practically possible to conduct a comparative experiment using the framework here proposed, and the effectiveness of the framework itself in comparing the performance of different systems.

7 Conclusions and Future Work

In this contribution we have seen the importance and feasibility of conducting a comparative experiment of recommender systems in TEL, towards a better understanding of their benefits for users. As result of the review of the literature, no comparative studies of such systems have been conducted in the field of TEL. Moreover, it is evident the lack of comparative evaluations of new systems against current solutions. Such evaluations are important when presenting a novel system in order to provide researchers, industries and even the end users with a clear improvement of the recommendation service provided by the novel system. The framework proposed in this contribution provides the stakeholders of recommender systems in TEL with a tool for comparing the accuracy performance of new systems against what they currently use. Even for researchers, this framework is fundamental for conducting comparative experiments for better insights of the performance of their work, which is the main goal of this paper.

In addition, an application of the framework in a popular case study is presented, namely the recommendation of educational resources for a Java Programming course (refer to Sect. 4 for more details). Using our framework, a comparative experiment of Google, Slideshare, Youtube, Connexions, MERLOT and ARIADNE has been conducted. Figure 6 summarises the results of the comparative experiment based on our framework, where those systems have been compared one another in a single experiment and in the same educational context. In that figure, MERLOT and ARIADNE are not reported because of their problems in performing the steps of the experiment (refer to Sect. 5.5 for more details).

Another important finding of this paper is the result of such experiment, which is a very significant benchmark when conducting the evaluation of future novel recommender systems in TEL. In fact, researchers can repeat the comparative experiment with the case study here analysed, and use the results of this experiment for demonstrating the actual contribution of their systems.

In conclusion, with the application of the proposed comparative framework, a comparative experiment has been successfully conducted for the comparison of accuracy performance of systems with different characteristics. We expect other applications of the framework for a better understanding of its effectiveness for the evaluation of other systems.

References

1. Anand, D., Mampilli, B.S.: Folksonomy-based fuzzy user profiling for improved recommendations. Expert Syst. Appl. **41**(5), 2424–2436 (2014)
2. Bobadilla, J., Ortega, F., Hernando, A., Alcalá, J.: Improving collaborative filtering recommender system results and performance using genetic algorithms. Knowl.-Based Syst. **24**(8), 1310–1316 (2011)
3. Bozo, J., Alarcón, R., Iribarra, S.: Recommending learning objects according to a teachers' contex model. In: Wolpers, M., Kirschner, P.A., Scheffel, M., Lindstaedt, S., Dimitrova, V. (eds.) EC-TEL 2010. LNCS, vol. 6383, pp. 470–475. Springer, Heidelberg (2010)
4. Brent, I., Gibbs, G.R., Gruszczynska, A.K.: Obstacles to creating and finding open educational resources: the case of research methods in the social sciences. J. Interact. Media Educ. 2012(1):Art-5 (2012)
5. Casali, A., Gerling, V., Deco, C., Bender, C.: A recommender system for learning objects personalized retrieval. In: Educational Recommender Systems and Technologies: Practices and Challenges, pp. 182–210. PA, Hershey, Information Science Reference (2012)
6. Cechinel, C., Ochoa, X.: A brief overview of quality inside learning object repositories. In: Proceedings of the XV International Conference on Human Computer Interaction, p. 83. ACM (2014)
7. Drachsler, H., Verbert, K., Santos, O., Manouselis, N.: Panorama of recommender systems to support learning. status: accepted (2015)
8. Herlocker, J.L., Konstan, J.A., Terveen, L.G., Riedl, J.T.: Evaluating collaborative filtering recommender systems. ACM Trans. Inf. Syst. (TOIS) **22**(1), 5–53 (2004)
9. Karampiperis, P., Koukourikos, A., Stoitsis, G.: Collaborative filtering recommendation of educational content in social environments utilizing sentiment analysis techniques. In: Manouselis, N., Drachsler, H., Verbert, K., Santos, O.C. (eds.) Recommender Systems for Technology Enhanced Learning, pp. 3–23. Springer, Heidelberg (2014)

10. Klerkx, J., Vandeputte, B., Parra, G., Santos, J.L., Van Assche, F., Duval, E.: How to share and reuse learning resources: the ARIADNE experience. In: Wolpers, M., Kirschner, P.A., Scheffel, M., Lindstaedt, S., Dimitrova, V. (eds.) EC-TEL 2010. LNCS, vol. 6383, pp. 183–196. Springer, Heidelberg (2010)

11. Liang, C.: User profile for personalized web search. In: 2011 Eighth International Conference on Fuzzy Systems and Knowledge Discovery (FSKD), vol. 3, pp. 1847–1850. IEEE (2011)

12. Limongelli, C., Lombardi, M., Marani, A., Sciarrone, F.: A teacher model to speed up the process of building courses. In: Kurosu, M. (ed.) HCII/HCI 2013, Part II. LNCS, vol. 8005, pp. 434–443. Springer, Heidelberg (2013)

13. Limongelli, C., Lombardi, M., Marani, A., Sciarrone, F.: A teaching-style based social network for didactic building and sharing. In: Lane, H.C., Yacef, K., Mostow, J., Pavlik, P. (eds.) AIED 2013. LNCS, vol. 7926, pp. 774–777. Springer, Heidelberg (2013)

14. Limongelli, C., Miola, A., Sciarrone, F., Temperini, M.: Supporting teachers to retrieve and select learning objects for personalized courses in the moodle_ls environment. In: 2012 IEEE 12th International Conference on Advanced Learning Technologies (ICALT), pp. 518–520. IEEE (2012)

15. Maloney, S., Moss, A., Keating, J., Kotsanas, G., Morgan, P.: Sharing teaching and learning resources: perceptions of a university's faculty members. Med. Educ. **47**(8), 811–819 (2013)

16. Mangina, E., Kilbride, J.: Evaluation of keyphrase extraction algorithm and tiling process for a document/resource recommender within e-learning environments. Comput. Educ. **50**(3), 807–820 (2008)

17. Manouselis, N., Drachsler, H., Vuorikari, R., Hummel, H., Koper, R.: Recommender systems handbook. In: Ricci, F., Rokach, L., Shapira, B., Kantor, P.B. (eds.) Recommender Systems in Technology Enhanced Learning, pp. 387–415. Springer, Heidelberg (2011)

18. Manouselis, N., Vuorikari, R., Assche, F.V.: Simulated analysis of maut collaborative filtering for learning object recommendation. In: Proceedings of the 1st Workshop on Social Information Retrieval for Technology Enhanced Learning, pp. 27–35 (2007)

19. Ochoa, X., Klerkx, J., Vandeputte, B., Duval, E.: On the use of learning object metadata: the globe experience. Towards Ubiquitous Learning, pp. 271–284. Springer, Heidelberg (2011)

20. Palavitsinis, N., Manouselis, N., Sanchez-Alonso, S.: Metadata quality in learning object repositories: a case study. Electron. Libr. **32**(1), 62–82 (2014)

21. Salehi, M.: Application of implicit and explicit attribute based collaborative filtering and bide for learning resource recommendation. Data Knowl. Eng. **87**, 130–145 (2013)

22. Sergis, S., Sampson, D.: Learning object recommendations for teachers based on elicited ICT competence profiles. IEEE Trans. Learn. Technol. (2015)

23. Shani, G., Gunawardana, A.: Evaluating recommendation systems. In: Ricci, F., Rokach, L., Shapira, B., Kantor, P.B. (eds.) Recommender Systems Handbook, pp. 257–297. Springer, Heidelberg (2011)

24. Shulman, L.S.: Those who understand: knowledge growth in teaching. Educ. Res. **15**(2), 4–14 (1986)

25. Sicilia, M.Á., García-Barriocanal, E., Sánchez-Alonso, S., Cechinel, C.: Exploring user-based recommender results in large learning object repositories: the case of merlot. Procedia Comput. Sci. **1**(2), 2859–2864 (2010)

26. Sosteric, M., Hesemeier, S.: When is a learning object not an object: a first step towards a theory of learning objects. Int. Rev. Res. Open Distance Learn. 3(2) (2002)
27. Spink, V., Jansen, B.J.: Searching multimedia federated content web collections. Online Inf. Rev. **30**(5), 485–495 (2006)
28. Tumer, D., Shah, M.A., Bitirim, Y.: An empirical evaluation on semantic search performance of keyword-based and semantic search engines: Google, yahoo, msn and hakia. In: Fourth International Conference on Internet Monitoring and Protection, ICIMP 2009, pp. 51–55. IEEE (2009)
29. Verbert, K., Manouselis, N., Ochoa, X., Wolpers, M., Drachsler, H., Bosnic, I., Duval, E.: Context-aware recommender systems for learning: a survey and future challenges. IEEE Trans. Learn. Technol. **5**(4), 318–335 (2012)
30. Wan, X., Okamoto, T.: Utilizing learning process to improve recommender system for group learning support. Neural Comput. Appl. **20**(5), 611–621 (2011)
31. Zapata, A., Menéndez, V.H., Prieto, M.E., Romero, C.: A framework for recommendation in learning object repositories: an example of application in civil engineering. Adv. Eng. Softw. **56**, 1–14 (2013)

An Affective and Cognitive Tutoring System for Learning Programming

María Lucía Barrón-Estrada[1], Ramón Zatarain-Cabada[1(✉)],
Francisco González Hernández[1], Raúl Oramas Bustillos[2],
and Carlos A. Reyes-García[3]

[1] Instituto Tecnológico de Culiacán, Juan de Dios Bátiz s/n, col. Guadalupe,
Culiacán, Sinaloa 80220, Mexico
{lbarron,rzatarain}@itculiacan.edu.mx
[2] Universidad de Occidente, Carretera a Culiacáncito, km. 1.5, Culiacán
Sinaloa 80054, Mexico
[3] Instituto Nacional de Astrofísica, Óptica Y Electrónica (INAOE), Luis Enrique
Erro no. 1, Sta. Ma. Tonanzintla, Puebla 72840, Mexico
kargaxxi@inaoep.mx

Abstract. In this paper, we present a multiplatform and Intelligent Tutoring System for learning Java (Java Sensei). The learning system combines state-of-the-art action selection, motivation through emotions, a modern recommendation mechanism, and multimodal instructional and selection learning. Java Sensei architecture works with a collection of modules and processes, each with its own effective representations and algorithms. The learning system was implemented under different learning methodologies like problem-solving for the pedagogical module, knowledge space for the expert module, and overlays for the student module. One of the main contributions of this work was the integration of cognitive and affective information in a behavioral graph which is used by a learning companion to show emotions and empathy to the student. Java Sensei was tested with different groups of university students with which we obtained positive results. In addition to providing a detailed description of the implementation and evaluation of Java Sensei, we also provide some proposals of future work in our intelligent tutoring systems.

Keywords: Intelligent tutoring systems · Affective computing · Artificial neural networks · Fuzzy logic · Mobile learning · Knowledge spaces

1 Introduction

Learning a programming language is the first big challenge for a student of computer science or a related field [1]. Some of the issues that contribute to this obstacle are: the teaching methods employed by the instructor, the difficult nature of computer programming, the study methods, abilities and attitudes employed by the student, the nature of the art of programming, the lack of prior knowledge of novice students, and the psychological influence that the student suffers from society [2–5].

Many researchers have proposed and developed methodologies and tools to help students learn programming. For example the ACM has SIGCSE (Special Interest

O. Pichardo Lagunas et al. (Eds.): MICAI 2015, Part II, LNAI 9414, pp. 171–182, 2015.
DOI: 10.1007/978-3-319-27101-9_12

Group on Computer Science Education) where issues related to the development, implementation and/or evaluation of programs and curricula are discussed [6].

Today, in the field of Artificial Intelligence, affect recognition is an emerging research area of significant theoretical and applied awareness to a number of academic fields including machine learning, computational linguistics, computer vision and speech and language, neuroscience, educational psychology, and pedagogy [7].

The link between affect computing and student learning has been a topic of increasing attention in recent years. Due to the importance of this connection of emotions and learning, one of the current aims of many intelligent tutoring systems is to recognize and manage student emotional states by means of affective mediations. Intelligent Tutoring Systems (ITS) try to simulate a human tutor to provide personalized instruction taking into account not only cognitive aspects of students [8] but also affective elements [9].

This paper presents the implementation of an Intelligent Learning Environment (ILE) for Java programming. This system works in a flexible and interactive multiplatform environment that considers both cognitive and affective states of students.

The paper is organized as follows: Sect. 2 describes related work of the main topics. Section 3 shows and explains the architecture of the ILE Java Sensei. Affect recognition and feedback is illustrated in Sect. 4. Section 5 presents the experiments and results produced with the system. Conclusions and future work are discussed in Sect. 6.

2 Related Work

Research on intelligent tutoring systems for programming language has focused on different programming languages like Java, C-C#, or PHP. Wiggins et al. [10] implemented The JavaTutor System, an affective tutoring system that uses natural language dialogues for human-to-human or human-to-computer dialogues using machine learning techniques. The system takes into account cognitive aspects, where it applies the ACT-R theory of cognition for knowledge representation. Affect focused on nonverbal behavior obtained through bodily expressions and detection is performed by different hardware tools. CSTutor is a tool [11] to help students learn programming in C#. The tool incorporates anchored instruction for the domain representation of the programming language and game theory, instead of affect recognition, for motivation improvement. The PHP ITS was developed to teach students to program in PHP scripting language [12]. The tutor makes an analysis written by the student and translates to the equivalent of an abstract syntax tree (AST) code. Then, the AST is used to create events or trigger actions. The facts that exist after all AST nodes are processed are called the final state. To check the correctness of a program, the tutor analyzes whether all predicates in the goal for a particular task are present in the final state. Through this method, the student writes the solution of the task defined in its own way, as long as the final state of his/her program meets the specified target.

CTutor [13] is an intelligent learning environment (ILE) where students perform exercises programming in C. The idea of this system is to facilitate the effectiveness of learning when students navigate through complex problems and thereby provide an advanced education system to enhance the learning process. This ILE allows teachers to create new programming exercises and manage them from the system interface. The domain in the system is adjustable for each solution of each exercise. From the perspective of a student the CTutor interface is a tool with controls to represent the solution of the exercises. The tool uses a constructivist pedagogical orientation where the authors give special weight to feedback as the main source of information; moreover, its domain is formed based on a constraint-based model. On the other hand, CTutor does not support affect recognition.

3 Java Sensei Architecture

In this section we present the main architecture of Java Sensei: the affective environment for learning Java programming. Figure 1 shows the different layers and components of our architecture. Sensei Java architecture is designed in seven layers with a client-server structure with a fat client. The aim of developing a thick client is to reduce the processing load on the server.

Next, we explain the function of each layer.

- *Web Layer:* The Web Layer is the layer of the client, and is made up of modules that need to run in the web browser when the user interacts with the system. This layer contains the following components:

  - *Web Interface:* This component represents the web user interface, so this component is responsible for interaction with the customer, the use of external libraries and centralizing interactions with other layers, mainly with the Service Layer.
    Example-Tracing Engine: This element is the semantic and visual interpretation of all courses in the system. Within this component, the following tasks are performed: creation of tracing trees, extraction of tree information, and interaction with the Web Interface to build the GUI. In addition, the events generated by the example-tracing logic and notification of state changes are managed.
    Pedagogical Agent: This component creates the visual representation of a learning companion and it is based on the pedagogical information obtained from the server layer. The actions performed are: extraction of pedagogical data for the visual representation of the agent and extraction of information of affective information from the student using the tree created by Engine Example-Tracing.
    Camera in Background: This component manages the capture of the array of photographs in the background during exercise sessions in the system. It is responsible for starting and stopping the photography sessions, clear the memory of a photograph queue, and manage the time between each capture; also it is responsible for converting the array of photographs into an understandable format for the Server Layer.
- *Service Layer:* It is the layer where the components related to the handling of external requests to the server are located. In this layer the components must be

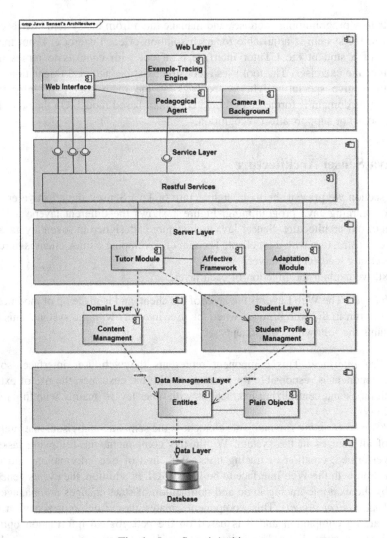

Fig. 1. Java Sensei Architecture

accessible from the Web and use the HTTP communication protocol. This layer holds the next components:

- *Restful Services:* This component is responsible for receiving incoming web requests from the Web Layer. Its role is to accept requests and ensure its integrity and completeness. It also gives them a format so they can be worked on by the components comprising the Server Layer.
- *Server Layer:* The Server Layer is the layer that contains the modules of the server, which is composed of modules that need a strong interaction with the Domain Layer and Student Layer; also it makes decisions using a high burden of processing and

memory resources. Within this layer there are some key components for making instructional decisions.

- *Tutoring Module:* It is responsible for taking appropriate cognitive and affective educational decisions for the student as: assessing the quality of student response, assessing the overall ability of the student and use the Affective Framework component for obtaining affective information.
- *Adaptation Module:* It uses the perceptions and preferences of the student in relation to the exercises and help resources to build a recommendation system.
- *Affective Framework:* This component represents the affective student assessment. It uses cognitive and affective information from the students provided by the Tutoring Model. It uses a back propagation neural network to recognize emotions through the face and uses a fuzzy logic system for affective pedagogical strategy.

- *Domain Layer:* This layer contains one component: The Content Manager, which is responsible for interacting with the Server Layer and Data Management Layer. The Content Manager represents the tutor domain or knowledge of the Java language. This knowledge is represented using the theory of knowledge spaces which is encoded using JSON files.
- *Student Layer:* It represents the student's knowledge compared to the domain model. This layer contains one component: The Student Profile Management. The tasks of the component are: calculate the overall ability of the student (the total number of correct exercises) and quality of the current response (the number of errors that the student makes in an exercise); verify changes in the domain model to upgrade the overlay student model; and store student preferences regarding exercises and resources. The component also interacts with the Data Management Layer to store/retrieve student data in JSON format.
- *Data Management Layer:* This layer contains two components: *Entities* and *Plain Objects*. The component *Entities* are data structures that encapsulate domain and student information that are used in the Data, Domain, and Student Layers respectively. The component *Plain Objects* contains information in plain text in JSON format.
- *Data layer:* This layer manages the data for the Domain and Student Modules represented in JSON and MongoDB formats.

4   Affective Recognition and Feedback

Figure 2 shows the steps followed in the recognition and affective feedback from the system. In the first step the ILE Java Sensei receives the data and the student's collection of images from the browser which are later sent to the ILE. In the second step the ILE starts a cycle with several student faces being sent to the neural network, and decides, at the end of the cycle, the current emotion. This current emotion is obtained based on the most frequent student emotion. In the third step the ILE sends the updated student model to the fuzzy system which performs the fuzzy rules to output the tutor actions. In the last step, the tutor actions are sent to the browser to build the actions of the pedagogical agent.

Pedagogical Agent: The pedagogical agent is responsible for transmitting messages that a human tutor would perform. For this, it has been provided with both facial expressions and dialogues that can communicate to the student.

These expressions are based on facial expressions investigated by Ekman [14]. Positions of the eyebrow, mouth, and eye opening are taken into account. These positions are entered as parameters in the FaceGen Modeller [15] software. In Fig. 3 we observe the four facial expressions made by the pedagogical agent of Java Sensei. These emotions were based on the pedagogical agent working with AutoTutor [16].

Fuzzy System and Neural Network: The fuzzy logic system seeks to represent the way a human tutor acts when he/she faces various scenarios related with cognitive and emotional situations of a student. These situations have to do with the predefined actions. The fuzzy system uses the emotional values obtained by the neural network which recognizes the affective state of the student when he/she works with the ILE Java Sensei. The fuzzy logic system works with four input fuzzy variables and three output ones. A total of 144 fuzzy rules were constructed. To define these rules we use *Fuzzy Control Language*, a standardized language for creation of fuzzy rules. The implementation was done with *jFuzzyLogic* [17].

The emotion recognition system was built in three steps: the first one was an implementation to extract features from face images in a corpus used to train the neural network. The second step was the implementation of the neural network. We used the Java-based algorithms implemented in NeuroPH [18] to implement classification by using a neural network (feed-forward method). The third step integrated feature extraction and emotion recognition with the fuzzy system. For training and testing the neural network, we used the corpus RAFD (Radboud Faces Database), which is a database with 8040 different facial expressions that contain a set of 67 models including men and women. In the training process we obtained a successful rate of 86 % which we consider is good enough for our system. Once the emotional state is extracted from the student, the emotional state is sent to the fuzzy system.

Adaptation Module: The ILE must be able to adapt to the student. The ILE collects the rating produced by the student concerning the exercises and resources that the student visits. The rating of one exercise is measured using Likert scale [19] where one indicates total disagreement with the exercise and five indicates total agreement. At the beginning all the exercises are rated with a value of two. We used a recommendation system created with Apache Mahout [20]. This tool helps to find the next problem the student must solve. The system implements the K-Nearest Neighbor (k-NN) approach and the Pearson Correlation. As more users are included, the rating system generates the best recommendations and thereby it gets more adapted to the changes.

Pedagogical Module: The system uses the pedagogical model known as "problem solving" [21] where the student learns as he solves problems with a certain structure. The system uses three types of strategies for solving problems. Type 1 is used to evaluate theoretical concepts with "true-false" exercises. Type 2 questions present a complete program or piece of code and ask the student to determine the output of the

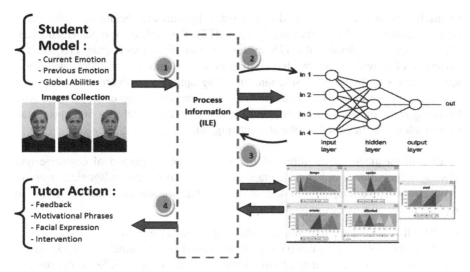

Fig. 2. Affect recognition and response

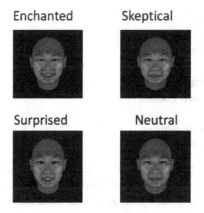

Fig. 3. Pedagogical agent

code. Type 3 is a combination of the two previous types and allows creating more complex exercises involving "*n*" number of steps to reach the solution.

Expert Module: This model contains the expert knowledge that the student wants to learn and practice. The system represents the knowledge using JSON files (a variation of XML files). Knowledge representation uses the knowledge space theory [22]. The expert model represents six basic skills that students must master to be modeled by a graph representing the Knowledge Space. These skills are: Introduction to Java, Variables and calculations, selection, iteration, methods, and arrays.

Example-Tracing Engine: An ILE combines hypermedia techniques with other methods used by Intelligent Tutoring Systems (ITS). We applied Example-Tracing [23, 24] in order to implement the ITS in Java Sensei. Example-Tracing ITS has the advantage of providing step-by-step guiding to the students and providing with multiple strategies to the problem solution, including optimal or sub-optimal solution or miss-conception management. Example-Tracing exercises can be easily adapted with the pedagogical model implemented with "problem solving" and they are represented by a graph that is traversed by the student (Fig. 4).

One of the main contributions of our work is the integration of cognitive and affective information in a behavior graph which is used by the pedagogical agent to show emotion and empathy to the student. Next, we describe the algorithm to implement the affective-example-tracing:

(a) The ILE loads the JSON file with the corresponding exercise.
(b) From the JSON file, a behavior graph is created and an initial step is executed.
(c) As students traverse the graph (by clicking with the mouse), different options can be performed and different paths are traversed. The options are:

  i. Initial step (IS)
  ii. Error step (ES)
  iii. Optimal step (OS)
  iv. Sub-optimal step (SOS)
  v. Final Optimal step (FOS)
  vi. Final Sub-optimal step (FSS)

(d) Every step triggers two events:

  i. Actual emotion evaluation.
  ii. Tutor action evaluation.

Every time a student chooses some of the options in the graph, the engine calls the fuzzy logic system to get the tutor action (feedback, intervention, etc.) and to get the emotion information so the pedagogical agent can build the graph. Figure 4 illustrates an example. At the left we can observe how the student solved the problem in an optimal way. At the right the student made a mistake.

5 Experiments and Results

In order to test the ILE, we made different experiments with different kind of students of the Instituto Tecnológico de Culiacán. The system was first tested with graduate students in our research lab. This test has the aim to test the functionality of the ILE. Next, we show (Fig. 5) a small session of a student browsing in the ILE. To access the ILE, the student must use a browser with a PC, laptop, or mobile device (e.g. a smartphone), and a Facebook account allowing the use of the Web cam. The left part of the example shows a problem with the student making a mistake, at the end of the code. In the right part of the problem the student finish successfully the exercise.

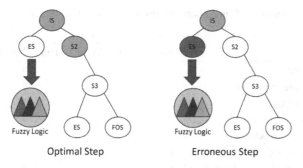

Fig. 4. Affective example-tracing

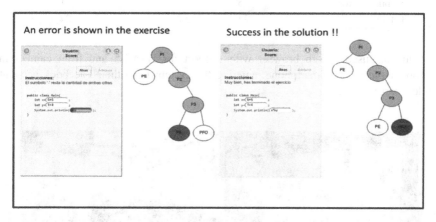

Fig. 5. Affective example-tracing

The following evaluation was applied to Computer Systems students (Engineering) taking currently a Java course. In this case we consider two aspects: the software functionality and the software effectiveness. With respect to software functionality we compared Java Sensei against three similar ILEs: JavaTutor System [25], JITS [26] y jLatte [27]. We considered 9 features to evaluate [6] and Likert scale from 1 to 5, where 1 represents an incomplete feature and 5 represents a complete feature the ILE accomplish. Table 1 shows the results obtained from the software functionality evaluation.

The results show that Java Sensei and JavaTutor System are the ILEs that get better results in the evaluation. The evaluated systems meet almost every feature of an ILE/ITS system except for three features (Mixed Initiative) and 6 (self-improvement). Feature 7 (Affect recognition and Handling) which is a recent area causing that few systems incorporate this feature. The same applies to features 8 and 9. It is expected that modern ITS migrate to the Web and Mobile platforms.

For evaluation of the effectiveness of the system, we conducted a test with a group of 20 students in the subject *Object Oriented Programming* (OOP), looking to measure the learning outcome of the ILE JavaSensei on the topic of inheritance. The selection of students was not performed randomly, but by availability of participants. To access the

Table 1. Comparisons results in software functionality.

Feature	JavaSensei	JavaTutor system	JITS	jLatte
Generativity	3	5	4	4
Student and expert modeling	5	5	5	5
Mixed initiative	2	2	1	1
Interactive learning	4	5	4	5
Instructional modeling	5	5	5	5
Self-improving	1	1	1	1
Affect recognition and handling	4	5	1	1
Web platform	5	5	1	1
Mobile platform	5	1	1	1
Total	34	34	23	24

ILE, students used a web browser with support for HTML5 and front camera in desktops, laptops, and smartphone, entering the system from their Facebook account (see left part of Fig. 6).

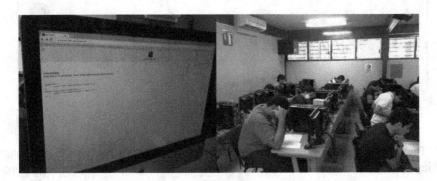

Fig. 6. Students using Java Sensei

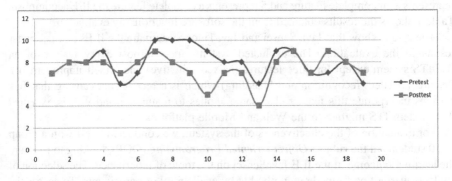

Fig. 7. Pretest and posttest results

The evaluation design methodology consisted of measuring the knowledge of two groups of student: one experimental group who learns by using the ILE and one control group who learns by using traditional teaching. The time given to the pretest was 15 min (see right part of Fig. 6), the time for the ILE session was 70 min, and the time for the posttest was 20 min. Figure 7 shows the evaluation of both tests. The results in the posttest indicate that the experimental group obtained better scores (in most cases) than the control group.

6 Conclusions and Future Work

The ILE has been implemented with open source code in programming languages and software libraries like Java, Javascript, MongoDB, JSON, jFuzzyLogic, Apache Mahout, Weka, jQuery, jQueryMobile among others, and can be accessed from different platforms (operating systems, web browser, computers, etc.). Right now, a group of programming Java professors is applying more tests to the ILE with students from our university (Instituto Tecnológico de Culiacán). For future work, we want to include gamification techniques in order to work more the motivational part of the system. We also want to work with emotions that affect the process of learning (engagement, boring, frustration, etc.). Last we are developing a new version oriented to more collaboration work among students and authoring new exercises by instructors.

Funding. The work described in this paper is fully supported by a grant from the DGEST (Dirección General de Educación Superior Tecnológica) in Mexico under the program "Projects of Scientific Research and Technological Innovation".

References

1. Rodrigo, M.M.T., Baker, R.S.J., Jadud, M.C., Amarra, A.C.M., Dy, T., Espejo-Lahoz, M.B. V., Lim, S.A.L., Pascua, S.A.M.S., Sugay, J.O., Tabanao, E.S.: Affective and behavioral predictors of novice programmer achievement. SIGCSE Bull. **41**, 156–160 (2009)
2. Matthíasdóttir, Á.: How to teach programming languages to novice students? Lecturing or not. In: International Conference on Computer Systems and Technologies-CompSysTech (2006)
3. Jenkins, T.: On the difficulty of learning to program. In: Proceedings of the 3rd Annual Conference of the LTSN Centre for Information and Computer Sciences (2002)
4. Gomes, A., Mendes A.J.: Learning to program-difficulties and solutions. In: International Conference on Engineering Education–ICEE (2007)
5. Bernard, M., Bachu, E.: Enhancing the metacognitive skill of novice programmers through collaborative learning. Metacognition: Fundaments, Applications, and Trends, pp. 277–298. Springer, Berlin (2015)
6. SIGCSE 2015 [cited 2015]. http://www.sigcse.org/
7. Picard, R.: Affective computing: from laughter to IEEE. IEEE Trans. Affect. Comput. **1**, 11–17 (2010)
8. Woolf, B.P.: Building Intelligent Interactive Tutors. Morgan Kaufmann Publishers, Amherst (2009)

9. Harley, J.M., Lajoie, S.P., Frasson, C., Hall, N.C.: An integrated emotion-aware framework for intelligent tutoring systems. In: Conati, C., Heffernan, N., Mitrovic, A., Verdejo, M. (eds.) AIED 2015. LNCS, vol. 9112, pp. 616–619. Springer, Heidelberg (2015)
10. Wiggins, J.B., Boyer, K.E., Baikadi, A., Ezen-Can, A., Grafsgaard, J.F., Ha, E.Y., Wiebe, E. N.: JavaTutor: an intelligent tutoring system that adapts to cognitive and affective states during computer programming. In: Paper Presented at the Proceedings of the 46th ACM Technical Symposium on Computer Science Education (2015)
11. Budi, H., Jim, R.: Incorporating anchored learning in a C# intelligent tutoring system. In: Paper presented at the Consortia Proceedings of the 21st International Conference on Computers in Education. Indonesia: Asia-Pacific Society for Computers in Education (2013)
12. Weragama, D., Reye, J.: Designing the knowledge base for a PHP tutor. In: Cerri, S.A., Clancey, W.J., Papadourakis, G., Panourgia, K. (eds.) ITS 2012. LNCS, vol. 7315, pp. 628–629. Springer, Heidelberg (2012)
13. Kose, U., Deperlioglu, O.: Intelligent learning environments within blended learning for ensuring effective C programming course. Int. J. Artif. Intell. Appl. 3(1), 20 (2012)
14. Ekman, P.: Facial expressions. Handb. Cognit. Emot. 16, 301–320 (1999)
15. Todorov, A., Oosterhof, N.N.: Modeling social perception of faces [social sciences]. IEEE Sig. Process. Mag. 28(2), 117–122 (2011)
16. D'Mello, S., et al.: AutoTutor detects and responds to learners affective and cognitive states. In: Workshop on Emotional and Cognitive Issues at the International Conference on Intelligent Tutoring Systems (2008)
17. Cingolani, P., Alcalá-Fdez, J.: jFuzzyLogic: a java library to design fuzzy logic controllers according to the standard for fuzzy control programming. Int. J. Comput. Intell. Syst. 6 (sup1), 61–75 (2013)
18. Sevarac, Z.: Neuroph-Java neural network framework. Accessed July 2015
19. Likert, R.: A method of constructing an attitude scale. Scaling: a Sourcebook for Behavioral Scientists, pp. 233–243. Aldine, Chicago (2012)
20. Anil, R., Dunning, T., Friedman, E.: Mahout in Action, pp. 145–183. Manning, Shelter Island (2011)
21. Kumar, R., et al. Comparison of algorithms for automatically building example-tracing tutor models. In: Educational Data Mining (2014)
22. Doignon, J.P., Falmagne, J.C.: Knowledge Spaces. Springer, Berlin (1999)
23. Aleven, V., et al.: A new paradigm for intelligent tutoring systems: example-tracing tutors. Int. J. Artif. Intell. Educ. 19(2), 105–154 (2009)
24. Aleven, V., McLaren, B.M., Sewall, J., Koedinger, K.R.: The cognitive tutor authoring tools (CTAT): preliminary evaluation of efficiency gains. In: Ikeda, M., Ashley, K.D., Chan, T.-W. (eds.) ITS 2006. LNCS, vol. 4053, pp. 61–70. Springer, Heidelberg (2006)
25. Wallis, M. JavaTutor-a remotely collaborative, real-time distributed intelligent tutoring system for introductory Java computer programming-a qualitative analysis (2011)
26. Sykes, E.R., Franek, F.: An intelligent tutoring system prototype for learning to program Java TM. IEEE Xplore. In: Proceedings of the 3rd IEEE International Conference on Advanced Learning Technologies (2003)
27. Holland, J., Mitrovic, A., Martin, B.: J-LATTE: a constraint-based Tutor for Java (2009)

Strategic Learning Meta-Model (SLM): Architecture of the Personalized Virtual Learning Environment (PVLE) Based on the Cloud Computing

Rafaela Blanca Silva-López[1(✉)], Iris Iddaly Méndez-Gurrola[1],
Oscar Herrera Alcántara[1], Mónica Irene Silva-López[1],
and Jalil Fallad-Chávez[2]

[1] Universidad Autónoma Metropolitana,
Av. San Pablo no. 180, Col. Reynosa Tamaulipas, Delegación Azcapotzalco,
02200, Distrito Federal, Mexico
{rbsl,oha}@correo.azc.uam.mx, iddalym@yahoo.com.mx,
msilva@correo.1er.uam.mx
[2] Universidad de Guadalajara, Centro Universitario de La Costa Sur,
Av. Independencia Nacional 151, 48900
Autlán de Navarro, Jalisco, Mexico
jfallad@cucsur.udg.mx

Abstract. In this paper a Personalized Virtual Learning Environment (PVLE) architecture is presented which integrates three components is as follows: (I) the Learning Management System (LMS); (II) the Virtual Learning Environment (VLE); and (III) the Ontological Model (OM). The components were implemented as a solution for Cloud Computing. The fieldwork considered two stages: a proof of concept that is used as a benchmark and test cases where the PVLE were applied. We observed during the performance of stage 1 the average scores for thought styles (logical processes, creative, relational) considerably remain unchanged. While in stage 2, we observed the scores average has increased, with a tendency to improve creative, logical and process styles. Therefore, there is a significant contribution in the development of students' cognitive profile to personalize its learning activities and the use of PVLE.

Keywords: Ontological model · Personalized virtual learning environment · Cloud computing · Strategic learning · Virtual learning environment

1 Introduction

The integration of an ontological model in virtual learning environments facilitates the organization of knowledge that allows the setting of recommendations of learning activities on a course, which fosters the development of cognitive skills in students and enables a strategic learning.

© Springer International Publishing Switzerland 2015
O. Pichardo Lagunas et al. (Eds.): MICAI 2015, Part II, LNAI 9414, pp. 183–194, 2015.
DOI: 10.1007/978-3-319-27101-9_13

1.1   Conceptual Framework

In recent years the research associated with the evaluation strategies of learning is approached from different perspectives by authors such as Smyth [1], Sangster [2], Cassidy [3], García-Ros and Pérez-González [4], Uğur et al. [5], Verhoeven et al. [6], Burnett [7], Farrell and Leung [8], Marshall [9], among others. They made interesting contributions that can be categorized into four approaches: (1) those related to learning style; (2) formative assessment practices; (3) interaction and learning communities; and (4) personalized learning assessment. Then works from points 1 and 4 directly related to our research are described.

1.2   Learning Evaluation and Learning Styles

Many authors who focus their research on adapting of learning assessment from the student's learning style point of view. Sangster, Cassidy, García-Ros and Pérez-González, Uğur et al., considered that to know the student's learning style might allows you to select appropriate strategies to improve their ability how to learn to learn [2–5]. Therefore, it is desirable that any investigation related to the students academic performance might include as independent variable the student learning styles [2].

Meanwhile, Uğur et al. analyze the students' vision in a blended learning environment (b-learning) with respect to their learning style [5]. They use Kolb's theory, based on experience which considers four types of learning styles: (a) concrete experience; (b) reflective observation; (c) abstract conceptualization; and (d) active experimentation [10].

Likewise, Verhoeven et al., identify a relationship between learning styles and ICT skills. They also consider learning styles may explain the differences among groups of students according to certain characteristics [6, 7].

These studies suggest that the student's learning style is a determinant element in learning and the learning assessment.

1.3   Personalization of Learning Assessment

Attention to diversity in assessment practices is an issue addressed in the researches of Coll et al. [11]. They identified the need to reconsider the common practices used to assess student learning. They propose an overall strategy that integrates the principles of adaptive education and attention to student diversity in schools. For them it is important to have an outline of an inclusive evaluation culture, incorporating the principles of diversification and flexibility (adaptive learning feature). They recognize the importance of a rigorous and systematic review of assessment practices [11].

Another interesting vision, environment evaluation as a mechanism of motivation and learning is presented by Dochy et al. They propose different mechanisms to make the assessment into a motivational tool, teaching and learning. They also conducted an analysis about differences between self-assessment, peer assessment and co-assessment [12].

While Guzman and Conejo pose a cognitive assessment model based on adaptive testing for diagnosis in intelligent tutoring systems that apply AI techniques to guide the student during instruction [13].

It is clear that there is concern to harness the knowledge of the learning style of the student to attend diversity and a more fair evaluation.

Other interesting vision, environment evaluation as a mechanism of motivation and learning, is presented by Dochy et al. Propose different mechanisms to make the assessment in a motivational tool, teaching and learning. Analyze the differences between self-assessment, peer assessment and co-assessment [12].

While Guzman and Conejo pose a cognitive assessment model based on adaptive testing for diagnosis in intelligent tutoring systems that apply AI techniques to guide the student during instruction [13].

It is clear that there is concern to harness the knowledge of the student's learning style in order to attend diversity and a more fair evaluation.

1.4 Research Focused in Evaluation of E-Learning

Learning assessment mediated by ICT is a subject in which authors as Mödritscher et al. [14], Odeh and Qaraeen [15], Tedman et al. [16] and Samarakou et al. [17] have worked. Focus their investigative work on issues associated with the teaching evaluation models [14], methods and techniques proposed for evaluation in E-Learning [15], addressing the evaluation of online learning as well as student assessment tools supported Artificial Intelligence of [17].

Harnessing ICTs as a mean to make a more specific assessment to support courses on e-learning, it has become a need.

1.5 Research Based on the Design and Application of Ontologies

In the last nine years, there have been studies in which the use of ontologies in e-learning and modeling of student profile is applied. Authors like Dahmani et al. [18], Rezgui et al. [19], Hosseini et al. [20], Hackelbusch [21], Capuano et al. [22], Mencke and Dumke [23] direct their research in the design and application of ontologies such as: E-learning resources modeling, ontologies based on learner profile [19], learning experiences based on semantics [22], didactic models [23], adaptive exercises using an automated evaluation and use of ontologies [18], ontologies for academic programs representation [21], customized E-learning ontologies [20].

An example of this is OMNIBUS, a declarative model belonging to learning theories and instructional design, from where an ontology based on learning states is constructed. It is focusing to build learning scenarios with a learning objects selection, which are suited to various states of learning. However, it does not consider two key points that must be present during the individual's learning: (1) motivation and (2) the learning individual preferences and cognitive skills to be developed during their learning experience [24].

1.6   Researches Focused on Learning Personalization and Teaching

We can consider some proposals around the learning personalization and teaching. Authors such as Colace et al. [25], Abik and Ajhoun [26], Jovanovic et al. [27], Saul and Wuttke [28], Swinke [29], have focusing their work on customizing learning situations [26], in customized E-assessment models generation [28], in customized learning tracking [25] and multidimensional models construction for personalized contents according to student profile [29].

A radical change in pedagogy is the learning personalization, such as Reload-LDE projects and ALFANET propose personalized learning platforms, but they do not consider all the individual characteristics of the participants. Abik and Ajhoun proposed a system that can transform a learning situation, depending on the context, into a more structured and customized learning situation [26]. This work is characterized by its flexibility, which allows you to manipulate the personalization criteria and the standardized profiles that provide the context of learning personalization in an LMS. To validate the model, they designed a normalization and personalization prototype for learning situations (NPLS) based on Java and XML.

Under the former scenario, it appears that the authors recognize the importance in consider the student learning style as a key element in the learning and learning assessment. Likewise, the concern arises to address the diversity and a more fair evaluation. Finally, from the computational standpoint, two authors applied the use of ontologies based on the profile of the learner [19] were located, and e-learning customization [20]. However, to attend diversity by customizing learning activities, applying a neuroscientific theory has not been studied.

1.7   Ontology for Personalized Learning Activities Based on a Cognitive Theory

Our research aims to determine the impact of customizing learning activities with cognitive development.

For this goal, we use the Ned Herrmann's Neuroscience Total Brain theory, which defines student thinking style on a brain metaphorical model, by dividing it into four quadrants: two upper corticals and two lower limbic. The model identifies how an individual perceives, learns, solves problems and makes decisions. Each brain areas or quadrants performs distinct functions: (a) left upper lobe is responsible for the logical, analytical, mathematical thinking and it based on concrete facts, so it focuses on the reasoning; (b) left lower lobe, it is characterized by a planned, controlled, organized, sequential and detailed thought style, it a very oriented on processes; (c) right lower lobe, maintains a humanistic, emotional and sensory thinking style it is symbolic, and it goes from the interpersonal to the spiritual; (d) right upper lobe, maintains a theoretical-conceptual, holistic and comprehensive way of thinking, it is responsible for integrating, while synthesizing, artistic, spatial, visual and creative [30]. With all of these, the student's thinking style is determined.

The works presented in this section addressing the student's learning style, but do not focus on the thinking style, neither applies a neuro-scientific theory. In addition, integrated architectures of type Virtual Learning Environment (VLE). In our work, we are incorporating the design and implementation of an ontological model that provides recommendations for personalizing learning activities based on Ned Herrmann's model, and therefore, a Virtual Learning Environment (VLE) personalized architecture is proposed.

2 Methodology

Methodology includes the architecture of Personalized Virtual Learning Environment (PVLE) design and an empirical work in two stages. The first stage focuses on the realization of a concept proof, for which is an empirical reference (Structured Programming course for engineering students at the Universidad Autónoma Metropolitana-Azcapotzalco) and an experimental unit, the factors considered, the information treatment for the parameters of evaluation and experiments for the fieldwork is established. This stage serves as a reference to align the test cases of the second stage.

At the conclusion of the first stage experiments, the model design and PVLE architecture and as well the ontology design for associated recommendations with customizing learning activities is carried out by applying the methodology for the Graphical Ontology Design Methodology (GODeM) [31].

GODeM the methodology comprises by the following steps:

1. Specify the domain of knowledge and scope of the ontology.
2. Identification of requirements ontology.
3. Validation of the possibility of using existing ontologies or metadata.
4. Ontological model design.
5. Implementation of the ontological model.
6. Populate classes.
7. Evaluation.
8. Document the ontology [31].

Finally, the ontological model is applied for personalizing learning activities for the Structured Programming course, and five experiments are performed in the second stage.

3 Personalized Virtual Learning Environment (PVLE) with a Ontological Model (OM)

The PVLE is an environment for learning, in it an ontological model, which enables recommendations for customizing activities learning, from cognitive skills you want to develop in students is integrated. In this section, the components of the architecture are described PVLE: Learning to Management System (LMS), the Virtual Learning Environment (VLE) and the Ontological Model (OM) [32]. The PVLE is part of the strategic learning meta-model [33] consists of a layer of infrastructure [32], an intelligent layer (OM) and a reactive layer.

3.1   LMS Architecture

LMS architecture includes the use of SAKAI (developed in Java) and is installed on virtualized servers to have a cloud solution. It requires a database server and an applications server, all deployed in a virtualization infrastructure as shown in Fig. 1.

3.2   VLE Architecture

VLE architecture consists of an application server and three frameworks; the first for the services centralization (Spring), the second for database mapping (Hibernate), and the third for controlling and Vista (Struts) implementation, implemented on a virtualized server, as is shown in Fig. 1.

Personalized Virtual Learning Environment (PVLE) that we are proposing is integrated by using the Ontological Model (OM) in the VLE, whose architecture is described in Sect. 3.3.

3.3   Ontological Model (OM) Architecture

The ontological model architecture integrates for an Apache Web Server, a Protégé framework for building intelligent system (open-source platform) and Pellet is using as reasoning, as shown in Fig. 1. OWL DL is used which is a standard description formal language for ontology specification. The ontology was modeled with OntoDesign Graphics [34]. In Sect. 4, the ontological model design is described by applying GODeM methodology [31].

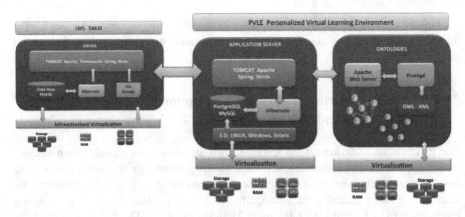

Fig. 1. PVLE architecture.

4 Study Case

The case study is comprised of two stages. In the first stage a concept testing is done, the objective of this is to have a reference point before applying the learning activities personalization. At this stage, two experiments are carried out in Fall 11 (11-F) and 12-Winter quarters (12-W).

The second stage integrates cases testing where the experiments are applying to engineering students during Structured Programming course (which aims to develop cognitive logic abilities, to active the creativity, encourage the students to learn how to analyze a problem and propose a solution by developing an algorithm and a program). In stage 2, 5 experiments were performed in the 12-Spring (12-S), 12-Fall (12-F), 13-Winter (13-W), 13-Spring (13-S) and 13-F (13-F) quarters. For model validity and for the proposed architecture, teaching modalities and no face-to-face course learning (CNP) and cooperative learning system (SAC) were used. Those courses were conducted to a large group of students (from 70 to 250 students per quarter).

The ontological model version 4, consists in four ontologies: profiles, students, courses and assessment activities. Those ontologies were designed by using GODeM and plotted with OntoDesign Graphics [34]. Finally, these ontologies were implemented by using Protégé.

4.1 Design of the Ontology Using the Methodology GODeM and OntoDesign Graphics Notation

The knowledge domain for personalizing learning activities is modeled based on two of the four ontologies: the ontology assessment activities; where different types of activities and technological tools sorted by the thinking style are integrated. And profiles ontology, where the Ned Herrmann's total brain cognitive theory is described and the description of the characteristics of each thinking style for dominant cerebral quadrant were stored, as is showing in Fig. 2.

4.2 Implementation of the Ontology Protégé

In order to build the knowledge domain model associated with learning activities personalization Protégé 5.0 was used. In Fig. 3, populated profiles data and assessment activities ontologies is shown.

4.3 Results

The results obtained in the concept test are shown in Table 1. The differences between the assessment initial values for the students' cognitive abilities in each quadrant seem to be very similar.

For the case tests, results show scores increase on student' cognitive skills assessment. In the first experiment no progress was presented. In the experiments two and three show significant improvement in all cognitive skills, with the highest scores on logic and process skills. While in the fourth and fifth experiment, scores show

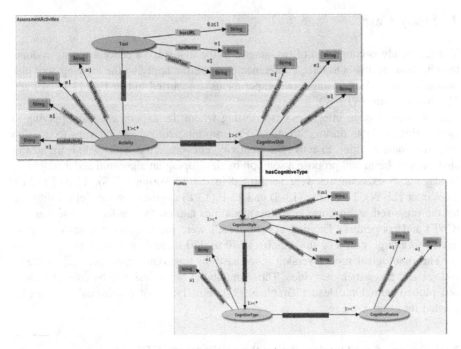

Fig. 2. Ontological model for the learning activities personalization designed by using OntoDesign Graphics.

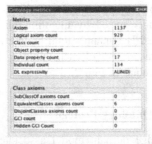

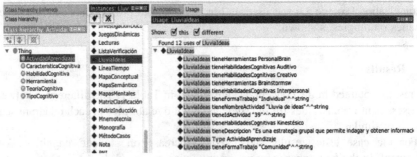

Fig. 3. Ontologies implementation by using Protégé.

Table 1. Results of the two experiments stage 1.

Period	11-Fall (11-O)		12-Winter (12-I)	
Thinking Style	Initial	Final	Initial	Final
Logic	10.5672	10.6213	10.3017	10.7743
Processes	10.4444	10.4319	10.8106	10.7782
Relational	10.9941	10.6331	11.5207	11.1128
Creative	11.4152	11.0473	11.2840	11.2062

Table 2. Results of experiments on stage 2.

Period	12-Spring (12-P)		12-Fall (12-O)		13-Winter (13-I)		13-Spring (13-P)		13-Fall (13-O)	
Thinking Style	Initial	Final	Initial	Final	Initial	Final	Initial	Final	Initial	Final
Logic	10.36	10.32	11.29	13.42	11.40	14.99	12.22	14.87	13.35	14.99
Processes	10.55	10.23	11.54	13.37	11.86	14.95	12.48	15.17	13.58	15.96
Relational	11.20	10.64	11.77	12.90	12.37	14.90	12.60	14.91	13.79	14.70
Creative	11.56	11.22	11.82	12.95	12.25	14.73	12.83	15.39	14.66	15.69

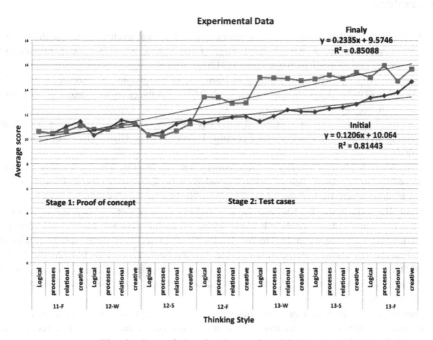

Fig. 4. Curve fitting for the results of fieldwork.

improvement in all cognitive students skills, obtaining a higher score on creative and process skills, as shown in Table 2.

Figure 4 shows adjusted curves for data experimental of experiment 7 made in fieldwork.

5 Conclusions

The results of two experiments in stage 1 of methodology (concept test), whereas learning activities personalization is not applied, the average scores for student's cognitive abilities were similar in both, initial and final stages. While for the last 4 experiments in stage 2 (test cases), where personalization of learning activities was applied, an increase in areas of creative, processing and logical thinking were observed.

Then, we can conclude that the personalization of learning activities has a positive impact on the development of cognitive skills of students. Our contribution is the incorporation of an OM; whose function is to recommend the types of learning activities and the technological tools, and the VLE architecture; which allows you to define a PVLE new architecture.

Future work will automate reactive layer meta-model of strategic learning, with the goal to provide an adaptive tracking learning activities personalization.

References

1. Smyth, K.: The benefits of students learning about critical evaluation rather than being summatively judged. J. Assess. Eval. High. Educ. **29**(3), 370–378 (2004). http://www.tandfonline.com/doi/pdf/10.1080/0260293042000197609
2. Sangster, A.: Objective tests, learning to learn and learning styles. J. Account. Educ. **5**(2), 131–146 (1996). https://www.academia.edu/1087355/Objective_tests_learning_to_learn_and_learining_styles
3. Cassidy, S.: Assessing 'inexperienced' students ability to self-assess: exploring links with learning style and academic personal control. J. Assess. Eval. High. Educ. **32**(3), 313–330 (2007)
4. García-Ros, R., Pérez-González, F.: Assessment preferences of pre-service teachers: analysis according to academic level and relationship with learning styles and motivational orientation. Teach. High. Educ. **16**(6), 719–731 (2011). doi:10.1080/13562517.2011.570434
5. Uğur, B., Akkoyunlu, B., Kurbanoğlu, S.: Students' opinions on blended learning and its implementation in terms of their learning styles. Educ. Inf. Technol. **16**(5), 5–23 (2011)
6. Verhoeven, J.C., Heerwegh, D., De Wit, K.: First year university students' self-perception of ICT skills: Do learning styles matter? Educ. Inf. Technol. **17**(1), 109–133 (2010). doi:10.1007/s10639-010-9149-1. http://download.springer.com/static/pdf/573/art%253A10.1007%252Fs10639-010-9149-1.pdf?auth66=1398547037_849a524bcd42be568e4d014600e5aea3&ext=.pdf
7. Burnett, C.: Medium for empowerment or a 'centre for everything': students' experience of control in virtual learning environments within a university context. Educ. Inf. Technol. **16**(3), 245–258 (2011)

8. Farrell, G., Leung, Y.: Innovative online assessment using confidence measurement. Educ. Inf. Technol. **9**(1), 5–19 (2004). http://link.springer.com/article/10.1023%2FB%3AEAIT. 0000024258.29560.3c#page-1

9. Marshall, G.: A trio of evaluation and assessment models from pre ICT innovations: lessons from the past. Educ. Inf. Technol. **15**(1), 37–50 (2010)

10. Kolb, D.: Experiential Learning. Prentice-Hall, Englewood Cliffs (1984)

11. Coll, C., Barberà, E., Onrubia, J.: La atención a la diversidad en las prácticas de evaluación. Infancia y Aprendizaje, GRINTIE **90**, 111–132 (2000)

12. Dochy, F., Segers, M.Y., Dierick, S.: Nuevas Vías de Aprendizaje y Enseñanza y sus Consecuencias: una Nueva Era de Evaluación. Revista de Docencia Universitaria, 2(2). Recuperado de http://revistas.um.es/redu/article/view/20051/19411

13. Guzmán, E., Conejo, R.: Self-assessment in a feasible. Adapt. Web-Based Test. Syst. IEEE Trans. Educ. **48**(4), 688–695 (2005)

14. Mödritscher, F., Andergassen, M., Lai-Chong, E., García-Barrios, V.: Application of learning curves for didactic model evaluation: case studies. Int. J. Emerg. Technol. Learn. **8**(4), 62–69 (2013)

15. Odeh, S., Qaraeen, O.: Evaluation methods and techniques for e-learning software for school students in primary stages. Int. J. Emerg. Technol. Learn. **2**(3), 1–8 (2007)

16. Tedman, R., Loudon, R., Wallace, B., Pountney, H.: Integrating regular, on-line evaluation by students into the curriculum review process in an Australian medical program. Int. J. Emerg. Technol. Learn. **4**(3), 59–66 (2009)

17. Samarakou, M., Papadakis, A., Fylladitakis, E., Hatziapostolou, A., Tsaganou, G., Gerrit, W.: An open learning environment for the diagnosis, assistance and evaluation of students based on artificial intelligence. Inter. J. Emerg. Technol. Learn. **9**(3), 36–44 (2014)

18. Dahmani, B., Mohammed, S., Catherine, C., Pierre, C.: Adaptive exercises generation using an automated evaluation and a domain ontology: the ODALA+ approach. Int. J. Emerg. Technol. Learn. **6**(2), 4–10 (2011)

19. Rezgui, K., Mhiri, H., Ghédira, K.: An ontology-based profile for learner representation in learning networks. Int. J. Emerg. Technol. Learn. **9**(3), 16–25 (2014)

20. Ali, S., Abdel-Rahman, T., Jahankhani, H., Yarandi, M.: Towards an ontological learners? Modelling approach for personalised e-learning. Int. J. Emerg. Technol. Learn. **8**(2), 4–10 (2013)

21. Hackelbusch, R.: Ontological representation of academic programs. Int. J. Emerg. Technol. Learn. **1**(3), 1–3 (2006)

22. Capuano, N., Mangione, G., Pierri, A., Salerno, S.: Personalization and contextualization of learning experiences based on semantics. Int. J. Emerg. Technol. Learn. **9**(7), 5–14 (2014)

23. Mencke, S., Dumke, R.: Didactical ontologies. Int. J. Emerg. Technol. Learn. **3**(1), 65–73 (2008)

24. Hayashi, Y., Bourdeau, J., Mizoguchi, R.: Using ontological engineering to organize learning/instructional theories and build a theory-aware authoring system. Int. J. Artif. Intell. Educ. **19**, 211–252 (2009)

25. Colace, F., De Santo, M., Greco, L.: E-learning and personalized learning path: a proposal based on the adaptive educational hypermedia system. Int. J. Emerg. Technol. Learn. **9**(2), 9–16 (2014)

26. Abik, M., Ajhoun, R.: Normalization and personalization of learning situation: NPLS. Int. J. Emerg. Technol. Learn. **4**(2), 4–10 (2009)

27. Jovanovic, D., Milosevic, D., Zizovic, M.: INDeLER: eLearning personalization by mapping student's learning style and preference to metadata. Int. J. Emerg. Technol. Learn. **3**(4), 41–50 (2008)

28. Saul, C., Wuttke, H.: An adaptation model for personalized e-assessments. Int. J. Emerg. Technol. Learn. **8**, 5–12 (2013)
29. Swinke, T.: A unique, culture-aware, personalized learning environment. Int. J. Emerg. Technol. Learn. **7**, 31–36 (2012)
30. Herrmann Ned, S.L.M.: The Creative Brain. Brain Books, Búfalo (1989)
31. Silva-López, R.B., Silva-López, M.I., Méndez-Gurrola, I., Bravo, M., Sánchez, V.: GODeM: a graphical ontology design methodology. Res. Comput. Sci. **84**(2014), 17–28 (2014)
32. Silva-López, R.B., Méndez-Gurrola, I.I., Herrera, O.: Metamodelo de aprendizaje estratégico (MAE): Arquitectura de la capa de infraestructura, solución basada en la cloud computing. Res. Comput. Sci. **93**(2015), 175–188 (2015)
33. Silva-López, R., Méndez-Gurrola, I., Sánchez-Arias, V.: Strategic learning, towards a teaching reengineering. Res. Comp. Sci. **65**(2013), 133–145 (2013)
34. Silva-López, R.B., Silva-López, M., Méndez-Gurrola, I.I., Bravo, M.: Onto design graphics (ODG): a graphical notation to standardize ontology design. In: Gelbukh, A., Espinoza, F.C., Galicia-Haro, S.N. (eds.) MICAI 2014, Part I. LNCS, vol. 8856, pp. 443–452. Springer, Heidelberg (2014)

Open Student Model for Blended Training in the Electrical Tests Domain

Yasmín Hernández[(✉)] and Miguel Pérez

Gerencia de Tecnologías de la Información,
Instituto de Investigaciones Eléctricas,
Reforma 113, Palmira, 62490 Cuernavaca, Morelos, Mexico
{myhp,mperez}@iie.org.mx

Abstract. Electrical tests are important because they anticipate problems. When they are erroneously performed, human accidents or equipment damage can occur; thus, efficient training is mandatory. Traditional training under supervision of human instructors has proved to be successful; but it is costly and takes a long time. We need to complement traditional training with computers systems which adapt the training to particular trainee and shorten the training time. We have defined a blended learning model to support adaptive and distance training for complementing traditional training. We have defined an open trainee model to represent how much trainees know and how they feel. The model is used by instructors to adapt instruction, and by trainees to know what needs to be reinforced. The trainee model is represented by Bayesian networks and the instruction is presented via a virtual reality system. This paper presents the open trainee model and current results on using it.

Keywords: Electrical tests · Bayesian networks · Blended learning · Open student model · Virtual reality

1 Introduction

Performing electrical tests in substations is very important because they allow foreseeing problems, which might otherwise end up damaging substation equipment and in turn originating power interruptions. When electrical tests are erroneously performed, they might originate human accidents or equipment damage. Thus, efficient training is mandatory in order to ensure optimal operation of the substations.

Traditional training includes two ingredients, namely classroom training and camp practice. However, it faces some problematic situations, for instance: the knowledge about electrical tests is not easily available to students and opportunity to practice in a real substation is limited. Moreover training might be unaffordable and could take a long time.

In traditional training, camp practice and face-to-face instruction are very important as they have proven to be efficient [4, 21]. However due to the need for training more electricians in less time and with less cost, we have complemented traditional training with computers systems.

O. Pichardo Lagunas et al. (Eds.): MICAI 2015, Part II, LNAI 9414, pp. 195–207, 2015.
DOI: 10.1007/978-3-319-27101-9_14

We have developed a virtual reality system (VRS) for supporting training in electrical tests. Trainees still attend classroom courses and have camp practice but they complement learning and practice aided by this VRS before attending the camp training [28].

The system allows self-training and has helped to improve training; moreover both costs and training time have been reduced. However, the system does not allow yet adaptive training. In this way the VRS represents the starting point of intelligent and adaptive training where the individual state of trainees is considered, in such a way that the instruction adapts to trainee' needs intelligently.

Thus, we have defined a blended learning model. Blended learning (b-learning) is a new term and an innovative model in education although the concept has already existed for a long time. It can take many forms and there are several definitions which include roughly the same elements. A general and perhaps the most accepted definition states that blended learning is learning that is facilitated by the effective combination of different delivery modes, models of teaching and styles of learning, and founded on transparent communication amongst all parties involved in a course [13].

The blended training process includes three actors which have a strong relationship, namely: trainees, instructors and the training platform [20]. The instructor and the training platform have to adapt to the needs of the trainee. In order to achieve an adaptive training, we have defined an open student model to represents how much trainees know. Open learner models are student models that are accessible to the user, usually the student being modeled, but sometimes also to other users [7].

In our proposal, instructors can see the trainee model in order to adapt their instruction, and also can design new training and testing material based on the trainee model. Trainees can see the model to know which electrical test, they need to reinforce. We are especially interested in providing trainees with tools for self-assessment, since it is one of the meta-cognitive skills necessary for effective learning. Students need to be able to critically assess their knowledge in order to decide what they need to study [23]. Also, we include in the trainee model the affective state of the student with the aim of adapting the instruction based on both the affective and the knowledge states.

In this paper we present the blended learning model and describe the trainee model. We also present the current results of applying the blended learning model in a Mexican utility. The rest of the paper is organized as follows: Sect. 2 describes some related work. Section 3 describes the blended training model and the virtual reality system. Section 4 presents the trainee model. Finally, some conclusions and future work are presented in Sect. 5.

2   Related Work

There are multiples examples of applications of blended learning, not only in Universities but also in companies, some few examples are: AulaWeb, a blended learning system, is a successful application in the Polytechnic University of Madrid, [5]. Positive appraisal in the acquisition of competences by the students is reported in [3]; so much in the comprehension of the purposes and processes of the learning as in the achievement of the competences planned. They applied an electronic portfolio as a tool to evaluate two courses in the Pedagogy program. In Centra, a software company, is exemplified the use of blended collaborative learning principles in a new employee orientation program [29]. Beyond the short initial kickoff session, the remainder of these events takes place in the employee's work context over an extended period of time - minimizing the employee's time- to productivity while fostering internalization and application of key learning in the job context [29].

In fact, the benefits of blended learning have originated a tendency in universities and institutes around the world to integrate it in their teaching/learning activities, some few examples are: Lancaster University, U. of Leeds, Babson in Massachusetts, IEEE BL Program in VLSI, Nipissing University in Canada, U. of de Air in Japan, Clark County School District in Las Vegas, U. of Yale, U. of Stanford, Waterloo university, U of Western Sydney, etc.

Regarding Virtual Reality (VR), it is a technology for which an extensive literature has presented diverse arguments and evidences as an excellent tool for teaching and training [6, 10, 27]. There are many applications of VR as a training tool reported in the literature, some of them fall within electrical substation environments, most of these are devoted to train on substation operation [2, 11, 12, 22]. Only some few are devoted to maintenance work in substations [1, 9, 28].

In other fields, such as in medicine, it is reported a comparative study in which two groups of novice students are trained in Laparoscopic Cholecystectomyce (LC) using Blended Learning (BL) [24]; where VR group completed the LC significantly faster and more often within 80 min than BL. The BL group scored higher than the VR group in the knowledge test and both groups showed equal operative performance of LC in the OSATS (Objective Structured Assessment of Technical Skills) score. These authors suggest that multimodality training programs should be developed that combine the advantages of both approaches. On this stance, there is also the term Blended Reality (BR), which is defined as an interactive mixed-reality environment where the physical and the virtual are intimately combined in the service of interaction goals and communication environments [19], where is intended to take advantage of the potentials in combining virtual worlds and face-to-face classes.

It makes sense that having two or more technologies, they all presenting benefits in the learning/teaching activities, a combination of them is expected to increment benefits for learning. This is also in accordance with the multidimensional model presented in [27].

3   Blended Training Model

Blended learning has emerged as a response to the need of having the benefits of face-to-face interaction with the advantages of new technologies. A general and perhaps the most accepted definition states that blended learning is learning that is facilitated by the effective combination of different modes of delivery, models of teaching and styles of learning, and founded on transparent communication amongst all parties involved with a course [13].

The training program on electrical tests is very detailed and very strict. A trainee has to accredit the classroom courses but he also must have camp practice with the close supervision of an instructor. In this traditional training the trainees spend a lot of time and also the training becomes costly.

We have developed a blended training model to train electricians which allows adapting the instruction to particular needs. The aim is to have efficient, fast and safe training, and also to reduce training costs.

In this blended model, the trainees learn through three elements: (i) an instructor in a face-to-face interaction, (ii) a VRS and (iii) camp practice.

The instructor teaches trainees in classroom based on a course plan which includes theoretical lessons and practice in the VRS. Separately, trainees can learn and practice with the VRS as much as they want; this is in a self-learning modality. When trainees have attended the appropriate courses they have to serve as auxiliary electrician to have camp practice in a real substation.

The training course is planned by an instructor; he decides topics and designs the course in the system. In classroom, the instructor explains theoretical concepts and shares its experience in the performance of electrical tests. Also, the instructor describes the electrical tests, its steps and sub-steps relying in the VRS system.

The trainee attends the course and practices the electrical tests included in the course by using the VRS, however he can use the VRS as distance self-training tool. The training and examination material were carefully developed and designed by a team of experts on electrical tests and training.

A key element of this blended model is a trainee model that is built based on the interaction of trainees with the three training elements. This model represents the knowledge and affective states of trainees. The information in the trainee model is useful for instructors to adapt the instruction in classroom, to plan the camp practice, to recommend attending other training courses or finally to grant a certification. This trainee model can be useful to design new courses and new examination materials and even to redesign training material.

Nevertheless, the aim of the open student model is to adapt the instruction, currently this is not the case; since the electrical tests have to be thought in a sequence of steps and it is hard to try adapting its strict structure. However, trainees and instructors adapt themselves according to the trainee model, in this way; we have an open trainee model.

The trainee affect is used by an empathic animated agent to present the instruction properly. We are using the characteristics of the operators for developing the agent, such as wearing the uniform and safety helmet, among other features. We believe that by representing the tutor as an electrician, operators will accept better the training environment. Empathy is the ability to perceive, understand and experience others' emotions, in other words, step into the shoes of another. This construct has been incorporated in animated agents with the aim to achieve credibility, social interaction and user engagement [18].

The b-model also includes the representation of the trainee's affect and it is used by an empathic agent which presents the instruction in a suitable way. The affective state of trainees is recognized by interaction with the VRS. The empathic agent shows facial expressions to motivate trainees. The blended training model is presented in Fig. 1.

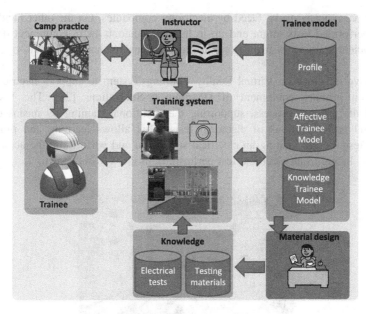

Fig. 1. Blended training model. The model has three components: classroom classes, VR system and camp practice. These three components can be adapted according to the open student model. The instruction is presented by means of an empathic agent.

3.1   VRS for Electrical Test Training

In an overall view, electrical tests consist of a sequence of steps where the equipment to be tested has to be bypassed so that is not energized. Then the testing equipment is connected to the primary equipment under test, and outcomes of the tests are recorded. If not other tests is performed, then the testing equipment is disconnected and removed, finally the primary equipment under test is connected again and reestablished. It should be mentioned that in every step safety regulations and measures must be observed [8]. Figure 2 shows the performance of an electrical test.

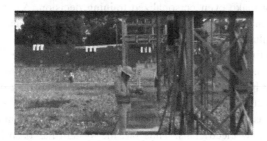

Fig. 2. Bypassing an interrupter. This works is previous to electrical tests performance.

Electrical tests in substations allow foreseeing possible problems, which might end up damaging substation equipment and in turn originating interruptions, which is the last situation expected to be faced by electricity companies. On the other hand, erroneously performed tests might end up in human accidents or in equipment damage. Thus, efficient training is mandatory in order to ensure that substations operate in optimally.

We have developed a Virtual Reality Training System to support electrical tests learning on primary equipment of Distribution Substations [28]. The VRS has improved the training process, supporting the traditional training by means of presenting 3D representations of electrical tests. This allows learning and practicing electrical tests before visiting an electrical substation and performing the actual electrical tests. In Fig. 3 an electrical test performing in the VRS is shown.

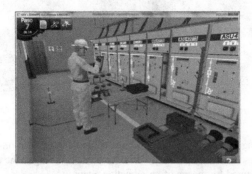

Fig. 3. Performing the electrical tests for metal clad switchboards.

The system includes 40 electrical tests to different primary equipment such as transformers, interrupters, capacitors bank, and so on. Among the tests, we can mention isolation resistance, power factor, and operation time.

This kind of systems provides advantages derived from 3D representations. For instance, the system contains different catalogs of 3D models of tools, equipment, materials and safety gear; it also includes a 3D virtual substation. Thus, trainees can visualize 3D tools and navigate virtually a substation. This allows students to familiarize with all items used when tests are performed. It allows self-learning and provides supports for classroom courses, since it is able to keep records of trainees' progress so that instructors can make even personalized training decision. As in real work, electrical tests are presented as sequences of steps. On each step, explanations are provided and activities are illustrated using 3D animations.

The main objective of the system is to complement and enhance traditional method of training. Nevertheless, the risk of electroshock or damage to equipment, still demands that only human experts can certify trainees, when they consider they are ready to realize electrical tests by themselves.

The system is installed in the 16 distribution areas across the country. This benefits some hundreds of new electricians. Thus far, the system has been helpful as a supporting tool to improve training. Nevertheless other technologies can be integrated to our VR systems, so that they can exhibit intelligent and adaptive behaviors which improve them as training tools. With this aim we propose an open student model and it is described in the next section.

4 Trainee Model

The core of the blended learning model is the trainee model which is a representation of the state of the trainee. The model is built as the trainee learns the theoretical concepts included in the classroom lessons, practices in the VRS and attends camp practice. The trainee model includes the knowledge of the trainee about the electrical tests included in the course, the affective state of the trainee and his profile. The trainee model is useful for the instructor and for the trainee; in modalities of self-learning and course. The trainee model is composed as shown in Fig. 4.

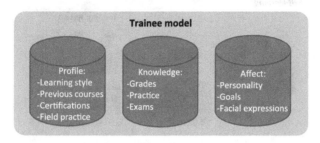

Fig. 4. Trainee model. The model represents the state of trainee, which includes the knowledge and affective states and the trainee's profile.

The profile contains information about previous courses that the trainee has attended and preferences on learning. The profile is built the first time the student visits the training system and is updated when the course is attended by the trainee, when the course is over and when the student gains a certification. The outcomes of the camp practice are registered by the instructor. Our proposal for detecting the affective state of the trainees is described in [16].

The knowledge model is updated when the trainee practices the electrical tests and when he solves theoretical exams. The affect model is updated as the trainee interacts with the training system; the emotions are modeled through the achievement of goals and with facial expressions.

In the course modality, the instructor can see the model in order to adapt the instruction, give recommendations to trainees and provide grades and certifications. Trainees can see the model to practice the electrical test that they have not learnt yet. Neither the instructor nor the trainee can see the affective model, because we do not know accurately if this is useful for learning. We need to conduct some studies to investigate what is the impact of the awareness of the trainee about what the training system knows about him, regarding his affective and knowledge states.

In the self-learning modality, trainees can practice all the time as they want. However, self-learning is separated from the course; that is, in self-learning modality a parallel trainee model is built. The model can be seen by trainee as in the course modality. Currently, instructors do not see this model and the trainee model in self-learning modality is not taken into account in the development of the course.

Besides to modeling the knowledge of the trainee, his affective state is also modeled. The trainee can see the representation of his knowledge but he cannot see the representation of his affect. We need more analysis about the effects of awareness the representation of the affect by trainees and instructors. Currently the affect is only used by the empathic agent to present the instruction accordingly to the trainee affective state. A description of the empathic agent is presented in [14]. In Fig. 5 the interaction with the trainee model in the self-learning modality is presented, and in Fig. 6 the interaction in the course modality is presented.

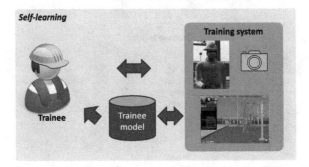

Fig. 5. Self-learning modality. The trainee can see the representation of his knowledge state in the trainee model, and so that he can reinforce its learning.

Since the electrical test is composed by many steps and many sub-steps, in the task of evaluating the knowledge of the student, there are many factors that impact the results of a practice or exam such as guesses and slips. In order to minimize this impact, we have modeled the impact of knowing a sub-step in knowing a step, and in turn its impact in knowing the electrical test, besides having the precise answer of the trainee.

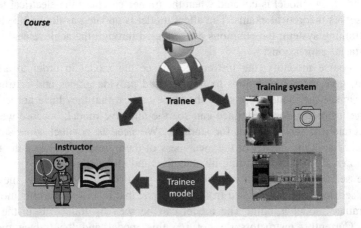

Fig. 6. Course modality. The trainee can see the representation of his knowledge state in the trainee model, and reinforce his learning. The instructor can see the representation of the trainee and so that adapt the instruction.

But this process involves uncertainty; therefore the model relies on Bayesian reasoning which provides strong mechanisms to work with any minimal evidence in order to manage uncertainty [26].

The Bayesian network is built when the instructor design a course. The Bayesian network is composed by a node for each electrical test included in the course and a node for an exam which comprises the items of the theoretical exam also designed by the instructor. In turn, each node of the Bayesian network representing a test is a Bayesian network composed by steps and sub-steps. This Bayesian network represents how trainees have performed the electrical tests. In Fig. 7 a test with four steps is shown; but most electrical tests have an average of 40 steps.

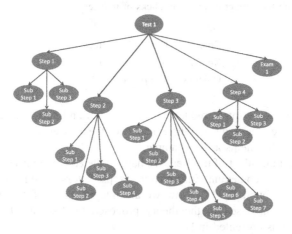

Fig. 7. Bayesian network for an electrical test with four steps. The knowledge about electrical test is impacted by the knowledge of each step and a theoretical exam.

Initially, each node representing a sub-step has two possible values: known and unknown which correspond to the possible result of performing the sub-step (to execute an instruction). The nodes representing steps have two possible values: learnt and not learnt and their probabilities are conditionally dependent on the probabilities of the sub-step nodes. Step nodes represent the probability that the trainee has learnt the step. Test nodes also have two values: acquired and not acquired and their probabilities are conditionally dependent on the probabilities of the step nodes.

The evidence for sub-steps nodes comes from the trainee' movements when he is practicing in the VRS, that is to say, the probability of knowing a sub-step comes from the correct or incorrect clicks. We have configured the conditional probabilities table (CPT) of sub-steps nodes with parameters p and q which are calculated based on the numbers of sub-step intents and numbers of test tries. Currently, we have the configuration for sub-steps showed at Fig. 8 and the CPT is shown in Table 1.

The theoretical exam is also represented by a Bayesian network composed by a number of items. The causal relationships between items and conditional probabilities for each node will be established when the exam is designed by the instructor. For the time being, we have not defined the complete structure and values of this Bayesian

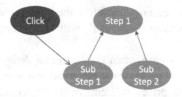

Fig. 8. Fragment of Bayesian network for an electrical test. The click node represents the evidence of knowing or not the sub-step.

Table 1. Conditional probabilities table for sub-step nodes. The probability of knowing a sub-step comes from the correct or incorrect clicks of trainees.

Sub-step		
Click	Correct	Incorrect
Known	p	$1 - q$
Unknown	$1 - p$	q

network. However we want to model trainee' guesses and slips on the basis of the relationships between the items and the evidence of the answers to questions. Figure 9 shows an exam with 8 items as an example.

We also model the affect of trainees. We have modeled emotions as stated by OCC [25], which use the contextual information as predictors of emotion. A detailed description can be found in [17]. Now we are integrating the facial expressions as indicators of emotion based in the theory proposed by Ekman. Our proposal for affective modeling is presented in [14].

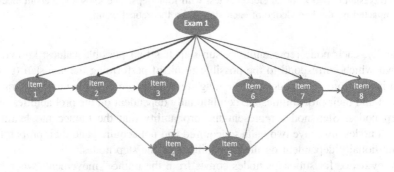

Fig. 9. Bayesian network for an exam including eight items. This structure represents only the relationship between topics of the items.

5 Conclusions and Future Work

There are domains where learners can self-learn using a system whose instructional content is comprehensive and really well done. In such cases the presence of instructor might not be determinant for trainees. Nevertheless, electrical tests procedures involve physical activity, which is not provided by a computer system. Computer systems, even

VR systems, are still limited with respect to the real electrical tests performance, there are physical actions such as claiming up a transformer, removing cables or taking care of safety regulations within specific circumstances, whose expertise cannot be obtained by using a system, but in the actual work. This is why, it is responsibility of a human instructor who will have to cover the physical and practical training and verify the skills of the trainees. Thus, the system is a helpful complementary training tool which can be used to enhance the traditional training but it cannot be used instead of it.

On the other hand, in order to have an efficient instruction, it is necessary an adaptive training to specific need of trainees. We model the knowledge and affect of trainees. Due to strict order in the performance of electrical tests, we do have a complete adaptable instruction, for the time being, we have composed an open student model which allows instructors to adapt the instruction to the progress of the trainees and it also allows trainees to know which electrical tests needs to be reinforced.

We are working in the adaptation of the instruction base on the student model. As future work we are planning to conduct a study to evaluate the open trainee model as a self-evaluation tool.

In the blended learning model, we include an empathic agent to present the instruction. We have conducted a study to evaluate the animated agent with encouraging outcomes [14], which will be used to guide the refining the agent.

In this paper we described our blended learning model for learning electrical tests, and we propose an open student model that models the progress of trainees on mastering the electrical tests. The aim of the model is to help trainees to improved learning and support instructors to know the progress of trainees, make recommendations and adapt his own instruction.

References

1. Akiyoshi, M., Miwa, S., Nishida, S.: The application of virtual reality technology to maintenance task of substations. Mitsubishi Denki Giho **70**(6), 34–38 (1996)
2. Arroyo, E., Los Arcos, J.L.: SRV: a virtual reality application to electrical substations operation training. In: IEEE International Conference on Multimedia Computing and Systems, vol. 1, pp. 835–839 (1999)
3. Barragán, R., García, R., Buzón, O., Rebollo, M.A., Vega, L.: E-portfolio in blended-learning processes: Assessment innovations in the European Credits Transfer System. RED Revista de Educación a Distancia, no. VIII (2009)
4. Bejerano, A.R.: Face-to-face or online instruction? Face-to-face is better. In: Communication Currents Knowledge for Communicating Well, vol. 3, no. 3. National Communication Association (2008)
5. Bravo, J.L., Sánchez, J.A., Farjas, M.: El uso de sistemas de b-learning en la enseñanza universitaria. Universidad Politécnica de Madrid (2004)
6. Burdea, G.C., Coiffet, P.: Virtual Reality Technology. Wiley Interscience, New York (2003)
7. Bull, S., Kay, J.: Open learner models. In: Nkambou, R., Bourdeau, J., Mizoguchi, R. (eds.) Advances in Intelligent Tutoring Systems. SCI, vol. 308, pp. 301–322. Springer, Heidelberg (2010)

8. CFE: Handbook of Electrical Test procedures, Comisión Federal de Electricidad. Technical report in Spanish (2003)
9. Chang, Z., Fang, Y., Zhang, Y., Hu, C.: A training simulation system for substation equipments maintenance. In: International Conference on Machine Vision and Human-Machine Interface, MVHI 2010, pp. 572–575 (2010)
10. Chen, C., Toh, S.C., Fauzy, W.M. The theoretical framework for designing desktop virtual reality-based learning environments. J. Interact. Learn. Res. (2004)
11. Frank, P.: Using simulations to provide safety and operations training in the electric power industry. IEEE Eng. Soc. Winter Meet. 2, 986–988 (1999)
12. Garant, E., Malowant, A.: A virtual reality training system for substation operators (1997)
13. Heinze, A., Procter, C.: Reflections on the use of Blended Learning. University of Salford (2004)
14. Hernández, Y., Pérez, M., Zatarain, R., Barrón, L., Alor, G.: Submitted to Special Issue on Intelligent and Affective Learning Environments: New trends and Challenges of Journal of Educational Technology and Society (2015)
15. Yasmín, H., Miguel, P.: A B-learning model for training within electrical tests domain. Res. Comput. Sci. 87, 43–52 (2014)
16. Hernández, Y., Rodriguez, G.: Learning styles theory for intelligent learning environments. In: Proceedings of CSEDU, pp. 456–459 (2011)
17. Hernández, Y., Sucar, L.E., Arroyo-Figueroa, G.: Affective modeling for an intelligent educational environment. In: Peña-Ayala, A. (ed) Intelligent and Adaptive Educational-Learning Systems: Achievements and Trends. Smart Innovation, Systems and Technologies, vol. 17, no. XII, pp. 3–24. Springer, Berlin (2012)
18. Hone, K.: Empathic agents to reduce user frustration: the effects of varying agent characteristics. Interact. Comput. 18(2), 227–245 (2006)
19. Hoshi, K., Pesola, U.M., Waterworth, E.L., Waterworth, J.: Tools, perspectives and avatars in blended reality space. Stud. Health Technol. Inform. 144, 91–95 (2009)
20. Martín, M., Álvarez, A., Ruiz, S., Fernández-Castro, I., Urretavizcaya, M.: Helping teachers to track student evolution in a B-learning environment. In: Proceeding of IEEE International Conference on Advanced Learning Technologies, pp. 342–346 (2009)
21. Means, B., Toyama, Y., Murphy, R., Bakia, M., Jones, K.: Evaluation of evidence-based practices in online learning: a meta-analysis and review of online learning studies. In: Center for Technology in Learning (2010)
22. Meng, F., Kan, Y.: An improved virtual reality engine for substation simulation. In: 2nd International Conference on Future Computer and Communication (ICFCC), vol. 1, pp. 846–849 (2010)
23. Mitrović, A., Martin, B.: Evaluating the effects of open student models on learning. In: De Bra, P., Brusilovsky, P., Conejo, R. (eds.) AH 2002. LNCS, vol. 2347, pp. 296–305. Springer, Heidelberg (2002)
24. Nickel, F., Brzoska, J.A., Gondan, M., Rangnick, H.M., Chu, J., Kenngott, H.G., Linke, G.R., Kadmon, M., Fischer, L., Müller-Stich, B.P.: Virtual reality training versus blended learning of laparoscopic cholecystectomy: a randomized controlled trial with laparoscopic novices. Medicine 94(20), 764 (2015)
25. Ortony, A., Clore, G.L., Collins, A.: The Cognitive Structure of Emotions. Cambridge University Press, Cambridge (1988)
26. Pearl, J.: Causality: Models, Reasoning, and Inference. Cambridge University Press, Cambridge (2000)
27. Pérez-Ramírez, M., Ontiveros-Hernández, N.J.: Virtual reality as a comprehensive training tool. In: Proceedings of Workshop on Intelligent Learning Environments WILE, pp. 203–215 (2009)

28. Pérez, M., Santiago, J., Zayas, B., Islas, E., Hernández, I., Rodríguez, Y., Espinoza, C.: Capacitación en Pruebas a Subestaciones de Distribución utilizando Realidad Virtual. In: Proceedings of CIINDET (2014)
29. Singh, H., Reed, C.: A white paper: achieving success with blended learning. Centra Software (2001)

Applying Data Mining Techniques to Identify Success Factors in Students Enrolled in Distance Learning: A Case Study

José Gerardo Moreno Salinas[1(✉)] and Christopher R. Stephens[2]

[1] Coordinación de Universidad Abierta y Educación a Distancia
(CUAED) – UNAM, Coyoacán, Mexico
gerardo_moreno@cuaed.unam.mx
[2] Centro de Ciencias de la Complejidad (C3) e Instituto de Ciencias
Nucleares – UNAM, Mexico City, Mexico
stephens@nucleares.unam.mx

Abstract. Distance learning is now a key component in higher level education. Given the high dropout rates and the important investments in distance learning it is of utmost concern to determine the most critical data in the success and failure of students. In this article we data mine enrollment profiles, educational background and students´ data from the Open University System and Distance Learning of the National Autonomous University of Mexico to determine the key factors that drive success and failure, creating a relevant predictive model using a Naive Bayes classifier. We have found that the number of subjects approved and their average qualification in the first semester are part of the most interesting predictors of student success.

Keywords: Distance learning · Keys to success · Data mining · Naive Bayes classifier

1 Introduction

The global population aged to study higher education is increasingly considering distance education as the first and best choice. At the same time, the number of universities that offer courses online is growing. Some of the main advantages of distance learning for a student are: (i) flexible learning hours better adapted to work and family life; (ii) ability to set their own pace of study; and, (iii) greater efficiency and less wasted time commuting to a fixed place of learning. On the other hand, distance education requires a greater commitment to self-management of study time. The benefit of group learning and social peer support is also lacking despite the existence of chats and other on-line social forums.

In 2012, the United States Department of Education reported that of 18,236,340 students enrolled in undergraduate education, 11 % were enrolled in distance education only and 14.2 % were enrolled in at least one distance learning course. In the case of Mexico, the Open University System and Distance Education (SUAyED, acronym in Spanish) of the National Autonomous University of Mexico (UNAM, acronym in

© Springer International Publishing Switzerland 2015
O. Pichardo Lagunas et al. (Eds.): MICAI 2015, Part II, LNAI 9414, pp. 208–219, 2015.
DOI: 10.1007/978-3-319-27101-9_15

Spanish), has registered approximately 27,000 students in a range of careers between 2005–2015.

Furthermore, the constant growth in the number of students in the system, there is also the data we get from them, for example: Entry profiles, educational background and enrollment data. The data may contain essential information to improve the quality of education, with the potential to customize the learning experiences of the students [1].

The school dropout and identifying success factors of students in higher education has been a concern for everyone involved in the education; in particular for the distance mode, [2] Which investigated that various authors said they agreed with "dropout rates from distance education that are generally higher than those in conventional education. Many students are easily leaving online learning courses and programs or finishing without satisfaction".

When we talk about the success that SUAyED students can achieve, we refer to the possibility of getting 100 % of the credits of their career in ten semesters (curriculum time). Since 2009 the SUAyED in distance learning started to have the first students with the success characteristics aforementioned. On average, 6 % of students who began their studies have completed total credits in curriculum time, which is worrying since many efforts in terms of human resources, development time and online courses implementation have been invested, as well as the technological infrastructure in order to provide high quality distance education.

As much as dropout rates are considered an indicator of quality in distance education [3, 4] if students completed all their credits in curricular times it will certainly help to improve quality indicators.

Therefore, it became necessary to identify from those who have already finished their studies, the success factors that determined the achievement of the 100 % of credits in curriculum time. A review in the literature was made to achieve this where many analyses and case studies describe the relevance of performing data mining over academic data. Even the term "Educational Data Mining" is already common [5].

Data mining algorithms examined with multiple data such as (gender, age, occupation and courses) from 510 online students who got the best results with Naive Bayes algorithm [6].

From a study made by [6], to address the problem of dropout in the Hellenic Open University, compared six data mining algorithms and concluded that Naive Bayes algorithm is the most appropriate technique for predicting dropout.

A good example of the potential of doing studies of data mining in education is the case presented by [7], they used a questionnaire of 37 questions in five sections which included demographics data and perspectives of students in online courses. In that study, researchers used data mining algorithms to predict the academic success of the students, and found that students who publish questions, answers and surf in the Internet tend to get higher scores.

The advantage of developing a data mining study instead of continue doing traditional statistics is to illustrate the following example: suppose John Smith is a minority student in the first year of college. Data mining asks the question, "Will John Smith return to college for his sophomore year?" A hypothesis based research question asks, "Are minority students liable as other students to return to college?" [1].

This means, data mining has the ability to provide very specific information, whereas the statistics will establish possibilities between more general data set.

The above mentioned examples strengthen the relevance of developing an analysis of data mining techniques where the Naive Bayes classification algorithm is implemented, with the purpose of developing the predictor model of the success factors of SUAyED students in distance education courses. All studies show that academic success depends on multiple factors of students, such as: qualifications, personality, expectations and sociological background [8].

2 Methodology

To identify the most important factors of the students' success, we used the following data mining methodology, which describes the steps to be followed for data selection, feature selection, model creation and model performance analysis (Fig. 1).

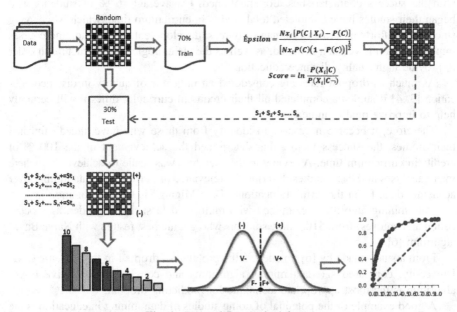

$$\acute{E}psilon = \frac{Nx_i\left[P(C\mid X_i)-P(C)\right]}{\left[Nx_iP(C)(1-P(C))\right]^{\frac{1}{2}}}$$

$$Score = \ln \frac{P(X_i\mid C)}{P(X_i\mid C\neg)}$$

Fig. 1. Data mining methodology

From the total number of students enrolled in distance learning at SUAyED we selected those who had been studying for ten semesters. It´s necessary to define the class for analysis and identify the entry profiles, educational background and enrollment data in the first semester. For a later integration of all of them into a relational database. The data was divided randomly into a training set (70 %) and a test set (30 %). On the training data the Epsilon and Score measures were calculated; these measures allowed to have another dimension of analysis for each descriptor of the students and their categories, thus making the identifying process and selection of variables easier to be considered for the classifier model.

Once the all the Score were selected by category, these were assigned to the 30 % of the test data. Subsequently all the Score by instances were added and the final results were sorted in a descending order to graph the distribution of the classifier model by deciles and see the discrimination made between classes. With the confusion matrix and their measure, the performance of the classification model was evaluated. Finally, the model was plotted in a ROC (Receiver Operating Characteristic) curve to examine the ability of the classifier model to identify and predict of the true positive rate against the false positive rate.

3 Data Collection

From the total number of students enrolled in distance education, only those with ten semesters concluded in the SUAyED were taken into consideration. The following figure shows the entry semesters that satisfy this condition (Fig. 2).

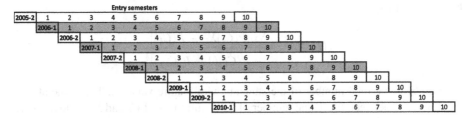

Fig. 2. Entry semester (In 2006-1, 2007-1 and 2008-1 there were no calls for distance learning)

The target population consists of 2,889 students, 6 % (177) out of which complied with all of their credits in the stipulated time frame. The next chart shows the distribution by entrance semester and class type (Table 1).

Table 1. Student by entry semester and class type

Entrance semester	Class		Total
	Yes	No	
2005-2	26	209	235
2006-2	12	240	252
2007-2	20	349	369
2008-2	21	353	374
2009-1	0	45	45
2009-2	26	313	339
2010-1	72	1,203	1,275
Total	**177**	**2,712**	**2,889**

The class is an identifier that classifies the students into two groups, the first group is made up of students who accumulated 100 % of the required credits after ten semesters (1) and the second refers to the students who did not accumulate the required credits in that time frame (0) (Table 2).

For each student we had access to the following data (displayed according to source, descriptor and category), which was analysed to determine its potential impact on academic success.

The Naive Bayes algorithm [9, 10] is a classification algorithm based on Bayes' theorem, which assumes that the predictors $X = \{X_1, X_2 \ldots X_m\}$ are conditionally independent. Thus, we write the posterior conditional probability $P(C_k|X)$ as

$$P(C_k|X) = \frac{P(X|C_k)P(C_k)}{P(X)} = \frac{\prod_{i=1}^{N} P(X_i|C_k)}{P(X)} \tag{1}$$

Where the product is over the N variables chosen by the feature selection process for the classifier. A useful diagnostic to determine the predictability of the X_i is a binomial test [9]

$$\varepsilon(C_k|X_i) = \frac{Nx_i[P(C_k|X_i) - P(C_k)]}{[Nx_jP(C_k)(1 - P(C_k))]^{\frac{1}{2}}} \tag{2}$$

Where Nx_j is the total number of the students with feature value X_i. The numerator is the difference between the actual number of co-occurrences of C_k and X_i, relative to the expected number if the class distribution were obtained by a binomial with sampling probability of $P(C_k)$. If we can approximate the binomial by a normal approximation then, $\varepsilon(C_k|X_i) = 1.96$ represents the 95 % significance level [9].

Epsilon determines which features to include in the score function that represents the classifier. Using the Naive Bayes approximation the score function is:

$$S(C_k|X) = \sum_{i=1}^{N} S(C_k|X_i) = \sum_{i=1}^{N} ln \frac{P(X_i|C_k)}{P(X_i|C_{k\neg})} + ln \frac{P(X_i|C_k)}{P(X_i|C_{k\neg})} \tag{3}$$

Where $C_{k\neg}$ is the complement of the set C_k. The score measures the degree that an instance X is a member of the class C_k. Therefore based on Score's higher values, the chances of complying with C_k will be higher. The Score function allows one to derive predictions based on a series of predictors X and is a monotonic function of Eq. (2). When the Score is zero, this means that the probability to find C_k is the same as it would be found if C_k were distributed randomly. If the Score is positive then there is a higher than random probability to find C_k present and on the contrary if the Score is negative [9].

Table 2. Data (source, descriptor and category)

Source	Descriptor	Category
Enrollment data (First semester)	Entrance semester	{Even semester, Odd semester}
	State headquarters	{Chiapas, DF, Edomex, Hidalgo, Oaxaca, Querétaro, Tlaxcala}
	Registered courses	{0, 1, 2, 3, 4, 5, 6, 7}
	Approved courses	{0, 1, 2, 3, 4, 5, 6, 7}
	Grade point average	{0, 5 - 5.4, 5.5 - 5.9, 6 - 6.4, 6.5 - 6.9, 7 - 7.4, 7.5 – 7.9, 8 - 8.4, 8.5 - 8.9, 9 - 9.4, 9.5 - 9.9, 10}
	Entrance cause[2]	{56, 58, 64, 67, 74, 76, 97}
	Gender	{Female, Male}
	Entrance age	{16 a 19, 19 a 22, 22 a 24, 24 a 26, 26 a 28, 28 a 31, 31 a 34, 34 a 38, 38 a 43, 43 a 63}. "Coarse graining"
	Nationality	{1 (Mexican), 2 (Foreign), NA.*}
	State of residence	{Aguascalientes, Chiapas, Chihuahua, Coahuila, Distrito Federal, Durango, Guanajuato... Zacatecas}
	Career	{Administration, Bibliotecology, Political science, Accounting, Law, Economy, Spanish, Informatics, English, Pedagogy, Journalism, Psychology, International relations, Sociology}
Entry profile	Marital status	{Married, Divorced, Widowed, NA, Single, Free union}
	Children	{NA, No, Yes}
	Work	{NA, No, Yes}
	Employment relationship	{Temporary, Permanent, No answer, NA.}
	Working hours per w	{10 or less, 11- 20, 21- 30, 31- 40, More than 40, No answer, NA}
	Relationship between studies and work	{No, Yes, No Answer, NA.}
	Number of people who depend on financial support (Family)	{1- 2, 3 - 4, 5 - 6, 7 or more, NA.}
	Number of people contributing to the family income	{1, 2 - 3, 4 or more, NA.}
	Mother's educational level	{No education, Elementary, Middle school, High school, Technical career, Undergraduate, Postgraduate, NA.}
	Father's educational level	{No education, Elementary, Middle school, High school, Technical career, Undergraduate, Postgraduate, NA.}
	Access to computer equipment	{No, Yes, NA.}
	Comprehension of English	{Good, Bad, Nothing, NA.}
	Spoken English	{Good, Bad, Nothing, NA.}
	Written English	{Good, Bad, Nothing, NA.}
Educational Background	Highest level of education	{High school, Undergraduate (finished), Undergraduate (not finished), NA., Postgraduate (finished), Postgraduate (not finished)}
	Grade point average in the highest level of education	{7 -7.9, 8 - 8.9, 9 - 10, NA.}
	Years without studying	{2 or less, 2 - 4, 5 - 8, 8 or more, NA.}
Score in the admission test		{33 - 40, 41- 48, 49 - 56, 57 - 64, 65 - 72, 73 - 80, 81- 88, 89 - 96, 97 - 104, NA.}

4   Results and Interpretation

The training data (70 % of students) were randomly selected and the Epsilon and Score were calculated. With the Epsilons in hand a feature selection step could be implemented. The selection criterion was for all those Epsilon higher or equal to two standard deviations (95 % confidence level). Those descriptors that comply with some of $\varepsilon(C_k|X_i) = 2$ categories are as follows (Table 3).

A conditional formatting for each descriptor was applied in the Epsilon column to identify those categories that have a higher representation in the model.

Once the Scores variables and measures have been selected, we assign each one of these to the relevant categories in the simple data, which means, the Score value obtained with the training date will replace the category according to the proof date. Afterwards, the total individual values are added to those of Score to obtain a total Score (St) for each instance[1], and these are ordered in a descending manner with its respective class (0/1). It is important to affirm that a positive value from Epsilon adds to the fulfillment of the class and a negative one does not. See the following Table 4.

The following chart was made considering all the complete fourth table and graph of the classifier model by deciles, in which the count of the class and its total respective distribution for each decile were presented (Table 5 and Fig. 3).

In the first two deciles almost 80 % of the class was added, demonstrating that the classifier model developed with the training data and using the Naive Bayes algorithm, complies with its predictive function and discriminates the testing data by "yes or no".

In order to measure the performance of the classifier model and to calculate the matrix of confusion it was necessary to define a threshold in the test data in order to establish the boundaries between the four categories of the confusion matrix: true positive (Tp), false negative (Fn), true negative (Tn) and false positive (Fp). This threshold is between a positive and negative value in St, but in fact the minor value in the list is zero, so we have to apply the next smoothing constant.

$$St\,fix = St + \ln\frac{Pc}{1 - Pc} \tag{4}$$

With this smoothing constant for each St, it was possible to identify the threshold in the new values of St fix, see Table 6.

The threshold was located between 0.001 and −0062 from the St fix column. This allowed to calculate the next confusion matrix and performance measures: sensitivity and specificity (Table 7).

Analyzing the performance measures, we see the probability of the model to correctly classify the true positive rate is of 79.3 % and the probability of correctly classifying the false positive rate is equal to 84.3 %.

In addition to the confusion matrix, the ROC (Receiver Operating Characteristic) graphs is an excellent technique to examine the performance of a binary classifier [11].

---

[1] Each instance refers to a student with his/her data entrance profile, educational background and enrollment data.

Table 3. Variables calculation (Epsilon and Score)

Descriptor	Category	Nx	Nxc=Ncx	N	Nc	Pc	P(xlc)	P(clx)	Epsilon	Score
Registered courses in first semester	0	896	4	2,022	114	0.06	0.04	0.00	-6.737	-2.384
Registered courses in first semester	1	167	1	2,022	114	0.06	0.02	0.01	-2.823	-1.624
Registered courses in first semester	2	118	1	2,022	114	0.06	0.02	0.01	-2.256	-1.276
Registered courses in first semester	3	139	1	2,022	114	0.06	0.02	0.01	-2.514	-1.440
Registered courses in first semester	4	107	1	2,022	114	0.06	0.02	0.01	-2.109	-1.178
Registered courses in first semester	5	164	17	2,022	114	0.06	0.16	0.10	2.625	0.694
Registered courses in first semester	6	289	58	2,022	114	0.06	0.51	0.20	10.636	1.432
Registered courses in first semester	7	142	31	2,022	114	0.06	0.28	0.22	8.366	1.549
Grade point average in first semester	0	542	2	2,022	114	0.06	0.03	0.00	-5.318	-2.394
Grade point average in first semester	5 - 5.4	394	2	2,022	114	0.06	0.03	0.01	-4.415	-2.074
Grade point average in first semester	5.5 - 5.9	65	1	2,022	114	0.06	0.02	0.02	-1.433	-0.680
Grade point average in first semester	6 - 6.4	109	1	2,022	114	0.06	0.02	0.01	-2.137	-1.197
Grade point average in first semester	6.5 - 6.9	88	2	2,022	114	0.06	0.03	0.02	-1.369	-0.566
Grade point average in first semester	7 - 7.4	168	7	2,022	114	0.06	0.07	0.04	-0.827	-0.207
Grade point average in first semester	7.5 - 7.9	125	8	2,022	114	0.06	0.08	0.06	0.369	0.228
Grade point average in first semester	8 - 8.4	163	24	2,022	114	0.06	0.22	0.15	5.029	1.079
Grade point average in first semester	8.5 - 8.9	118	20	2,022	114	0.06	0.18	0.17	5.327	1.251
Grade point average in first semester	9 - 9.4	174	34	2,022	114	0.06	0.30	0.20	7.951	1.408
Grade point average in first semester	9.5 - 9.9	61	10	2,022	114	0.06	0.09	0.16	3.642	1.248
Grade point average in first semester	10	15	3	2,022	114	0.06	0.03	0.20	2.412	1.623
Entry age	16 - 19	192	10	2,022	114	0.06	0.09	0.05	-0.258	-0.010
Entry age	19 - 22	208	6	2,022	114	0.06	0.06	0.03	-1.722	-0.566
Entry age	22 - 24	201	12	2,022	114	0.06	0.11	0.06	0.204	0.119
Entry age	24 - 26	211	7	2,022	114	0.06	0.07	0.03	-1.461	-0.442
Entry age	26 - 28	208	12	2,022	114	0.06	0.11	0.06	0.082	0.083
Entry age	28 - 31	209	5	2,022	114	0.06	0.05	0.02	-2.034	-0.730
Entry age	31 - 34	196	10	2,022	114	0.06	0.09	0.05	-0.325	-0.032
Entry age	34 - 38	201	16	2,022	114	0.06	0.15	0.08	1.427	0.409
Entry age	38 - 43	202	17	2,022	114	0.06	0.16	0.08	1.712	0.466
Entry age	43 - 63	194	19	2,022	114	0.06	0.17	0.10	2.510	0.627
State of residence	Chiapas	23	0	2,022	114	0.06	0.01	0.00	-1.172	-0.377
State of residence	Chihuahua	1	0	2,022	114	0.06	0.01	0.00	-0.244	2.108
State of residence	Distrito Feder	336	16	2,022	114	0.06	0.15	0.05	-0.696	-0.137
State of residence	Durango	3	1	2,022	114	0.06	0.02	0.33	2.080	2.396
State of residence	Guanajuato	4	0	2,022	114	0.06	0.01	0.00	-0.489	1.192
State of residence	Guerrero	3	0	2,022	114	0.06	0.01	0.00	-0.423	1.415
State of residence	Hidalgo	201	11	2,022	114	0.06	0.10	0.05	-0.102	0.034
State of residence	Jalisco	3	0	2,022	114	0.06	0.01	0.00	-0.423	1.415
State of residence	México	347	23	2,022	114	0.06	0.21	0.07	0.800	0.195
State of residence	Michoacán	7	1	2,022	114	0.06	0.02	0.14	0.992	1.549
State of residence	Morelos	15	2	2,022	114	0.06	0.03	0.13	1.292	1.261
State of residence	Oaxaca	404	23	2,022	114	0.06	0.21	0.06	0.048	0.034
State of residence	Puebla	60	3	2,022	114	0.06	0.03	0.05	-0.214	0.127
State of residence	Querétaro	12	1	2,022	114	0.06	0.02	0.08	0.405	1.010
State of residence	Quintana Roc	1	0	2,022	114	0.06	0.01	0.00	-0.244	2.108
State of residence	San Luis Pot(	3	0	2,022	114	0.06	0.01	0.00	-0.423	1.415
State of residence	Tamaulipas	3	0	2,022	114	0.06	0.01	0.00	-0.423	1.415
State of residence	Tlaxcala	583	31	2,022	114	0.06	0.28	0.05	-0.336	-0.048
State of residence	Veracruz	10	2	2,022	114	0.06	0.03	0.20	1.969	1.703
State of residence	Yucatán	1	0	2,022	114	0.06	0.01	0.00	-0.244	2.108
State of residence	Zacatecas	2	0	2,022	114	0.06	0.01	0.00	-0.346	1.703

(*Continued*)

Table 3. (*Continued*)

Descriptor	Category	Nx	Nxc=Ncx	N	Nc	Pc	P(x|c)	P(c|x)	Epsilon	Score
Career	Administratio	98	4	2,022	114	0.06	0.04	0.04	-0.668	-0.143
Career	Bibliotecology	29	1	2,022	114	0.06	0.02	0.03	-0.511	0.127
Career	Political science	153	6	2,022	114	0.06	0.06	0.04	-0.920	-0.250
Career	Counting	224	18	2,022	114	0.06	0.16	0.08	1.556	0.413
Career	Law	521	47	2,022	114	0.06	0.41	0.09	3.348	0.509
Career	Economy	75	2	2,022	114	0.06	0.03	0.03	-1.116	-0.404
Career	Spanish	2	0	2,022	114	0.06	0.01	0.00	-0.346	1.703
Career	Informatics	29	1	2,022	114	0.06	0.02	0.03	-0.511	0.127
Career	English	0	0	2,022	114	0.06	0.01	0.00	0.000	0.000
Career	Pedagogy	187	1	2,022	114	0.06	0.02	0.01	-3.026	-1.737
Career	Journalism	120	6	2,022	114	0.06	0.06	0.05	-0.303	0.002
Career	Psychology	518	26	2,022	114	0.06	0.23	0.05	-0.610	-0.103
Career	International	47	1	2,022	114	0.06	0.02	0.02	-1.043	-0.356
Career	Sociology	19	1	2,022	114	0.06	0.02	0.05	-0.071	0.550
Marital status	Married	554	45	2,022	114	0.06	0.40	0.08	2.536	0.395
Marital status	Divorced, Wi	111	8	2,022	114	0.06	0.08	0.07	0.717	0.354
Marital status	NA.	367	14	2,022	114	0.06	0.13	0.04	-1.514	-0.360
Marital status	Single	846	43	2,022	114	0.06	0.38	0.05	-0.700	-0.104
Marital status	Free Union	144	4	2,022	114	0.06	0.04	0.03	-1.488	-0.538
Children	NA.	479	21	2,022	114	0.06	0.19	0.04	-1.190	-0.237
Children	No	748	35	2,022	114	0.06	0.31	0.05	-1.137	-0.186
Children	Yes	795	58	2,022	114	0.06	0.51	0.07	2.026	0.275
Working hours per week	10 or less	150	7	2,022	114	0.06	0.07	0.05	-0.516	-0.089
Working hours per week	11-20	118	12	2,022	114	0.06	0.11	0.10	2.134	0.693
Working hours per week	21-30	163	8	2,022	114	0.06	0.08	0.05	-0.404	-0.051
Working hours per week	31-40	360	22	2,022	114	0.06	0.20	0.06	0.389	0.111
Working hours per week	40 o more	576	29	2,022	114	0.06	0.26	0.05	-0.628	-0.104
Working hours per week	No answer	266	20	2,022	114	0.06	0.18	0.08	1.330	0.336
Working hours per week	NA.	389	16	2,022	114	0.06	0.15	0.04	-1.304	-0.290
Access to computer equipment	NA.	393	16	2,022	114	0.06	0.15	0.04	-1.347	-0.300
Access to computer equipment	No	95	10	2,022	114	0.06	0.09	0.11	2.066	0.745
Access to computer equipment	Yes	1,534	88	2,022	114	0.06	0.77	0.06	0.168	0.013
Years without studying	2 or less	457	29	2,022	114	0.06	0.26	0.06	0.656	0.141
Years without studying	2 - 4	432	20	2,022	114	0.06	0.18	0.05	-0.909	-0.178
Years without studying	5 - 8	282	11	2,022	114	0.06	0.10	0.04	-1.265	-0.320
Years without studying	8 or more	386	37	2,022	114	0.06	0.33	0.10	3.362	0.581
Years without studying	NA.	465	17	2,022	114	0.06	0.16	0.04	-1.853	-0.415

Table 4. Class and Score total

Number	Class	St
1	1	5.014
2	1	4.948
3	1	4.561
..	..	..
865	0	0.000
866	0	0.000
867	0	0.000

Table 5. Class by deciles

Rank	Deciles	Counts	Relatives
1 - 87	1	33	0.524
88 - 174	2	17	0.270
175- 261	3	8	0.127
262 - 348	4	2	0.032
349 - 435	5	0	0.000
436 - 522	6	0	0.000
523 - 609	7	1	0.016
610 - 696	8	2	0.032
697 - 783	9	0	0.000
784 - 870	10	0	0.000
Total		**63**	**1**

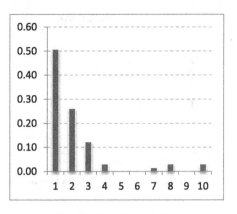

Fig. 3. Classifier model

Table 6. Threshold

Number	Class	St	St fix	
175	0	2.610	0.024	
176	0	2.587	0.001	**Threshold**
177	0	2.525	-0.062	
178	0	2.511	-0.076	

Table 7. Confusion matrix and performance measures

Confusion matrix		Performance measures	
Tp — 50 Fp — 126 Tn — 678 Fn — 13		Sensitivity	$\dfrac{Tp}{Tp + Fn}$ = 0.793
Where: Tp: If the instance is positive and it is classified as positive Fp: If the instance is negative and it is classified as positive Tn: If the instance is negative and it is classified as negative Fn: If the instance is positive and it is classified as negative *(Tp)+(Fn) = Class (1); (Fp)+(Tn) = Class(0)*		Specificity	$\dfrac{Tn}{Tn + Fp}$ = 0.843

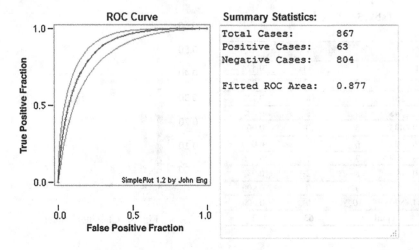

Fig. 4. ROC Curve

ROC graphs display the distribution of different pairs (false positives and true positives) for each interaction in the threshold. The point (0,1) shows a perfect classification, this means that it correctly classified all true positives and none of false positives. In contrast, the point (1,0) shows the worst classifier model. In the next graph[2] shows the ROC curve that determines the performance of our classifier model (Fig. 4).

The shape of the ROC curve has a closer approximation to the upper left corner (0, 1) and the area under the curve (AUC) is an important measure, which through a scale value between 0 and 1, determines the performance of the classifier model. The AUC of a classifier is equivalent to the probability that the classifier will rank a randomly chosen positive instance higher than a randomly chosen negative instance [12]. In our particular case, the AUC is equal to 0.877 and therefore demonstrates the good predictive ability of our model.

5   Conclusions

By analysing data from students involved in distance learning at SUAyED using data mining techniques we developed a model for predicting student success, success being defined as completing 100 % of all required credits within 10 semesters. We have shown that the Naive Bayes classifier used here is a good predictor of student success that the factors that influence it. The model achieved a sensitivity of 52 % and 27 % in the first two first two score deciles, respectively. The model performance as calculated from the ROC curve corresponded to an AUC of 0.88 when using feature selection and 0.85 for the model with all variables included. Using Epsilon we were able to identify

---

[2] The graph was generated with the web calculator ROC analysis of the school of medicine at Johns Hopkins University. URL: http://bit.ly/1eWFAnC.

the main predictors that contribute to the success of students. The most representative factors are that students pass at least five subjects in the first semester of their career with an average greater than or equal to eight. It was also found that students with an entrance age of 43 or more, enrolled in a law career and claimed at the moment of starting their studies to be: married, with or without children, working 11–20 h per week, not having a computer and counting more than eight years without studying, are those who are more likely to meet 100 % of credits in ten semesters.

Knowing that the classification model is predictive, the next project will be about making a program of this predictive model, which can constantly measure the performance interactions between variables that lead students toward academic success. In this way the SUAyED will be able to provide more personalized and actionable student information to decision makers, thereby improving student learning and increasing student retention and therefore the number of students completing their studies on time and, most of all, allowing for more efficient educational resource planning to maintain and improving the quality of distance education at the UNAM.

References

1. Zhao, C.-M., Luan, J.: Data mining: going beyond traditional statistics. New Dir. Inst. Res. **131**(2), 7–16 (2006)
2. Yukselturk, E., Ozekes, S., Türel, Y.: Predicting dropout student: an application of data mining methods in an online education program. Eur. J. Open Distance E-Learn. **17**(1), 118–133 (2014)
3. Lykourentzou, I., Giannoukos, I., Nikolopoulos, V., Mpardis, G., Loumos, V.: Dropout prediction in e-learning courses through the combination of machine learning techniques. Comput. Educ. **53**(3), 950–965 (2009)
4. Willging, P.A., Johnson, S.D.: Factors that influence students' decision to dropout of online courses. J. Asynchronous Learn. Netw. **13**(3), 115–127 (2004)
5. Lile, A.: Analyzing E-learning systems using educational data mining techniques. Mediterranean J. Soc. Sci. **2**(3), 403–419 (2011)
6. Kotsiantis, S., Pierrakeas, C., Pintelas, P.: Preventing student dropout in distance learning using machine learning techniques. Knowl.-Based Intell. Inf. Eng. Syst. **2774**, 267–274 (2003)
7. Zang, W., Lin, F.: Investigation of web-based teaching and learning by boosting algorithms. In: Proceedings of IEEE International Conference on Information Technology: Research and Education (ITRE 2003), pp. 445–449 (2003)
8. Dekker, G., Pechenizkiy, M., Vleeshouwers, J.: Predicting student drop out: a case study. In: Barnes, T., Desmarais, M., Romero, C., Ventura, S. (eds.), Proceedings of the 2nd International Conference on Educational Data Mining, (EDM 2009), pp. 41–50 (2009)
9. Stephens, C.R., Heau, J.G., González, C., Ibarra-Cerdeña, C.N., Sánchez-Cordero, V., et al.: Using biotic interaction networks for prediction in biodiversity and emerging diseases. PLoS ONE **4**(5), e5725 (2009). doi:10.1371/journal.pone.0005725
10. Mitchell, T., Machine Learning, Generative and Discriminative Classifiers: Naive Bayes and Logistic Regression (Draft Version). McGraw Hill (2005)
11. Swet, J.A.: Measuring the accuracy of diagnostic systems. Science **240**, 1285–1293 (1988)
12. Fawcett, T.: An introduction to ROC analysis. Pattern Recogn. Lett. **27**(8), 861–874 (2006)

Automatic Evaluation of Music Students

Antonio Camarena-Ibarrola$^{(\boxtimes)}$ and Sonia Morales-Pintor

Universidad Michoacana de San Nicolas de Hidalgo, Morelia, Mexico
camarena@umich.mx, smorales@dep.fie.umich.mx

Abstract. Music Schools would greatly benefit from a tool that would reduce the time teachers spend evaluating students while those teachers would be confident that evaluation is still a reliable and perhaps more transparent process. We propose a method for evaluating students by asking them to play a specific piece of music, then we transform the audio-signal into a sequence of feature vectors. We align this sequence to a reference to determine how well the student played. We found that Dynamic Time Warping works better than Levenshtein distance or the Longest Common Subsequence distance to determine the similarity between the music played by the student and the reference. We tested our system with 28 musical performances played by music students and compare the grades determined by our system with the actual grades given to them by their teacher getting very encouraging results.

1 Introduction

Since the benefits of music learning for the cognitive processes of the brain are well known, teaching how to play a musical instrument has become quite common and even mandatory in public and private schools. A tool for automatic evaluation of music students would help the teaching-learning process. Nowadays music teachers spend many hours evaluating their students in a one-by-one fashion, even worse, to avoid favoritism it is common practice to designate several teachers to evaluate each student. Using computers to evaluate music students not only discharge teachers from such time consuming task but might also increase confidence in the process since computers would not favor a student over another. Students could also use the evaluation tool to practice before the actual examination date. Robine *et al.* introduced in [4] a software tool which analyses the technical ability of saxophonists. They estimate pitch using autocorrelation for evaluating the performer by considering the evolution of the fundamental frequency during the performance of specially designed exercises. Their method is however intended only for monophonic music. The IMUTUS project [1,5] introduced an interactive multimedia system for training students using MIDI (Musical Instrument Digital Interface) instruments. This system has a score performance matching module to detect spurious or missing note onsets and offsets, however, it is not intended for advanced students but for beginners. Beginners play monophonic music, that is music played one note at a time. In order to evaluate piano students, Vila *et al.* in [8] extract discrete histograms

© Springer International Publishing Switzerland 2015
O. Pichardo Lagunas et al. (Eds.): MICAI 2015, Part II, LNAI 9414, pp. 220–231, 2015.
DOI: 10.1007/978-3-319-27101-9_16

of occurrences of the different note durations at low level from MIDI files to evaluate the rhythmic *correctness* of various performances of the same piano piece and compare it to a performance considered as the *correct performance*. No aligning technique was used in that work, the performances are evaluated only by comparison of the histograms.

For MIDI instruments the evaluation problem is easier, instead of an audio signal the stream consists of symbolic data and string matching techniques might be used. However, most musical instruments such as flutes and violins have no MIDI Ports, so we have to capture the audio-signal through a microphone and an A/D converter included in almost every modern computer. The digitalized audio-signal must be processed in order to extract features from it and observe how these features evolve in time. Spectrograms for example show how energy distribute in frequency and also how its frequency components change in time. The spectrogram should next be compared to a reference which ideally should be the music score but could also be another spectrogram which could be synthesized from the score or instead it could be extracted from a well-played performance of the same music, for example played by the teacher.

Chromagrams are preferred over spectrograms for characterizing music signals specifically. There are 12 chromas in an octave which correspond to the tones and semitones (i.e. white and black keys) normally found in the keyboard of a piano within an octave. A Chromagram shows the level of energy in each chroma for each short period of time. In [2] Hu *et al.* proposed to synthesize chromagrams from MIDI files and align them to chromagrams extracted from audio signals for music retrieval purposes.

2   Feature Extraction

A chromagram is a sequence of vectors of chroma values, the Constant Q transform may be used to determine the chroma values of a segment of audio.

2.1   The Constant Q Transform

The constant Q transform (CQT) can be visualized as a filter bank where the filters are logarithmically separated The k-th filter has a bandwidth given by

$$\Delta f_k = 2^{\frac{1}{b}} \Delta f_{k-1} \tag{1}$$

where b is the number of filters per octave

Each octave has b filters so the filter numbered $b-1$ is the last filter of the first octave, the b-th filter is the first filter of the second octave and so forth. The bandwidth of the first filter of an octave is twice the bandwidth of the first filter of the previous octave. And half the bandwidth of the first filter of the next octave. The bandwidth of the k-th filter is related to the bandwidth of the very first filter of the filter bank by Eq. (2)

$$\Delta f_k = \left(2^{\frac{1}{b}}\right)^k \Delta f_0 \tag{2}$$

The *Quality factor Q* which remains constant for all the filters in the filter bank is defined in Eq. (3)

$$Q = \frac{f_k}{\Delta f_k} \tag{3}$$

where f_k is the center frequency of the k-th filter defined in Eq. (4)

$$f_k = f_0 2^{\frac{k}{b}} \quad \forall\, k = 0, 1, ..., K \tag{4}$$

where K is the number of filters $K = \left\lceil \left(b \log_2 \left(\frac{f_{max}}{f_0} \right) \right) \right\rceil$

The bandwidth of the k-th filter is then determined as in Eq. (5)

$$\Delta f_k = f_{k+1} - f_k = f_k 2^{\frac{1}{b}} - f_k = f_k (2^{\frac{1}{b}} - 1) \tag{5}$$

Combining Eqs. (3) and (5) we obtain Eq. (6) for the quality factor Q

$$Q = \frac{f_k}{\Delta f_k} = (2^{\frac{1}{b}} - 1)^{-1} \tag{6}$$

So the ratio of frequency to resolution (the quality factor) does not depend on the frequency, it is constant. What makes the Constant Q transform so interesting is that by choosing appropriate values of f_0 and b, the center frequencies correspond to musical notes or semitones. Another important characteristic of the Constant Q transform is that it uses more samples of the signal for the lower frequencies than for the higher ones, it resembles the human auditory system which needs more time to perceive the lower frequencies than the higher ones. The Constant Q Transform (CQT) is defined as in Eq. (7).

$$x[k] = \frac{1}{N_k} \sum_{n < N_k} x[n] W_{N_k}[n] e^{-2\pi n Q/N_k} \quad \forall\, k = 0, 1, 2, ..., K \tag{7}$$

where N_k is the number of samples used in the k-th filter
$N_k = \left\lceil \left(Q \frac{f_s}{f_k} \right) \right\rceil$ and f_s is the sampling rate
W_{N_k} is a window function (i.e. The Hamming window) of length N_k.

3   Aligning Techniques

A chromagram is a sequence of chroma vectors determined as explained in the previous section. Once a chromagram has been extracted from the audio-signal of a music piece it should be aligned to the chromagram of a correct version of the same music in order to compare it and determine how similar these chromagramas are, the more similar the higher the grade assigned to the student is. We will now explain several aligning techniques which are at the same time a way of establish how similar those time series are.

3.1   Dynamic Time Warping (DTW)

Aligning two performances $R(n)$, $0 \leq n \leq N$ and $T(m)$, $0 \leq m \leq M$ is equivalent to finding a warping function $m = w(n)$ that maps indexes n and m so that a time registration between the time series is obtained. Function w is subject to the boundary conditions $w(0) = 0$ and $w(N) = M$ and might be subject to local restrictions, an example of such restriction is that if the optimal warping function goes through point (n, m) it must go through either $(n - 1, m - 1)$, $(n, m - 1)$ or $(n - 1, m)$, a penalization of 2 is charged when choosing $(n - 1, m - 1)$.

Let $d_{n,m}$ be the distance between frame n of performance R and frame m of performance T, then the optimal warping function between R and T is the one that minimizes the accumulated distance $D_{n,m}$ as in (8).

$$D_{n,m} = \sum_{p=1}^{n} d_{R(p),T(w(p))} \qquad (8)$$

$D_{N,M}$ can be computed using the recurrence defined in Eqs. (9), (10) and (11). Based on this recurrence $D_{N,M}$ can be obtained using dynamic programming.

$$D_{i,0} = \sum_{k=0}^{i} d_{i,0} \qquad (9)$$

$$D_{0,j} = \sum_{k=0}^{j} d_{0,j} \qquad (10)$$

$$D_{i,j} = min \begin{cases} D_{i-1,j-1} + 2d_{i,j} \\ D_{i-1,j} + d_{i,j} \\ D_{i,j-1} + d_{i,j} \end{cases} \qquad (11)$$

An alternative and new way of aligning time series is using flexible string matching techniques. We will now give a brief introduction beginning with the most general string edit distance also called *Levenshtein distance*.

3.2   Levenshtein Distance

The string edit distance between two strings is defined as the number of operations needed to convert one string into the other, the considered operations are *insertions*, *deletions* and *substitutions*. A different cost maybe assigned to each operation. If only substitutions are allowed and the cost is 1.0, the *Hamming distance* is obtained. If only insertions and deletions are allowed and for both operations the cost is 1.0 then the *Longest common subsequence* (LCS) distance is obtained [3].

To compute the Levenshtein distance between string t of length N and string p of length M, Eqs. (12), (13) and (14) can be used. Note that to all considered operations (insertion, deletions and substitutions) the same cost of 1.0 has been assigned.

$$L_{i,0} = i \quad \forall \quad i = 0..N - 1 \tag{12}$$

$$L_{0,j} = j \quad \forall \quad j = 0..M - 1 \tag{13}$$

$$L_{i,j} = \begin{cases} L_{i-1,j-1} & t_i = p_j \\ min[L_{i-1,j-1}, L_{i,j-1}, L_{i-1,j}] + 1 & t_i \neq p_j \end{cases} \quad j = 1..M - 1 \; ; \; i = 1..N - 1 \tag{14}$$

The classical approach for computing the Levenshtein distance relies in Dynamic Programming, for instance, the Levenshtein distance between the string *hello* and the string *yellow* is 2 as can be seen on location $(5,6)$ of matrix (15) corresponding to two operations (i.e. substitute "h" by a "y" and add "w" at the end)

		y	e	l	l	o	w
	0	1	2	3	4	5	6
h	1	1	2	3	4	5	6
e	2	2	1	2	3	4	5
l	3	3	2	1	2	3	4
l	4	4	3	2	1	2	3
o	5	5	4	3	2	1	2

$$(15)$$

There is no need for keeping the whole dynamic programming table in memory. The Levenshtein distance can be computed in just one column. To compute the Levenshtein distance between string t of length N and string p of length M using only one column, initialize the column as $L_i^0 = i$ for $i = 0..N - 1$ and then update it using (16).

$$L_i^j = \begin{cases} L_{i-1}^{j-1} & \forall \, t_i = p_j \\ min[L_{i-1}^{j-1}, L_{i-1}^j, L_i^{j-1}] + 1 & \forall \, t_i \neq p_j \end{cases} \quad j = 1..M - 1 \; ; \; i = 0..N - 1 \tag{16}$$

where L^j stands for L once j characters of string p have been read.

3.3   The LCS Distance

The computation of the LCS distance is done just as the computation of the Levenshtein distance, except that only insertions and deletions are allowed. The LCS distance was designed to report a low value where the same sequence of symbols are present in both strings as is usually the case with speech signals, in this context, a symbol represents an acoustic event. For example, the Levenshtein distance can not tell that the strings *computer* and *curtain* are any more different than the strings *computer* and *cooommpuuuteeer*. The LCS distance can however, report that the first couple of strings are more different than the second couple of strings as can be seen on Table 1.

Table 1. LCS distance for strings that contain the same sequence of symbols and for strings that do not

x	y	$Levenshtein(x, y)$	$LCS(x, y)$
Computer	Cooommpuuuteeer	7	7
Computer	Curtain	7	10

The recurrence defined in (17), (18) and (19) is used with dynamic programming to compute the LCS distance. Of course, LCS can also be computed using a single vector.

$$C_{i,0} = i \qquad \forall \quad i = 0..N - 1 \tag{17}$$

$$C_{0,j} = j \qquad \forall \quad j = 0..M - 1 \tag{18}$$

$$C_{i,j} = \begin{cases} C_{i-1,j-1} & t_i = p_j \\ min[C_{i,j-1}, C_{i-1,j}] + 1 & t_i \neq p_j \end{cases} \quad j = 1..M - 1 \,;\, i = 1..N - 1 \tag{19}$$

4 Description of the Automatic Evaluation System

For evaluating a music student, the student plays his instrument in front of a microphone connected to a computer running the evaluation program. The student selects the piece he is about to perform among a list of musical pieces known to the system as well as the instrument he is going to use for that purpose, then he starts playing whenever he is ready. After he finishes he asks the computer for his grade. The system has two modules, the front-end module extracts features from the audio-signal and the evaluation module compares the performance of the student to a correct performance of the music selected by the student.

4.1 Front-End Module

The Front-end module captures the audio-signal with a sampling frequency of 44,100 samples per second, with a precision of 16 bits per sample in mono-aural and linear scalar quantization. After the student has selected the piece he is about to perform, there is a space of time before he really starts playing the instrument. In a similar way, after he finishes to play his instrument and before he requires for the computer to assign him a grade there is also a space of time. For this reason, the front-end module needs to locate the beginning and the end of the performance in the audio-signal, this process is called segmentation of the signal or localization of the Region Of Interest (ROI). The signal is analyzed in short segments of time called frames, our frames for are 30 ms long and are overlapped by 2/3 so the frames are shifted along the signal by 10 ms with respect to its previous position. Let N be the number of samples that fit in a frame, in our case $N = 1323$ samples. To locate the beginning of the performance, we use three features extracted in time domain:

1. Short time Energy. It is determined using the following equation:

$$E_n = \sum_{m=n-N+1}^{n} x^2(m) \tag{20}$$

where n is the location of the frame, so E_n is the energy of the frame that ends in sample n and $x(m)$ is the m-th sample of the audio-signal inside that frame.

2. Short time Zero Crossings Rate (ZCR). It is an estimation of the frequency of the signal and it is determined using:

$$Z_n = \sum_{m=n-N+1}^{n} |sign[x(m)] - sign[x(m-1)]| \tag{21}$$

where Z_n is the ZCR of the frame that ends in sample n and:

$$sign[x(m)] = \begin{cases} 1 & x(m) \geq 0 \\ -1 & x(m) < 0 \end{cases} \tag{22}$$

3. Short time Entropy. According to Claude Shannon [6], entropy measures the amount of information content in a signal, it is determined with Boltzman Eq. (24). To determine the entropy we first estimate the probability distribution function using a histogram as follows:

$$p_i = \frac{f_i}{N} \tag{23}$$

where f_i is the number of times a sample falls within the range of the i-th bin

$$H(x) = -\sum_{i=1}^{B} p_i ln(p_i) \tag{24}$$

where B is the number of bins in the histogram, we use $B = 36$.

We determine all three short time features described above for every frame starting at the beginning of the signal and if E_n, Z_n, and H_n are all above their respective threshold values, then the frame ending in sample n is declared to belong to the ROI, that is the student has begun playing his instrument. We proceed in a similar way to detect the end of the performance starting with a frame at the end of the recorded signal and proceed backwards to detect the end of the student's performance.

Once the audio signal has been segmented, we apply a pre-emphasis filter defined with the following difference equation:

$$y(n) = x(n) - 1.95x(n-1) \tag{25}$$

That is, each sample of the signal at the output of the pre-emphasis filter is determined with a combination of two samples of the signal at the input of the filter, this filter with only two coefficients (the length of the filter) emphasizes the higher frequencies of the signal. After the preprocessing of the signal, we frame the signal in the same way that we do in the segmentation phase, except now we use a frame size of about 92 ms, which correspond to $N = 4096$ with an overlap of 50 % between frames and extract a chroma vector for every frame so we will end with a feature vector for each 46 ms of music approximately.

To every frame we apply a Hamming window to reduce the spectral leakage. The Hamming window is defined as:

$$hamming(n) = 0.54 + 0.46cos(2\pi n/N) \tag{26}$$

Instead of using the constant Q transform as described in Subsect. 2.1 for extracting the chroma-values for the short segment of audio inside a frame, we extract the chroma values using the Fast Fourier Transform (FFT) since using CQT directly would make the feature extraction a very slow process. After applying the FFT we locate the spectral coefficients within bands with center frequency f_k given by Eq. (27) and bandwidth Δf_k given by Eq. (28):

$$f_k = f_0 2^{\frac{k}{b}} \quad \forall\, k = 0, 1, ..., K \tag{27}$$

where $K = \left\lceil \left(b \log_2 \left(\frac{f_{max}}{f_0} \right) \right) \right\rceil$

$$\Delta f_k = \frac{f_k}{Q} \quad \forall\, k = 0, 1, ..., K \tag{28}$$

We use $b = 12$ and so $Q = (2^{\frac{1}{12}} - 1)^{-1} = 16.817$ and $f_0 = 261$ Hz and $f_{max} = 8372$ Hz, that is the frequencies between C4 and C9 (i.e. five full octaves starting with note DO), and $K = 72$.

The sets of spectral coefficients within bands numbered $k + mb$ belong to the same k-th chroma so instead of K bands we are left with only b chromas, then we determine the arithmetic average of the magnitude of the spectral coefficients that belong to each chroma and that is how we obtain each chroma vector of twelve values each one. As we said before, extracting the chroma vector for each frame we end up with a chromagram with a constant height (i.e. the value of b) and a length that depends on the duration of the musical performance.

4.2   Evaluation Module

To evaluate a student we compare the chromagram extracted as explained in the previous subsection from the music played by the student with a goal chromagram, that is a chromagram that is considered correct since it was extracted from a well played performance of the same music piece, such well played performance could be stored in a CD accompanying the student's learning book or could simply be played by the teacher. If the two chromagrams are very similar it means the student played very well and should get the higher grade. To establish how similar the chromagrams are, we use the aligning techniques explained in Subsect. 3.1, 3.2 and 3.3 (DTW, Levenshtein distance, and LCS) these techniques not only align time series (i.e. chromagrams) but also deliver a distance between them. The lower the distance the more similar the chromagrams are. In order to convert distances to grades, the distances have to be normalized so they do not depend on the length of the musical performances under comparison, this is done by dividing the distance by the sum of the lengths of the performances in terms of number of vectors of chroma, also, by establishing the dynamic range of the distances, which is done off-line, the distances between vectors of Chroma are normalized as well to the range [0–1], after all, not even the teacher can play the music exactly the same twice. Normalization against lengths of chroma vectors under comparison which is related to the amount of energy content is unnecessary since we use the cosine distance to compare these vectors. Finally The grades are determined using Eq. (29).

$$grade = 10 * (1.0 - d) \tag{29}$$

where d is the distance between the performance and the correct performance of the piece of music selected for the test which is in the range of 0 and 1.

5   Experiments

Our experimental set consists of 38 musical performances recorded with a smartphone at the music school named *Conservatory of the Roses in Mexico*. Students taking piano lessons played ten different music pieces, they are shown in Table 2, in the same table, the number of performances for each piece and the average duration is also shown and at the end of the table the total recording time was added. The compressed versions in mp3 may be downloaded from http://dep.fie.umich.mx/~camarena/conservatory/.

For each music piece of Table 2 there are several performances, one of them was considered correct since it was played by the teacher, by comparing the

Table 2. Set of performances for automatic evaluation tests

Music piece name	Number of performances	Average duration
Chun	4	16 s
Extra	5	30 s
Fugue VI, The art of the Fugue (J.S. Bach)	4	160 s
Für Elise (L.V. Beethoven)	3	180 s
The Flea Waltz	3	40 s
Mikrokosmos Lesson 2 (B. Bartok)	4	18 s
Minuet in G Major (J.S. Bach)	6	32 s
Des pas sur la neige, Praeludium VI (C. Debussy)	3	110 s
Praeludium I (J.S. Bach)	3	150 s
Praeludium VI (J.S. Bach)	3	100 s
Total	38	47 min: 38 s

rest of the performances of the same piece with the correct one a distance was determined using DTW, Levenshtein distance, and LCS distance. The automatic evaluation system assigns a grade to the student based on the distance between the performance played by the student and the correct performance played by the teacher, the larger the distance the lesser the grade.

In Table 3 the grades assigned to the students by the system using the aligning techniques explained above and the actual grade given by the teacher. In Table 3 column labeled G_T is the grade assigned by the teacher, column G_{DTW} is the grade assigned by the system using DTW for comparing the student performance to the reference, column G_L is the grade assigned by the system using the Levenshtein distance, and G_{LCS} is the grade assigned by the system using LCS distance. In the same table the absolute differences between the grades assigned by the teacher and the grades assigned by the system for the three metrics used are also shown in columns $|G_T - G_{DTW}|$, $|G_T - G_L|$, $|G_T - G_{LCS}|$.

Taking the grades assigned by the teacher as the ground truth, then the best evaluation method is the one that assigned grades that were closest to the grades assigned by the teacher and were most highly correlated with the grades assigned by the teacher. At the end of Table 3 the sum of the absolute differences between the grades assigned by the teacher and those assigned by the system. We can see there that $\sum |G_T - G_{DTW}| = 18.0$, $\sum |G_T - G_L| = 26.0$, and $\sum |G_T - G_{LCS}| = 51.7$. The correlation r_{xt} between method x (i.e. DTW, Levenshtein, or LCS) and the teacher t is determined using

$$r_{xt} = \frac{S_{xt}}{S_x S_t} \tag{30}$$

where S_{xt} is the covariance between the grades assigned by method x and the grades assigned by the teacher, S_x is the standard deviation of the grades assigned by method x and S_t is the standard deviation of the grades assigned by the teacher.

The correlation obtained by the three considered evaluation methods in our experiment is shown in Table 4. As Table 4 shows, Dynamic Time Warping turned out to be the best evaluation method assuming the grades assigned by the teacher to be the ground truth. this is confirmed by the fact that the least total absolute differences between the grades assigned by the teacher and those assigned by the system occurred when DTW was used. All three methods compare chromagrams by temporal alignment but DTW does not consider the sequences of chroma vectors to be sequences of symbols as edit distances do, even thought the cost of substitution in Levenshtein distance was taken as proportional to the difference between the chroma vectors being replaced one by the other (normalized to the range between 0 and 2), the cost of insertion and deletion was 1.0. Also in computing the LCS distance where no substitutions are allowed, the vectors were considered different if the normalized distance (in the range [0,1]) between them was below 0.25, several tests were conducted and this value appeared to be the most adequate.

Table 3. Grades obtained in automatic evaluation tests

Student	G_T	G_{DTW}	$|G_T - G_{DTW}|$	G_L	$|G_T - G_L|$	G_{LCS}	$|G_T - G_{LCS}|$
1	10	10.0	0.0	10.0	0.0	10.0	0.0
2	8	8.3	0.3	7.7	0.3	9.6	1.6
3	4	3.7	0.3	4.0	0.0	4.0	0.0
4	10	10.0	0.0	10	0.0	10.0	0.0
5	9	9.5	0.5	9.3	0.3	8.3	0.7
6	4	4.4	0.4	6.0	2.0	3.9	0.1
7	7	7.6	0.6	2.0	5.0	2.0	5.0
8	10	10.0	0.0	10.0	0.0	10.0	0.0
9	7	7.3	0.3	9.3	2.3	9.9	2.9
10	2	3.5	1.5	2.0	0.0	2.0	0.0
11	9	8.8	0.2	8.0	1.0	10.0	1.0
12	9	10.0	1.0	10.0	1.0	8.0	1.0
13	9	8.2	0.8	8.0	1.0	10.0	1.0
14	9	10.0	1.0	10.0	1.0	10.0	1.0
15	10	10.0	0.0	10.0	0.0	10.0	0.0
16	2	2.8	0.8	2.0	0.0	7.9	5.9
17	8	8.5	0.5	7.9	0.1	2.0	6.0
18	9	10.0	1.0	10.0	1.0	2.0	7.0
19	7	9.4	2.4	7.4	0.4	9.4	2.4
20	8	8.8	0.8	9.7	1.7	10.0	2.0
21	5	5.7	0.7	2.0	3.0	7.1	2.1
22	2	3.6	1.6	3.9	1.9	9.0	7.0
23	9	10.0	1.0	10.0	1.0	10.0	1.0
24	4	4.2	0.2	4.0	0.0	4.0	0.0
25	9	9.3	0.3	10.0	1.0	10.0	1.0
26	9	10.0	1.0	9.0	0.0	10.0	1.0
27	10	10.0	0.0	10.0	0.0	10.0	0.0
28	6	6.8	0.8	8.0	2.0	4.0	2.0
			Sum 18.0		Sum 26.0		Sum 51.7

Table 4. Correlation between the grades determined by the automatic evaluation module and the grades assigned by the teacher

DTW	Levenshtein	LCS
0.969	0.864	0.501

6   Conclusions and Future Work

Both the feature extraction and the evaluation module of a system that automatically evaluates music students were described in detail in this paper, even thought we are glad with the results of the experiments reported here, we know both modules may be improved. Regarding the feature extraction module, we intend to improve it by determining the chromagrams from the Harmonic Product Spectrum as in [7]. As for the evaluation method we intend to use a Hidden Markov Model to perform the comparison between the chromagram extracted from the music produced by the student and a correct performance of the same music, such correct performance would be used to build the Hidden Markov Model using the EM algorithm and the comparison would be performed by the forward procedure. We intend to use continuous Markov Models since using discrete ones would require vector quantization techniques that might affect the results.

References

1. Fober, D., Letz, S., Orlarey, Y., Askenfelt, A., Hansen, K.F., Schoonderwaldt, E.: Imutus: an interactive music tuition system. In: The Sound and Music Computing Conference (SMC 2004), 20–22 October 2004, pp. 97–103. IRCAM, Paris (2004)
2. Hu, N., Dannenberg, R.B., Tzanetakis, G.: Polyphonic audio matching and alignment for music retrieval. In: IEEE Workshop on Applications of Signal Processing to Audio and Acoustics (2003)
3. Navarro, G.: A guided tour to approximate string matching. ACM Comput. Surv. **33**(1), 31–88 (1997)
4. Robine, M., Percival, G., Lagrange, M.: Analysis of saxophone performance for computer-assisted tutoring. In: Proceedings of the International Computer Music Conference (ICMC 2007), vol. 2, pp. 381–384 (2007)
5. Schoonderwaldt, E., Askenfelt, A., Hansen, K.F.: Design and implementation of automatic evaluation of recorder performance in imutus. In: Proceedings of the International Computer Music Conference (ICMC), pp. 97–103 (2005)
6. Shannon, C., Weaver, W.: The Mathematical Theory of Communication. University of Illinois Press, Urbana (1949)
7. Stein, M., Schubert, B.M., Gruhne, M., Gatzsche, G., Mehnert, M.: Evaluation and comparison of audio chroma feature extraction methods. In: 126th Audio Engineering Society Convention. Audio Engineering Society (2009)
8. Vila, A.T., Cifre, B.S., Llabrs, B.M.: Objective rhythmic performance evaluation tool (o.r.p.e.t.): a numerical method to evaluate the accuracy of a musical performance. J. Music Technol. Educ. **6**(1), 61–80 (2013)

On the Extended Specific Objectivity of Some Pseudo–Rasch Models Applied in Testing Scenarios

Joel Suárez–Cansino[1](✉), Luis R. Morales–Manilla[2],
and Virgilio López–Morales[1]

[1] Information and Systems Technologies Research Center, Autonomous University
of the State of Hidalgo, Mineral de la Reforma, Hidalgo, Mexico
jsuarez@uaeh.edu.mx
[2] Applied Software Development Research Group, Engineering Division,
Polytechnic University of Tulancingo, Tulancingo, Hidalgo, Mexico

Abstract. The design of a Computer Adaptive Testing (CAT) system
assumes the existence of an item pool containing properly calibrated
items. The calibration is based on an Item Characteristic Curve (ICC).
In this paper two mathematical ICC models, and how these models properly
fit into the concept of extended Rasch specific objectivity, are under
analysis. The results make clear that the comparison between two items
depends on subdomains of the complete domain of the corresponding
ICC's. The introduced models are also useful to describe the characteristics
of skewness and bimodality in the population, where classical models
commonly fail.

Keywords: Computer Adaptive Testing · Specific objectivity · Item
Characteristic Curve · Skewness · Bimodality

1 Introduction

Computer Adaptive Testing (CAT) is an example of a Computer Based Test
(CBT) and is one of the main trending topics in the area of knowledge testing [1]
and, more recently, in e–learning or in Intelligent Tutoring Systems scenarios [2].
The Item Response Theory (IRT) defines the theoretical basis of a CAT implementation
[3], which assumes the existence of a repository of items that is used
during the testing process of a particular examinee. Every item in the repository
must be calibrated at the initial steps of the implementation of the CAT system,
based on the specification of a psychometric model. The calibration process is
achieved to determine the parameters values defined by a psychometric model
previously defined and, in general, the parameters values change from one item
to another. In fact, the calibration stage can be compared with the learning stage
of an artificial intelligent system, and this is one of the main reasons to make a
reliable calibration process.

© Springer International Publishing Switzerland 2015
O. Pichardo Lagunas et al. (Eds.): MICAI 2015, Part II, LNAI 9414, pp. 232–248, 2015.
DOI: 10.1007/978-3-319-27101-9_17

The psychometric model used in the process depends on the specific scenario where the CAT system is applied. Usually, its structure is defined by a sigmoidal or logistic function, which depends on the examinee's ability and contains one or more parameters. Hence, an item designer could find models of one, two, three or four parameters, depending on the chosen model called 1PL, 2PL, 3PL and 4PL model, respectively.

For 1PL model, also known as the Rasch's model, ideal experimental conditions are assumed, while for the remaining models some additional item properties are highlighten which are useful to describe the item's capability to clearly distinguish among the examinees' abilities, the degree of item guessing and the degree of item inattention.

However, when considering some simulated or real experimental results, these models can have a lower performance when skewed and/or multimodal behaviors are included in the statistical characteristics of the population. The knowledge of the distribution behavior becomes a very important question when student achievement is involved. A distribution with bimodality in this kind of context can be useful to predict failures of the lower sub–population in future testing processes, and to make more reliable item calibrations. There are some interesting examples in the literature where dealing with these failures is a very important question for solving several academic problems [4–6].

The choose of a suitable psychometric model structure and its parameters is a *sine qua non* condition in order to provide reliable information concerned with the examinee's ability, item's and test's difficulty, among others.

Furthermore, the values of the item's parameters are related to this kind of information, and once that the parameters values are obtained, they are very useful in e–learning scenarios, Intelligent Tutoring Systems or Computer Adaptive Testing Systems, where an immediate and reliable diagnostic is required for giving a support to the teaching–learning or testing process [7].

The finding of meaningful interpretations of the parameters in the model can be also very useful to make the best decisions in this sense. The constraint models (for instance, 2PL/MML framework), nonparametric function estimates and others flexible models, such as Ramsay–curves and splines, do not provide a direct way of doing this. On the other hand, the cited examples are real contexts where constraint models like 2PL/MML are not enough to describe them.

As a matter of fact, it is well known that traditional psychometric models provide an interpretation of every item's parameter in terms of the item's difficulty, item's discriminant, degree of item guessing, and so on [8]. In this paper, the properties of two generalized sigmoidal psychometric models are analyzed and shown to be more flexible than the previous ones, meaning that they could be applied in more complex testing scenarios, where some aspects of skewness and bimodality can be included.

The analysis of our models is made on the basis of the mathematical behavior, which is described not only by the latent trait variable or examinee's ability, but by the parameters, as well. The concept of specific objectivity is also used as a mean of validation of our models.

1.1   Standard Psychometric Models and Specific Objectivity

The 1PL model is the simplest psychometric model and is defined by the Equation (1)

$$p_i(x = 1|\theta, \mu_i) = \frac{1}{1 + e^{-(\theta - \mu_i)}} \tag{1}$$

where $p_i(x = 1|\theta, \mu)$ denotes the probability of a correct response of the examinee to the i–th item, given that θ is the examinee's ability and μ_i is the item's difficulty. An important characteristic of this model is that the specific objectivity is verified, since it allows a comparison of both the performance of any two examinees and of any two items in one test [9,10].

In order to state a formal definition of specific objectivity, let us recall the following. The psychometric model verifies $p : E \times I \longrightarrow (a, b)$, where E and I are the sets of examinees and items in the test, respectively, and $(a, b) \subseteq [0, 1]$. The specific objectivity of the model assumes the existence of a function, $\chi : (a, b) \times (a, b) \longrightarrow \mathbb{R}$, and defines a multivariable vector function $\boldsymbol{p} : (E \times I) \times (E \times I) \longrightarrow (a, b) \times (a, b)$, where $\boldsymbol{p}((r, u), (s, v)) = (p(r, u), p(s, v))$, such that the composition of functions $c = \chi \circ \boldsymbol{p} : (E \times I) \times (E \times I) \longrightarrow \mathbb{R}$ compares the pair (r, u) with the pair (s, v) under one of the following conditions [9,10],

1. The comparison of any two objects $r, s \in E$ is independent of the choice $u, v \in I, u = v$, and of any other element $t \in E, t \neq r, s$.
2. The comparison of any two objects $u, v \in I$ is independent of the choice $r, s \in E, r = s$, and of any other element $w \in I, w \neq u, v$.

Comparing function c is specifically objective within the frame of reference defined by E, I and p. The function c of the first condition does not need to be equal to the function c of the second condition; *i.e.*, the function χ of the first condition can be quite different of the function χ of the second condition. However, the psychometric model p is always the same.

1.2   Generalized Models

Some authors have explained the reasons for proposing more sophisticated alternatives formulations to the Rasch model, with the main intention of including the possible skewness of the experimental data [11]. In [9] it is proposed an extension of the specific objectivity concept, giving the possibility of comparing three or more elements in the sets E or I, and even in [10] the specific objectivity concept is excluded as a necessary requirement, which leads to the idea of pseudo–Rasch models.

Example 1. A relatively simple general model can be proposed, which is a slight modification of another function by [12],

$$p(x = 1|\theta, \mu, \alpha, a, c, d, g) = d + (a - d)p^g \left(x = 1 \bigg| \theta, \mu + \frac{1}{\alpha} \mathrm{lnc}, \alpha \right) \tag{2}$$

where the Cumulative Distribution Function (CDF), p, on the right hand side of (2), is given by the 2PL model, as defined by (3),

$$p(x = 1|\theta, \mu, \alpha) = \frac{1}{1 + e^{-\alpha(\theta - \mu)}}. \tag{3}$$

2 Analysis of the Proposed Models

In this scenario, several alternatives of psychometric models are possible. However, in order to keep the strength of Rasch's model [13,14] some constraints are introduced. For instance,

(i) the proposed model must be part of a frame of reference with specific objectivity, even with the extended one, which admits the comparison among two, three or more elements of E or I,

(ii) the model also must be quite flexible to admit skewness and some multimodality that the ability could possibly show and,

(iii) finally, the proposed model must verify the Rasch's model as a particular case.

The model given by (2) contains six parameters μ, α, a, c, d and g, and it verifies the constraints mentioned before. As a matter of fact, the interpretation of parameters μ, α, a and d, coincides with that given to the parameters in the very well known 1PL, 2PL, 3PL and 4PL models [12,15]. In addition to that, the Rasch's model, along with the 2PL, 3PL and 4PL models, are particular cases of the more general 6PL model defined by (2).

Furthermore, with the model given by (2), hereafter called extended 6PL Rasch's model, the interpretation of the new parameters c and g includes the concept of skewness of the experimental data, since the parameter c implies a correction term to the difficulty μ. However, it can be proved that the model does not produce symmetrical skews (the left skew is not a mirror image of the right skew).

2.1 Behavior of the Extended 6PL Rasch's Model

The change of concavity and the symmetrical behavior relative to the upper and lower asymptotes, respectively defined by the equations (4),

$$\lim_{\theta \to \pm\infty} p(x = 1|\theta, \mu, \alpha, a, d, c, g) = \begin{cases} a \\ d \end{cases} \tag{4}$$

are two important points to be considered in the behavior of the extended 6PL Rasch's model. At this stage of the discussion, let us analyze conditions to successfully apply this CDF as a proper psychometric model, mathematically speaking.

In order to do so, in the analysis of the function behavior first and second derivatives are involved and it can be easily proved that the CDF (2) is an increasing function. On the other hand, the change of concavity occurs at the single point

$\theta = \mu + \frac{1}{\alpha}\ln(cg)$ in the domain of the CDF (2) and $d + \frac{a-d}{(1+g^{-1})^g}$ is the value of the function at this point. Now, the condition of rapid growing of the CDF is established through the definition of a positive parameter κ such that,

$$\frac{\kappa}{\alpha g(a-d)} \le p^g \left(x=1\,\middle|\,\theta, \mu + \frac{1}{\alpha}\ln c, \alpha\right) - p^{g+1}\left(x=1\,\middle|\,\theta, \mu + \frac{1}{\alpha}\ln c, \alpha\right) \quad (5)$$

Then, the set of abilities θ satisfying this inequality becomes the interval where the CDF (2) grows rapidly. Since this CDF is an increasing function, then the roots of the equality in inequation (5) define the *infimum* and *supremum* of the interval. Inequality (5) can also be seen as the specification of the lower bound given by $\frac{\kappa}{\alpha g(a-d)}$ to the polynomial $f(x) = x^g - x^{g+1}$ in the real unit interval $(0,1)$, with real power $g, 0 < g$. The derivative of this polynomial is given by (6)

$$\frac{d}{dx}f(x) = (g+1)x^{g-1}\left(\frac{g}{g+1} - x\right), \quad (6)$$

which is always positive in the interval $\left(0, \frac{g}{g+1}\right)$ (increasing function f) and negative in the interval $\left(\frac{g}{g+1}, 1\right)$ (decreasing function f).

If $0 < g < 1$, then the function f does not have a change of concavity and is always concave downward (since its second derivative is always negative). On the other hand, if $1 < g$, then the function f changes from being concave upward to be concave downward at the critical point $\theta = \frac{g-1}{g+1}$. The point $\theta = \frac{g}{g+1}$ in the domain of f is a critical point where the function f has a *maximum* value for arbitrary values of the parameter $g, 0 < g$. This means that the function defined by the equality in (5) has only two real roots if the constant $\frac{\kappa}{\alpha g(a-d)}$ satisfies the conditions (7),

$$0 < \frac{\kappa}{\alpha(a-d)} < \left(\frac{g}{g+1}\right)^{g+1} \quad (7)$$

The asymmetrical behavior of the function f ensures that the two roots are asymmetrical with respect to the point $\frac{g}{g+1}$. This behavior of f implies the possibility of obtaining a skewed Probability Density Function (PDF) for the CDF (2); however, the behavior of this skewness is not completely symmetrical, in the sense already explained at the beginning of this section.

The prove of the existence of an asymmetrical skewness for the extended 6PL Rasch's model considers the value of this function at the point $\theta = \mu + \frac{1}{\alpha}\ln(cg)$, where the change of concavity appears. The distance between the point $(\mu + \frac{1}{\alpha}\ln(cg), d)$ on the lower asymptote and the point where the change of concavity appears is given by the expression $\frac{a-d}{(1+g^{-1})^g}$, which means that the distance is proportional to $a - d$, where the proportion is defined by the expression $\frac{1}{(1+\frac{1}{g})^g}$.

Note that the parameter g has a lower bound equal to zero, but it can grow without limit, so that it is interesting to know the bounds of this proportion. By using the definition of the basis of the natural logarithm and the L'Hopital's rule, it is relatively easy to notice that these limits are 1 and $\frac{1}{e}$, when $g \to 0$ and $g \to +\infty$, respectively.

Thus, the distance between the point on the lower asymptote, $(\mu + \frac{1}{\alpha}\ln(cg), d)$, and the point on the CDF where the change of concavity occurs, can be as long as $a - d$ or as short as $\frac{1}{e}(a - d)$, which means that the right skewness of the CDF is not necessarily symmetrical to the left skewness of the same model of the CDF.

2.2 The Extended 6PL Rasch's Model and Specific Objectivity

The behavior of this model is quite complex, and it is difficult, if not impossible, to handle in a direct way the concept of specific objectivity. However, the function can be approximated by the piecewise function (8), which is defined in some interval of abilities,

$$
p(x = 1|\theta, \mu, \alpha, a, c, d, g) \approx
\begin{cases}
\frac{1}{1+\exp\left(-\alpha\left(\theta-\mu-\frac{1}{\alpha}\ln c\right)\right)}, & \text{if } \mu + \frac{1}{\alpha}\ln c \ll \theta \\[2ex]
\frac{1}{\exp\left(-\alpha g\left(\theta-\mu-\frac{1}{\alpha}\ln c\right)\right)}, & \text{if } \theta \ll \mu + \frac{1}{\alpha}\ln c \\[2ex]
\frac{1}{2^g\left(1-\frac{1}{2}g\right)} \cdot \frac{1}{1+\exp\left(-\alpha\left(\theta-\mu-\frac{1}{\alpha}\ln\frac{cg}{2\left(1-\frac{1}{2}g\right)}\right)\right)}, & \text{otherwise}
\end{cases}
\tag{8}
$$

The piecewise definition of the function $p(x = 1|\theta, \mu, \alpha, a, c, d, g)$ and the idea of an extended specific objectivity permit to compare three arbitrarily chosen abilities and two arbitrarily chosen items. It should be noticed that the choice of any two expressions of the piecewise definition of the function $p(x = 1|\theta, \mu, \alpha, a, c, d, g)$ represents to exactly the same CDF, so that the concept of specific objectivity is properly applied in this sense.

Hence, the comparison of three abilities can be made by means of the following definition of the function $\chi : (0,1) \times (0,1) \times (0,1) \longrightarrow \mathbb{R}$,

$$
\chi(x_1, x_2, x_3) = \frac{\ln\left(\frac{x_1}{1-x_1} \cdot \frac{1-x_2}{x_2}\right)}{\ln\left(\frac{x_1}{1-x_1} \cdot \frac{1-x_3}{x_3}\right)}
\tag{9}
$$

and through the assumption that the specific objectivity gets rid of any scale factor in any expression of the piecewise definition of the CDF. So, for example, $c((r, u), (s, u), (t, u)) = \frac{\theta_r - \theta_s}{\theta_r - \theta_t}$. Similarly, two items can be compared through the following definition of the function $\chi : (0,1) \times (0,1) \times (0,1) \times (0,1) \longrightarrow \mathbb{R}$,

$$
\chi(x_1, x_2, x_3, x_4) = \frac{\ln\left(\frac{x_1}{1-x_1} \cdot \frac{1-x_2}{x_2}\right)}{\ln\left(\frac{x_3}{1-x_3} \cdot \frac{1-x_4}{x_4}\right)}
\tag{10}
$$

and the idea of specific objectivity already suggested. Therefore, two items can be compared considering the same expression, or any two expressions, of the piecewise definition of the CDF, as follows, $c((r, u), (s, u), (r, v), (r, v)) = \frac{\alpha_u}{\alpha_v}$ or $c((r, u), (s, u), (r, v), (r, v)) = \frac{\alpha_u g_u}{\alpha_v}$.

These results imply that one single item can be compared with itself through subdomain definitions, making clear that one item can have different discriminant capabilities. Therefore, two different items (u, v) can be compared taking some of the following indexes $\frac{\alpha_u}{\alpha_v}, \frac{\alpha_u g_u}{\alpha_v}, \frac{\alpha_v}{\alpha_u g_u}, \frac{\alpha_v}{\alpha_u}$ and one single item u with the indexes $g_u, \frac{1}{g_u}$.

2.3   An Improved and More Flexible 6PL Model

The authors in reference [16] propose another CDF with six parameters in a different context, and this function is defined as follows,

$$p(x = 1|\theta, \mu, \alpha, \beta, k, a, d) = d + \frac{a - d}{1 + \frac{e^{-\alpha(\theta-\mu)}}{1+e^{k(\theta-\mu)}} + \frac{e^{-\beta(\theta-\mu)}}{1+e^{-k(\theta-\mu)}}} \tag{11}$$

where the definition $k = \frac{2\alpha\beta}{|\alpha+\beta|}$ specifies a constraint on the possible values of k. However, the model discussed in this work only requires that $0 \leq d < a \leq 1, \mu \in (-\infty, +\infty)$ and does not impose constraints on the possible values of k. Notice also that the model satisfies the two asymptotic behaviors when $\theta \to \pm\infty$ and that the Rasch's model can be obtained as a particular case when $a = 1, d = 0, k = 0$ and $\alpha = \beta$. The possible values of α and β are deduced from an analysis of the asymptotic behavior of the function (11). This analysis shows that $0 < \alpha$ and $0 < \beta$.

2.4   The Flexible 6PL Model and Specific Objectivity

The condition of specific objectivity is in some way intimately related to the concept of inverse function. So that, given the CDF (11), one possible means to find the proper transformation, leading to the property of specific objectivity, consists in finding the roots of the equation (12)

$$1 + \frac{1}{1 + e^{k(\theta-\mu)}} e^{-\alpha(\theta-\mu)} + \frac{1}{1 + e^{-k(\theta-\mu)}} e^{-\beta(\theta-\mu)} = \frac{a - d}{p(x = 1|\theta, \mu, \alpha, \beta, k, a, d) - d} \tag{12}$$

which comes after some manipulation over the Equation (11).

At first sight, it might be quite difficult to find an analytical expression of the possible roots of (12). However, the asymptotic analysis shed some light on the behavior of the left side of (12) in the limits $k \longrightarrow \pm\infty$ and $\theta \longrightarrow \pm\infty$.

Conditions specified by Table 1 say that, for some proper parameters α, β, k, there are regions in the domain of the function $p(x = 1|\theta, \mu, \alpha, \beta, k, a, d)$ where the specific objectivity is achieved. So, for example, the conditions $\alpha > 0, \beta > 0$ and $k \gg 1$ define the asymptotic behavior $1 + e^{-\alpha(\theta-\mu)}$ of the left side of (12) in an interval $(-\infty, \theta^*)$, where $\theta^* < \mu$.

A similar analysis on some interval $(\theta^{**}, +\infty)$, where $\mu < \theta^{**}$, shows the existence of specific objectivity, as well. By symmetry, one should expect similar results when $k \ll -1$, with the asymptotic behavior specified by the second row of the Table 1. So, three regions in the domain of definition of the CDF (11) specify the approximated behavior of the model.

Table 1. The asymptotic behavior of the left side of the Equation (12). Although ur means 'unrestricted value', it is assumed that $\alpha > 0$ and $\beta > 0$ to satisfy the asymptotic behavior of the function (11).

k	θ	α	β	Asymptotic behavior	Comments
$+\infty$	$-\infty$	$+$	ur	$1 + e^{-\alpha(\theta-\mu)}$	These conditions imply the existence of
	$+\infty$	ur	$+$	$1 + e^{-\beta(\theta-\mu)}$	intervals to the left and right of $\theta = \mu$ where the CDF given by (11) becomes increasing and with complex behavior in a neighborhood of $\theta = \mu$
$-\infty$	$-\infty$	ur	$+$	$1 + e^{-\beta(\theta-\mu)}$	Similar comments to previous row
	$+\infty$	$+$	ur	$1 + e^{-\alpha(\theta-\mu)}$	

Thus, the flexible 6PL model can be approximated by the piecewise exponential function (13),

$$p(x = 1|\theta, \mu, \alpha, \beta, k, a, d) \approx \begin{cases} \frac{1}{1+e^{-\alpha(\theta-\mu)}} & \text{if } \theta \in I_\alpha(\mu, k), \\ \frac{1}{1+e^{-\frac{\alpha+\beta}{2}(\theta-\mu)}} & \text{if } \theta \in I_{\frac{\alpha+\beta}{2}}(\mu, k), \\ \frac{1}{1+e^{-\beta(\theta-\mu)}} & \text{if } \theta \in I_\beta(\mu, k), \end{cases} \quad (13)$$

where the intervals $I_\alpha(\mu, k), I_{\frac{\alpha+\beta}{2}}(k), I_\beta(\mu, k)$ depend on the parameters μ and k. Note that $I_\alpha(\mu, k) \cap I_{\frac{\alpha+\beta}{2}}(\mu, k) = \emptyset, I_\alpha(\mu, k) \cap I_\beta(\mu, k) = \emptyset, I_\beta(\mu, k) \cap I_{\frac{\alpha+\beta}{2}}(\mu, k) = \emptyset$ and also $I_\alpha(\mu, k) \cup I_{\frac{\alpha+\beta}{2}}(\mu, k) \cup I_\beta(\mu, k) = \mathbb{R}$. This representation suggests that the item contains three discriminant parameters, as given by α, β and $\frac{\alpha+\beta}{2}$.

Thus, the comparison function is similar to the function of the extended Rasch 6PL model and three abilities and two items can be compared by using the functions defined in the Equation (9) and the Equation (10), respectively. Let $\mu_u, \alpha_u, \beta_u, k_u$ be the parameters of the item u and $\theta_r, \theta_s, \theta_t$, which are the abilities of three arbitrary and different examinees. Then the comparison function is evaluated as follows,

$$c((r, u), (s, u), (t, u)) = \frac{\theta_r - \theta_s}{\theta_r - \theta_t} \quad (14)$$

Similarly, in order to compare two items, let us consider only the examinees r and s and the items u and v. Then,

$$c(p(r, u), p(s, u), p(r, v), p(s, v)) = \frac{\gamma_u}{\gamma_v}, \quad (15)$$

compares two arbitrary items, without considering the examinee's characteristics. The comparisons can be obtained as follows, $\frac{\alpha_u}{\left(\frac{\alpha_v+\beta_v}{2}\right)}, \frac{\beta_u}{\left(\frac{\alpha_v+\beta_v}{2}\right)}, \frac{\alpha_u}{\alpha_v}, \frac{\beta_u}{\beta_v},$ $\frac{\left(\frac{\alpha_u+\beta_u}{2}\right)}{\beta_v}, \frac{\left(\frac{\alpha_u+\beta_u}{2}\right)}{\alpha_v}, \frac{\alpha_u}{\alpha_v}, \frac{\beta_u}{\beta_v}, \frac{\left(\frac{\alpha_u+\beta_u}{2}\right)}{\left(\frac{\alpha_v+\beta_v}{2}\right)}$ or even within the same item it could be there comparisons by regions, $\frac{\alpha_u}{\left(\frac{\alpha_u+\beta_u}{2}\right)}, \frac{\beta_u}{\left(\frac{\alpha_u+\beta_u}{2}\right)}, \frac{\alpha_u}{\beta_u}, \frac{\beta_u}{\alpha_u}, \frac{\left(\frac{\alpha_u+\beta_u}{2}\right)}{\beta_u}, \frac{\left(\frac{\alpha_u+\beta_u}{2}\right)}{\alpha_u}.$

3 Simulation Results

In order to get a glimpse of the possible conclusions coming from the theoretical analysis of both models, in the following, a discussion of some results obtained by a numerical simulation, is given.

The simulation can be implemented in two ways that assume the definition of the samples of examinees and items. The examinees' abilities and items' parameters represent the examinees and items, respectively. Given an examinee and an item, the probability of correct response is computed through the *a priori* definition of the psychometric model, as well.

However, these definitions are given with simulation purposes, since in a real calibration process they are unknown and need to be determined. Both approaches have some advantages and drawbacks and proceed as follows.

3.1 Complete Simulation Process

The experimental setting of the simulation considers the number of examinees, M, and items, N, as two variables running into proper sample sizes. The simulation defines a test with these examinees and items, whose abilities and parameters, respectively, are unknown. However, for simulation purposes, their values are randomly generated by a normal or uniform distribution, within *a priori* bounded real intervals or just considering some well–known finite sets of real numbers, *cf.* [17–19].

After defining the mechanism to generate the unknown variables and parameters, the definition of another mechanism to generate the items' responses is performed. This kind of simulation can involve the generation of examinees' responses based on the application of the CDF (11) along with uniformly and randomly generated values in the unit interval $(0, 1)$.

Given an examinee and an item, which are respectively represented by θ and a set of the parameter's values $(\mu, \alpha, \beta, k, a, d)$, the probability of successful response is computed through the model (11). So, the result is compared against r, which is a number randomly selected with uniform distribution from the unit interval $(0, 1)$. If $r \leq p$, then the response is assumed correct, otherwise the response is incorrect.

Responses are then processed to obtain the experimental values of the examinee's abilities, the item's difficulties and the probabilities of successful responses. However, this procedure does not necessarily ensure that the experimental probabilities of successful response are properly fitted into the generating CDF (11). Nevertheless, the acquisition of simulated experimental raw data is one of the main advantages of this procedure. These data can then be fitted into a proper psychometric model to obtain the estimated items' parameters.

3.2 Partial Simulation Process

Unlike the complete simulation process, the partial simulation does not require to generate items' responses. The probabilities of correct responses are not experimentally computed, but they are directly given by the CDF (11), and slightly modified through a normal or uniformly distributed random noise. In other words, the procedure assumes that a set of responses are previously given and that a calibration process has been made to get the experimental probabilities of a successful response.

For a given simulated ability θ, the corresponding noised probability $p(\theta)$ of a correct response is a random variable with normal distribution $\mathcal{N}(p(\theta), \sigma_c)$ in some subinterval of the unit interval $[0, 1]$, or a random variable with skewed normal distribution $\mathcal{N}(0, \sigma_l)$ in a neighborhood of 0, or a random variable with skewed normal distribution $\mathcal{N}(1, \sigma_r)$ in a neighborhood of 1. The Fig. 1 shows this kind of behavior in the experimental probability with error.

The lack of a specific set of experimental responses, to explain where these probabilities are coming from, is one of the main inconvenience of this method. However, there are some possibilities to analyze the fit of the data to others different psychometric models, by making some comparisons against the generating function $p(x = 1 | \theta, \mu, \alpha, \beta, k, a, d)$.

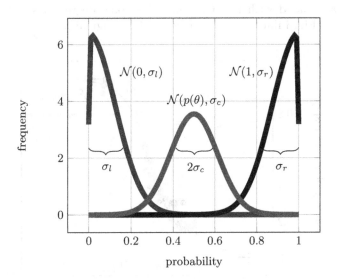

Fig. 1. Experimental probabilities are produced with three different PDF's. The probabilities closer to the asymptotes of the ICC are produced with skew normal distributions.

3.3   Presentation of Experimental Results

Based on some previous results in the literature on the topic [17, 19], the examinees' abilities are assumed to have a normal distribution $\mathcal{N}(0, 1)$ and a sample size of 80 examinees has been chosen. Nevertheless, in a real situation, skewness and multimodality appear. Then, the function $p(x = 1 | \theta, \mu, \alpha, \beta, k, a, d)$ should be adopted during the simulation. Hereafter, the comparison between the 2PL model, the extended 6PL Rasch model and the flexible 6PL model considers the data produced by a partial simulation process.

Within ideal circumstances, the experimental data should fit properly the 2PL, the 6PL extended Rasch and the 6PL flexible models. The ideal situation assumes the lack of skewness and multimodality, and this situation is precisely considered by any of the different versions of the original Rasch model (1PL, 2PL, 3PL and 4PL models). Furthermore, in Subsection *Behavior of the extended 6PL Rasch's model* and Subsection *An improved and more flexible 6PL model* it is shown that some kind of skewness and multimodality in experimental data coming from a population, can be properly represented into the extended 6PL Rasch and the flexible 6PL models. In Fig. 2 this behavior is shown, where simulated data were generated with the CDF

$$p(x = 1|\theta) = \frac{1}{1 + \left(1 - \frac{1}{1+e^{-10\theta}}\right)e^{-\theta} + \frac{e^{-5\theta}}{1+e^{-10\theta}}} \tag{16}$$

The PDF associated with this CDF contains some degree of skewness and a bimodality as Fig. 3 illustrates (curve with label 'original').

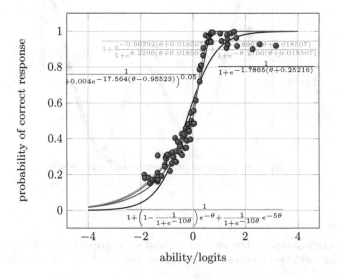

Fig. 2. Experimental simulated probabilities are generated with the CDF (16) and random noise given by PDF in Fig. 1.

Notice that in Fig. 3 the 'flexible' 6PL model with four fixed parameters $(\beta = 5, k = 10, a = 1, d = 0)$, and two parameters (μ, α) determined by curve fitting, achieves a better approximation than 2PL and extended 6PL Rasch's models.

On the other hand, the 'extended' 6PL Rasch's model with four fixed parameters $(a = 1, d = 0, c = 0.004, g = 0.05)$, and two parameters (μ, α) determined

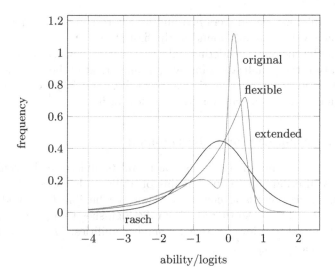

Fig. 3. The PDF's of the corresponding CDF's shown by the Fig. 2. The PDF coming from the fitted 6PL flexible CDF exactly fits the PDF coming from the CDF (16).

by curve fitting, performes better than 2PL Rasch's model, but does not improve over the 'extended' 6PL with four fixed parameters.

Finally, in Fig. 3 it is also shown that the simulated data fit better to the PDF from the flexible 6PL model, which contains skewness and bimodality. On the other hand, the extended 6PL Rasch's model contains the skewed behavior of the experimental data. The 2PL Rasch's model cannot predict these kind of behaviors.

The Akaike Information Criterion (AIC) and the Bayesian Information Criterion (BIC) are two importante statistical methods to test the performance of fit [20–22]. The first method includes a penalization for overparameterization and, along with BIC, respectively produce the results 151.7, 151.18 and 151.29, when the 2PL Rasch's model, the flexible model and the extended 6PL Rasch's model consider only the two parameters (μ, α), while the rest of the parameters are fixed.

However, the 2PL Rasch's model is outperforming when, in the parameter estimation, the fitting of the whole set of parameters is considered. The 2PL Rasch's model produce similar results by using both AIC and BIC. Since AIC includes a penalization for overparameterization, it should be expected that the 2PL Rasch's model is more efficient. This result changes through the application of the following three steps, where the inattention and guessing parameters are set to 1 and 0, respectively

1. Fit the models with the presence of the corresponding set of fitting parameters; in other words, the fitting process must consider as unknown two parameters for the 2PL Rasch model and four parameters for the extended 6PL Rasch's model, and the flexible 6PL model.

2. Keep the unknown parameters μ, α and fix the rest of the unknown parameters to their values already found in the first step.
3. Fit again the models considering only the parameters μ, α as unknown. In this situation the penalization for overparameterization becomes identical in the three models, and the statistical tests AIC and BIC consider only the mean square error as a criterion for goodness of fit.

3.4 Computation of Item's Discriminant

The results of the simulation can also be useful to illustrate the computation of the item's discriminant in subdomains of abilities. For example, the Fig. 2 shows an item characteristic curve based on the flexible 6PL model, where $\alpha = 0.96792, \beta = 4.8961$, so that the item distinguishes to a greater degree for higher abilities and to a lower extent for smaller abilities; $i.e.$, $\frac{\beta}{\alpha} = 5.0584, \frac{\beta}{\gamma} = 1.6699, \frac{\gamma}{\alpha} = 3.0292$, where $\gamma = \frac{\alpha+\beta}{2}$.

3.5 Abilities and Parameters Estimation

The proposed models can actually be estimated and the number of observations needed to make the estimation can be acceptably good, since the maximum likelihood method leads to a system of decoupled nonlinear equations; namely, M equations for abilities $\boldsymbol{\theta}$ need to be solved, where some seeds are required for the $6N$ parameters, and $6N$ equations involving the parameters μ, α, β, k, a and d, need to be solved assuming the abilities' values already found in the first step,

Particularly, the estimated ability of the i–th examinee can be computed by finding the roots of the equation i–th in the given system of decoupled nonlinear equations. Of course, the standard assumptions given in the literature must be also applied to get the required results (for instance, every examinee provide a correct response and one incorrect response, at least, to one pair of items in the set of items) [3, 23, 24].

The decoupled aspect of the nonlinear system of equations concerning the parameters of the items, leads to similar comments to those given at the end of the previous paragraph, although a system of six coupled nonlinear equations per item needs to be solved. In this case, it is very useful to know that the parameters α_i, β_i, a_i and d_i for item i–th need to satisfy the constraints $0 < \alpha_i, 0 < \beta_i$ and $0 \le d_i < a_i \le 1$.

Although the topic on root finding is currently under research by the authors of this paper, it is possible to get some information about this problem, based on the comments already made in the previous paragraphs, and the realization of relatively simple simulated examples. One example considers the case where 45 is the number of examinees and items. Assuming that the items' parameters are known, a single iteration estimates the abilities with an rms error equal to 0.03. The second example considers the case where 20 is the number of examinees and 15 is the number of items. The example applies two iterations to estimate the examinees' abilities, assuming that at the first iteration the items' parameters are known. The estimate of the abilities at the first iteration produces an rms error equal to 0.01 in the values, while the estimate of the parameters in the same iteration produces an rms error equal to 0.09 in the values. Finally, the second iteration produces an estimate of abilities with an rms error equal to 0.07 in the values. The correlation coefficient between the estimated abilities in the first and the second iterations acquires the value 0.93, which is acceptably fine. Figure 4 shows the results after the second iteration in the abilities values for the case of 20 examinees and 15 items.

The extended 6PL Rasch's model has an identifibiality problem for its ability and difficulty parameter θ and $\mu + \frac{1}{\alpha}\ln c$, respectively, since the CDF remains the same when they are substituted by the corresponding expressions $\theta + \delta$ and $\mu + \frac{1}{\alpha}\ln c + \delta, 0 < \delta$ [25]. This is a location identifiability, but there is a scale identifiability as well, since the CDF also remains the same through the scaling $\frac{\alpha}{\kappa}, \theta\kappa, \left(\mu + \frac{1}{\alpha}\ln c\right)\kappa$, where $0 < \kappa$. A popular practice to solve the problem of identifiability defines the mean and standard deviation of the parameters θ's equal to zero and one across the test takers in the sample, respectively [25]. This procedure is usually applied in the cases of the 2PL and 3PL models, where a similar expression as a function of the ability θ and the parameters α and μ produce the identifiability problem, as well. However, there are some other possibilities of useful restrictions giving equally good estimates [25]. On the other hand, the approximation of the flexible 6PL model suggests also that the same set of restrictions should yield acceptable results.

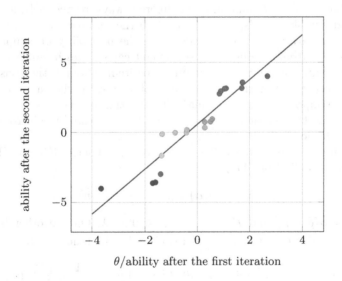

Fig. 4. Correlation between the abilities' estimates in first and second iterations in the case of 20 examinees and 15 items. The correlation coefficient is equal to 0.93 and the linear fit is given by the function $1.6\theta + 0.57$, where θ is the ability after the first iteration.

4   Conclusion

In addition to the possibility of the item's difficulty, the item's discriminant, the item guessing and the item inattention, some complex testing scenarios need to be considered in contexts where multimodality and skewness can be found. Thus, traditional psychometric models are not useful any more to cope with this problem. Particularly, two well–known psychometric models have been analyzed here. Every model is defined by six parameters, where four parameters are associated with the difficulty, discriminant, guessing and inattention, and the others could be associated with distribution skewness and bimodality from population under analysis. A direct extension of the usual psychometric 1PL, 2PL, 3PL and 4PL models is introduced, and the new models so defined use parameters to control the characteristics of bimodality and skewness in the distribution functions.

Naturally, the models performance depend on the accomplishment of a specific objectivity. In this sense, the concept of specific objectivity is also modified giving models that satisfy the specified requirements, at least in some intervals of ability in the worst case, as represented by the extended 6PL Rasch's model. Furthermore, as a drawback, the degree of skewness is constrained under the extended 6PL Rasch's model, which is avoided with the flexible 6PL model.

The identification of two and three values of the item's discriminant for a single item is an interesting result arising from the extended 6PL Rasch's model and the flexible 6PL model, respectively. Another result is that the value of the item's discriminant is found to depend on the interval where the ability belongs to. The redefinition of a specific objectivity suggests that two arbitrary items can be compared in four and nine different ways, respectively, for the 6PL Rasch's and flexible models, which depend on the selected values of the items' discriminants. Particularly, both models give the possibility of comparing one single item with itself, through its discriminant capabilities by subdomains.

The possibility of comparing examinees or items through the constraint of specific objectivity, even though they do not belong to the same asymptotic region, is one important point to remark. The partial specific objectivity in some models, or even the absence of this property, has suggested the introduction of pseudo–Rasch models [10].

The authors of the reference [26] introduce less restrictive ICC's to IRT models through the definition (17),

$$p(x = 1|\theta, \mu, \alpha) = d + (a - d)F(m) \tag{17}$$

where $m = \alpha(\theta - \mu)$ and $F(x) = \frac{1}{(1+e^{-x})^\lambda}, 0 < \lambda$. On the other hand, the proposed extended 6PL Rasch's model is given by the function (18),

$$p(x = 1|\theta, \mu, \alpha, a, c, d, g) = d + (a - d)p^g\left(x = 1 \bigg| \theta, \mu + \frac{1}{\alpha}\ln c, \alpha\right), 0 < g, c \tag{18}$$

where $p(x = 1|\theta, \mu, \alpha)$ is defined through the equation (3).

The value of the item's difficulty is the main difference between the two models. The authors of reference [26] assume that μ is the item's difficulty, while the extended 6PL Rasch's model assumes that the difficulty is given by the expression $\mu + \frac{1}{\alpha}\ln c$. The presence of the parameter c implies the existence of right or left skewness in the PDF. So that, in this work, just one function for the CDF contains the left and right skewed behavior reported by Bolfarine et. al., who uses two CDF's to describe it. On the other hand, the parameter g plays exactly the same role in both models, which means that the two lead to similar conclusions about the comparison of items or examinees in subdomains.

References

1. Guzmán, E., Conejo, R.: A model for student knowledge diagnosis through adaptive testing. In: Lester, J.C., Vicari, R.M., Paraguaçu, F. (eds.) ITS 2004. LNCS, vol. 3220, pp. 12–21. Springer, Heidelberg (2004)
2. Kozierkiewicz-Hetmańska, A., Nguyen, N.T.: A computer adaptive testing method for intelligent tutoring systems. In: Setchi, R., Jordanov, I., Howlett, R.J., Jain, L.C. (eds.) KES 2010, Part I. LNCS, vol. 6276, pp. 281–289. Springer, Heidelberg (2010)
3. van der Linden, W.J., Hambleton, R.K.: Handbook of Modern Item Response Theory. Springer, Heidelberg (1997)
4. Yadin, A.: Using unique assignments for reducing the bimodal grade distribution. Stand. Art. Sect. J. ACM Inroads **4**(1), 38–42 (2013)
5. Bonisegni, M.: Bimodal Distributions of Student Achievement. Consulted in 20 January 2015. https://expbook.wordpress.com/page/21/, 14 September (2008)
6. Robins, A.: Learning edge momentum: a new account of outcomes in CS1. Comput. Sci. Educ. **20**(1), 37–71 (2010)
7. Lazarinis, F., Green, S., Pearson, E.: Creating personalized assessments based on learner knowledge and objectives in a hypermedia Web testing application. Comput. Educ. **55**, 1732–1743 (2010)
8. Magis, D.: A note on the item information function of the four-parameter logistic model. Appl. Psychol. Meas. **37**(4), 304–315 (2013)
9. Irtel, H.: An extension of the concept of specific objectivity. Psychometrika **60**(1), 115–118 (1995)
10. Scheiblechner, H.H.: Rasch and pseudo-Rasch models: suitableness for practical test applications. Psychol. Sci. Q. **51**(2), 181–194 (2009)
11. Bazán, J.L., Branco, M.D., Bolfarine, H.: A skew item response model. Bayesian Anal. **1**(4), 861–892 (2006)
12. Gottschalk, P.G., Dunn, J.R.: The five-parameter logistic: a characterization and comparison with the four-parameter logistic. Anal. Biochem. **343**, 54–65 (2005)
13. Rasch, G.: An individualistic approach to item analysis. In: Lazarsfeld, P.F., Henry, N.W. (eds.) Reading in Mathematical Social Science, pp. 89–107. MIT Press, Cambridge (1996)
14. Rasch, G.: On Objectivity and Models for Measuring. In: Stene, J. (ed.) Lecture notes (1960)
15. Hambleton, R.K.: Item Response Theory: The Three-Parameter Logistic Model. In: Graduate School of Education, University of California, Los Angeles. Center for the Study of Evaluation Report No. 220 (1982)
16. Ricketts, J.H., Head, G.A.: A five-parameter logistic equation for investigating asymmetry of curvature in baroreflex studies. Am. J. Physiol. **277**, 441–454 (1999)

17. Engelhard, G. Jr.: A Simulation Study of Computerized Adaptive Testing with a Misspecified Measurement Model. In: Proceedings of the Section on Survey Research Methods 1986. American Statistical Association, pp. 631–636, 18–21 August 1986

18. van Rijn, P.W., Eggen, T.J.H.M., Hemker, B.T., Sanders, P.F.: A Selection Procedure for Polytomous Items in Computerized Adaptive Testing. In: Measurement and Research Department Reports 2000–5, 2000. Central Institute for Test Development - Cito, September 2000

19. Thorpe, G.L., Favia, A.: Data analysis using item response theory methodology: an introduction to selected programs and applications. Psychology Faculty Scholarship, Paper 20, The University of Maine, DigitalCommons@UMaine, July 2012

20. Akaike, H.: A new look at the statistical model identification. IEEE Trans. Autom. Control AC **19**(6), 716–723 (1974)

21. Maydeu-Olivares, A., García-Forero, C.: Goodness-of-Fit Testing. In: International Encyclopedia of Education 2010, vol. 7, pp. 190–196. Elsevier (2010)

22. Kang, T., Cohen, A.S.: IRT model selection methods for dichotomous items. Appl. Psychol. Meas. **4**(31), 331–358 (2007)

23. Olea, J., Ponsoda, V.: Tests Adaptativos Informatizados. Universidad Nacional de Educación a Distancia, Madrid (2003)

24. Muñiz, J.: Introducción a la Teoría de Respuesta a los Ítems. Psicología Pirámide, Madrid (1997)

25. van der Linden, W.J.: Linking response - time parameters onto a common scale. J. Educ. Meas. **47**(1), 92–114 (2010)

26. Bolfarine, H., Bazan, J.L.: Bayesian estimation of the logistic positive exponent IRT model. J. Educ. Behav. Stat. **35**(6), 693–713 (2010)

Algorithms and Machine Learning Techniques in Collaborative Group Formation

Rosanna Costaguta[✉]

Facultad de Ciencias Exactas y Tecnologías (FCEyT),
Instituto de Investigación en Informática y Sistemas de Información (IIISI),
Universidad Nacional de Santiago del Estero (UNSE), Avda. Belgrano (S) 1912,
Santiago del Estero 4200, Argentina
rosanna@unse.edu.ar

Abstract. Computer Supported Collaborative Learning (CSCL) is an emerging interdisciplinary research area that deals with the formation of students groups to work and to learn together in an educational context. One of the factors that affect successful collaborative learning is the group composition. This paper surveys the most relevant researches carried out in this field to date. For each one it describes the applied criterion to form learning groups and the way in which the grouping criterion is applied. These researches are compared and some conclusions are outlined.

1 Introduction

Collaborative learning (CL) can be seen as teaching methods in which students work in small groups to help them learn from each other [1]. The technological advance occurred in recent decades allowed the CL adopt computational tools that facilitate collaboration, coordination and communication transforming it in Computer Supported Collaborative Learning (CSCL). Today its use is diffused in the area of education, and there are numerous studies showing that can be advantageously applied.

A learning group is defined as a structure formed by people who interact to achieve specific learning objectives through their participation [2]. In CSCL there are different approaches to form groups, it is possible randomly select the members, let them self-select themselves, or choose them by certain criterion established by the teacher, and also do it manually (by the teacher) or automatic (by the system). Each of these alternatives has certain disadvantages. Randomization can generate very unbalanced groups that are unlikely to be effective; the self-selection can cause discrimination among students with poor social relationship; and manually creating unviable when the number of students is high or when the selection criterions are complex.

The objective of this work is to present some background on proposed approaches to the formation of groups in CLSL, analyzing in them the algorithms and machine learning techniques that apply. This paper is organized as follows: Sect. 2 describes the experiences surveyed in the formation of groups, Sect. 3 performs an analysis and comparison of the same, and finally, Sect. 4 presents some conclusion.

O. Pichardo Lagunas et al. (Eds.): MICAI 2015, Part II, LNAI 9414, pp. 249–258, 2015.
DOI: 10.1007/978-3-319-27101-9_18

2 Applied Approches in Collaborative Group Formation

The Supnithi *et al.* [3] suggest the formation of opportunistic group using two ontologies, one of negotiation and other collaborative learning. For authors opportunistic group is one that is dynamically generated when a situation where it is desirable that the student migrate individual learning to collaborative, there formed a group with members who share a goal of learning is detected. In this proposal the students start working individually with a software agent that monitors the actions of the student and updates his student profile. This agent is able to recognize when your student would benefit by changing to the mode of collaborative work. In such cases, the agent initiates a process of negotiation with the agents of other students of the course to form a group. The agent begins by setting goal of learning for the group and a role for the student group. The agents of all other students negotiate with him using the ontology created for it (each agent considers the information contained in the profile of the student and estimate the benefits that could get, if it participate of the group that it was called). If negotiation is successful every student is informed about the target of the group learning and the role which must assume, and a communication channel is opened for the use of members. When one of the students affirms to have reached the goal, the agents close the communication channel and update the student profile. The authors claim to have developed the ontologies but still no experimental data.

Balmaceda *et al.* [4] suggest the use of an assistant agent to form collaborative groups based on three characteristics that may affect the group performance: the psychological styles, team roles and social relationships. The psychological styles considered are those proposed by Myers-Briggs (extroversion/introversion, sensing/ intuitive, thinker/sentimental, judgment/perception). Respect to roles, they take the life cycle phases of collaborative work and the eight team roles proposed by Mumma, respecting the paired appearance of these by phase. Zheong [5] consider that the formation of groups is a constraint satisfaction problem; they take every place in the group as a variable, the list of course students as the domain of these variables, and derived from Mumma roles and the styles from Myers-Briggs the restrictions that them have to satisfy. Some examples of restrictions proposed by the authors are: the student may participate in only one group in each group all roles must appear, psychological styles must be balanced. The preferences of each student regarding the manifestation of roles and psychological styles are stored in your student profile. To validate the proposal's authors developed a pilot without assessing the performance of the groups created experience.

Zheong [5] proposes a generator groups by applying data mining techniques (clustering), analyzes the interactions of students to extract interaction patterns. These patterns and the rating assigned by the teacher are used to differentiate between effective and weak groups. Based on this distinction, and using decision trees, establish composition rules of groups used by the generator groups. Students are represented by a set of personal characteristics, and the first cluster is carried out considering these characteristics. Then, by having the teacher's grade and the level of interaction revealed new patterns that allow you to refine the formation of groups and produce new groupings are extracted. The authors plan to implement and validate the proposal.

Henry [6] describes a program that automatically performs the grouping of students. Initially students are surveyed to capture information necessary for the creation of his student profiles (preferred programming language, number of postponements, subject notes, whit which partner it prefer to work and which not, etc.). The teacher must indicate the desired size for the groups, and whether homogeneous or heterogeneous want based on a particular feature. The authors state that they use the described software for years but they do not have experimental results.

Hoppe [7] establishes three criterions to perform the grouping: a complementary criterion where a student with high competence in a topic is grouped with other of low competition, a competitive approach where students are grouped with similar profiles, and finally, a selection criterion of problem where no member of the group can solve the problem alone but a group integrating with other members who possess the knowledge as required. There is little documentation of experimentation by the author.

Wessner and Pfister [8] present a group formation process composed of three stages: initiation, pairs identification and negotiation. The initiation of a collaborative situation can arise for student choice or decision of the teacher. When the student proposes the initiative, the system searches the profiles of students other pupils who meet the requirements to work with him, providing a list of these or telling you that there are no matches. The student can choose his partner from the list, or cancel the training. In the case where a candidate selected, the system will consult whether to accept it. If the group agree is created, but rather the student may choose another candidate. The group created a communication channel opens. Wessner and Pfister [8] also propose the concept of point of cooperation (PoC), understood as an opportunity to collaborate included in the system. Also, classify PoC in: generic PoC (GPoC), which are all the facilities of cooperation provided by the system that may or may not be used by students (mail, chat, etc.); spontaneous PoC (SPoC), incorporated into the course but not linked to a particular position (seek help from the teacher, find a partner for dialogue, etc.) activities, and intentional PoC (IPOC), logical collaborative activities and didactically integrated course in a given thereof (forum enabled by the teacher after the development of certain units, chat to discuss a given concept, etc.) point. The authors implemented their concept of PoC in the L3 environment. There is a working mode in collaboration that allows synchronous and asynchronous POCI with formation of groups by the teacher manually or automatically by the system. For automatic formation the system considers the course as a sequential list of units and calculates the learning distance among students by calculating the difference between the units in which students find themselves.

Duque Medina et al. [9] suggest identifying indicators of collaboration and then apply some of these criterions to form groups: concentration, grouping students who have similar values in certain indicators, and dispersion, grouping students differ in the values of certain indicators. Obviously, while a criterion generates homogeneous groups the other produces heterogeneous groups. However, the authors experimented with the combination of both criterions in the COLLECE system. For this they calculated indicators of the student: work (it measures the dedication) and discussion (it measures the level of participation), indicators of the group: coordination (it measures the extent to which students agree to share the charge and the workspace), and speed (it measures the time taken on the task), and indicators of solution: correctness and validity. Then they generated the groups considering the concentration criterion for indicators for student and dispersion criterion for indicators of the solution, achieving homogeneous groups in some aspects and heterogeneous in others.

Cocea and Magoulis [10] proposed case-based reasoning combined with data mining techniques (clustering) to form the groups. The authors experimented with the proposal by using the learning environment eXpresser in the field of mathematics generalization. With case-based reasoning can recognize solving strategies applied and the clustering can detect students who applied similar strategies. With this information the teacher defines the constitution of the groups.

Sukstrienwong [11] proposes the use of a genetic algorithm for forming hetero-geneous groups. The author considers each student attributes defined by the current rating and score on the previous year, by way of representing the academic and edu-cational skills of the student, respectively. Averaging the values of the members for the two attributes it is calculated by a chromosome also two attributes per group. The authors describe an experiment and they analyze the results.

Lin et al. [12] consider the formation of collaborative groups as a problem of multi-grouping and to fix propose using the particle swarm optimization. For this purpose define two grouping criterions: the level of understanding of each student on a given topic, and the level of student interest on that topic. With these criterions, the authors calculate the difference in the level of understanding between groups and the maximum distance in the level of interest among groups. The first time the indicators are calculated on historical data and are updated for later groupings. Experimental data show the viability of the proposal.

Yannibelli and Amandi [13] propose setting up well-balanced groups to the nine roles of equipment known as Belbin roles. An unbalanced group is one where these roles do not appear naturally or where the same role is manifested by different members. The authors suggest the existence of three indicators and the implementation of a genetic algorithm. The first indicator shows whether each of the roles appear naturally in each group. The second indicator is applied to each group and calculate the balance level roles based on the first indicator. The third indicator maximizes the average balance levels in all groups, and is taken as evaluation function indicator for the genetic algo-rithm. The constitutive genes of chromosome correspond to students of the course. The initial population is given by random permutations of the value of the genes, that is, with the same students positioned at various locations within different chromosomes.

Martin and Paredes [14] propose using learning styles by Felder and Silverman as a main feature for grouping students. The authors propose the creation of groups which combine different styles in the same proportion, making a temporary shape with a criterion of homogeneous styles and then regrouping with a criterion of heterogeneous styles. There are no experimental results.

Carro et al. [15] propose the use of grouping rules looking for students with similar characteristics to integrate the same group. Initially to form the groups is considered one of the following characteristics: learning style, knowledge level and frequency of interaction. Then there is the possibility of sub-groupings within groups formed, considering some of the other characteristics or other criterions (for example, consid-ering the collaboration wishes of students, with whom they want to work or with who do not want to).

Liu *et al.* [16] propose perform an intelligent grouping of students based on their learning styles. For this, first they get the learning style of each student using the styles of Felder and Silverman. The teacher provides the necessary grouping parameters (number of groups to form and number of members per group). Students are arranged in descending order according to the score obtained for the style, and then the ranked list is segmented into as many equal parts as students should have each group, and finally, the groups are generated by assigning randomly from each segment to one student group. There are no experimental results.

Barati Jozán *et al.* [17] propose the use of a genetic algorithm and two evaluation functions: one intragroup and intergroup other. While the first measures the quality of each group, the second compares the competition between groups created. The authors seek heterogeneity intergroup and intragroup homogeneity. The genetic algorithm considers each group as a chromosome and students as genes. The length of chromosome indicates the number of group members. For define the initial population the students are randomly distributed within groups to form. The experiences analyzed are on simulated data.

Razmerita and Brun [18] propose perform homogeneous groupings using data mining techniques (clustering) on the data of students who are judged adequate. The authors suggest evaluating the performance (individual and group) of these groups to make changes to the groupings made. There are no experimental results.

Ounnas *et al.* [19] propose to create well-balanced groups to the nine roles of Belbin, which implies a certain presence of roles in the group. The authors using ontologies for modeling the characteristics of the students, which includes personal, social and academic data (learning style, favorite subjects, preferred partners, leading role, supporting role, etc.). The negotiation is presented as a constraint satisfaction problem, for example, looking for heterogeneity in learning style or homogeneity in the favorite subjects. The teacher shows how many students want to group. The authors conducted experiences with real students and also with simulated data.

Wang *et al.* [20] introduce a heterogeneous grouping system called DIANA. This system uses a genetic algorithm to form groups heterogeneous with same size and same level of diversity. For this genetic algorithm one chromosome represents one group and each gene within a chromosome represents one student. The tool uses the students thinking styles collected from questionnaires to create groups with 3 to 7 members. DIANA was tested with real students.

3   Analysis and Comparison of the Applied Approaches

To make the comparison between the different approaches of clusters of students in CSCL environments, the following questions were raised: 1 - What students features involved in the grouping process are considered?, 2 - What techniques or algorithms are applied especially for grouping?, 3 - Form groups is the decision of one person (teacher or student) or the same system?, 4 – In the formed groups, the characteristics of the students assume similar values (homogeneous groups), different (heterogeneous groups), or there are some with similar characteristics and other with differing values (mixed groups)?, 5 – The used algorithm raises the possibility of regrouping looking for improvement ?, 6 - Are there experimental results?.

Considering the first question, we can say that all the approaches analyzed use own characteristics of the students involved. In some cases there are similarities in the aspects evaluated, in [3, 4, 13, 19] are considered the team roles, in [4, 14–16] learning styles, in [3, 5, 9, 11, 17] teacher qualifications, in [12, 18] the topic or level of interest, in [7, 8, 12, 15, 17, 18] the level of knowledge or understanding, in [6, 7, 18, 19] private personal data, and in [4, 5, 9, 15, 17] social relations, the level of interaction or communication. In other cases there are no similarities, for example, only in [3] takes the target learning feature, in [10] the style of problem solving, and in [20] the thinking style. It was also noted that in [3–6] the authors identify in their proposals a student model as the place where all these characteristics are stored.

Considering the second question, we can say that the techniques and algorithms applied are varied, although in some cases there are similarities. In [3, 19] ontologies are proposed, in [3, 4] software agents are used, in [5, 10, 18] clustering is used, in [7–9, 12, 15] rules or specific grouping criterions are defined, in [4, 12, 19] grouping is solved as a constraint satisfaction problem, in [14, 18] segmentation system is applied, and in [11, 13, 17, 20] genetic algorithms are proposed. The decision trees are used only in [5].

Considering the third question, we can say that most of the analyzed approaches perform the formation of groups at the request of teacher organizes the course of CSCL [4–20]. Only in [3, 8] there are possibilities of automatic grouping initiative (by systems), and in [8] the possibility of forming groups on the initiative of the students themselves are also offered.

Considering the fourth question, we can say that the approaches of heterogeneous groups and approaches of homogeneous groups exist in the same amount. The proposed approaches in [3, 5, 7, 11, 16, 19, 20] only generate heterogeneous groups, whereas in [8, 10, 13, 17, 18] only homogeneous, and in [6, 9, 12, 15] it is possible to choose between the two categories. Furthermore, in particular, in [4, 9, 12, 14, 15] exists the possibility of forming mixed groups, using simultaneously criterions to homogeneity and heterogeneity.

Considering the fifth question, we can say that only in [5, 12] there are possibilities of iterative regrouping looking for more efficient formation of groups.

Finally, considering the sixth question, we can say that considerable number of analyzed approaches does not support their proposals with experimental results; this occurs in [3, 5, 6, 8, 14–16, 18].

In Table 1 the questions and answers are synthetized.

Table 1. Comparison of grouping approaches

Ref.	Questions					
	1	*2*	*3*	*4*	*5*	*6*
[3]	Team roles, Qualifications, Learning goals	Ontologies, Agents	System	Heterogeneous	No	No

(*Continued*)

Table 1. (*Continued*)

Ref.	Questions					
	1	*2*	*3*	*4*	*5*	*6*
[4]	Psychologies styles, Team roles, Social, relationships	Agents, Constraints satisfaction	Professor	Mixed	No	Yes
[5]	Qualifications, Interaction level	Clustering, Decision trees	Professor	Heterogeneous	Yes	No
[6]	Collaboration preferences, Personal information	Grouping criterions	Professor	Homogeneous Heterogeneous	No	No
[7]	Knowledge, Capacities	Grouping criterions	Professor	Heterogeneous	No	Yes
[8]	Knowledge	Grouping criterions	Professor, Students, System	Homogeneous	No	No
[9]	Communication level, Quality	Grouping criterions	Professor	Homogeneous Heterogeneous Mixed	No	Yes
[10]	Style of problem resolution	Clustering, Case-based reasoning	Professor	Homogeneous	No	Yes
[11]	Qualifications	Genetic algorithms	Professor	Heterogeneous	No	Yes
[12]	Interest level Learning level	Grouping criterions	Professor	Homogeneous Heterogeneous Mixed	Yes	Yes
[13]	Team roles	Genetic algorithms	Professor	Homogeneous	No	Yes
[14]	Learning styles	Rank and segmentation	Professor	Mixed	No	No
[15]	Learning styles, Knowledge level, Interaction style, Opinions, Collaboration preferences	Grouping criterions	Professor	Homogeneous Heterogeneous Mixed	No	No
[16]	Learning styles	Rank and segmentation	Professor	Heterogeneous	No	No
[17]	Social characteristics, Qualifications	Genetic algorithms	Professor	Homogeneous	No	Yes

(*Continued*)

Table 1. (*Continued*)

Ref.	Questions					
	1	*2*	*3*	*4*	*5*	*6*
[18]	Interest topics, Knowledge level, Country	Clustering	Professor	Homogeneous	No	No
[19]	Team roles Sex	Ontologies, Constraint satisfaction	Professor	Heterogeneous	No	Yes
[20]	Thinking styles	Genetic algorithms	Professor	Heterogeneous	No	Yes

4 Conclusions

In many areas of science and industry success depends on individual skills to be a productive member of a group that people can demonstrate, this is also true for ACSC. So far, the formation of collaborative groups are made based on personal information of the students of the course which is available on systems, and is usually contained in the profiles or student models (data such as sex, age, level of knowledge, main interests, preferences, learning styles, grades obtained, level of participation, etc.). Thus, these data are evaluated to select the members of the group so that everyone benefits potentially working together. In making this selection sometimes complementarity is encouraged (when there is heterogeneity in the group), in other cases competitiveness (when there is homogeneity among members), and others are looking for both (when there is homogeneity between some characteristics of the members and heterogeneity in others).

Several approaches of group formation have been proposed and machine learning techniques that are varied include: genetic algorithms, agents, clustering, optimization of restrictions, individual grouping criterion, etc. The factors that guide the grouping are also varied: psychological styles, learning styles, social relations, level of knowledge, level of participation, etc. Many of the proposed approaches to the formation of groups have been tested, but most points to validate the effectiveness of clustering algorithm rather than evaluating the effects on the performance of the group formed with this algorithm.

Predominantly the formation of groups in CSCL is performed at the request of the teacher who also indicates the parameters under which the grouping algorithm will perform its task. In general, these parameters are the number of groups to be formed, the number of members that each group should have. In some cases the teacher should indicate the type of group to form (homogeneous or heterogeneous) and the student characteristics for the selection of members. The examples in which these tasks are performed automatically or delegated to software agents are few.

The current perspectives for ubiquitous computing and its relationship to intelligent systems augur the emergence of new approaches to the formation of groups of CSCL including components related to the context of the student. Examples of contextual variables in CSCL that could be considered in future grouping algorithms are: emotional parameters, noise, climate, temperature, availability of devices, proximity of others, etc.

Acknowledgements. This study was partially supported by research projects PICTO UNSE 2012-0016 and SECYT UNSE 23-C089.

References

1. Slavin, R.: Cooperative Learning: Theory, Research and Practice. Pearson, London (1995)
2. Souto, M.: Didáctica de lo grupal. Ministerio de Educación y Justicia. In: INPAD (1990)
3. Supnithi, T., Inaba, R., Ikeda, M., Toyoda, J., Mizoguchi, R.: Learning goal ontology supported by learning theories for opportunistic group formation. In: Proceedings of 9th World Conference on Artificial Intelligence in Education, France (1999)
4. Balmaceda, J., Schiaffino, S., Diaz-Pace, J.: Using constraint satisfaction to aid group formation in CSCL. Revista Inteligencia Artif. **17**(53), 35–45 (2014)
5. Zheong, Z.: A dynamic group composition method to refine collaborative learning group formation. In: Proceedings of 6th International Conference on Educational Data Mining, pp. 360–361 (2013)
6. Henry, T.: Creating effective student groups: an introduction to groupformation.org. In: Proceeding of 44th. ACM Technical Symposium on Computer Science Education, pp. 645–650, USA (2013)
7. Hoppe, H.: The use of multiple student modeling to parametrize group learning. In: Proceedings of 7th World Conference on Artificial Intelligence in Education, USA (1995)
8. Wessner, M., Pfister, H.: Group formation in computer-supported collaborative learning. In: Proceedings of International ACM SIGGROUP Conference on Supporting Group Work, pp. 24–31, USA (2001)
9. Duque Medina, R., Gómez-Peréz, D., Nieto-Reyes, A., Bravo Santos, C.: A method to form learners groups in computer-supported collaborative learning systems. In: Proceedings of First International Conference on Technological Ecosystem for Enhancing Multiculturality, pp. 261–266, Spain (2013)
10. Cocea, M., Magoulis, G.: User behaviour-driven group formation throuh case-based reasoning and clustering. Expert Syst. Appl. **39**, 8756–8768 (2012)
11. Sukstrienwong, A.: A genetic algorithm approach for forming heterogeneous groups of students. Int. J. Appl. Eng. Res. (IJAER) **9**(3), 297–311 (2014)
12. Lin, Y., Huang, Y., Cheng, S.: An automatic group composition system for composing collaborative learning groups using enhanced particle swarm optimization. Comput. Educ. **55**, 1483–1493 (2010)
13. Yannibelli, V., Amandi, A.: A deterministic crowding evolutionary algorithm to form learning teams in a collaborative learning context. Expert Syst. Appl. **39**, 8584–8592 (2012)
14. Martin, E., Paredes, P.: Using learning styles for dynamic group formation in adaptive collaborative hypermedia systems. In: Proceedings of First International Workshop on Adaptive Hypermedia and Collaborative Web-based Systems (AHCW), pp. 188–198 (2004)
15. Carro, R.M., Ortigosa, A., Martín, E., Schlichter, J.: Dynamic generation of adaptive web-based collaborative courses. In: Favela, J., Decouchant, D. (eds.) CRIWG 2003. LNCS, vol. 2806, pp. 191–198. Springer, Heidelberg (2003)

16. Liu, S., Joy, M., Griffiths, N.: iGLS: intelligent grouping for online collaborative learning. In: Proceedings 9th IEEE International Conference on Advanced Learning Technologies (ICALT), Latvia (2009)
17. Barati Jozán, M., Taghiyareh, F., Faili, H.: An inversion-based genetic algorithm for grouping of students. In: Proceedings of 7th International Conference on Virtual Learning, pp. 152–161, Rumania (2012)
18. Razmerita, I., Brun, A.: Collaborative learning in heterogeneous classes. towards a group formation methodology. In: Proceedings of 3rd International Conference on Computer Supported Education, The Netherlands (2011)
19. Ounnas, A., Davis, H., Millard, D.: A framework for semantic group formation in education. Educ. Technol. Society 12(4), 43–55 (2009)
20. Wang, D., Lin, S., Sun, C.: DIANA: a computer-supported heterogeneous grouping system for teachers to conduct successful small learning groups. Comput. Hum. Behav. 23, 1997–2010 (2007)

Biomedical Applications

An Architecture Proposal Based in Intelligent Algorithms for Motifs Discovery in Genetic Expressions

Augusto G. Schmidt$^{(\boxtimes)}$, Frederico S. Kremer, Vinícius S. Pazzini,
Michel S. Pedroso, and Marilton S. de Aguiar

Centro de Desenvolvimento Tecnológico,
Universidade Federal de Pelotas (UFPEL), Pelotas, Brazil
`augustgs@gmail.com`, `marilton@inf.ufpel.edu.br`

Abstract. Motifs are not random entities found in DNA chains. A motif can also be defined as not a single phenomenon. Already motifs, besides having recurring patterns in the analyzed sequence, also have a biological function. Intelligent algorithms are search techniques widely used to find approximate solutions to optimization and search patterns in the science area of computing. Finding motifs in gene sequences is one of the most important problems in bioinformatics and belongs to the class NP-Complete. Therefore, it is plausible to investigate the hybridization of consolidated tools, but limited in their performance, in combination with intelligent systems techniques. This work has the premise to show a research of the main techniques and concepts of intelligent algorithms used in discovery of patterns (motifs) in gene expression and also an in-depth study of the major bioinformatics algorithms that are used for this function in recent years by researchers. It is understood that such techniques in combination, can achieve interesting results for research in bioinformatics. Thus proposing an optimized architecture for motifs discovery in genetic expressions of promoter regions of a bacteria. Using as many intelligent algorithms such as bioinformatics algorithms and refining techniques of its main data provided by the algorithms used. Thus forming an architecture with better performance due to hybridization of consolidated tools to search for patterns in genetic expressions.

Keywords: Bioinformatics · Genetic algorithm · Neural networks · Motif discovery

1 Introduction

Bioinformatics is a new and developing science and both has grown exponentially in recent years, showing that bioinformatics is now a need for data analysis in molecular biology [1].

One of the primary tools used today for local sequence alignment is BLAST (basic local alignment search tool) is a set of bioinformatics algorithms for sequence

© Springer International Publishing Switzerland 2015
O. Pichardo Lagunas et al. (Eds.): MICAI 2015, Part II, LNAI 9414, pp. 261–269, 2015.
DOI: 10.1007/978-3-319-27101-9_19

comparison mounted to exploit all the information contained in database DNA and protein sequences from a database that has similarity to be analyzed [4].

For multiple alignment algorithms we use a package called MUSCLE (multiple sequence comparison by log-expectation) that is very fast and efficient based on an approach, in general, progressive (analysis hand in hand, tree guide construction and alignment) However performs subsequent refinements to improve the initially created alignment [5].

HMMER [6] is used to search for protein sequences that have been cataloged in various databases and uses probabilistic techniques hidden Markov models [7].

But these tools are used separately at the discretion of the researcher who is analyzing the data. Finding motifs in gene sequences is one of the most important problems in bioinformatics and belongs to the class NP-Complete. Therefore, it is plausible to investigate the hybridization of consolidated tools, but limited in performance, along intelligent systems techniques. In this context, this proposal is based, aiming to improve the technology currently available to the bioinformatics researchers.

2 Motifs

Motifs are not-random entities found in DNA chains. A pattern can also be defined as not a single phenomenon. Already motifs, besides having recurring patterns in the analyzed sequence, also have a biological function. One can define motifs as a short segment shared by multiple DNA sequences that can contain information about evolution, structure or function [2].

The recognition of these motifs is often only based on shared patterns it is hardly possible to obtain information of 3D structures, details of chemical reactions, changes or features. Taking into account all these points is noted that not all patterns found in DNA strands are motifs. Then most of existing algorithms presents possible motifs. Within the recognition motifs can elicit two types intra sequences and between sequences. The second information having a higher load, since the probability that patterns that are maintained in several different individuals have more relevant motifs functionality need not be exactly equal, they may have some difference between them. These differences are possible because the affinity reduction at this point can be compensated in one point ahead in its structure [2].

2.1 Deterministic Model

Within the group of deterministic models have become regular expressions and consensus sequence. Regular expressions used in motifs discovery is a subset of regular languages, usually using symbols unambiguous and ambiguous, fixed and variable spacing. The use of regular expressions enables an easier representation of complex patterns with large or multiple spacing [2].

The consensus sequence that represents a set of possible motifs sequences, which are at a maximum distance x from the consensus. This distance x is the number of different characters between the two sequences. Each instance of this set is consensus occurrence of call. Usually the number of differences between an occurrence of consensus and the consensus sequence is defined and is directly proportional to the size consensus [3].

The two above approaches may be combined so that the characters presented in the regular expressions to be a consensus derived from all instances, may also allow for differences between the consensus and occurrences. However, these expressions can become very complex and difficult to be handled, in fact some existing tools enable the use of an even smaller subset of regular expressions.

2.2 Probabilistic Model

The simplest probabilistic model is a matrix score or PWM (position weight matrices). Its main advantage compared to the deterministic model is the ability to express different amounts for each symbol. While the deterministic model if a consensus position i have the occurrence of two symbols, both are equally important. The scoring matrix is a representation of a set of sequences without gaps, for each position of the sequence defines the frequency of each possible symbol. The calculation is given by Eq. 1.

$$F_{xi} = \frac{N_{xi}}{N} \tag{1}$$

In Eq. 1, F_{xi} is the frequency of the symbol x at position i, N_i is the number of x instances of the symbol at position i of all occurrences, and N is the total number of

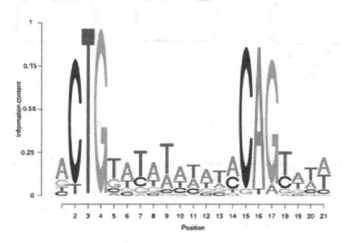

Fig. 1. Probabilistic model of a PWM.

occurrences. Thus the scoring matrix has dimensions $4 \times N$. Figure 1 shows a PWM of the probabilities of each nucleotide at each position is repeated [3].

2.3   Motif Recognition

Motifs are sets of DNA sequences that can be represented in different ways presented above. Usually the sequence is analyzed using sliding window. The window size is set to the size of the motif and the window is slid by the sequence one base at a time until the end thereof. A hit occurs if the subsequence in the window matches the motif being examined under the user considerations [3].

3   Implementation of the Architecture

Implementation were used all the concepts discussed earlier, where each execution flow returns the input of the next stage. The implementation of other programs were implemented and built on the Linux system. All programs from the Genetic Algorithm

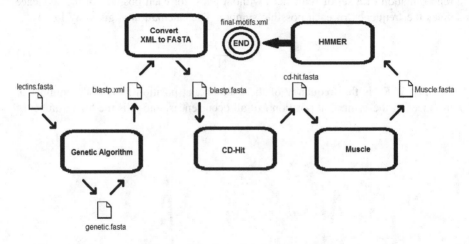

Fig. 2. Data flow of the architecture.

were used and arranged in the Python language, where BioPython library is used. The difficulty with this implementation is the large number of sequences generated through every step of executing, so it was necessary the use of a filter when converting from one format to another and the use a refining tool [8]. The Fig. 2 shows the data flow of the architecture and its modules.

3.1   Genetic Algorithm

The genetic algorithm (GA) was implemented using techniques found in several previous works and was written in the Java programming language. The score is implemented manually in the GA so that there was greater control and understanding of the operation of the code. Although the algorithm theory is simple various considerations and decisions needed to be taken.

Given a set of M sequences width 1 of the alphabet $\sum\{A, R, N, D, C, E, Q, G, H, I, L, K, M, F, P, S, T, W, Y, V, U, O, B, Z, J, X\}$ the algorithm must find a combination with one or more subsequence candidates motifs of size W. However, the difficulty of the problem grows when freedom is given to motifs to have differences, and these differences are from one nucleotide or length of the motif.

Shown in Eq. 1 the total number of possible motifs in a given sequence i, one realizes that test all possibilities becomes unviable.

$$\prod_i 26^{l-w+1} \tag{2}$$

Two methods for the generation of initial population were implemented. The first and simplest is a random generator, in this method are created as many individuals as specified by the user, typically between 100 and 200. Although this method is simple, it can take the GA to take more to find the optimal solution or in the worst case to get stuck in a maximum place. The second approach used was a simple clustering technique based hashed, the size of the hash is given by following formula $Top = Log_4 Size$, $Size$ is a user input. This hash size defines how many of the N characters of each motif can be used for clustering, after setting this size are randomly selected N positions that will be used to calculate the hash of every possible motif. Thus two sequences that have the same characters in these positions randomly selected will be grouped in the same cluster. Although this technique is not complex or deterministic she accelerated speed at which the GA is the solutions.

As it is not possible to say, in this problem, that the optimal solution was found we needed to define a method stop. The approach used was simple in this work, the algorithm continues to search as the number of generation grows and the best suited individual that changed is less than twenty percent of the maximum set by the user. If it was decided that the maximum number of generations is 1000 and for 200 generations the best individual has not changed is considered that there will be no more changes and the process is terminated.

The crossover is the function in the algorithm responsible for combining two individuals and generating one or more new individuals. Here we used two crossover functions, the first can be subdivided into two: one and two crossover points. These two approaches function entry of individuals are divided and reunited. The second crossover technique used may be called the "best each", in this approach we used a PMF (positive matrix factorization) of each of the two individuals and the nucleotide which has the highest conservation value is used to generated individual. The mutation is another part that belongs to the generation of new individuals to the population.

During all crossovers there is a small chance that one nucleotide is changed randomly, this process also aims to escape from local maxima generating individuals who could not be created using crossover only. There is only an addendum to be done on the mutation, it never occurs in a position that is retained absolute.

It used the roulette selection method with weights, this method all individuals of the population is likely to be chosen but the chance is greater higher the fitness of that individual, thereby allow the best of them prevail, but also allow diversity.

The fitness was calculated using the conservation of the formula which is given in Eq. 3.

$$RE_{(a)}(i) = P_{ci} * \log \frac{P_{ci}}{\pi_c} \qquad (3)$$

Where P_{ci} is the probability to have a nucleotide c in the position i, and π_c is the probability to have a nucleotide c in the background. It is understood as background the remainder of all sequences where there was an instance when withdrawing the portion of the occurrence. So using this formula, a higher value to nucleotides that have less frequently in background, assuming as they are less likely to be a random organization bases. Finally the individual's fitness can be represented by the sum of the score of N motif positions, as can be seen in Eq. 4.

$$RE_a' = \sum_{i=1}^{N} RE_{(a)}(i) \qquad (4)$$

While this is a good fitness calculation method it still does not take into account the size and the motif number of occurrences, which can lead to an individual with a perfect occurrence have a higher fitness than an individual with ten non-perfect events. To resolve this problem formula was adapted to Eq. 5.

$$F(a) = RE_a' - 3 * \frac{NS}{NM} \qquad (5)$$

Where NS is the number of input sequences and NM the number of hits found by the individual. Using this formula the individuals who have few occurrences suffer greater penalty, but it is still possible that an individual with less occurrences receives a score higher than another with more occurrences.

A new occurrence is added to the individual when it reaches values that exceed the limits set by the user. The first compared value is the similarity corresponding to how much is a new sequence similar to the set of sequences present in the individual. The similarity calculation is performed as follows, the individual frequencies matrix is calculated and using this matrix are summed values of each nucleotide corresponding to a new sequence. Thereby calculating the similarity ceases to be the sum of the matches and becomes the sum of the probabilities, which allows sequences that previously would not be added would becomes added. Having a value of similarity and the same being larger than the defined threshold, is then calculated relative entropy (*RE*) of the new sequence joint with the sequences present in the individual, Eq. 3 shows the formula of the relative entropy. Finally, subsequences that present the greatest value of relative entropy are added to the set of occurrences of the individual.

One of the difficulties was because the algorithm does not converge to a single response and was trapped in a local maximum. Trying to solve this problem two operations are conducted at the end of each iteration, these operations has the goal to remove exact or near duplicates, thereby maintaining individuals well adapted and ensuring the diversity of the population. The first operation use an operation of similarity previously described, using a limit of 70 % of similarity, so if two sequences are 70 % or more similar the only one with largest fitness will be saved to the next generation. The second function uses the Smith Waterman alignment algorithm. As this algorithm returns an integer value which it's maximum is twice the size of the threshold sequence and was calculated as 70 % of its maximum value. And because at removing all duplicates the population starts to get smaller than it was specified and it is filled with individuals randomly generated.

The parallelism can be easily explored in this algorithm, since the calculation of the motif which is one of the heaviest tasks is also unique, just an individual's fitness calculation does not interfere in the calculation of others. Using the Java IntStream

$i \leftarrow 0$
$G \leftarrow 100$
Read the input file
Generate all the random sequences
and group them together
repeat
$\quad i \leftarrow i + 1$
Evaluates all individuals
Orders the population
Remove Duplicates
Fills the gaps in the population
Performs Crossover + Mutation
until $i > G$ or Converge
Select the best individuals

Fig. 3. Flow of execution of the genetic algorithm.

function was possible to create the desired competition with ease, two hundred tests were rotated eat without competition and the results showed an improvement of 67.8 % at runtime when using a machine with four physical cores and eight cores logical. It is shown in Fig. 3, the basic flow of execution of the genetic algorithm developed. Note that the operation of the algorithm is quite simple, considering the complexity lies in the more specific approach of operations in this case complexity in this part of evaluating (calculating the fitness) for individuals.

3.2 BlastP

The basic local alignment search tool protein (BlastP) is a program for finding similarities between sequences. This extension is only for proteins, which uses a local database generated from the sequence to be analyzed, also calculates statistics for hits [4].

At this stage the BlastP input is the output of Genetic Algorithm, which is contained all random motifs previously generated. In this step, the output format is .xml, will only take some necessary information from this file for the purpose of this article. This format was chosen for its ease of use tags to capture this information.

3.3 Conversion .XML to .FASTA

This procedure is performed using the Blast NCBIXML function module from the BioPython library to load the .xml file information generated by BlastP. To separate the necessary information, were used Python commands. At the end of the conversion is used a filter of the aligned sequences where only be utilized the sequences with a percentage greater or equal to 70 % (the ratio between the ID value, and the size of the sequence to be analyzed). Thus, the aligned sequences will only be used locally and which have a high probability of being valid. After conversion, the information is saved in a .FASTA file containing a header with your ID and the sequence.

3.4 CD-Hit

After execution of the steps above, even with filtering Conducted, the number of sequences is extremely high. Having the necessity to use the tool for these specific situations [8].

To reduce the amount of sequences in a satisfactory mannered and contains high probability of validity, the filter was 70 %. Thus, not only relevant sequences and sequences containing redundant results will be eliminated, with less promising sequences.

3.5 MUSCLE

Muscle [5] is a tool for performing multiple alignments of protein sequences. The sequence is aligned with the other sequences of the same input file. This tool performs peer-to-peer analysis, building tree guide and alignment tree. In this step the aligned sequence is the result of previously performed refining implementation, as in .FASTA one of the input files supported by the tool. Due to realization of filtering in the conversion step, it was not necessary to use parameters that limit the number of interactions due to the fact the information already being optimized and previously guaranteed.

Table 1. Motifs found in each step.

GA.fasta	BlastP.xml	BlastP.fasta	CD-hit.fasta	Muscle.fasta	% Valid *motifs*
1.757 seqs	174.914 seqs	17.283 seqs	28 seqs	28 seqs	1.59 %

3.6 HMMER

This tool does not generate new findings or modify the sequences already found. This step uses the result of the multiple alignment (Muscle) held previously. The role of this step is to generate a static model of multiple sequence alignments, or even individual sequences. This model contains specific information for each column of alignment, it is possible to analyze from basic information to model definitions, facilitating the visualization of the results performed before this step [7].

4 Conclusion and Future Work

The overall architecture execution time was 2 min and 51.956 s. After all executions and filters used, the result was considerable. Using lectins.fasta file as initial input, a quantity of 28 protein motifs was found. Considering the initial amount of 1,757 random motifs generated we can say that 28 sequences of motifs are likely to be correct motifs.

As we can see in the table above, we find that a gain of minus 98.40 % over the amount sequences first found in the GA.fasta archive (Table 1).

Among the aspects raised to continue the work, we need to improve the following:

- Development of a computational tool for motifs discovery.
- Optimization of the genetic algorithm.
- Create a database of already noted motifs for future testing.
- Provide a dataset template to search promoter regions in bacteria.
- Make download of the architecture available to the academic community.

References

1. Prosdoscimi, F., et al.: Bioinformática: manual do usuário. Biotecnologia Ciência and Desenvolvimento **29**, 12–25 (2002)
2. Yi-Ping, P.C.: Bioinformatics Technologies. Springer Science and Business Media, Berlin (2005)
3. Parida, L.: Pattern Discovery in Bioinformatics: Theory and Algorithms. CRC Press, Boca Raton (2007)
4. Altschul, S.F., et al.: Basic local alignment search tool. J. Mol. Biol. **215**(3), 403–410 (1990)
5. Edgar, R.C.: MUSCLE: multiple sequence alignment with high accuracy and high throughput. Nucleic Acids Res. **32**(5), 1792–1797 (2004). doi:10.1093/nar/gkh340. PMC 390337. PMID15034147
6. Durbin, R., Eddy, S.R., Krogh, A., Mitchison, G.J.: Biological Sequence Analysis: Probabilistic Models of Proteins and Nucleic Acids. Cambridge University Press, Cambridge (1998)
7. Finn, R.D., Clements, J., Eddy, S.R.: HMMER web server: interactive sequence similarity searching. Nucleic Acids Res. Web Server Issue **39**, W29–W37 (2011)
8. Li, Weizhong, Godzik, Adam: Cd-hit: a fast program for clustering and comparing large sets of protein or nucleotide sequences. Bioinformatics **22**(13), 1658–1659 (2006)

A Kernel-Based Predictive Model
for Guillain-Barré Syndrome

José Hernández-Torruco[1], Juana Canul-Reich[1(✉)], Juan Frausto-Solis[2],
and Juan José Méndez-Castillo[3]

[1] División Académica de Informática y Sistemas, Universidad Juárez Autónoma de
Tabasco, Cunduacan, Tabasco, Mexico
{jose.hernandezt,juana.canul}@ujat.mx
[2] Instituto Tecnológico de Ciudad Madero, Av. 1o. de Mayo esq. Sor Juana Inés de la
Cruz s/n, Col. Los Mangos, 89440 Ciudad Madero, Tamaulipas, Mexico
juan.frausto@gmail.com
[3] Hospital General de Especialidades Dr. Javier Buenfil Osorio, Av. Lázaro Cárdenas
208, Col. Las Flores, 24097 San Francisco De Campeche, Campeche, Mexico
juanmdzdr-neuro@yahoo.com.mx

Abstract. The severity of Guillain-Barré Syndrome (GBS) varies among
subtypes, which can be mainly Acute Inflammatory Demyelinating
Polyneuropathy (AIDP), Acute Motor Axonal Neuropathy (AMAN),
Acute Motor Sensory Axonal Neuropathy (AMSAN) and Miller-Fisher
Syndrome (MF). In this study, we use a real dataset that contains clinical, serological, and nerve conduction tests data obtained from 129 GBS
patients. We apply Support Vector Machines (SVM) using four different kernels: linear, Gaussian, polynomial and Laplacian to predict four
GBS subtypes. We compare SVM results with those of C4.5. We evaluated performance under both 10-FCV and train-test scenarios. Experimental results showed performance of both classifiers are comparable. SVM
slightly outperformed C4.5 with Polynomial kernel in 10-FCV. And it did
with Laplacian, polynomial and Gaussian kernels in train-test. This is an
ongoing research project and further experiments are being conducted.

Keywords: SVM kernels · Classification · Performance evaluation · AUC

1 Introduction

Guillain-Barré Syndrome (GBS) is an autoimmune neurological disorder characterized by a fast evolution, usually it goes from a few days up to four weeks. The
severity of GBS varies among subtypes, which can be mainly Acute Inflammatory Demyelinating Polyneuropathy (AIDP), Acute Motor Axonal Neuropathy
(AMAN), Acute Motor Sensory Axonal Neuropathy (AMSAN) and Miller-Fisher
Syndrome (MF). Currently, the identification of AIDP, AMAN, and AMSAN
subtypes is made according to electrodiagnostic criteria applied after nerve conduction studies [13]. These three subtypes are known as electrophysiological

Note: The first three authors equally contributed to this paper.

© Springer International Publishing Switzerland 2015
O. Pichardo Lagunas et al. (Eds.): MICAI 2015, Part II, LNAI 9414, pp. 270–281, 2015.
DOI: 10.1007/978-3-319-27101-9_20

subtypes. On the other hand, Miller-Fisher (MF) subtype is characterized by the clinical triad: ophthalmoplegia, ataxia and areflexia [8]. Reason why MF is considered a clinical subtype.

Hospitalization time and the cost of treatments vary according to the severity of the specific GBS subtype. The ultimate goal of a physician is to get patients to a full recovery. This can be more effectively achieved when an early diagnosis of the case is performed using a minimum number of medical features. In this study, we investigate the predictive power of a reduced set of only 16 features selected from an original dataset of 365 features. This dataset holds data from 129 Mexican patients and contains the four aforementioned GBS subtypes.

Our goal in this study is to build a predictive model for the four GBS subtypes present in our dataset. For this model, we applied Support Vector Machines (SVM) using four different kernels: linear, Gaussian, polynomial and Laplacian. We compare SMV results with those of C4.5. SVM is one of the most widely used classifiers due to its high performance in classification problems of diverse nature. We selected C4.5 as a benchmark classifier due to its competitive performance in classification applications as well as its implementation simplicity. Further experiments with other algorithms will follow.

The experimental results showed a good performance of the methods and allowed us to obtain a predictive model for GBS subtypes using machine learning techniques.

2   Materials and Methods

2.1   Data

The dataset used in this work comprises 129 cases of patients seen at Instituto Nacional de Neurología y Neurocirugía located in Mexico City. Data were collected from 1993 through 2002. There are 20 AIDP cases, 37 AMAN, 59 AMSAN, and 13 Miller-Fisher cases. Hence, there are four GBS subtypes in this dataset. The identification of subtypes was made by a group of neurophysiologists based on the clinical and electrophysiological criteria established in the literature [8,11,13].

Originally, the dataset consisted of 365 attributes corresponding to epidemiological data, clinical data, results from two nerve conduction tests, and results from two Cerebrospinal Fluid (CSF) analyses. The second nerve conduction test was conducted in 22 patients and the second CSF analysis was conducted in 47 patients only. Therefore, data from these two tests were excluded from the dataset.

The formal diagnostic criteria for GBS [8,11,13] were considered to determine which variables from the original dataset could be important in the characterization of the four subtypes of GBS. We made a pre-selection of variables based on these criteria. After pre-selection, it was left with 156 variables: 121 variables from the nerve conduction test, 4 variables from the CSF analysis and 31 clinical variables.

In a previous work [2], we identified a set of 16 relevant features out of the 156 features. In this study, we investigate these features to create a predictive model for GBS. The features are listed in Table 1. The first four features are all clinical and the remaining features come from a nerve conduction test.

Table 1. List of features used in this study

Feature label	Feature name
v22	Symmetry (in weakness)
v29	Extraocular muscles involvement
v30	Ptosis
v31	Cerebellar involvement
v63	Amplitude of left median motor nerve
v106	Area under the curve of left ulnar motor nerve
v120	Area under the curve of right ulnar motor nerve
v130	Amplitude of left tibial motor nerve
v141	Amplitude of right tibial motor nerve
v161	Area under the curve of right peroneal motor nerve
v172	Amplitude of left median sensory nerve
v177	Amplitude of right median sensory nerve
v178	Area under the curve of right median sensory nerve
v186	Latency of right ulnar sensory nerve
v187	Amplitude of right ulnar sensory nerve
v198	Area under the curve of right sural sensory nerve

2.2 Multiclass Classification

In this study, we face a multiclass classification problem (n number of classes > 2). SVM tackles multiclass classification using either OVA (One vs All) or OVO (One vs One) strategy. In this study, we use OVO strategy as it is proven to show higher performance than that of OVA for SVM classifications [5]. OVO strategy consists of building $n(n-1)/2$ binary classifiers, the appropriate class is found by a voting scheme. The implementation of this process was out-of-the-box in the R versions of SVM we used in this study [1,10]. As for C4.5, multiclass classification is intrinsically supported.

2.3 Support Vector Machines (SVM)

SVM was first introduced by Vapnik and colleagues [14]. Given a set of training instances (input space), where each instance belongs to class A or class B, SVM uses a mapping function (kernel) to transform the input space into a higher dimension space (feature space), that is, if input space is 2-D, then it is mapped into a 3-D space. In the feature space, SVM finds a hyperplane that gives the largest separation between classes, named maximum marginal hyperplane. The maximum margin hyperplane has the largest distance from the hyperplane to the closest training instances. The instances located in the boundaries of the hyperplane are called support vectors. However, the largest margin is not always the best solution since it can compromise the generalization of the model to new instances. For the sake of flexibility, SVM introduces a parameter C that creates a soft margin that allows for some errors in classification but at the same time it penalizes them. A tuning procedure is necessary for finding the best value of C.

In this study, we use four different kernels: linear, Gaussian, polynomial and Laplacian. Each of these kernels has particular parameters and they must be tuned in order to achieve the best performance. Table 2 shows the parameters of each kernel used in this study.

Table 2. Kernel parameters

Kernel	Parameter
Linear	C
Polynomial	C, degree, σ (γ), coef
Gaussian	C, σ (γ)
Laplacian	C, σ (γ)

C4.5. C4.5 builds a decision tree from training data using recursive partitions. In each iteration, C4.5 selects the attribute with the highest gain ratio as the attribute from which the tree branching (splitting attribute) is performed. This results in a more simplified tree (fewer subtrees). C4.5 is widely used in classification problems of diverse nature.

2.4 Performance Measures

Average Accuracy. A more suitable measure for multiclass classification problems is the average accuracy [12]. It assesses the accuracy individually for each class without distinguishing between the other classes. The original n x n confusion matrix obtained from the multiclass problem is transformed in n 2 × 2 confusion matrices. From each binary confusion matrix, a per-class accuracy is computed. All individual per-class accuracies are averaged to give a final accuracy. Formally:

$$Average Accuracy = \frac{\sum_{i=1}^{l} \frac{TP_i + TN_i}{TP_i + FN_i + FP_i + TN_i}}{l} \qquad (1)$$

where TP_i = True Positive for class i, TN_i = True Negative for class i, FP_i = False Positive for class i and FN_i = False Negative for class i.

For the sake of simplicity, we will refer to this measure as accuracy throughout this paper.

Sensitivity. Sensitivity measures the proportion of true positives, which were correctly identified by a predictive model. For a diagnostic test, sensitivity measures the ability of a test to detect ill subjects.

Specificity. Specificity measures the proportion of true negatives, which were correctly identified by a predictive model. For a diagnostic test, specificity measures the ability of a test to detect healthy subjects.

Multiclass Area Under the Curve (AUC). A ROC (Receiver Operating Characteristic) curve measures the performance of the classifier based on how well it separates the group being tested into those belonging to one class and another. Performance is measured by the AUC. AUC from a ROC graph ranges [0,1] where 1 is a perfect classification. An AUC of 0.5 represents a random classification. Hand et al. [7] derived an AUC for multiclass problems, which measures the pairwise discriminability of classes. Formally:

$$AUC_{total} = \frac{2}{|C|\,(|C|-1)} \sum_{\{C_i, C_j\} \in C} AUC(C_i, C_j) \tag{2}$$

where $AUC(C_i, C_j)$ is the area under the two-class ROC curve involving classes C_i and C_j. The summation is calculated over all pairs of distinct classes, regardless of order [6].

Kappa Statistic. Kappa statistic, introduced by Cohen [3], measures the agreement between the classifier itself and the ground truth corrected by the effect of the agreement between them by chance. Formally:

$$kappa = \frac{P(A) - P(E)}{1 - P(E)} \tag{3}$$

where $P(A)$ is the proportion of agreement between the classifier and the ground truth, $P(E)$ is the proportion of agreement expected between the classifier and the ground truth by chance.

Train-Test. Train-test consists of separating the original complete dataset into two independent new datasets. These two datasets contain both the predictor features and the outcome variable. The first dataset, named train, used for a classification algorithm to discover relationships or patterns among data, that is, to train or to fit a model. The second dataset, named test, used for the model fitted to estimate its performance on completely unseen data. In this study we used two-thirds of the original dataset for train and one-third for test.

Cross-Validation. Cross-validation divides the original complete dataset into k independent new datasets (k folds). Then, it performs k loops in which $k - 1$ partitions of the original dataset is used for training and the rest for testing. For each fold, the measure of evaluation of the model obtained from the confusion matrix is calculated and summed. When all the k loops have ended, the cross-validation accuracy is obtained. In this study, we use a 10-fold cross-validation (10-FCV).

3   Experimental Design

We used the 16-feature subset, described in Sect. 2.1, for experiments. We added the class variable to this subset, that is, the GBS subtype. Finally, we created a dataset containing the 129 instances and 17 features. As mentioned in Sect. 2.1, our dataset has 4 classes, identified with numbers 1 to 4, where 1 is AIDP, 2 is AMAN, 3 is AMSAN, and 4 is MF.

We used two model evaluation schemes: train-test and 10-FCV. For each of these schemes, we performed 30 runs where we applied each of the kernels described earlier. In each run, we set a different seed. The same seeds were used for each kernel. These seeds were generated using Mersenne-Twister pseudo-random number generator [9]. The use of a different seed for each run ensures producing different splits of train and test sets in both evaluation schemes.

3.1   10-FCV

For each run, we performed a 10-FCV. For each fold, we computed accuracy, sensitivity, specificity, Kappa statistic and multiclass AUC. After the 10 folds, we calculated 10-FCV accuracy and the average of each of the other measures. Finally, we averaged each of these quantities across the 30 runs.

3.2   Train-Test

For each run, we computed accuracy, sensitivity, specificity, Kappa statistic and multiclass AUC. Finally, we averaged each of these quantities across the 30 runs.

3.3   C4.5

We applied the experimental design described above for C4.5. C4.5 was applied with pruning.

3.4   SVM Parameter Optimization

An effective and simple method of tuning C and σ simultaneously is given by Hsu et al. [4]. This method consists of an exhaustive grid search using growing values for C and σ. The C values used in this study for all kernels were 1, 10, 50, 80 and 100. The σ (γ) values were exponentially growing values from 0.001 to 100.

The tuning procedure for the rest of Polynomial parameters was to try different values for degree (from 2 to 10), and 0–1 for coef. We analyzed the behavior of accuracies across polynomial degrees. As for coef, these are the typical values used in the literature.

For each combination of parameter values, we performed 30 SVM runs both the 10-FCV and train-test process with different seeds each. We calculated the accuracy of each run and the average accuracy over 30 runs. We selected the combination of parameters that obtained the highest accuracy.

4   Results and Discussion

The results of the linear kernel optimization for both train-test and 10-FCV are shown in Table 3.

Table 3. Linear kernel optimization. The units of the results are shown in average accuracy over 30 runs. The highest value appears in bold.

C	train-test	10-FCV
1	**0.9175**	**0.9069**
10	0.8965	0.8890
50	0.8969	0.8890
80	0.8969	0.8890
100	0.8969	0.8890

The results of the polynomial kernel optimization for both train-test and 10-FCV are shown in Table 4. We show only the best results for each degree.

Table 4. Polynomial kernel optimization. The units of the results are shown in average accuracy over 30 runs. The highest value appears in bold.

degree	coef	train-test			10-FCV		
		γ	C	accuracy	γ	C	accuracy
2	1	0.001	50	0.9110	0.01	10	0.9178
3	1	0.001	100	0.9110	0.01	10	0.9176
4	1	0.001	80	0.9126	0.001	100	0.9175
5	1	0.01	1	0.9118	0.01	1	0.9213
6	1	0.01	1	**0.9142**	0.01	1	**0.9235**
7	1	0.01	1	0.9126	0.01	1	0.9232
8	1	0.001	50	0.9122	0.001	80	0.9218
9	1	0.001	10	0.9114	0.001	80	0.9214
10	1	0.001	10	0.9110	0.001	50	0.9194

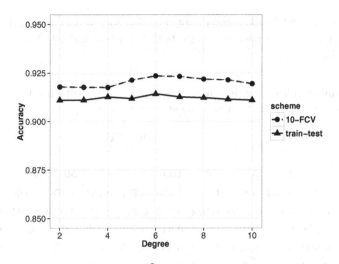

Fig. 1. Accuracies vs degrees in polynomial kernel

In Fig. 1, we show the behavior of accuracies for each degree in polynomial kernel both in 10-FCV and train-test. As shown in Fig. 1, accuracies grow as degrees increases until reaching a maximum accuracy of 0.9235 (train-test) and 0.9175 (10-FCV) at degree equal 6. For degrees above 6, accuracies decrease. The optimal parameters for both train-test and 10-FCV were degree = 6, coef = 1, C = 1 and $\gamma = 0.01$.

The results of SVM parameters optimization for Gaussian kernel are shown in Table 5. The first row shows C values. The first column represents γ values. Each entry of the table is the accuracy averaged across 30 runs using both train-test and 10-FCV, as described in Sect. 3. The optimal parameters for both train-test and 10-FCV were C = 10 and $\gamma = 0.001$.

Table 5. Gaussian kernel optimization. The units of the results are shown in average accuracy over 30 runs. The highest value appears in bold.

	train-test					10-FCV				
	C					C				
γ	1	10	50	80	100	1	10	50	80	100
0.001	0.733	0.887	0.911	0.910	0.909	0.736	0.885	0.913	0.915	0.915
0.01	0.885	**0.913**	0.904	0.902	0.903	0.882	**0.919**	0.915	0.910	0.912
0.1	0.910	0.900	0.896	0.896	0.896	0.910	0.895	0.893	0.893	0.893
1	0.809	0.814	0.814	0.814	0.814	0.799	0.809	0.809	0.809	0.809
10	0.732	0.734	0.734	0.734	0.734	0.726	0.729	0.729	0.729	0.729
100	0.732	0.732	0.732	0.732	0.732	0.727	0.727	0.727	0.727	0.727

The results of SVM parameters optimization for Laplacian kernel are shown in Table 6. The optimal parameters for both train-test and 10-FCV were C = 50 and $\sigma = 0.01$.

Table 6. Laplacian kernel optimization. The units of the results are shown in average accuracy over 30 runs. The highest value appears in bold.

	train-test					10-FCV				
	C					C				
σ	1	10	50	80	100	1	10	50	80	100
0.001	0.732	0.732	0.893	0.898	0.905	0.727	0.752	0.878	0.895	0.903
0.01	0.732	0.905	**0.916**	0.912	0.913	0.745	0.901	**0.920**	0.911	0.913
0.1	0.898	0.913	0.913	0.913	0.913	0.891	0.913	0.913	0.913	0.913
1	0.880	0.884	0.884	0.884	0.884	0.875	0.875	0.875	0.875	0.875
10	0.732	0.732	0.732	0.732	0.732	0.727	0.727	0.727	0.727	0.727
100	0.732	0.732	0.732	0.732	0.732	0.727	0.727	0.727	0.727	0.727

The optimal parameters for each kernel were used for further classification experiments with SVM.

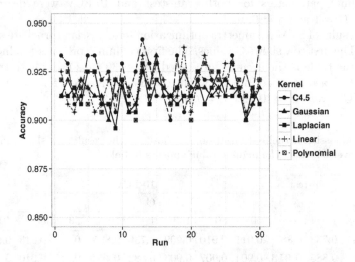

Fig. 2. Accuracy across 30 runs using 10-FCV for SVM kernels.

In Fig. 2, we show the average accuracy of the four GBS subtypes across 30 10-FCV runs for linear, polynomial, Gaussian and Laplacian kernels as well as C4.5. Accuracy of linear kernel ranged from 0.9042 to 0.9375 (s = 0.0096). Accuracy of polynomial kernel ranged from 0.9000 to 0.9292 (s = 0.0080). Accuracy of Gaussian kernel ranged from 0.9000 to 0.9333 (s = 0.0067). Finally, accuracy of Laplacian kernel ranged from 0.8958 to 0.9292 (s = 0.0072). Accuracy of C4.5 ranged from 0.9000 to 0.9417 (s = 0.0109). Gaussian kernel showed the most stable behavior across the 30 runs.

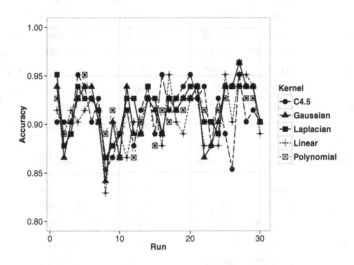

Fig. 3. Accuracy across 30 runs using train-test for SVM kernels.

In Fig. 3, we show the average accuracy of the four GBS subtypes across 30 train-test runs for linear, polynomial, Gaussian and Laplacian kernels as well as C4.5. Accuracy of linear kernel ranged from 0.8293 to 0.9512 (s = 0.0282). Accuracy of polynomial kernel ranged from 0.8659 to 0.9834 (s = 0.0230). Accuracy of Gaussian kernel ranged from 0.8415 to 0.9634 (s = 0.0292). Finally, accuracy of Laplacian kernel ranged from 0.8659 to 0.9512 (s = 0.0233). Accuracy of C4.5 ranged from 0.8537 to 0.9512 (s = 0.0283). Polynomial kernel showed the most stable behavior across the 30 runs.

Table 7 shows the prediction results of linear, polynomial, Gaussian and Laplacian kernels as well as C4.5 across 30 10-FCV runs. The standard deviation (sd) of each measure is also shown. Polynomial kernel slightly outperformed the rest of the kernels in accuracy. C4.5 obtained the second best accuracy, above Laplacian, Gaussian and linear kernels.

Table 8 shows the prediction results of linear, polynomial, Gaussian and Laplacian kernels as well as C4.5 across 30 train-test runs. The standard deviation (sd) of each measure is also shown. Laplacian kernel slightly outperformed the rest of the kernels in accuracy. Also, Laplacian, Polynomial and Gaussian outperformed C4.5 in accuracy.

Overall, no major differences were observed in the results obtained across different kernels and C4.5 both in train-test and 10-FCV. An important fact is

Table 7. Performance measures averaged across 30 10-FCV runs

kernel/classifier	Accuracy	Multiclass AUC	Sensitivity	Specificity	Kappa
Polynomial	0.9235	0.8985	0.8308	0.9481	0.7648
(sd)	(0.0080)	(0.0199)	(0.0287)	(0.0058)	(0.0265)
C4.5	0.9211	0.8857	0.8136	0.9446	0.7567
(sd)	(0.0109)	(0.0242)	(0.0421)	(0.0081)	(0.0321)
Laplacian	0.9201	0.8712	0.7952	0.9466	0.7554
(sd)	(0.0072)	(0.0240)	(0.0457)	(0.0051)	(0.0195)
Gaussian	0.9193	0.8897	0.8212	0.9448	0.7515
(sd)	(0.0067)	(0.0221)	(0.0316)	(0.0049)	(0.0214)
Linear	0.9175	0.8632	0.7831	0.9415	0.7423
(sd)	(0.0096)	(0.0232)	(0.0461)	(0.0076)	(0.0317)

Table 8. Performance measures averaged across 30 train-test runs

kernel/classifier	Accuracy	Multiclass AUC	Sensitivity	Specificity	Kappa
Laplacian	0.9163	0.7913	0.7753	0.9432	0.7523
(sd)	(0.0233)	(0.0844)	(0.0764)	(0.0159)	(0.0675)
Polynomial	0.9142	0.8361	0.7858	0.9390	0.7452
(sd)	(0.0230)	(0.0717)	(0.0674)	(0.0163)	(0.0677)
Gaussian	0.9126	0.8210	0.7884	0.9397	0.7427
(sd)	(0.0292)	(0.0672)	(0.0704)	(0.0200)	(0.0827)
C4.5	0.9114	0.8085	0.7727	0.9356	0.7348
(sd)	(0.0283)	(0.0827)	(0.0727)	(0.0218)	(0.0850)
Linear	0.9069	0.7751	0.7572	0.9355	0.7246
(sd)	(0.0282)	(0.0830)	(0.0822)	(0.0198)	(0.0810)

that all different kernels reached an accuracy above 0.90 and so did C4.5. This indicates that the 16 features used in this study constitute a good predictor subset for the four GBS subtypes. On the other hand, it was observed a higher variability in accuracy in train-test than in 10-FCV.

5 Conclusions

In previous clustering research [2], we found 16 features identifying four GBS subtypes with a purity of 0.8992 (from a range [0,1]). We investigated the predictive power of these features in this study. The results obtained in the prediction model confirm that we identified a good feature subset using the method we proposed. Further analysis is being conducted as to the relevance of each feature in the context of data classification. Experimental results showed performance of both classifiers are comparable. SVM slightly outperformed C4.5 with Polynomial kernel in 10-FCV. Also, it performed better than C4.5 with Laplacian, polynomial and Gaussian kernels in train-test. We will further apply other classification methods.

The final 16 relevant feature subset included 4 clinical variables and 12 variables related with nerve conduction studies, no variable from the CSF test was selected by our method. From the medical point of view, the reduced number of features used to predict the four GBS subtypes could guide physicians to design a faster, simpler and cheaper diagnosis of the case. However, a predictive model using only clinical variables would be more effective for both patients and physicians since additional studies would be avoided. Currently, we are investigating the building of such model.

References

1. Hornik, K., Karatzoglou, A., Smola, A., Zeileis, A.: kernlab - an S4 package for kernel methods in R. J. Stat. Softw. **11**(9), 1–20 (2004)
2. Canul-Reich, J., Hernández-Torruco, J., Frausto-Solis, J., Méndez-Castillo, J.J.: Finding relevant features for identifying subtypes of guillain-barré syndrome using quenching simulated annealing and partitions around medoids (in review)
3. Cohen, J.: A coefficient of agreement for nominal scales. Educat. Psychol. Meas. **20**(1), 37–46 (1960)
4. Chang, C.C., Hsu, C.W., Lin, C.J.: A practical guide to support vector classification. Technical report, Department of Computer Science, National Taiwan University (2003)
5. Lin, C.J., Hsu, C.W.: A comparison of methods for multiclass support vector machines. IEEE Trans. Neural Netw. **13**, 1045–1052 (2002)
6. Fawcett, T.: An introduction to roc analysis. Pattern Recogn. Lett. **27**(8), 861–874 (2006)
7. Hand, D.J., Hill, R.J.: A simple generalisation of the area under the roc curve for multiple class classification problems. Mach. Learn. **45**(2), 171–186 (2001)
8. Kuwabara, S.: Guillain-barré syndrome. Drugs **64**(6), 597–610 (2004)
9. Matsumoto, M., Nishimura, T.: Mersenne twister: a 623-dimensionally equidistributed uniform pseudo-random number generator. ACM Trans. Model. Comput. Simul. **8**(1), 3–30 (1998)
10. Meyer, D., Dimitriadou, E., Hornik, K., Weingessel, A., Leisch, F.: e1071: Misc Functions of the Department of Statistics (e1071), TU Wien (2014). R package version 1.6-3
11. Pascual, S.I.P.: Protocolos Diagnóstico Terapéuticos de la AEP: Neurología Pediátrica. Síndrome de Guillain-Barré. Asociación Espanola de Pediatría, Madrid (2008)
12. Solokova, M., Lapalme, G.: A systematic analysis of performance measures for classification tasks. Inf. Process. Manage. **45**, 427–437 (2009)
13. Uncini, A., Kuwabara, S.: Electrodiagnostic criteria for guillain-barré syndrome: a critical revision and the need for an update. Clin. Neurophysiol. **123**(8), 1487–1495 (2012)
14. Vapnik, V.: Statistical Learning Theory. Wiley, New York (1998)

Feature Selection in Spectroscopy Brain Cancer Data

Félix F. González-Navarro[1]([⊠]), Lluìs A. Belanche-Muñoz[2],
Brenda L. Flores-Ríos[1], and Jorge E. Ibarra-Esquer[1]

[1] Instituto de Ingeniería, Universitad Autonóma de Baja California,
Blvd. Benito Juárez y Calle de la Normal s/n, 21280 Mexicali, México
{fernando.gonzalez,brenda.flores,jorge.ibarra}@uabc.edu.mx
[2] Dept. de Llenguatges i Sistemes Informàtics, Universitat Politècnica de Catalunya,
Ω-Building, North Campus, 08034 Barcelona, Spain
belanche@lsi.upc.edu

Abstract. In cancer diagnosis, classification of the different tumor types is of great importance. An accurate prediction of different tumor types provides better treatment and toxicity minimization on patients. Predicting cancer types using non-invasive information –e.g. ^{1}H-MRS data– could avoid patients to suffer collateral problems derived from exploration techniques that require surgery. Two Feature Selection Algorithms specially designed to be use in ^{1}H-MRS Proton Magnetic Resonance Spectroscopy data of brain tumors are presented. These two algorithms take advantage of two distinctive aspects: first, metabolite levels are quite different between types of tumors and two, ^{1}H-MRS data possess a quasi-temporal series shape. Experimental readings on an international data set show highly competitive models in terms of accuracy, complexity and medical interpretability.

Keywords: Cancer research · Feature selection · Classification

1 Introduction

Hydrogen 1 Magnetic Resonance Spectroscopy (^{1}H-MRS) has been used extensively in biochemistry for *in vitro* chemical analysis of small samples for several years. As a technique for *in vivo* sampling of biological tissue, it provides a quantified biochemical fingerprint of metabolite[1] concentrations [25]. ^{1}H-MRS data has the appearance of a plot of peaks along the x-axis, with the peak position depending on the resonant frequency of the associated metabolite [21]. In Fig. 1 it is shown an example of ^{1}H-MRS data set.

Nowadays, it has been proven its value as a powerful tool in the clinical assessment of several pathologic conditions –e.g. epilepsy, multiple sclerosis, cancer– specially neurological affections [2,9]. Framed as a minimal invasive technic, its application in brain tumor oncologic diagnosis carries tremendous benefits to

---

[1] Metabolites are resulting products of metabolic processes.

© Springer International Publishing Switzerland 2015
O. Pichardo Lagunas et al. (Eds.): MICAI 2015, Part II, LNAI 9414, pp. 282–296, 2015.
DOI: 10.1007/978-3-319-27101-9_21

patients, relieving them from complicated surgical procedures and minimizing trauma to normal tissue surrounding the particular lesion or other vital elements.

The use of systematic approaches based on ^{1}H-MRS data for the diagnosis and grading of adult brain tumors is subject of an extensive scientific research. One of these growing approaches takes as backbone well established machine learning techniques acting as intelligent engines to discern between several classes of brain tumor [6,22,24].

This particular task is quite challenging, obeying to its scarce data values and its high dimensionality. Therefore, the use of dimensionality reduction methods becomes amendable in order to present low complexity and interpretable models to oncologists. In this study, experimental work is shown in which two different feature selection strategies are used as a way to generate relevant subsets of spectral frequencies. These two algorithms take advantage of two distinctive aspects: first, metabolite levels are quite different between types of tumors and two, ^{1}H-MRS data possess a quasi-temporal series shape. This later feature could lead us to design algorithms that explore spectral data sweeping very specific region of interest.

This paper is organized as follows: Section two describes scientific papers related to the task at hand. In sections three and four, the two FS algorithms will be detailed described. Section five gives the experimental settings, data description, validation method and a few experimental considerations. Section six analyzes the FS and performance results given by the two FS algorithms, as long as metabolic interpretations. Finally, some conclusions and final thoughts are given.

2 Literature Review

First attempts using ^{1}H-MRS data in assessing human brain tumors *in vivo* are back to [2]. It was found that spectra differ significantly from normal brain spectra and between tumors by detecting the presence/absence of different metabolites. Even though no ML analysis of spectra was done in establishing these differences, it was concluded that ^{1}H-MRS spectroscopy may help to differentiate tumors for diagnostic and therapeutic purposes, limiting the need for invasive and risky diagnostic procedures such as biopsies.

At this point, ML techniques arise in order to *automate* the classification tasks. Artificial neural networks (e.g. [1,23]) and Linear discriminant analysis (LDA) (e.g. [18,22]) are commonly used methods. Later studies perform dimensionality reduction, either considering the *peak* signals, ratios between peak signals or *feature extraction* (FE) based in Principal Components or Independent Components [4,11,16]. First studies in performing explicit Feature Selection (FS) used well-known algorithms to select subset of spectral points: the Forward Selection [19], the Fisher criterion and the Relief algorithm [17].

Most recent works in FS properly speaking are found in [7,14,20,24], which address a multi-class problem on the same data set analyzed in this work. Dominant techniques are basic neural networks definitions as dimensionality reduction

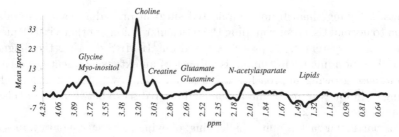

Fig. 1. Long echo ^{1}H-MRS data set example. Some of the metabolites found in this spectra are for example the Choline, which is a combination of multiple metabolites and is elevated in all brain tumors; the creatine, a marker of oxidative metabolism of cells; the N-acetylaspartate, a neuronal density marker; the Lipids, seen in condition of necrosis; etc.

method –aliencies measures of features– and custom-made feature selection algorithms using several classifiers on which linear discriminant solutions yield best models.

In the next sections, the two FS algorithms will be described. Both algorithms explore subsets of spectral points assuring the confidence about which features posses enough merit to be considered as relevant trough bootstrap resampling. Thereby, certainty readings in performance (standard errors) at *step by step search* for the best subset are generated with such a quantity of information that stability of solutions is as much rigorous as the end-user requires in its particular domain and demands.

3 Class-Separability Feature Selection

It is known that metabolites (spectral points or features) in ^{1}H-MRS data present notorious differences among tumors. For example, theoretically, meningiomas do not contain n-acetyl aspartate (NAA) and present the choline (CHO) elevated (up 300 times normal). Metastases present a moderate reduction in NAA and a decreased creatine (CR) signal. These *fingerprints* that distinguish each tumor could lead us to try to establish a measure of physical distance between kinds of tumors that measures the separability between classes.

To capture the aforementioned behavior, the CSFS algorithm (which briefs for *Class-Separability Feature Selection*) is designed and outlined in Algorithm 1. The rationale behind such idea rests in the calculation of a distance value for each metabolite, given its membership to a specific tumor class. Taking as primary data a bootstrap distribution, stable estimations of such distances from the original ^{1}H-MRS could be computed, a metric or centroid m for every spectral point within each tumor is computed (lines 2–5). Thus, a $\bar{m}$-subspace of centroids is generated by averaging them over the B bootstrap samples (line 6). In order to asses the separability degree of metabolites with respect to each tumor, the cumulative difference between pair of elements –i.e. between tumors– is computed (lines 7–9), obtaining a new feature vector based on distances named DS

Algorithm 1. $CSFS$ Class Separability Feature Selection

```
input  : B: Bootstrap samples M: Metric
output: BSS: Best Spectral Subset
```
1 $space \leftarrow 1 \ldots TotalSpectralPoints$
2 **foreach** *sample* $b \in B$ **do**
3   **foreach** *spectral point* s **do**
4   **foreach** *class* c **do**
5        $m(b, s, c) \leftarrow CalculateMetric(M)$

6 Average on $b | m(b, s, c)$ becomes $\bar{m}(s, c)$
7 **foreach** *spectral point* s **do**
8   **foreach** *possible combination* $(c_i, c_j) | i \neq j$ **do**
9      $DS(s) \leftarrow DS(s) + |\bar{m}(s, i) - \bar{m}(s, j)|$

10 Sort DS descendently
11 $BSS \leftarrow \varnothing$
12 $Jbest \leftarrow 0$
13 $space \leftarrow DS$
14 **repeat**
15   ***Forward Stage***
16   **for** $i = 1 : |space|$ **do**
17   **foreach** *sample* $b \in B$ **do**
18        $J(b) \leftarrow PF(BSS \cup \{space(i)\})$
19   Average on $b | J(b)$ becomes $\bar{J}$
20   **if** $\bar{J} > Jbest$ **then**
21        $Jbest \leftarrow \bar{J}$
22        $BSS \leftarrow BSS \cup space(i)$
23   Remove element i from $space$
24   ***Backward Stage***
25   **repeat**
26   **foreach** *sample* $b \in B$ **do**
27        $J(b) \leftarrow PF(BSS \setminus \{BSS(j)\})$
28   Average on $b | J(b)$ becomes $\bar{J}$
29   **if** $\bar{J} \geq Jbest$ **then**
30        $Jbest \leftarrow \bar{J}$
31   Remove element j from BSS
32   **until** *No more Backward improvement*
33 **until** *No more Forward and Backward improvement*

(sorted in descendent order in line 10). It is hypothesized that the direction that best separates tumors taking as basis the metabolites that present abnormal values is partly expressed in DS vector.

Once completed the metric evaluation a simple Forward-Backward Search Strategy is implemented being feed by DS vector as follows: a Forward step is given taking the first element in the ranked list DS (lines 15–23) and its performance (line 18, PF function) is evaluated again on each bootstrap sample, and averaging over B samples (line 19). Taking into account that ^{1}H-MRS data could be considered as a time-series, in the sense that spectral points could be ordered, it is likely that contiguous spectral points offer similar separability values and hence being indexed in consecutive positions in DS. To exemplify, Creatine peak, located at 3.03 ppm[2] in the spectrum could have a separability value similar to 3.01 ppm spectral point which *almost* define the same metabolite.

---

[2] parts per million.

Algorithm 2. $BCFS$ Block-Contiguous Feature Selection

---

input : B: Bootstrap samples T: Block size
output: BSS: Best Spectral Subset
1    $space \leftarrow 1 \ldots TotalSpectralPoints$
2   **foreach** *sample* $b \in B$ **do**
3   **foreach** *spectral point* s **do**
4          $m(b, s) \leftarrow PF(space(s))$

5   Average on $b|m(b, s)$ becomes $\bar{m}(s)$
6    $BSS \leftarrow argmax\bar{m}(s)$
7    $Jbest \leftarrow \bar{m}(argmax\bar{m}(s))$
8    $space \leftarrow space \setminus BSS$
9   **for** $i = 1 : |space|$ **do**
10   **for** $j = 1 : min(T, space - i + 1)$ **do**
11   ***Forward Stage***
12   **foreach** *sample* $b \in B$ **do**
13            $J(b) \leftarrow PF(BSS \cup \{space(i \ldots i + j - 1)\})$

14   Average on $b|J(b)$ becomes $\bar{J}$
15   **if** $\bar{J} > Jbest$ **then**
16            $Jbest \leftarrow \bar{J}$
17            $BSS \leftarrow BSS \cup \{space(i \ldots i + j - 1)\}$

18   ***Backward Stage***
19   **repeat**
20   **foreach** *sample* $b \in B$ **do**
21               $J(b) \leftarrow PF(BSS \setminus \{BSS(k)\})$

22   Average on $b|J(b)$ becomes $\bar{J}$
23   **if** $\bar{J} \geq Jbest$ **then**
24               $Jbest \leftarrow \bar{J}$
25   Remove element k from BSS

26   **until** *no Backward improvement*

In order to avoid the inclusion of redundant features, a Backward-Stage (BWS) is embedded right after Forward-Stage (FWS), but with the difference that the BWS is executed as much as necessary, in other words, until no improvement is achieved (line 29). Such arrangement of FS stages assures the removal of any possible redundancy.

4 Block-Contiguous Feature Selection

The CSFS Algorithm takes advantage of abnormal presence of certain metabolites that allows to identify some specific tumor. As a consequence, the ones that present higher separability degree in a ranked list guide its operation. Algorithm presented in this section finds subsets of spectral points in a complete different fashion, exploiting the sequential property of spectral points.

The Block-Contiguous Feature Selection algorithm (named BCFS and shown in Algorithm 2) implements a *blockwise* Forward-Backward search strategy which is feed by blocks of consecutive spectral points. It starts by selecting the most relevant feature (evaluated in PF, line 4). Such a strategy forces the BCFS to set an initial threshold that next subsets must surpass (lines 1–4). Following the same guessing of gaining stability in performance readings, the average of B bootstrap samples is computed for each spectral point (line 5).

At any given position of the continuous spectrum (from spectral point 1 to 195), a block starting at $i - position$ and having size of T is analyzed. Every subset of consecutive spectral points of size $\leq T$ is evaluated. To illustrate the mechanism, let suppose that $N = 7$ features must be explored. Given a block of size $T = 3$, an a starting position $i = 1$, the subsets exploration is as follows: In the first shift-cycle (given by the outer for-loop in line 9 of BCFS algorithm) the subsets $\{\{1\}, \{1, 2\}, \{1, 2, 3\}\}$ are generated (for-loop in line 10) and evaluated over the B bootstrap samples (lines 12–13); at the second shift $\{\{2\}, \{2, 3\}, \{2, 3, 4\}\}$; at the third shift $\{\{3\}, \{3, 4\}, \{3, 4, 5\}\}$; at forth shift $\{\{4\}, \{4, 5\}, \{4, 5, 6\}\}$ ... until the N-space is explored. Complexity of BCFS algorithm calculated in $\frac{1}{2}NT(T + 1)\mathcal{O}(PF)$ seems to be prohibitive with block sizes near N, but it is expected that keeping small block sizes assure us reasonable performance demands. Each time a block is added to the current best solution BSS (line 17) in the Forward stage, the Backward stage is applied under the same policy described in algorithm CSFS (lines 19–26).

In the next section, experimental conditions applied on both algorithms are outlined. The ^{1}H-MRS data set employed is described jointly with the brain pathologies involved. Several well known classifiers are used to measure the subsets performance as long as statistical tests to asses certainty about comparisons between models.

5   Experimental Settings

An essential variable in the acquisition of ^{1}H-MRS spectra is the choice of echo time. With short echo times (around 20 ms), larger numbers of metabolites are detected (myoinositol, glutamate, glutamine), but it is more likely that peak superimposition will occur, causing difficulty in spectroscopic curve interpretation. By using long echo times (>135 ms), most metabolites in the brain are lost (except that of choline, creatine, N-acetyl aspartate and lactate), but with better definition of peaks, thereby facilitating graphic analysis [3]. There are a few studies comparing the classification potential of the two types of spectra (see e.g. [6,18]). These works seem to give a slight advantage to using SET information or else suggest a combination of both types of spectra.

The targeted ^{1}H-MRS data is drawn from a database belonging to the *International Network for Pattern Recognition of tumors Using Magnetic Resonance* (INTERPRET). An European research project aimed to develop systematic tools to enable radiologists and other clinicians without special knowledge or expertise to diagnose and grade brain tumors routinely using magnetic resonance spectroscopy [12]. The data set is constructed by single voxel ^{1}H-MR spectra acquired *in vivo* from brain tumor patients in two configurations: Long Echo Time (PRESS 135–144 ms), named LET, and Short Echo Time (PRESS 30–32 ms), named SET. Brain pathologies that conform both configurations are distributed as following:

- LET: 195 cases which include 55 meningiomas, 78 glioblastomas, 31 metastases, 20 astrocytomas grade II, 6 oligoastrocytomas grade II and 5 oligodendrogliomas grade II.
- SET: 217 cases with: 58 meningiomas, 86 glioblastomas, 38 metastases, 22 astrocytomas grade II, 6 oligoastrocytomas grade II, and 7 (SET) oligodendrogliomas grade II.

Both spectra were grouped into three super-classes: high-grade malignant tumors (metastases and glioblastomas), low-grade gliomas (astrocytomas, oligodendrogliomas and oligoastrocytomas) and meningiomas. A third configuration was prepared in order to explore the discriminative power of the merged LET and SET data resulting in 195 common observations of the two previous data sets, and labeled as LSET.

To obtain *reliably* relevant features we advocate for the use of *bootstrapping* techniques in the feature selection process. Bootstrap resampling techniques are used to yield mean performance estimates and their variability, and thus a more reliable measure of predictive ability. The original ^{1}H-MRS data sets $S = \{LET, SET, LSET\}$ were used to generate $B = 1,000$ bootstrap samples $S_1, \ldots, S_B$ that play the role of *training sets* in the feature selection process: each *Performance Function PF* in the both algorithms trains a classifier on the S_i sample and its performance is assesed on the test sample $S \setminus S_i$ –recall that bootstrap resampling definition requires to be done with replacement–, and *averaged* across the B bootstrap samples.

Once the final subset is obtained with both algorithms, the final performance by means of six classifiers in 10 times 10-fold Cross Validation fashion (10x10cv) in the original ^{1}H-MRS data sets is assessed: a *nearest-neighbor* (kNN) with parameter k (number of neighbors), the *Logistic Regression* (LR), a *Linear and Quadratic Discriminant classifier* (LDC, QDC), *Support Vector Machine* with *linear* kernel (lSVM) and parameter C (regularization constant) and *Support Vector Machine with* radial *kernel* (rSVM) and parameters C and σ^2 (amount of smoothing in the kernel)[3]. Wilcoxon signed rank test is applied in order to give statistical significance in performance between the models.

Table 1. CSFS Feature selection results and final performance. Cell in table contains the FS information as follows: Left number, final BSS performance rendered by CSFS; exponent of left number, final size of BSS; right number, 10x10xv accuracy in the original ^{1}H-MRS data.

	NN		LDC		QDC		LR		lSVM		rSVM	
LET	87.47^{11}	89.70	91.72^{15}	93.51	86.12^9	89.09	88.64^7	91.48	88.13^9	91.82	$\mathbf{90.46^{10}}$	**93.88**
SET	89.79^8	92.21	91.94^{16}	93.34	86.86^6	87.40	88.86^8	90.48	90.57^{12}	93.14	$\mathbf{91.89^8}$	**94.48**
LSET	93.59^{17}	96.14	$\mathbf{95.76^{26}}$	**98.27**	90.66^8	92.83	89.54^7	92.07	92.79^{14}	94.83	92.14^{12}	94.77

---

[3] C and σ^2 are optimized via a grid search.

Table 2. BCFS Feature selection results and final performance. Cell in table contains the FS information as follows: Left number, final BSS performance rendered by BCFS; exponent of left number, final size of BSS; right number, 10x10xv accuracy in the original ^{1}H-MRS data.

	NN		LDC		QDC		LR		lSVM		rSVM	
LET	89.09^{19}	91.74	$\mathbf{91.97^{15}}$	**93.90**	84.78^8	86.89	86.69^8	89.10	89.10^{14}	91.55	87.92^{11}	90.01
SET	86.29^8	88.58	90.49^{10}	90.89	86.75^5	87.97	87.56^9	90.00	88.21^9	89.72	$\mathbf{90.06^7}$	**93.22**
LSET	88.39^{18}	91.83	94.33^{20}	95.85	88.39^8	90.83	89.31^{10}	92.09	$\mathbf{94.08^{22}}$	**96.44**	90.24^{14}	92.68

6 Experimental Results

6.1 CSFS Results

CSFS algorithm were tested with two metrics: the median and the harmonic mean. Imputable to space regulations and to experimental results (best accuracy), only median records are supplied. In Table 1, CSFS feature selection process is displayed. Among the seven classifiers in LET data, LDC observes the best performance, giving a 91.72 % of accuracy with only 15 spectral points. The rSVM is placed at second position with a decay of almost 1 % of accuracy and 5 spectral points less than LDC. But, this later model achieves the best 10x10xval accuracy, 93.88 %. Wilcoxon signed rank test p-values at 95 % level show significative results comparing rSVM against all, excepting with LDC (p-value = 0.16016). SET experiments shows exactly the same tendency as LET results, but offering higher values. rSVM reaches 94.48 % 10x10xval accuracy with only 8 spectral points and its first place in this data configuration is significative supported (all p-values $\leq$ 0.00195).

LSET experiments render the best results in both algorithms. FS final performance were set at 95.76 % of accuracy under 26 spectral points. 10x10xval accuracy in the original ^{1}H-MRS data yields a respectable 98.27 % value. This is one of the best values achieved using this data set with this particular configuration of super-classes (see [4,6,7,13,16,22]). A recent work published a similar accuracy performance [14], claiming a 98.46 % of 5x5xval accuracy with 18 spectral points by means of a Single-Layer Perceptron Artificial Neural Network. Despite offering a solution with a better but small difference in performance (0.19 %) and less spectral points, CSFS-LSET-LDC solution requires no parameter tuning in training phase. Wilcoxon test p-values give statistical confirmation to this competitive model.

6.2 BCFS Results

In the present section, BCFS experimental results are reported. To this end, the block size T was to be assessed ir order to obtain a value which gives a good compromise between size of final subset, total time of processing and accuracy. Several block sizes were tested ($T = 2 \ldots 15$) using only the half of bootstrap samples. This condition was chosen because the T-value process would consume a considerable amount of time. Two classifiers were selected to be the performance measure, the kNN (with parameter $k = 1$) and the LDC. In Figs. 2 and 3 are shown the response of their accuracy (recall that BCFS algorithm averages the test set accuracy over 500 bootstrap samples), the size of the BSS yielded and computational time demand (measured in hrs.) to the gradually variation of T. The all measures were obtained in the three data sets.

1NN accuracy chart on Fig. 2 –top-left– shows a slightly decreasing tendency with respect to the increasing value of T on LET and LSET data. Almost similar behavior is shown in LDC classifier –Fig. 3, top-left chart– equally in the same types of data. Congruently in both classifiers, the 1NN and the LDC, by using the SET data, a clear conclusion can not be made.

On assessing the impact of T on BSS size measure $-|BSS|-$, a similar but opposite tendency than accuracy described above is observed -i.e. the higher T values the higher $|BSS|$ size–. 1NN best values –Fig. 2 top-right– are on SET and LSET data which is $T = 4$ for both sets and 89.98 % and 91.17 % respectively, however their $|BSS|$ values are quite uneven, 9 and 27 in the same order. LET value reaches its best performance in $T = 7$ with 25 spectral frequencies and 88.93 % of accuracy.

Once assured the T value, experimental results with the full set of samples are given as following: On LDC LET data –Fig. 3 top-right chart– a $T = 5$ block size gives a higher accuracy –92.48 %– with $|BSS| = 18$, compared with a $T = 6$ configuration that gives a better accuracy, but worst $|BSS|$ reading –25 features–. SET data offers a good arrangement $-accuracy = 90.37$ % and $|BSS| = 12$– with $T = 5$, finally on LSET data a $T = 3$ setting gives a very good accuracy value, 96.09 % with $|BSS| = 21$.

It could be briefed that on 1NN experiment $T = 4$ dominates the setting, and on LDC, $T = 5$ does its corresponding contribution. Time consumption with these two values is neglectable –see Figs. 2 and 3 bottom charts– in the sense that this measure does not incline the final selection of T value. As a consequence, $T = 5$ was selected as the one to be used in the complete experiments, given that with this value offers on the one hand good accuracy values, but on the other hand a more stable differences between the three data sets in their respective performance measure –i.e. accuracy and $|BSS|$ value–.

Table 2 readings are not as high as the offered by CSFS algorithm. For the LET data set, LDC gives the best values, 91.97 % of accuracy with 15 spectral frequencies, and 93.90 % 10x10xval accuracy on the original data set. On SET configuration lowest results are achieved. However its best result, the rSVM, sets a 90.06 % of accuracy with only 7 features and 93.22 % 10x10xval accuracy.

LSET experiments give highest accuracy values in BCSF algorithm, having lSVM model its best representative, whose records are 94.08 % of accuracy with 22 features and carrying out a 96.44 % 10x10xval accuracy. It is worth it to mention that this result represents almost 3 times in size with respect to SET-rSVM model with an attenuation of only 3 % of 10x10 xval accuracy. Such a situation tell us to be caution in concluding which model gives the best balanced solution in terms of accuracy, complexity and interpretability.

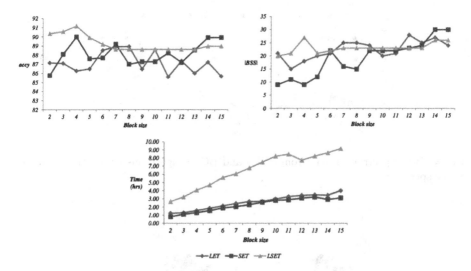

Fig. 2. Accuracy, size of BSS and computational time demand variation given several block sizes T in BCFS algorithm using the Nearest Neighbor classifier with parameter k=1 as performance measure.

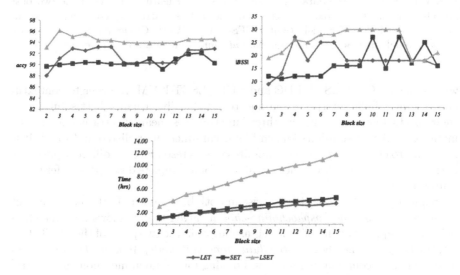

Fig. 3. Accuracy, size of BSS and computational time demand variation given several block sizes T in BCFS algorithm using the Linear Discriminant classifier as performance measure.

6.3 Metabolic Interpretation

In Fig. 4 is pointed out the best spectral subsets as positioned in the whole spectrum –i.e. 390 x-values for LSET data given that best models come from this data set configuration– for the winner models using CSFS and BCFS algorithms, which

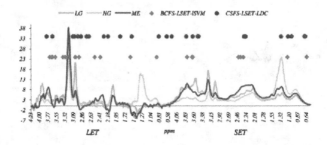

Fig. 4. Best Spectral Subsets from CSFS and BCFS algorithms as positioned in the whole spectrum.

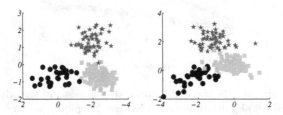

Fig. 5. Projection of the data sets (using the *selected* feature subsets of the two best models) onto the first three eigenvectors of the scatter matrices as coordinate system. Left: CSFS-LSET-LDC model, Right: BCFS-LSET-lSVML. Circles represent low-grade *gliomas*; filled squares high-grade *malignant tumors* and stars *meningiomas*.

will be named CSFS-LSET-LDC and BCFS-LSET-lSVM. In order to contextualize the metabolic interpretation and to graphically visualize best solutions in their spectral environment, the three super-classes mean spectra is added. The metabolites detected and its known biological function are listed in Table 3. It is necessary to clarify that some metabolites posses resonances at different positions in the spectrum –e.g. Threonine or Valine–. For a complete description refer to the source at [8].

Some metabolites consistently arise in both best models: Particular comment deserves the *Glycerol-phosphocholine-choline*, given that it shows an interesting behavior in appearing in both models as long as in the two parts of the LSET data set, the Long and the Short echo. *Glutathione-glutamate*, *Alanine*, *Threonine* and *Valine* are also common metabolites. Looking for common metabolites with [14] (previously discussed in literature review) the following were found: Alanine, Myo-Inositol, Taurine, Choline, Glutamate and Glutamine.

Data visualization in a low-dimensional space may become extremely important to radiologists, helping them to gain insights into what undoubtedly is a complex domain. We use in this work a method based on the decomposition of the scatter matrix with the property of maximizing the separation between the projections of compact groups of tumor classes –see [15]–. Such visualization is illustrated in Fig. 5. These are scatter plots of 3-D projections of the three classes (using the first three eigenvectors of the scatter matrices). It is seen that the three supper-classes are notoriously clustered by the best models of both algorithms.

Table 3. Metabolic interpretation in best models. For reading purposes the first group on each metabolite labeled as *A* corresponds to CSFS-LSET-LDC model, and the second labeled as *B* to BCFS-LSET-lSVM model. Prefix *L*, *S* signal which part belong to and all values are ppm expressed.

Metabolite	Biological interpretation
Glycerol-phosphocholine-choline	An end product of membrane phospholipid degradation and increased concentrations have been associated with cerebral ischemia, seizures and traumatic brain injury. A={L3.66 S3.66} B={L3.66 S3.66}
Glutathione-glutamate	An anti-oxidant, essential for maintaining normal red-cell structure. Altered levels have been reported in Parkinsons's disease and other neurodegenerative diseases. A={L2.18} B={L2.54}
Alanine	A nonessential amino acid that has been observed in increased levels in meningiomas. A={L1.55} B={L1.59 S3.79}
Threonine	A large neutral amino acid essential to the diet. A={S4.19 S1.32} B={L3.58}
Valine	An essential amino acid necessary for protein synthesis observed in brain abscesses. A={S2.25 S1.04} B={L0.89}
Ethanolamine	Increased levels of this metabolite has been observed in ischemic brain tissue of rats and gerbils. A={L3.81 S3.81}
Phenylalanine	An aromatic amino acid that presents elevated readings in phenylketonuria, an abnormal phenylalanine metabolization. A={L3.11 L3.07}
Glutathione-cysteine	See Glutathione-glutamate. A={L2.98 L2.90}
Aspartate	An exitatory amino acid that performs as a neurotoxin in elevated concentrations [5]. A={L2.75}
NAA-Aspartate	A free amino acid whose function is poorly understood, but is commonly believed to provide a marker of neuronal density. A={L2.69}
GABA	A primary inhibitory neurotransmitter whose altered concentrations are associated with neurological disorders. A={L2.29 L1.86 S2.29}
Myo-inositol	Its function is not enough understood, although it is believed to be a requirement in cell growth. Altered levels have been linked with Alzheimer's disease, hepatic encephalopathy and brain injury. A={S3.53}
Choline	A combination of multiple metabolites and is elevated in all brain tumors. Its required for the synthesis of neurotransmitters constituents of membranes. A={S3.49}

(Continued)

Table 3. (*Continued*)

Metabolite	Biological interpretation
Glutamate	See Aspartate. B={L3.74 S2.31}
Glycerol-phosphocholine-glycerol	Metabolite associated with cerebral ischemia, seizures and traumatic brain injury. B={L3.68}
Scyllo-inositol	An isomer associated in high levels with Alzheimer's disease [10]. B={L3.38 L3.32}
Taurine	Amino acid reported to have a number of biological functions including osmoregulation en modulation of neurotransmitters. B={L3.24}
Histidine	A neutral amino acid essential for the synthesis of proteins. B={L3.22}
Tyrosine	An important precursor of epinephrine, norepinephrine and dopamine. It may have some clinical use for treatment of Parkinson's disease and depression. B={L3.05}
Homocarnosine-GABA	Elevated levels of this dipeptide in brain tissue are characteristic of homocarnosinosis, a metabolic disorder associated with spastic paraplegia, mental retardation and retinal pigmentation. B={L2.96}
Succinate	Increased levels of succinate have been reported in brain abcesses. B={L2.39 S2.39}
Phosporyl choline	It is often referred, jointly with Choline and glycerophosphorylcholine as "Total Choline". See Choline. B={S3.64}
Glutamine	Plays a role in detoxification and regulation of neurotransmitter activities. B={S2.44}
Not identified	A={L0.83 L0.62 S1.13 S0.70 S0.66} B={S1.15 S0.64}.

7   Conclusions

In this work, two Feature Selection algorithms are introduced as a strategy to select subsets of spectral points from a ^{1}H-MRS spectral data of brain tumors. Both algorithms take advantage from two attractive –in algorithmic sense– and distinctive aspects underpinned in biochemical definitions and spectral data morphology. The models convenience arisen from using algorithms proposed in this work are considerable competitive in terms of accuracy, complexity of the algorithmic solution and medical interpretability. The CSFS Algorithm performance assessed in this contribution is one of the highest regarding the use of an international data set as explained above. Aside from this, its independency from the metric used to measure the class separability jointly with the resampling strategy, make this proposal a suitable mechanism to test other mathematical definitions.

The BCFS algorithm as novel search strategy, is intend to explore in a parsimoniously fashion data sets that posses a quasi-temporal series shape, given that consecutive spectral points may reflect the presence of the same metabolite with a certain and neglectable small difference –i.e. redundancy–. Despite not offering a higher performance than CSFS Algorithm –only 1.8 % less– its design permits to be adapted to more complex search strategy. For example, it could be implemented to run in a parallel way to explore simultaneously different regions on data sets of considerable size.

Even tough its usefulness in biochemistry analysis of brain tissue, ^{1}H-MRS is not strengthen as a standard method for clinical diagnosis. Machine learning proposals on this field must be robust and highly reliable taking account the scarcity of data towards to be recurrent and solicited tool by medical experts. In this tenor, the provided solution in this paper gives a drastic reduction in dimensionality with competitive performance and interpretable models.

References

1. Ala-Korpela, M., et al.: Artificial neural network analysis of 1H nuclear magnetic resonance spectroscopic data from human plasma. Neurocumputing **13–15**, 3085–3097 (2009)
2. Bruhn, H., et al.: Noninvasive differentiation of tumors with use of localized H-1 MR spectroscopy in vivo: initial experience in patients with cerebral tumors. Radiology **172**, 541–548 (1989)
3. Castillo, M., Kwock, L., Mukherji, S.: Clinical applications of proton MR spectroscopy. AJNR **17**, 1–15 (1996)
4. Devos, A.: Quantification and classification of MRS data and applications to brain tumour recognition. Ph.D. Thesis, Katholieke Univ. Leuven (2005)
5. Farooqui, A., Ong, W., Horrocks, L.: Glutamate and Aspartate in Brain. Springer, New York (2008)
6. Garcia, J., et al.: On the use of long te and short TE SV MR. Spectroscopy to improve the automatic brain tumor diagnosis. Technical report (2007). ftp://ftp.esat.kuleuven.ac.be/pub/SISTA/ida/reports/07-55.pdf
7. Gonzalez, F., et al.: Feature and model selection with discriminatory visualization for diagnostic classification of brain tumors. Neurocomputing **73**, 622–632 (2010)
8. Govindaraju, V., Young, K., Maudsley, A.: Proton NMR chemical shifts and coupling constants for brain metabolites. NMR Biomed. **13**(3), 129–153 (2000)
9. Hansen, J., et al.: ^{1}H-MR spectroscopy of the brain: absolute quantification of metabolites. Radiology **246**(2), 318–332 (2006)
10. Hollander, J., Stewart, C., Evanochko, W., Buchthal, S., Harrell, L., Zamrini, E., Brockington, J., Marson, D.: Elevated brain scyllo-inositol concentrations in patients with Alzheimer's disease. NMR Biomed. **20**(8), 706–716 (2007)
11. Huang, Y., Lisboa, P., El-Deredy, W.: Tumour grading from magnetic resonance spectroscopy: a comparison fo feature extraction with variable selection. Stat. Med. **22**, 147–164 (2003)
12. INTERPRET: International network for pattern recognition of tumours using magnetic resonance project (2002). http://azizu.uab.es/INTERPRET
13. Ladroue, C.: Pattern Recognition Techniques for the Study of Magnetic Resonance Spectra of Brain Tumours. Ph.D. Thesis, St. George's Hospital Medical School (2003)

14. Lisboa, P., et al.: Classification, dimensionality reduction, and maximally discriminatory visualization of a multicentre 1h-mrs database of brain tumors. In: ICMLA 2008: Proceedings of the 2008 Seventh International Conference on Machine Learning and Applications, pp. 613–618. IEEE Computer Society (2008)

15. Lisboa, P., et al.: Cluster based visualisation with scatter matrices. Pattern Recogn. Lett. **29**(13), 1814–1823 (2008)

16. Lukas, L., et al.: Brain tumor classification based on long echo proton MRS signals. Artif. Intell. Med. **31**, 73–89 (2004)

17. Luts, J., et al.: A combined MRI and MRSI based multiclass system from brain tumour recognition using LS-SVMs with class probabilities and feature selection. Artif. Intell. Med. **40**, 87–102 (2007)

18. Majos, C., et al.: Brain tumor classification by proton MR spectroscopy: comparison of diagnostic accuracy at short and long TE. Am. J. Neuroradiol. **25**, 1696–1704 (2004)

19. Nikulin, A., et al.: Near-optimal region selection for feature space reduction: novel preprocessing methods for classifying MR spectra. NMR Biomed. **11**, 209–216 (1998)

20. Romero, E., Vellido, A., Sopena, J.M.: Feature selection with single-layer perceptrons for a multicentre ^{1}H-MRS brain tumour database. In: Cabestany, J., Sandoval, F., Prieto, A., Corchado, J.M. (eds.) IWANN 2009, Part I. LNCS, vol. 5517, pp. 1013–1020. Springer, Heidelberg (2009)

21. Sibtain, N.: The clinical value of proton magnetic resonance spectroscopy in adult brain tumours. Clin. Radiol. **62**, 109–119 (2007)

22. Tate, A., et al.: Development of a decision support system for diagnosis and grading of brain tumours using in vivo magnetic resonance single voxel spectra. NMR Biomed. **19**, 411–434 (2006)

23. Usenius, J., et al.: Automated classification of human brain tumors by neural network analysis using in vivo 1H magnetic resonance spectroscopic metabolite phenotypes. Neuroreport **7**(10), 1597–1600 (1996)

24. Vellido, A., et al.: Outlier exploration and diagnostic classification of a multi-centre ^{1}H-MRS brain tumour database. Neurocomputing **72**, 3085–3097 (2009)

25. Zamani, A.: Proton MR Spectroscopy. In: Minimal Invasive Neurosurgery, pp. 75–86. Humana Press (2005)

Towards Ambient Intelligent Care and Assistance Systems for Patients with Dementia

Jesús Emeterio Navarro-Barrientos$^{(\boxtimes)}$, Daniel Herfert,
and Alfred Iwainsky

Gesellschaft zur Förderung angewandter Informatik e. V. (GFaI) –
Society for the Promotion of Applied Computer Science,
Volmerstr. 3, 12489 Berlin, Germany
jenavarrob@gmail.com, {herfert,iwainsky}@gfai.de

Abstract. This paper presents a monitor assistant system for detection of dangerous events and health diagnostics for patients with dementia. The proposed framework brings together three different types of ambient intelligence: (i) sensors for detecting life-threatening events that can occur at home, like falls and anomalies in vital signs predicting risk of myocardial infarction; (ii) sensors placed under bed-posts for detecting unhealthy poor movement while patients are lying on the bed which can cause bedsores (decubitus); and (iii) analysis of the current cognitive state of patients with dementia by means of serious computer games. This paper presents the framework, methods and sensors used by our system to assist patients with dementia by triggering different type of alarm signals informing which patient needs what and how some help could be provided.

Keywords: Ambient intelligence · Ambient assisted living · Decubitus ulcers · Dementia · Serious computer games · Ubiquitous computing and wearable sensors

1 Introduction

The recent advances in sensor technology surrounding our homes lead to different intelligent systems tracking activities, events and health conditions of house residents. One of the aims of the research area "ambient assisted living" is basically to develop smart and flexible sensors (clients), to investigate smart sensor communication protocols as well as to perform smart management and analysis (server) of the information sensed [1, 2]. A central paradigm when conceiving solutions for ambient assisted living systems is the privacy of the data collected. Another important aspect is the user-friendliness of the devices and the system, as well as their robustness, especially if the intended users are elderly, nursing staff and medical doctors [2].

Ambient assisted living systems that monitor especially the activity of elderly people have not a large presence in homes for the elderly. This is especially needed,

---

J.-E. Navarro-B. was with the GFaI, and is now with moovel GmbH.

© Springer International Publishing Switzerland 2015
O. Pichardo Lagunas et al. (Eds.): MICAI 2015, Part II, LNAI 9414, pp. 297–309, 2015.
DOI: 10.1007/978-3-319-27101-9_22

given that the percentage of elderly people in the world population increases every year. For example, the World Health Organization (WHO) reported in 2010 that the percentage of population over 65 years old was estimated to be 8 % and forecasts an increase in this percentage to 11 % in 2025 and to 16 % in 2050 [3]. This occurs given the improvements in life expectancy over the last years. Moreover, one of the most important situations where it is important to monitor activities of old people is when they suffer from dementia. In Germany, for example, around 1.4 Million people over the age of 65 are currently suffering from the consequences of dementia, with approximately 200,000 people developing the disorder each year [4].

Different type of events and situations are important to monitor for the well-being of senior citizens, especially those suffering of dementia. Some of the most important events is to register abnormal movements like reporting the fall of a senior citizen. Also important it is to track the daily vital signs to predict risk of myocardial infarction. Furthermore, it is also important to assess enough movement during sleep to avoid the appearance of pressure bedsores (decubitus ulcers). Bedsores are very frequent and have a long-term stage. According to the Medical Commission of the SHI Association (MDS - Medizinischer Dienst des Spitzenverbandes Bund der Krankenkassen e.V.) bedsores are present in 5–10 % of patients in hospitals, 30 % of patients in geriatric clinics and residents of nursing homes, as well as, 20 % of patients in home care [5]. The prevention and therapy of pressure sores is usually done by regularly changing the body position of the patient. For immobile patients that stay most of the time on their beds, the process of changing the body position is done mainly by the nurses and represents usually a major challenge [6]. Moreover, not only is the state of the physical body important to monitor but also the emotional and mental state. However, it is not practical to assess the mental state of a person suffering with dementia. Recently, it has been determined by means of clinical trials and psychological tests that parameters like reaction-time and form-recognition are the most relevant parameters to determine the mental state of a patient with dementia [7, 10]. For many of these situations and potential problems that can arise during the daily life activities, there are different type of sensors that can be used together with computer systems to assist senior citizens to trigger for example an alarm signal in case of an emergency.

This paper presents the methods and preliminary results of an assistant system developed to track the information of sensors (bed-post sensors, fall sensor and heart beat sensor) positioned near patients with dementia. The proposed server/client network architecture reduces the flow of data information from the sensors providing also an appropriate management of the information [8]. An important component of our assistant system is a serious games jump-and-run computer program developed to track the reaction time of patients with dementia to analyze the current mental state of the patients. To our knowledge there exists no computer system like ours that focuses on assisting patients with dementia.

This paper is organized as follows. Section 2 presents the monitor assistant system, information infrastructure and the sensors used to assist patients with dementia. Section 3 presents the bed-posts sensor system for detecting unhealthy poor movement while lying in bed which can cause bedsores (decubitus). Section 4 presents our system for automated analysis of the current mental state of patients with dementia by means of jump-and-run serious computer games. And finally, in Sect. 5 we present our conclusions and further work.

2 Monitor Assistant System

2.1 Goals

The assistant system conducts the analysis and interpretation of raw data received from the sensors, it also manages and visualizes this processed data to trigger alarm signals when needed. Table 1 presents a summary of the different practical problems and sensor solutions that the monitor assistant system offers for patients with dementia.

Our monitor assistant system manages information from wearable sensors for fall detection and heart rate measurement, as well as information from bed-post sensors and results from serious computer games. Figure 1 shows schematically the system design and basic architecture of the system. For this purpose, the system offers a software component to receive the raw sensor data (patient-client), a component to analyze the data (server) and two components to visualize the information (browser application for data and GUI application for the visualization of patient events).

2.2 Methods

The assistant system is composed of the following component modules: patient-client, server, data and event browsers, and the associated database.

The patient-client is the interface between the wireless wearable sensors (fall and heart beat sensors), as well as the bed-post sensors. The patient-client consists of a gateway radio receiver for data-telegrams coming from sensors for fall-detection and bed-posts and a sender of information to the server via TCP/IP. The fall of a person can be detected by means of integrating together an accelerometer sensor and a position sensor. The heart rate can be measured using a finger-placed pulse oximeter [1]. The bed-post sensors consist of pressure sensors that track changes in the position of a person lying on the bed.

Table 1. Summary of the different practical problems and technical solutions our system offers

Practical problem	Technical offers
Fall: Ensuring promptly assistance to reduce danger of subsequent damages	Interface for communication with fall-sensors based on both an accelerometer sensor and a position sensor
Decubitus ulcers: To prevent the appearance of bedsores and also to assist nursing staff to avoid unnecessary turn overs of the patient in bed	Interface for communication with pressure sensors placed under on the four bed-posts of the bed to track changes in the position of a person lying on the bed. Evaluation of the raw data from the sensors to determine the risk for bedsores
Myocardial infarction: Ensuring promptly assistance to save the life of the patient	Interface for communication with devices for measuring the heart rate of the patient

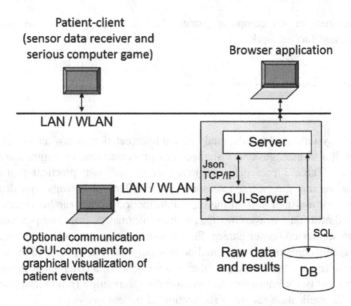

Fig. 1. Basic architecture of the system.

The data browser is a graphical user interface for nursing personal for the visualization of the sensor data and alarm signal events. The data browser provides also functionality for the acknowledgement of events and confirmation of having assisted the patient. Figure 2 shows the browser application AMENAMIN, which is used for managing the events and also for registering new patients and to assign sensors to patients. AMENAMIN is the abbreviation in German for the project "Ambient Energy und Ambient Intelligence für hilfsbedürftige Senioren" which translated to English reads "Ambient Energy and Ambient Intelligence for senior citizens with special needs" [8]. The browser application is also used by nurses or by medical doctors to analyze the processed data from the bed-post sensors to assess healthy enough movement of the patient while lying in bed. The data browser application is also used by medical doctors to analyze the results of the serious games computer game for the analysis of the mental state of the patient, this is discussed more in detail in Sect. 4.

Finally, the server is used for transferring and saving raw sensor data and processed sensor data for further analysis. The database is a component for saving data from the sensors and for loading saved data to the browser application for managing events by the nursing staff and for further analysis by the medical doctors.

2.3   Preliminary Results

The absolute difference between pressure measurements on the bedpost is tracked over time, processed and analyzed to answer the following question: Has the patient moved, turned around, waked-up or laid down? The main goal of this component is to give the nursing staff a clear overview of the last time the patient has successfully changed

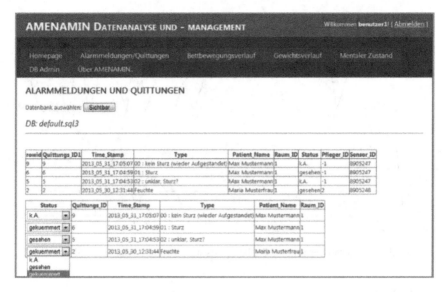

Fig. 2. Browser application (in German) to be used by nursing staff and medical doctors for: managing life-threatening events (Alarmmeldungen/Quittungen), sensor data analysis (Bettbewegungsverlauf) and current mental state of the patients (Mentaler Zustand)

position while lying in bed. The component also informs the nursing staff which beds are empty and which beds are occupied. Thus, the nursing staff is informed of the status of skin-health of the patients, knowing at any time when, where and who needs some help to be turned over in order to avoid the development of bedsores.

The infrastructure of the whole system gives the possibility to include other type of wearable sensors, for example humidity sensors, to determine if the patient has not managed to go in time to the bathroom and has become wet, this is especially helpful for patients with incontinence problems. Other type of wearables sensors that can be included in the system are discussed in our conclusions in Sect. 5.

3 Bed-Posts Sensor System

3.1 Goals

In this project, one of the goals was to develop a method to prevent and help the treatment of decubitus ulcers (also known as bedsores) [5]. The goal of the system is to turn on an alarm signal to inform the nursing staff when there has not been enough healthy movement of the patient after lying some time in bed. For this, the system tracks turns of the patient in bed as well as getting in and out of bed. This is done with help of not invasive pressure sensors placed on the bottom of each bed-posts. In this manner, the privacy of the patient remains unaffected. The pressure sensor can be energy self-sufficient sensors leading to a cheap daily indirect analysis of the sensor data.

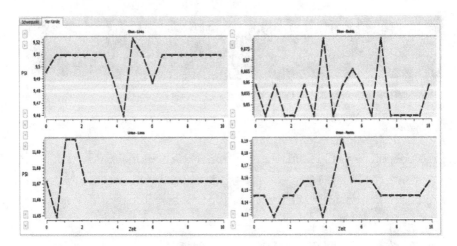

Fig. 3. Raw data over time of the bed-posts air pressure sensors (in PSI units).

3.2   Methods

The air pressure sensors placed under the bed-posts send every half second a data-telegram with the given pressure measurement on each bed-post. The difference over time of the pressure measurements on each bed-post has been used to detect turn overs and movement in bed. More in detail, the raw data from the pressure sensors was processed to track the differences over time of the center of mass of the weight (pressure) on the bed, see Fig. 3. Note that other type of pressure sensors can also be used for this task. The following algorithm was implemented to determine the different movements of a patient while lying on a bed. The first step is to determine the changes over time of the center of mass. For this, the center of mass of the bed is computed from the raw sensor data as shown in Eq. 1; where i represent each of the pressure measurements in each bed-post (i goes from 1 to 4, for four bed-posts); x and y are the corresponding coordinates of the pressure sensors (bed-posts); and M represents the sum over all measured masses $\sum m_i$, respectively.

$$\bar{x} = \frac{\sum_{i=1}^{4} m_i x_i}{M}; \bar{y} = \frac{\sum_{i=1}^{4} m_i y_i}{M} \tag{1}$$

A two-dimensional coordinate system is projected onto the bed, where the horizontal coordinate corresponds to lateral displacements and the vertical coordinate corresponds to elongated displacements on the bed. In order to detect turn overs on the bed, the forward-differences of two subsequent in time center of mass measurements are computed. For this, a time lag Δt should be fixed (typically from one second for very fast patients to ten seconds for very slow patients). Note that the forward differences should be computed separately for the vertical (y-axis) $\Delta \bar{y}$ and the horizontal (x-axis) $\Delta \bar{x}$ as it is shown in Eq. 2.

$$\Delta \bar{x} = \bar{x}(t + \Delta t) - \bar{x}(t); \Delta \bar{y} = \bar{y}(t + \Delta t) - \bar{y}(t) \qquad (2)$$

Given that the horizontal component has a much larger influence in the detection of turn overs than the vertical component, the horizontal and vertical components of the center of mass are weighted differently for the analysis of turn overs on the bed. For this, the time-weighted Euclidean forward difference of the center of mass (FWDM) is computed as shown in Eq. 3. [9].

$$FWDM = \sqrt{w \cdot \Delta \bar{x}^2 + (1 - w) \cdot \Delta \bar{y}^2} \qquad (3)$$

To detect if a patient has turned over his position on the bed, the FWDM is used together with a threshold value, which has been previously calibrated for different type of patients. If the FWDM is larger than this threshold then this means that the patient has changed the position on the bed. To detect if a patient is getting in or out of the bed, the weight of the patient is compared with the weight on the bed. For this, the weight of the patient has to be registered in the system together with the weight of the empty bed assigned to this patient. Finally, a threshold value has to be calibrated for both cases when the bed is empty and when the bed is occupied.

3.3   Preliminary Results

Figure 4 shows both the software for detection of movement on the bed as well as the visualization of alarm signals and events on a graphical user interface which was

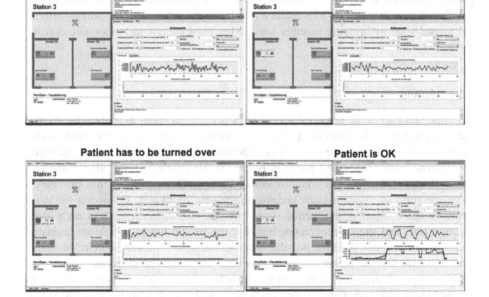

Fig. 4. Analysis of the bed-post pressure sensor measurements to detect bed movements.

especially designed for this hospital by the company Akktor GmbH. The communication between the software for detection of movement and the visualization component was done by means of TCP/IP messages. The system was successfully used to detect turn overs on the bed as well as when patients were getting in and out of the bed. The feedback obtained with this system was positive, and it was pointed out by medical doctors that the detection of other sleep related movement disorders could be also of interest. This means, however, that computer experiments should be done in a sleep laboratory and this also means that the simple threshold-based method presented in Sect. 3.2 may no longer adequately detect more complex movements. For this, more complex methods could be implemented, for example methods based on computer-based learning approaches for movement pattern recognition together with extra external Knowledge provided from an expert system.

4 Automated Analysis of the Current Mental State

4.1 Goals

The goal of this system component is to automatically analyze the mental state of patients with dementia by means of serious computer games. According to experts, the following two parameters are the most important parameters to determine the current mental state of a patient with dementia: reaction time and shape recognition. One of the goals of this project was to integrate these two parameters into a jump-and-run serious computer game. A second important criteria to determine the current mental state of a patient with dementia is the comparison between current and retrospective historical data. According to experts, tracking the chronological trend of the results of subsequent games can help to determine the current mental state of patients with dementia [7, 10]. Another important goal is to implement a rule-based system to automatically determine the mental state by bringing together knowledge from experts and automatic classification algorithms.

4.2 Methods

An important part of the project AMENAMIN is the component to analyze the mental state of patients with dementia. For this, a serious computer game has been implemented of the type jump-and-run. The specifications for the computer game were given by medical doctors from the Charité in Berlin (St. Hedwig's Hospital, Berlin Institute of Psychiatry, Charité – Universitätsmedizin Berlin). This type of games provides a large spectrum of different tasks keeping the patient motivated. Following the main goals for the analysis of the mental state, there are two different tasks in each level, reaction time and shape recognition. Initially, the patient has to choose an animated character, represented by three possible shapes: triangular, squared and circled shape. The first task for the patient is to manage that the animated character jumps over different type of obstacles: stones, bushes or holes. As the obstacle is approaching to the animated character there is besides a graphical signal, also an acoustic signal indicating to promptly press the jumping pushbutton. If the patient has jumped over the

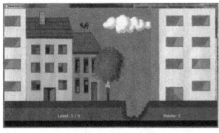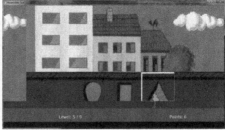

Fig. 5. Jump-and-run serious computer game: (left) first task, to jump over the obstacles, (right) second task, to choose the appropriate door according to the shape of the animated character.

obstacle successfully there is a positive feedback sound which motivates and assists the patient in the interaction with the serious computer game, see Fig. 5 (left).

The following parameters are considered the most relevant ones influencing the course of the computer game, defining the difficulty of each level: the number of obstacles in each level, the size of the obstacle and the time between two obstacles.

Both, the success ratio and the reaction times for jumping over obstacles provides basic information to analyze the current metal state of the patient. Furthermore, at the end of each level there is an extra task for the patient, which consists in choosing one door from three possible shapes: triangular, squared, or circled shape. The task is completed successfully if the shape of the door chosen by pressing a pushbutton corresponds to the shape of the animated character chosen by the patient in the beginning of the game, see Fig. 5 (right).

Once the game has finished, the results of the game are sent to the server and saved for further analysis, which is then performed afterwards by experts together with graphical software tools for statistical analysis of the time series. The main goal is to facilitate the analysis, providing software tools for an automatic classification of the mental state of a patient. For this, different algorithms for clustering and classification of the data could be implemented. This is further discussed in our conclusion in Sect. 5.

4.3 Preliminary Results

Firstly, the patients used an ergonomic medically certified interaction device push button from the company Spectronics (see Fig. 6 top-left) for the interaction with the computer game. The following interaction devices were also tested. An interaction ball developed by our project partner alpha-board GmbH, see Fig. 6 (left-middle), which consists on a self-sufficient interaction ball with a large number of pushbuttons energized with four solar cells and protected by an impermeable transparent cover. Figure 6 (left-bottom) shows a self-sufficient miniaturized switch module from the company EnOcean GmbH, which is powered by a built-in electro-dynamic power generator.

Some illustrative results for a series of computer games are shown in Fig. 6 (right). Initially, a medium level of difficulty was assigned (difficulty values range is from 1 to 10, where 1 is the lowest and 10 the highest level of difficulty, resp.). Figure 6

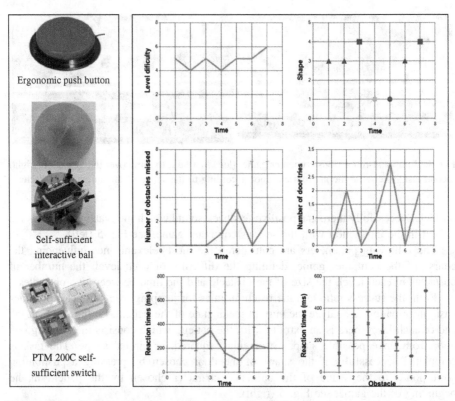

Fig. 6. (left) Different type of interaction devices: (top-left) ergonomic push button from the company Spectronics, (middle-left) self-sufficient interactive ball from the company and project partner alpha-board GmbH, and (bottom-left) PTM 200C self-sufficient switch module from the company EnOcean GmbH. (right) Results of the jump-and-run serious computer game used for analyzing the mental state of patients with dementia: (top-right) the difficulty level reached at the end of each game (time) and the animated character shape chosen by the patient in each game, (middle-right) the number of obstacles that the patient missed to jump over and the number of tries to match the door shape to the shape of the animated character at the end of each game, and (bottom-right) the mean and standard deviation of the reaction times in milliseconds for jumping over obstacles. The plot on the left shows the results for each level, whereas the plot on the right shows the results for each obstacle, in this case seven obstacles at each level.

(top-right) shows the level reached over time (games) and the shape of the animated character chosen by the patient. Moreover, Fig. 6 (middle-right) shows the number of obstacles successfully jumped over by the patient, as well as, the number of times needed to find the correct shape of the door matching the shape of the animated character. It can be seen that as the difficulty of the level increased over time, also the number of obstacles missed increased together with the number of tries needed to match the doors at the end of the game. Finally, Fig. 6 (bottom-right) shows the course of the reaction times for jumping over obstacles as well as the mean reaction times at the position of the obstacles in the game. It can be seen that the reaction times improve over time, meaning that the reaction is much faster every time, as the patient gets trained in the game. It can be seen that in the beginning there is a large standard deviation for the reaction times for jumping over obstacles. This probably indicates that the patient is not very prepared to the task, however over time the patients get used to the game and both the mean and the standard deviation of the reaction times decrease. Interestingly, note that the last obstacle has a very large mean reaction time, probably because the patient got distracted by the fact that a different task is approaching, or maybe the patient got bored from the task of jumping over obstacles only.

5   Conclusions

All sensors, analysis, procedures and component systems presented in this paper are state of the art and they are intended to assist particularly patients with dementia. To our knowledge there exists no assistant system like the one presented in this paper. Note also that our system is also in line with wearable sensor systems for health care, meaning that they can be also used by senior citizens not necessarily suffering problems of dementia. In some cases, we may need to increase the complexity of the procedures, for example in the case of the serious computer games, a simple jump-and-run computer game can be boring after playing two or three games the same scenario with the same tasks. The methods presented in this paper and their implementation were tested first within a facility in the psychiatric clinic of the Charité in the hospital St. Hedwig in Berlin. Some of the components of our system were also installed and tested in the show house AMINA in the Sunpark of the Evangelisches Johannesstift [11, p. 47]. Privacy and confidentiality of the data was assured by the architecture of our system and the encrypted protocols used for the wireless transmission of sensor data.

In Sect. 2.3 it was mentioned that the infrastructure of the whole system gives the possibility to include other type of sensors, for example humidity sensors for patients with incontinence problems. Other type of wearable sensors and devices that can be included in the monitoring systems include sensors for tracking physical activity to count the daily steps, body weight scales, and the like. The flexibility and versatility of the system proposed in this paper allows to include also sensors for home and building automation. For example, sensors to track when someone opens or closes a window or door; sensors to keep rooms at a given desired temperature; and sensors for turning lights on/off depending on the presence of persons in the rooms or corridors. All these type of sensors can be included in our system and the corresponding data can be also visualized in our browser application for turning on/off alarm signals, as well as, for further data processing and analysis. Section 3.2 presents a method for bed movement detection based on differences in center of mass over time. The AI community can provide more elaborated approaches, for example to train a neural network with the weight changes to predict the type and amount of movement on the bed. For this, the input data to the neural networks could variate from raw sensor data, to forward weighted differences (Eq. 2) for different Δt. This means, however, that different movements should be gathered and labelled for different type of patients, which could be a laborious task, given the variety of patient profiles and type of movements. Section 4.2 presented the properties of the jump-and-run serious computer game implemented in our system. Data resulting from the serious computer games together with expert knowledge and labelling of the data, could be used to train some algorithms for an automatic classification of the mental state of a patient. Moreover, the serious computer game presented in this paper could be also used to train the reaction and shape recognition of the patients towards a healthier mental state. This can be done, by means of implementing an automated system which takes into account the results of each patient and the set-up parameter values. If the patient performs well, the difficulty could be automatically adapted according to the performance of the patient. For this, different approaches could be consider, from reinforcement learning to rule-based systems.

Acknowledgements. We gratefully acknowledge support from the German Federal Ministry for Economic Affairs and Energy (Bundesminesterium für Wirtschaft und Energie) for financial supporting the ZIM-KF project AMENAMIN - ambient energy and ambient intelligence for senior citizens in need of assistance [8]. We thank Dr. H.-M. Voigt and Dr. W. Harder, both former heads of the department of Adaptive Modelling and Pattern Recognition at the GFaI, for their leadership, support and contribution throughout the project AMENAMIN. We thank also Prof. J. Gallinat, (former professor of the Charité, Universitätsmedizin Berlin) for his contribution to the project AMENAMIN. We also thank our partners involved in the AMENAMIN project: the Charité Universitätsmedizin Berlin, EnOcean GmbH, alpha-board GmbH, SHK Spree Hybrid &Kommuniationstechnik GmbH and SMI GmbH. Finally, special thanks to Prof. Friedrich Porsdorf (Kunsthochschule Berlin) for the graphical design of the serious computer game.

References

1. Pantelopoulos, A., Bourbakis, N.G.: A survey on wearable sensor-based systems for health monitoring and prognosis. IEEE Trans. Syst. Man Cybern. Part C Appl. Rev. **40**(1), 1–12 (2010)
2. Rashidi, P., Mihailidis, A.: A survey on ambient assisted living tools for older adults. IEEE J. Biomed. Health Inform. **17**(3), 579–590 (2013)
3. United Nations: World Population Prospects: The 2010 Revision. http://esa.un.org/unpd/wpp
4. Bundesministerium für Familie, Senioren, Frauen und Jugend; Welt-Alzheimertag: Bundesfamilienministerium startet weitere Lokale Allianzen für Menschen mit Demenz. http://www.bmfsfj.de/BMFSFJ/Presse/pressemitteilungen,did=200434.html. Accessed 20 Sep 2013
5. Anders, J., Heinemann, A., Leffmann, C., Leutenegger, M., Pröfener, F., von Renteln-Kruse, W.: Dekubitalgeschwüre-Pathophysiologie und Primärprävention. Dtsch Arztebl Int **107** (21), 371–382 (2010). doi:10.3238/arztebl.2010.0371
6. Rothgang, H., Müller, R., Unger, R., Weiß, C., Wolter, A.: BARMER GEK Pflegereport (2012)
7. Basak, C., Boot, W.R., Voss, M.W., Kramer, A.F.: Can training in a real-time strategy video game attenuate cognitive decline in older adults? Psychol. Aging **23**(4), 765 (2008)
8. Iwainsky, A.: AMENAMIN: Ein Verbundprojekt im Grenzbereich von AAL und Micro Energy Harvesting. GFaI-Informationen **3**, 3–4 (2012)
9. Maurer, R., Qi, R., Raghavan, V.: A linear algorithm for computing exact euclidean distance transforms of binary images in arbitrary dimensions. IEEE Trans. Pattern Anal. Mach. Intell. **25**, 265–270

10. Kühn, S., Gleich, T., Lorenz, R., Lindenberger, U., Gallinat, J.: Playing Super Mario induces structural brain plasticity: grey matter changes resulting from training with a commercial video game. Mol. Psychiatry **19**, 265–271 (2014)
11. Erbstößer, A.-C.: Smart Home Berlin – von der Komfortzone zum Gesundheitsstandort. Technologiestiftung Berlin, Report (2015)

Analysis of Neurosurgery Data
Using Statistical and Data Mining Methods

Petr Berka[1,2]([✉]), Josef Jablonský[1], Luboš Marek[1], and Michal Vrabec[1]

[1] University of Economics, W. Churchill Sq. 4, Prague, Czech Republic
{berka,jablon,marek,vrabec}@vse.cz
[2] University of Finance and Administration, Estonska 500, Prague, Czech Republic

Abstract. The data concerning the outcomes of surgical clipping and endovascular treatment in acute aneurysmal subarachnoid hemorrhage (SAH) patients have been analyzed to reveal relations between subjective neuropsychological assessments, measurable characteristics of the patient and the disease, and the type of treatment the patient had undergone one year before. We build upon results of previous analyses where have been found that the differences in neuropsychological assessment of the patients treated by either coiling or clipping was small and slightly in favor of surgical group. Using this data, we compare the "classical" statistical and data mining approach. While statistics offers techniques based on contingency tables, where the compared variables have to be manually selected, data mining methods like association rules, decision rules or decision trees offer the possibility to generate and evaluate a number of more complex hypotheses about the hidden relationships. We used SAS JMP to perform the statistical analysis and LISp-Miner system for the data mining experiments.

1 Introduction

A subarachnoid hemorrhage (SAH) is bleeding into the subarachnoid space, the area between the arachnoid membrane and the pia mater surrounding the brain. This may occur spontaneously, usually from a ruptured cerebral aneurysm, or may result from head injury. In most Western societies rupture of an intracranial aneurysm causing SAH occurs with a frequency of 5-11/100 000/ year. Improvement in SAH management such as superior and fast diagnostics, microscope introduction, clip sophistication, triple H therapy, etc. has led to morbidity/mortality decrease as assessed by neurological scales. Two treatment options are possible for these patients: surgical clipping or coil embolization. Clipping is a surgical procedure where under general anesthesia an opening is made in the skull. A tiny clip is then placed across the neck of the aneurysm to stop or prevent an aneurysm from bleeding. Coil embolization is less invasive treatment than surgery. In embolization procedures, physicians place small, soft metal coils within the aneurysm, where it helps block the flow of blood and prevents rupture of the aneurysm.

© Springer International Publishing Switzerland 2015
O. Pichardo Lagunas et al. (Eds.): MICAI 2015, Part II, LNAI 9414, pp. 310–321, 2015.
DOI: 10.1007/978-3-319-27101-9_23

The aim of this work is to compare the outcomes of surgical clipping and endovascular treatment in acute (< 72 hours) aneurysmal subarachnoid hemorrhage (SAH) one year after. Using this data, we compare the "classical" statistical and data mining approach. We build upon results of previous analyses [8] but use more advanced algorithms.

The rest of the paper is organized as follows. Section 2 discusses the relationship betwen statistical data analysis and data mining, Sect. 3 describes the used data, Sect. 4 shows the used statistical method, Sect. 5 presents the used data mining method, Sect. 6 shows some related work and Sect. 7 concludes the paper.

2 Statistics, Machine Learning and Data Mining

Statistics, machine learning and data mining are three disciplines that all deal with data analysis, i.e. with the process of inspecting, cleaning, transforming, and modeling data with the goal of highlighting useful information, suggesting conclusions, and supporting decision making. The conceptual difference between statistics on one side and machine learning and data mining on the other side is the fact that statistical analysis is hypothesis driven and model oriented while machine learning and data mining are data driven and algorithm oriented [6]. When doing statistical data analysis we have to start by formulating one or more hypotheses about a model, then collect the data (in a controlled way that preserves the expected theoretical characteristics of the data), then perform the analysis, and then interpret the results. Statisticians also usually analyze small volumes of numerical data with known statistical properties (they usually expect data to be drawn from a known distribution and to be stationary). When doing data mining, we are faced with huge heterogeneous amounts of data with a lot of missings and inconsistencies that may contain some interesting novel knowledge. This data is usually collected for completely different reasons than to provide representative training set for machine learning algorithms. We thus know nothing about the underlying distribution, about its properties (such as stationarity) and we very often do not know what models (dependencies) can be hidden in the data or what are the relevant characteristics (attributes) that will help us to uncover these models. We usually start by formulating a possible task (rather than a hypothesis), where some tasks (such as classification or prediction) are more related to statistical data analysis, while others (such as pattern discovery) are not. Then we try to find a relevant subset of available data to solve the task, then "play" with various algorithms (machine learning or statistical) and then interpret the results. Nevertheless, there is a lot of common ground in both areas and machine learning and statistics do converge in ideas and procedures. For example, algorithms for building decision trees from data were concurrently proposed in both the statistical community (CART by Breiman et al. [3]) and machine learning community (ID3 and C4.5 by Quinlan [9]), neural networks are very close to regression methods, nearest neighbor methods are used for classification in both areas, and purely statistical methods such as cross-validation or χ^2 test have been incorporated into many machine learning algorithms.

3   Used Data

During the study period total of 152 patients harboring cerebral aneurysm were treated by either surgical or interventional means. Of these 48 were able to undergo also psychological assessment one year later. 25 patients were treated by surgical clipping (9 men and 16 women), 23 patients were managed by coil embolization (7 men and 16 women). Remaining patients either died, refused to enter the study, were lost for 1-year follow-up or had neurological deficit preventing the neuropsychological evaluation.

The data collected for these patients at the time of treatment contain the basic socio-demographic info about the patients (age, sex), basic information about the findings (localization of aneurysma, their number and size), basic info about the surgery (type of treatment, urgency, complications, outcome). Characteristics of some of these attributes are shown in Table 1. The follow up assessment one year after SAH treatment include Trail Making test (A+B), Auditory Verbal Learning test, Wechsler Adult Intelligence Scale (WAIS-III), Subjective Memory Scale, SQUALA (Subjective Quality of Life Questionnaire), structured interview focused on subjective evaluation of health status, Beck Depression Inventory (BDI-II) and Temperament and Character Inventory.

4   Statistical Approach

We used descriptive statistics and decision trees to perform statistical analysis of the data. As stated earlier, decision trees are also widely used as machine learning and data mining methods. From the statistical point-of-view decision trees are a powerful form of multiple variable analysis. They provide unique capabilities to supplement, complement, and substitute for traditional statistical forms of analysis such as multiple linear regression.

Table 1. Attribute characteristics

Attribute	Clip	Coil
average Age (years)	41.48	45.95
Male/female	9/16	7/16
average Aneurysm size category	1.96	2.34
Ruptured/unruptured	9/16	11/12
Localization ACOM	5	6
Localization M1_2	12	0
Localization PCOM	4	2
Localization ICA	23	12

4.1 CART and Its Application

In our experiments, we used the CART decision tree algorithm [3]. CART creates a binary tree using Gini index as splitting criterion for categorical target and sum of squares for numeric target. We used trees to find criteria that mainly contribute to differentiation between coil (value "T" in a node) and clip (value "F" in a node) treatment. So we used decision trees for concept description and not for classification and thus we do not report the classification accuracies of the trees. As can be seen in Fig. 1, the key criterion is M1_2 localization followed by the size of aneurysma (SIZE) and the number of aneurysma (NO_ANEU). When omitting the M1_2 localization, ICA localization became the key criterion followed by urgency of the surgery (SURGERY), days from bleeding (INT_SAH_), sex, number of aneuryasma and age (AGE_PRI_) - see Fig. 2.

5   Data Mining Approach

We used association rules mining as an data mining method in our study. Instead of using "standard" association rules as presented by Agrawal [1], we are using association rules based on the GUHA method [5]. The statistical counterpart would be analysis of contingency tables, where each contingency table need to be created manually.

5.1   LISp-Miner System

LISp-Miner consists of several procedures that mine for different types of associations between conjunctions of literals [10, 12]. In our study, we will focus on two of them.

4 ft-Miner. The 4 ft-Miner procedure mines for association rules of the form

$$\phi \approx \psi \tag{1}$$

and for conditional association rules of the form

$$\phi \approx \psi/\gamma \tag{2}$$

where ϕ (antecedent), ψ (succedent) and γ, (condition) are conjunctions of literals and symbol $\approx$ denotes the relation between ϕ and ψ on the subset of examples, that satisfy the condition γ. If the condition is empty then the procedure analyzes the whole data table. The relation $\approx$ is defined using frequencies a, b, c, and d from a corresponding four-fold contingency table. Here a denotes the number of examples, that are covered both by ϕ and ψ, b denotes the number of examples, that are covered by ϕ but not covered by ψ, c denotes the number of examples, that are covered by ψ but not covered by ϕ and d denotes the number of examples that are covered neither by ϕ, nor by ψ. Table 2 gives some examples of different types of relations.

Literals are in the form $A(coef)$ or $\neg A(coef)$. In 4FT-Miner, $coef$, the list of possible values of an attribute A can be:

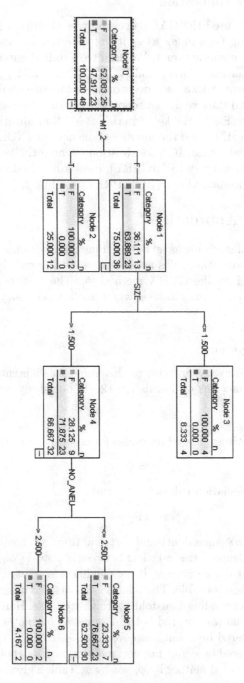

Fig. 1. Tree no 1.

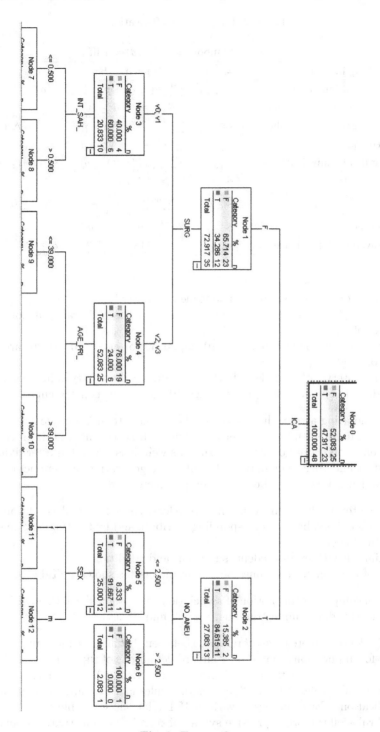

Fig. 2. Tree no 2.

Table 2. Examples of 4 ft-relations

Name	Symbol	$\approx (a,b,c,d) = 1$ iff
Founded implication	$\Rightarrow_{p,B}$	$\frac{a}{a+b} \geq p \wedge a \geq B$
Lower critical implication	$\Rightarrow^!_{p,\alpha,B}$	$\sum_{i=a}^{r} \binom{r}{i} p^i (1-p)^{r-i} \leq \alpha \wedge a \geq B$
Founded double implication	$\Leftrightarrow_{p,B}$	$\frac{a}{a+b+c} \geq p \wedge a \geq B$
Lower critical double implication	$\Leftrightarrow^!_{p,\alpha,B}$	$\sum_{i=a}^{n-d} \binom{n-d}{i} p^i (1-p)^{n-d-i} \leq \alpha \wedge a \geq B$
Founded equivalence	$\equiv_{p,B}$	$\frac{a+d}{a+b+c+d} \geq p \wedge a \geq B$
Lower critical equivalence	$\equiv^!_{p,\alpha,B}$	$\sum_{i=a+d}^{n} \binom{n}{i} p^i (1-p)^{n-i} \leq \alpha \wedge a \geq B$
Simple deviation	$\sim_{\delta,B}$	$\frac{ad}{bc} > e^\delta \wedge a \geq B$
Fisher	$\approx_{\alpha,B}$	$\sum_{i=a}^{\min(r,k)} \frac{\binom{k}{i}\binom{n-k}{r-i}}{\binom{r}{n}} \leq \alpha \wedge a \geq B$
χ^2 quantifier	$\sim^2_{\alpha,B}$	$\frac{(ad-bc)^2}{rkls} n \geq \chi^2_\alpha \wedge a \geq B$
Above average dependence	$\sim^+_{q,B}$	$\frac{a}{a+b} \geq (1+q)\frac{a+c}{a+b+c+d} \wedge a \geq B$

- one category, this is simply single value of an attribute A,
- subset of given length (e.g. city(London, Paris) is a literal that contains a subset of length 2),
- interval of given length (e.g. age(10–20, 20–30) or age(0–10, 10–20) are intervals of length 2),
- cut, i.e. interval of given length, that contains the boundary value (e.g. age(0–10, 10–20) is a cut of length 2 but age(10–20, 20–30) is not a cut).

When generating a rule, the system starts to generate an antecedent (as a conjunction of literals) and then generates all possible succedents to this antecedent. If the condition should occur in the rules as well, it is generated after fixing the antecedent and succedent part of the rule. The generating of conjunctions proceeds in depth-first way. The user given parameters are:

- list of literals that can occur in antecedent, succedent and condition; each literal is defined by the corresponding attribute and by the type and maximal length of coef,
- maximal length of antecedent, succedent and condition,
- type of relation $\approx$ and values of its parameters (as shown in Table 2).

When comparing this notion of association rules (we will call them 4FT rules) with the "standard" understanding, we will find, that:

- 4FT rules offer more types of relations between Ant and Suc; we can search not only for implications (based on standard definitions of support and confidence of a rule), but also for equivalences or statistically based relations. In the sense of 4FT rules "classical" association rules can be considered as founded implications (for examples of various 4FT relations see Table 2).
- 4FT rules offer more expressive syntax of ϕ and ψ; ϕ and ψ are conjunctions of literals (i.e. expressions in the form $A(coef)$ or $\neg A(coef)$, where A is an

attribute and *coef* is a subset of possible values), not only of attribute-value pairs (which are literals as well). If e.g. the analysed data contain attribute A with values a, b, c, attribute B with values x, y, z, and attribute C with values k, l, m, n, then a 4 ft-rule can be e.g.

$$A(b) \wedge B(x \vee y) \Rightarrow_{p,B} \neg C(k)$$

- a 4FT rule consists not only of antecedent ϕ and succedent ψ but can contain also a condition γ; this condition is generated during the rule learning process as well.

SD4FT-Miner. The SD4FT-Miner procedure mines for patterns of the form

$$\phi \approx \psi/(\alpha, \beta, \gamma) \tag{3}$$

A true SD4FT pattern refers to a situation when an 4FT association rule $\phi \approx \psi$ found for a subset of the analyzed data defined by conjunction of literals α differs (according to the parameters of relation $\approx$) from the (same) association rule found for a subset of the analyzed data defined by conjunction of literals β. Again, the analyzed data may or may not be restricted by a condition γ.

There is a number of SD4FT relations, that measure the difference between the two 4FT association rules in question. These measures are defined for two contingency tables, i.e. for the values a, b, c, d (the values for one rule) and a', b', c', d' (the values for the other rule). An example of such a measure that measures the difference between confidences of two rules and the condition that must be fulfilled is shown in Eq. 4.

$$\left| \frac{a'}{a' + b'} - \frac{a}{a + b} \right| \geq p. \tag{4}$$

This condition means that the absolute value of the difference of confidence of association rule $\varphi \approx \psi$ computed for examples that satisfy $\alpha \wedge \gamma$ and the confidence of this association rule computed for examples that satisfy $\beta \wedge \gamma$ is at least p.

5.2   Performed Analyzes

Using 4 ft-Miner and SD4FT-Miner procedures, we performed following three tasks:

1. Find 4FT rules, that relate up to three conditions of a patient before the treatment with the type of treatment (clip/coil).
   The input parameters were as follows:
   - ϕ: characteristics of the patient and of the aneurysma
   - ψ: type of treatment
   - $\approx$: founded implication (see Table 2) with $p = 0.75$ and *Base* $= 10\%$.

We found 162 4FT rules with support $a/(a + b + c + d)$ greater than 10 % and confidence $a/(a + b)$ greater than 0.75. These rules show, that the type of treatment (coil vs. clip) is determined mainly by the localization and by the urgency of the treatment (see Fig. 3).

2. Find 4FT rules, that relate the type of treatment (clip/coil) to the states of the patient (objective or subjective) one year after the surgery.

The input parameters were as follows:
  - ϕ: type of treatment
  - ψ: results of follow-up assessment of up to three characteristics (neuropsychological and personality ones)
  - $\approx$: founded implication (see Table 2) with $p = 0.75$ and $Base = 10$ %.

We found 162 4FT rules with support $a/(a + b + c + d)$ greater than 10 % and confidence $a/(a + b)$ greater than 0.75. The found rules show slightly but non-significantly better results for patients treated by surgical clipping (see Fig. 4).

3. Find SD4FT patterns between conditions of a patient before the treatment and the state of patient one year after the surgery, that show different characteristics with respect to the type of treatment (clip/coil).

The input parameters were as follows:
  - ϕ: one or no characteristic of the patient and of the aneurysma
  - ψ: results of follow-up assessment of up to three characteristics (neuropsychological and personality ones)
  - α: coil
  - β: clip
  - $\approx$: so called interestingness defined by the Eq. 4 with $p = 0.3$, $Base_1 = 10$ % and $Base_2 = 10$ %.

131 hypotheses that fulfill the given parameters have been found. The found patterns show that the subjective feeling of patients was often in favor of surgical clipping. See e.g. hypothesis no. 89, where 10 out of 17 patients treated by coiling suffered from health complications and problems with memory that the patients related to the treatment, while only 6 out of 24 patients treated by clipping had similar feelings (Fig. 5).

6   Related Work

The research presented in out paper is not the only example of using statistical and data mining analysis of data related to aneurysmal subarachnoid hemorrhage (SAH). Dumont, Rughani and Tranmer used artificial neural networks to predict the occurrence of symptomatic cerebral vasospasm after SAH. The resulting neural network, created for data about 91 patients was then compared with a multiple regression model [4]. De Toledo et al. analysed 441 SAH cases using different classification algorithms to generate decision trees and decision rules with the goal to distinguish between favourable and poor outcome. The authors argue in favor of these methods against less interpretable regression models [11]. Bisbal et al. report a development of several classifiers predicting whether a given

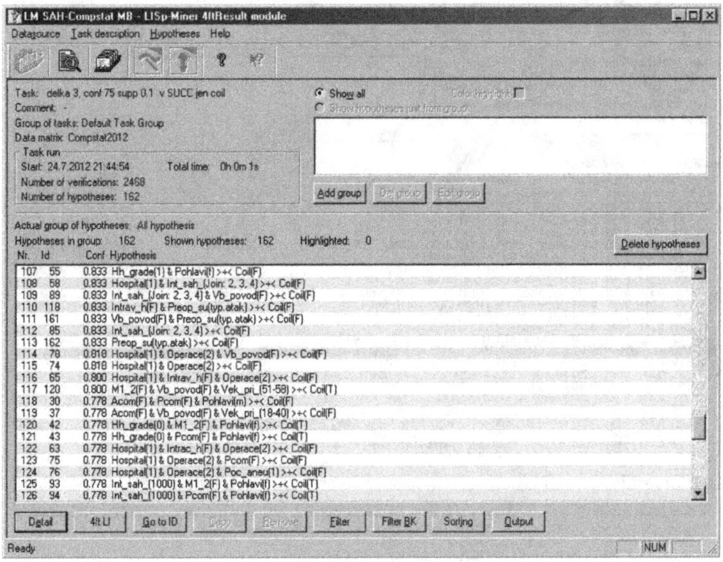

Fig. 3. 4FT Task no. 1

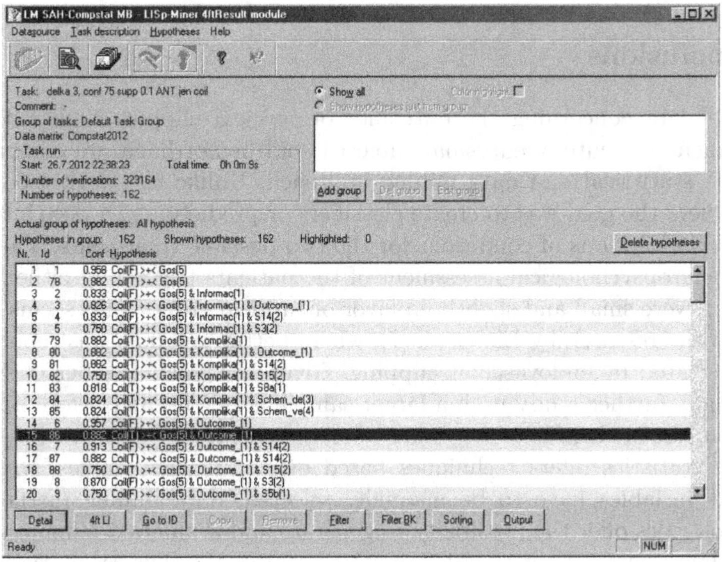

Fig. 4. 4FT Task no. 2

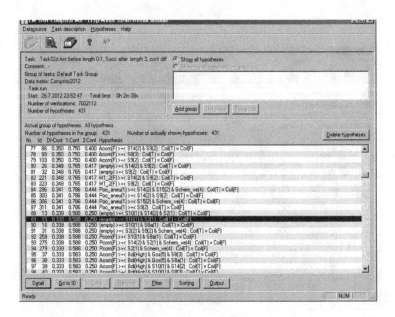

Fig. 5. SD4FT Task

clinical case is likely to rupture taking into account available information of the patient and characteristics of the aneurysm. Theused dataset included 157 cases with 294 features [2].

7   Conclusions

Using the data concerning the outcomes of surgical clipping and endovascular treatment in acute aneurysmal subarachnoid hemorrhage, we compare the "classical" statistical and data mining approach. Unlike the work reported in Sect. 6, where the goal was to create classifiers or predictors, we were interested in finding descriptions of conditions for the two possible treatments. The differences in neuropsychological assessment of the patients treated by either coiling or clipping were small and slightly in favor of surgical group. This seems to contradict to the research by Lin et al. [7], where better outcome was reported for patients treated by endovascular clipping. Given the small number of subjects in our study, further study with a larger sample size is needed before a reliable conclusion can be drawn.

While statistics offers techniques based on contingency tables, where the compared variables have to be manually selected, data mining methods like association rules offer the possibility to generate and evaluate a number of more complex hypotheses about the hidden relationships. We thus see statistical and data mining methods as complementary tools for analyzing the data. When comparing the results obtained by CART with the results obtained by LISp-Miner, we can see, that both methods have found the key factors like size of aneurysma or localization. But unlike the results obtained by decision trees that recursively split the feature space (and thus smaller and smaller number of examples is used to choose the splitting attribute), association rules are repeatedly created from the whole data, i.e. offer different viewpoints on the dependencies in data (and thus will find more relationships).

References

1. Agrawal, R., Imielinski, T., Swami, A.: Mining association rules between sets of items in large databases. In: SIGMOD Conference, pp. 207–216 (1993)
2. Bisbal, J., Engelbrecht, G., Villa-Uriol, M.-C., Frangi, A.F.: Prediction of cerebral aneurysm rupture using hemodynamic, morphologic and clinical features: a data mining approach. In: Hameurlain, A., Liddle, S.W., Schewe, K.-D., Zhou, X. (eds.) DEXA 2011, Part II. LNCS, vol. 6861, pp. 59–73. Springer, Heidelberg (2011)
3. Breiman, L., Friedman, J.H., Ohlsen, R.A., Stone, P.J.: Classification and Regression Trees. Wadsworth, Belmont (1984)
4. Dumont, T.M., Rughani, A.I., Tranmer, B.I.: Prediction of symptomatic cerebral vasospasm after aneurysmal subarachnoid hemorrhage with an artificial neural network. Neurosurgery **75**(1), 57–63 (2011)
5. Hájek, P., Havránek, T.: Mechanising Hypothesis Formation, Mathematical Foundations for a General Theory. Springer, Heidelberg (1978)
6. Hand, D.: Data mining: statistics and more? Am. Stat. **52**(2), 112–118 (1998)
7. Lin, N., Cahill, K.S., Frerichs, K.U., Friedlander, R.M., Claus, E.B.: Treatment of ruptured and unruptured cerebral aneurysms in the usa: a paradigm shift. J. NeuroIntervent Surgery **4**, 182–189 (2012)
8. Preiss, M., Beneš, V., Dragomirecká, E., Koblihová, J., Netuka, D., Kramář, F., Charvát, F., Klose, J., Vrabec, M.: Quality of life in patients treated with neurosurgical clipping versus endovascular coiling. In: Monduzzi (ed.) 12th European Congress of Neurosurgery. pp. 269–274 (2003)
9. Quinlan, J.R.: C4.5: Programs for Machine Learning. Morgan Kaufmann Publishers, San Francisco (1993)
10. Rauch, J.: Observational Calculi and Association Rules. Springer, Heidelberg (2013)
11. Toledo, P., Rios, P.M., Ledezma, A., Sanchis, A., Alen, J.F., Lagare, A.: Predicting the outcome of patients with subarachnoid hemorrhage using machine learning techniques. Am. Stat. **13**(5), 794–801 (2009)
12. Šimůnek, M.: Academic KDD project LISp-Miner. In: Abraham, A., Franke, K., Koppen, K. (eds.) 12th European Congress of Neurosurgery, pp. 263–272. Springer, Heidelberg (2003)

Image Processing and Computer Vision

Massively Parallel Cellular Matrix Model for Superpixel Adaptive Segmentation Map

Hongjian Wang$^{(\boxtimes)}$, Abdelkhalek Mansouri, Jean-Charles Créput, and Yassine Ruichek

IRTES-SeT, Université de Technologie de Belfort-Montbéliard, 90010 Belfort, France
hongjian.wang@utbm.fr

Abstract. We propose the concept of *superpixel adaptive segmentation map*, to produce a perceptually meaningful representation of rigid pixel image, with higher resolution of more superpixels on interesting regions according to the density distribution of desired attributes. The solution is based on the self-organizing map (SOM) algorithm, for the benefits of SOM's ability to generate a topological map according to a probability distribution and its potential to be a natural massive parallel algorithm. We also propose the concept of parallel cellular matrix which partitions the Euclidean plane defined by input image into an appropriate number of uniform cell units. Each cell is responsible of a certain part of the data and the cluster center network, and carries out massively parallel spiral searches based on the cellular matrix topology. Experimental results from our GPU implementation show that the proposed algorithm can generate adaptive segmentation map where the distribution of superpixels reflects the gradient distribution or the disparity distribution of input image, with respect to scene topology. When the input size augments, the running time increases in a linear way with a very weak increasing coefficient.

Keywords: Superpixel · Image segmentation · Self-organizing map · Cellular matrix model · Graphics processing unit

1 Introduction

Superpixels have become an essential tool to the vision community. As building blocks of many vision algorithms, superpixels divide raw image into perceptually meaningful atomic regions which can be employed to substitute the rigid structure of the pixel grid [1–3]. Therefore, these atomic regions should represent or reflect some local properties with respect to some attribute distributions of the raw image. However, most of the existing algorithms produce uniformly distributed superpixels. In this paper, we aim to generate adaptive segmentation, called *superpixel adaptive segmentation map* (SPASM), where the distribution (density) of superpixels coincides with the distribution of some desired attribute of input image, such as edges, textures, and depths. In order to implement the parallel level, on which parallel SPASM algorithm will take place, we also design

© Springer International Publishing Switzerland 2015
O. Pichardo Lagunas et al. (Eds.): MICAI 2015, Part II, LNAI 9414, pp. 325–336, 2015.
DOI: 10.1007/978-3-319-27101-9_24

a massively parallel computation model. Unlike most work of the *general-purpose computing on graphics processing units* (GPGPU) for image processing applications, where usually one thread deals with one pixel, we propose the concept of cellular matrix decomposition at different levels for (1) massive parallelism implementation under different topologies of the plane and (2) optimized load balancing computing with size-configurable cells. Each cell, assigned to one thread in our GPU implementation, is a basic parallel operation unit and performs *spiral search* [4] for closest point finding, e.g. from pixel to cluster center and vice versa. Then one important feature of the model is that it proceeds from a cellular decomposition of the input data in 2D space, such that each processing unit represents a constant and small part of data. Since the cellular matrix division is proportional to input data, and the processing units correspond one-to-one with the cells respectively, then, both the memory and the processing units needed are in linear correspondence of $O(N)$ to the input image size N. Hence, as more and more multi-cores will be available in a single chip in the future, the approach should be more and more competitive, especially when dealing with very large size inputs. This property is what we call "massive parallelism".

Numerous superpixel algorithms have been proposed in the literature and they could be roughly classified into graph-based methods and gradient ascent methods. Algorithms in the first category usually treat each pixel as a node in a graph where edge weights between two nodes are proportional to the similarity between neighboring pixels. Superpixels are then created by minimizing a cost function defined over the graph [5–8]. Gradient ascent approaches, on the other hand, usually start from a rough initial clustering of pixels and then iteratively refine the clusters until some convergence criterion is met to form superpixels. Examples in this category include *mean shift* [9], *quick shift* [10], watershed approach [11], and *Turbopixel* method [12]. Also, there exist some methods [13,14] that use depth as an additional feature to perform segmentation on *RGB-D* images. A comprehensive survey and comparison study of superpixel algorithms can be found in [1], where a fast algorithm called *simple linear iterative clustering* (SLIC) is proposed to adapt k-means clustering to generate superpixels with good adherence to image boundaries. Our proposed algorithm extends the state-of-the-art SLIC algorithm, using our adaptive meshing tool to add compression abilities, with respect to the density distribution of image attributes and the topological relationship of cluster centers. Different from SLIC which performs a restricted nearest point search within a square region, through our cellular matrix model, we can conduct the true closest point finding in a massively parallel way, using the efficient spiral search algorithm under different topologies.

2   SPASM Algorithm

The *superpixel adaptive segmentation map* (SPASM) algorithm is a superpixel segmentation algorithm. By the word "adaptive" we mean in the final segmentation map of input image, (1) the distribution (density) of superpixels is adaptive

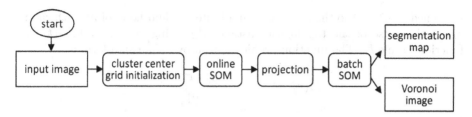

Fig. 1. Flowchart of the SPASM algorithm.

and (2) the size of superpixel is adaptive. As illustrated in Fig. 1, at the beginning of the SPASM algorithm, we initialize a regular (uniformly distributed) 2-dimensional grid of nodes, in the Euclidean plane defined by input image. Each node is the cluster center of a superpixel. Then we apply the online version of the Kohonen's self-organizing map [15] (SOM) algorithm on the grid of nodes, in order to deploy the nodes according to the distribution of some desired attribute of input image, such as edges, textures, and depths. Once the online SOM learning is finished, a projection procedure is carried out where each node searches its closest non-edge point (pixel) with spiral search under special conditions, and then all attributes (coordinates, color, density value, etc.) of nodes are copied from their closest points. After that, the batch version of SOM algorithm, using a new designed distance measure which considers the specific input image attribute, is applied to the deformed/adapted grid of nodes, for the final segmentation map. Meanwhile, a Voronoi color image is generated by filling the color of each point with the color of its cluster center node.

Now we give detailed explanations about how the online SOM and the batch SOM work in the SPASM algorithm. SOM deals with visual patterns that move and adapt themselves to brute distributed data in space. It is often presented as a non supervised learning procedure performing a non parametric regression that reflects topological information of the input data. The standard SOM works on a non directed graph $G = (V, E)$ of topological grid, where each vertex (node) $v \in V$ has a synaptic weight vector $w_v = (x, y) \in \Re^2$. Here a node corresponds to a superpixel cluster center.

When the online SOM is applied to the SPASM algorithm, the training procedure consists of a fixed amount of t_{max} iterations that are applied to the grid, with the node coordinates being initialized according to a regular topology. At each iteration t, firstly, a point (pixel) $p(t) \in \Re^2$ is randomly extracted from the image (**extraction step**) according to a roulette wheel mechanism depending on different density values of different pixels. Then, a competition between nodes against the input point $p(t)$ is performed to select the winner node n^* (**competition step**). Usually, it is the closest node to $p(t)$ in the Euclidean plane. Finally, the learning law (**triggering step**)

$$w_n(t+1) = w_n(t) + \alpha(t) \times h_t(n^*, n) \times (p(t) - w_n(t)) \qquad (1)$$

is applied to n^* and to the nodes within a finite neighborhood of n^* with radius σ_t, in the sense of the topological distance d_G, using learning rate $\alpha(t)$ and function profile h_t. The function profile is given by a Gaussian form of

$$h_t(n^*, n) = exp(-\frac{d_G^2(n^*, n)}{\sigma_t^2}) \tag{2}$$

Here, the learning rate $\alpha(t)$ and radius σ_t are geometric decreasing functions of time. To perform a decreasing run within t_{max} iterations, at each iteration t, the coefficients $\alpha(t)$ and σ_t are multiplied by $exp(ln(\chi_{final}/\chi_{init})/t_{max})$ with respectively $\chi = \alpha$ and $\chi = \sigma$, χ_{init} and χ_{final} being respectively the values at the starting and the final iteration.

The incremental-learning online SOM is a stochastic algorithm which updates the values of weight vectors sequentially iteration by iteration. Its deterministic batch equivalent, the batch SOM, uses all the data at each step. Instead of only one point being randomly extracted, at each iteration t of batch SOM, all points of the input image are taken into account, each of them being associated to its closest node according to a combined distance measure. The distance measure consists of spatial proximity, color, and density value, as

$$D(i, j) = \tau_s \|\boldsymbol{x}_{spa}(i) - \boldsymbol{x}_{spa}(j)\| + \tau_c \|\boldsymbol{x}_{rgb}(i) - \boldsymbol{x}_{rgb}(j)\| + \tau_d \|\boldsymbol{x}_{den}(i) - \boldsymbol{x}_{den}(j)\| \tag{3}$$

where $\boldsymbol{x}_{spa}$, $\boldsymbol{x}_{rgb}$, and $\boldsymbol{x}_{den}$ respectively correspond to 2D coordinate, 3D RGB color, and 1D density value, while τ_s, τ_c, and τ_d are their corresponding normalized coefficients. Note that this distance measure is an extension to the SLIC distance measure [1] with a third component of density. Therefore our superpixel segmentation algorithm should have the same ability of boundary adherence as the SLIC algorithm [1], meanwhile considering the peculiar density attribute for distance computation between points and cluster centers. At the triggering step of the batch SOM, nodes update the three attributes according to the learning law of

$$w_n(t + 1) = w_n(t) + \alpha(t) \times h_t(n^*, n) \times (\frac{\sum_{i=1}^k p_{n(i)}(t)}{k} - w_n(t)) \tag{4}$$

where k is the number of points $p_{n(i)}$ which are associated to node w_n. Note that the batch SOM is a generalization of the k-means algorithm with topological relationship among cluster centers. If we set $\alpha_{init} = \alpha_{final} = 1$ and $\sigma_{init} = \sigma_{final} = 0$, then the batch SOM degenerates into the k-means algorithm.

3   Parallel Cellular Matrix Model

In order to implement the parallel level, on which parallel SPASM algorithm will take place, we design a massively parallel cellular matrix model which partitions data. The input image (low level), along with the two-dimensional grid (base level) of superpixel cluster centers, which is deployed in the Euclidean plane defined by the input image, are partitioned into uniformly sized cells with rigid topologies. The topology of the cellular matrix (dual level) and the grid could be *quad*, *rhombus*, and *hexagonal*, as shown in Fig. 2. The role of the cellular matrix is to memorize data in a distributed fashion and authorize massively parallel operations. Suppose the input image is with size $W \times H$, and suppose both the grid of cluster centers and the cellular matrix are with quad topology. Then the initial grid of cluster centers is with size $W/Rg \times H/Rg$, where the parameter Rg is the distance (measured by pixel) between two neighboring nodes on the base level. The cellular matrix is with size $W/2Rc \times H/2Rc$, where the parameter Rc is the radius (measured by pixel) of cell on the dual level. Hence, Rc controls the degree of parallelism, and we assume a linear association from input data to memory as the problem size increases. Each uniformly sized cell in the cellular matrix is a basic training unit and will be handled by one parallel processing unit, here a thread in our GPU implementation, during the iterations of the SOM processing. This is the level on which massive parallelism takes place. Since the cellular matrix division is proportional to the input image size, and the processing units correspond one-to-one with the cells respectively, then, the processing units are also in linear relationship to the input image size.

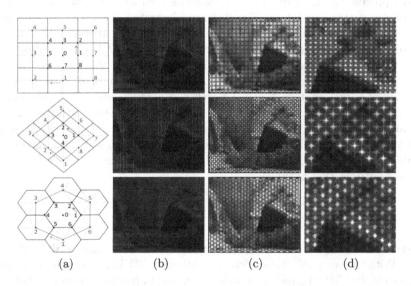

(a)   (b)   (c)   (d)

Fig. 2. Parallel cellular matrix model with different topologies. Rows: (upper) quad; (middle) rhombus; (lower) hexagonal. Columns: (a) traversal sequence - the black nodes denote the anticlockwise spiral traversal sequence on the low level or the base level while the red nodes denote the clockwise spiral traversal sequence on the dual level; (b) base level grid; (c) dual level cellular matrix; (d) zoom in of the dual level cellular matrix (Color figure online).

Under the cellular matrix model, each cell, which is assigned to one parallel processing unit, performs in parallel the iterative online SOM training. At the beginning of every iteration, a particular cell activation formula

$$pra_i = \frac{S_i}{\max\{S_1, S_2, \ldots, S_{num}\}} \times \delta \qquad (5)$$

is employed to decide if the cell will execute or not at the considered iteration. Here pra_i is the probability that the cell i will be activated, S_i is the sum of density values of all the pixels in the cell i, and num is the number of cells. The empirical preset parameter δ is used to adjust the degree of activity of cells, in order to avoid too many memory access conflicts. Equation 5 allows many data points, extracted at the first step of the online SOM at a given parallel iteration, to reflect the input data density distribution. As a result, the higher density value a cell contains, the higher is the probability this cell to be activated to carry out the SOM execution at each parallel iteration. In this way, the cell activation depends on a random choice based on the input data density distribution. In the parallel extraction step of the online SOM, each activated cell performs a local roulette wheel mechanism in the cell itself, in order to get the extracted pixel.

In the closet node/point finding procedure of the SPASM algorithm, each parallel processing unit carries out the spiral search as stated in [16], based on the cellular matrix model. In Fig. 2(a) are illustrated the traversal sequences of spiral searches at different levels based on cellular matrices with different topologies. Note that a single spiral search process takes $O(1)$ computation time on the average for a bounded distribution according to the instance size [4]. Then, one of the main interests of the cellular matrix model is to allow the execution of approximately N spiral searches in parallel, where $N (= W \times H)$ is the input size, and thus transforming an $O(N)$ sequential search algorithm into a parallel algorithm with theoretical constant time $O(1)$ in the average case for bounded distributions. This is what we call "massive parallelism", the theoretical possibility to reduce computation time by factor N, when solving a Euclidean NP-hard optimization problem.

4   Experimental Results

We use GPU to implement the cellular matrix model for parallel SPASM algorithm. With the *compute unified device architecture* (CUDA) programming interface, we employ GPU threads as processing units, to handle cells in parallel, and use CPU (host code) for flow control and the entire thread synchronization. The main CUDA algorithm is shown in Algorithm 1, where underscored lines are implemented with CUDA kernel functions that will be executed by GPU threads in parallel.

In line 4, of Algorithm 1, cells' activation probabilities are computed according to the activation formula of Eq. 5. The three steps (extraction step, competition step, and triggering step) of the online SOM are implemented in the kernel function of line 9. In this kernel function, after the cell locates its position in

Algorithm 1. CUDA SPASM algorithm

1: Initialize input density map, node grid, and cellular matrix;
2: Calculate cells' density values;
3: Find the max cell density value;
4: Calculate cells' activated probabilities;
5: **for** $ite \leftarrow 0$ to $t_{maxCons}$ **do**
6:     **if** $ite == 0 \ || \ ite \ \% \ CellRefreshRate == 0$ **then**
7:         Refresh cells;
8:     **end if**
9:     Parallel online SOM process;
10:     Modify online SOM parameters;
11: **end for**
12: Cluster center projection;
13: **for** $ite \leftarrow 0$ to $t_{maxImpr}$ **do**
14:     Refresh cells;
15:     Parallel batch SOM process;
16:     Modify batch SOM parameters;
17: **end for**
18: Voronoi superpixel image generation;
19: Save results;

the cellular matrix by *threadId* and *blockId* [17], it will firstly check if itself being activated or not. Only if being activated will the cell continue to perform local roulette wheel point extraction. Otherwise the cell finishes at this iteration. In the parallel batch SOM kernel function of line 15, there is no activation check and random extraction procedures. All cells perform spiral searches for all the points lie in them.

After the segmentation process is finished, a Voronoi color image is generated by filling the color of each pixel with the color of its cluster center node, through the kernel function of line 18.

Each cell has data structures where are deposited information of the number and indexes of the nodes this cell contains. This information may change during each iteration, but it appears that, during the online SOM learning phase, it can be sufficient to make the refreshing based on a refresh rate coefficient called *CellRefreshRate*. All the nodes' locations are stored in GPU global memory which is accessible to all the threads. Like other multi-threaded applications, different threads may try to modify a same node's location at the same time, which causes race conditions. In order to guarantee a coherent memory update in this situation, we use the CUDA atomic function which performs a read-modify-write atomic operation without interference from any other threads [17,18].

In our experiments, the online SOM parameters are fixed as $(\alpha_{init}, \alpha_{final}, \sigma_{init}, \sigma_{final}, t_{max}) = (1, 0.01, 20, 0.5, 100)$, while the batch SOM parameters are fixed as $(\alpha_{init}, \alpha_{final}, \sigma_{init}, \sigma_{final}, t_{max}) = (1, 0.1, 1.5, 0.5, 5)$.

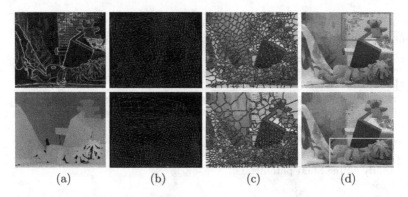

(a)   (b)   (c)   (d)

Fig. 3. Results obtained with image gradient (upper row) and disparity (lower row): upper (a) image gradient, lower (a) disparity map, (b) online SOM training result, (c) superpixel segments, (d) Voronoi image. The *Teddy* image from [19] is used.

We utilize two kinds of image attributes, as the density distributions which the online SOM is trained with. The first attribute is image gradient. In this case, at the beginning of the algorithm, we initialize input density map with color gradient values. Here we compute gradient through Sobel operator, which gives us a fast approximation of the edge distribution of input image, as shown in Fig. 3 upper (a). The activation possibility of each cell is then computed according to Eq. 5, where S_i is now the sum of gradient values of all the pixels inside the cell i. However in the point extraction step, we transfer the gradient g of each pixel into $1/(1 + g^2)$ for the local roulette wheel extraction. The reason is to make edge points (with high gradient values) less likely to be extracted. Therefore, the image gradient distribution is preserved on the cell level, meanwhile inside activated cells, situations of nodes being moved onto edge points are reduced. In Fig. 3 upper (b) of the adapted grid after the online SOM learning phase, areas with high image gradient present high density of nodes, with respect to the topology of the scene. Then these areas generate more superpixels after the batch SOM phase, as shown in Fig. 3 upper (c), and hence in the Voronoi superpixel image they have higher resolution and their details are more finely represented, as the example in the red box of Fig. 3 upper (d).

The second image attribute we have tested as the density distribution is the disparity map. Figure 3 lower (a) gives an example of the disparity map for input image, where brighter regions are nearer to the camera view point and they have higher disparity values. As expected, these regions demonstrate higher density of superpixels in the segmentation result of Fig. 3 lower (c) and accordingly their details are better represented in the Voronoi image, such as the example in the yellow box of Fig. 3 lower (d). Our algorithm's ability of generating adaptive superpixels with respect to user-specified density distribution can be proved through these two tests and the comparison of their results.

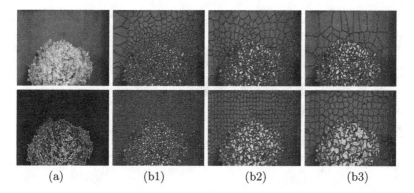

(a)   (b1)   (b2)   (b3)

Fig. 4. Comparison between SPASM (upper row) and SLIC (lower row). Upper (a) is input image and lower (a) is image gradient. The image size is 584×388. From (b1) to (b3), for both algorithms, the number of initial cluster centers is 2266, 566, 252. The *Hydrangea* image from [20] is used.

5 Comparison with SLIC Superpixel Algorithm

We compare the SPASM algorithm with the state-of-the-art SLIC superpixel algorithm [1] using publicly available source code[1]. The image gradient, as shown in Fig. 4 lower (a), is used as density map. For SPASM, we respectively set R_g to 10, 20, 30, which makes the initial superpixel size (with quad topology) is 100, 400, 900 and the number of initial cluster centers is $N/100$, $N/400$, $N/900$ (N being the input image size). For SLIC we set the initial superpixel size accordingly, in order to make the two algorithms work with same number of initial cluster centers. As shown in the upper row of Fig. 4, in all cases the SPASM algorithm produces a high density of fine superpixels in the edge-dense area (the flower clump) while the background is covered with relatively coarse superpixels sparsely. On the other hand as illustrated in the lower row of Fig. 4, no matter how the initial superpixel size is set, the SLIC algorithm will always generate uniformly distributed segments. This is because the SLIC algorithm is a tailored k-means approach with no function of distribution learning like the SPASM algorithm. Therefore, the superpixel resolution of SLIC correlates with the number of initial cluster centers, while SPASM has the tendency of better matching the finer-resolution regions that are selected by the density map attribute, meanwhile obtaining finer segmentation results in such regions, regardless of the number of initial cluster centers. This property of the SPASM algorithm could be employed for many computer vision tasks, which usually need to treat different areas of input image differently according to some underlying attribute distribution, such as edges or textures.

To provide a quantification of segmentation quality, we evaluate the results of these two algorithms according to the standard *mean color distortion* (MCD)

---

[1] http://ivrl.epfl.ch/research/superpixels.

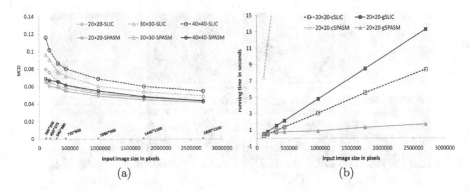

Fig. 5. (a) Comparison between SPASM and SLIC with different input sizes and different initial superpixel sizes. (b) Running time results of CPU SLIC (cSLIC), GPU SLIC (gSLIC), CPU SPASM (cSPASM), and GPU SPASM (gSPASM), with different input sizes. The *Cones* image from [19] is used. Experiment platform consists of an Intel Core 2 Duo CPU E8400 processor (only one core used) and a Nvidia GeForce GTX 570 Fermi graphics card endowed with 480 CUDA cores.

as defined in

$$MCD = \frac{1}{N}\sum_{i=1}^{N}(\|\boldsymbol{x}_{rgb}(i) - \bar{\boldsymbol{x}}_{rgb}(center(i))\|) \tag{6}$$

where N is the input image size, $\boldsymbol{x}_{rgb}(i)$ is the ground truth 3D RGB color of the ith pixel, and $\bar{\boldsymbol{x}}_{rgb}(center(i))$ is the color of the ith pixel's cluster center. We test input images of seven different sizes (360×300, 450×375, 640×480, 720×600, 1080×900, 1440×1200, 1800×1500) and set different initial superpixel sizes (20×20, 30×30, 40×40). For a good adherence to image boundaries, the distance parameters of SPASM are fixed as $(\tau_{spa}, \tau_{rgb}, \tau_{den}) = (1/2Rg^2, 1/3, 1/100)$ and the distance parameter (m parameter in [1]) of SLIC is set to 20. The iteration number of SLIC is set to the default of 10. Experimental results are depicted in Fig. 5(a). Note that all results are the mean values of 10 runs. Results from SPASM have smaller MCD values in all the tested cases when compared with results from SLIC. Also the MCD of SPASM results is steadier either with respect to different input image sizes, or with respect to different initial superpixel sizes. This shows the "adaptive" ability of our proposed SPASM which produces similar results regardless of the number of initial cluster centers and the input image size.

In order to make a running time comparison, we test four versions, the SLIC CPU implementation (cSLIC) with the raw public source code, the SLIC GPU implementation (gSLIC) in [21] with the raw public source code[2], the SPASM CPU implementation (cSPASM) which is a sequential simulation of parallel SPASM algorithm, and the SPASM GPU implementation (gSPASM). The initial superpixel size is set to 20×20 for the four versions. The running time results are

---

[2] https://github.com/carlren/gSLICr.

reported in Fig. 5(b). For small size images (360×300 and 450×375), the running time of cSLIC, gSLIC, and gSPASM is similar. For other larger size images, gSPASM runs faster than all the other three versions, especially for the largest image. cSPASM runs much slower than others for all images. This is because the sequential simulation of the iterative online SOM learning is time consuming. gSLIC runs slower than cSLIC for all images. This is because the gSLIC library we use is specifically optimized for high-end GPU cards, with a lot of shared memory employment, while the platform we use is a relatively out-dated GPU card. In spite of the absolute running time results of different implementations on different platforms (CPU and GPU), we think what is more important is that the running time of our GPU implementation of the parallel SPASM algorithm increases in a linear way with a very weak increasing coefficient. The results verify the "massive parallelism" characteristic of our proposed cellular matrix model, in a practical way by GPU implementation. We consider that such results are encouraging when solving very large scale problems.

6   Conclusion

The proposed SPASM algorithm extends the state-of-the-art SLIC superpixel algorithm, using our adaptive meshing tool to add compression abilities, with respect to the density distribution of image attributes while preserving the topological relationship of cluster centers. Experimental results support these merits, and they have better quality in the light of mean color distortion, when compared with the results of SLIC. This is attributed to (1) the "adaptive" ability of SPASM and (2) the true k-means clustering it employs by the efficient parallel spiral search under the cellular matrix model, rather than the restrained k-means that SLIC uses. The running time of our GPU implementation increases in a linear way with a very weak increasing coefficient according to the input size, which is encouraging to solve very large scale problems, under the proposed parallel cellular matrix model.

Future work should include comparisons with other state-of-the-art superpixel methods, by general benchmarks and standard quality evaluation criterions. Another important following work is to use the parallel SPASM algorithm based on the cellular matrix model, as a preprocessing tool and make possible fast and accurate visual correspondence applications such as stereo matching, optical flow, and scene flow.

References

1. Achanta, R., Shaji, A., Smith, K., Lucchi, A., Fua, P., Susstrunk, S.: Slic superpixels compared to state-of-the-art superpixel methods. IEEE Trans. Pattern Anal. Mach. Intell. **34**, 2274–2282 (2012)
2. Ren, X., Malik, J.: Learning a classification model for segmentation. In: 2003 Proceedings of the Ninth IEEE International Conference on Computer Vision, pp. 10–17. IEEE (2003)

3. Malisiewicz, T., Efros, A.A.: Improving spatial support for objects via multiple segmentations. In: BVMC (2007)
4. Bentley, J.L., Weide, B.W., Yao, A.C.: Optimal expected-time algorithms for closest point problems. ACM Trans. Math. Softw. (TOMS) **6**, 563–580 (1980)
5. Shi, J., Malik, J.: Normalized cuts and image segmentation. IEEE Trans. Pattern Anal. Mach. Intell. **22**, 888–905 (2000)
6. Felzenszwalb, P.F., Huttenlocher, D.P.: Efficient graph-based image segmentation. Int. J. Comput. Vision **59**, 167–181 (2004)
7. Moore, A.P., Prince, S., Warrell, J., Mohammed, U., Jones, G.: Superpixel lattices. In: 2008 IEEE Conference on Computer Vision and Pattern Recognition, CVPR 2008, pp. 1–8. IEEE (2008)
8. Veksler, O., Boykov, Y., Mehrani, P.: Superpixels and supervoxels in an energy optimization framework. In: Daniilidis, K., Maragos, P., Paragios, N. (eds.) ECCV 2010, Part V. LNCS, vol. 6315, pp. 211–224. Springer, Heidelberg (2010)
9. Comaniciu, D., Meer, P.: Mean shift: a robust approach toward feature space analysis. IEEE Trans. Pattern Anal. Mach. Intell. **24**, 603–619 (2002)
10. Vedaldi, A., Soatto, S.: Quick shift and kernel methods for mode seeking. In: Forsyth, D., Torr, P., Zisserman, A. (eds.) ECCV 2008, Part IV. LNCS, vol. 5305, pp. 705–718. Springer, Heidelberg (2008)
11. Vincent, L., Soille, P.: Watersheds in digital spaces: an efficient algorithm based on immersion simulations. IEEE Trans. Pattern Anal. Mach. Intell. **13**, 583–598 (1991)
12. Levinshtein, A., Stere, A., Kutulakos, K.N., Fleet, D.J., Dickinson, S.J., Siddiqi, K.: Turbopixels: fast superpixels using geometric flows. IEEE Trans. Pattern Anal. Mach. Intell. **31**, 2290–2297 (2009)
13. Weikersdorfer, D., Gossow, D., Beetz, M.: Depth-adaptive superpixels. In: 2012 21st International Conference on Pattern Recognition (ICPR), pp. 2087–2090. IEEE (2012)
14. Hasnat, M.A., Alata, O., Trmeau, A.: Unsupervised RGB-D image segmentation using joint clustering and region merging. In: Proceedings of the British Machine Vision Conference. BMVA Press (2014)
15. Kohonen, T.: Self-Organizing Maps, vol. 30. Springer Science & Business Media, The Netherlands (2001)
16. Wang, H., Zhang, N., Creput, J.C., Moreau, J., Ruichek, Y.: Parallel structured mesh generation with disparity maps by GPU implementation. IEEE Trans. Visual Comput. Graphics **21**, 1045–1057 (2015)
17. NVIDIA: CUDA C Programming Guide 4.2, CURAND Library, Profiler User's Guide (2012). http://docs.nvidia.com/cuda
18. Sanders, J., Kandrot, E.: CUDA by Example: An Introduction to General-Purpose GPU Programming. Addison-Wesley Professional, Upper Saddle River (2010)
19. Scharstein, D., Szeliski, R.: High-accuracy stereo depth maps using structured light. In: 2003 Proceedings IEEE Computer Society Conference on Computer Vision and Pattern Recognition, vol. 1, pp. I-195. IEEE (2003)
20. Baker, S., Scharstein, D., Lewis, J., Roth, S., Black, M.J., Szeliski, R.: A database and evaluation methodology for optical flow. Int. J. Comput. Vision **92**, 1–31 (2011)
21. Ren, C.Y., Reid, I.: gSLIC: a real-time implementation of SLIC superpixel segmentation. Technical report, Department of Engineering, University of Oxford (2011)

Feature Extraction-Selection Scheme for Hyperspectral Image Classification Using Fourier Transform and Jeffries-Matusita Distance

Beatriz Paulina Garcia Salgado[✉] and Volodymyr Ponomaryov

Instituto Politecnico Nacional, ESIME Culhuacan, Mexico-City, Mexico
bgarcias1404@alumno.ipn.mx, vponomar@ipn.mx

Abstract. Hyperspectral Image Classification represents a challenge because of their high number of bands, where each band represents a random variable in the classification system. In the first place, the computational cost can be higher because of large data volume during processing. In addition, some information can be redundant or irrelevant; furthermore, it maybe not a discriminatory. Consequently, a classifier has a little biased information related to the classes resulting in lower accuracy rates. In this work, we describe a novel methodology in performing feature extraction in classification as well as in efficient feature selection based on coefficients obtained via Discrete Fourier Transform (DFT) for signals by linking the bands of the images and making a selection by Jeffries-Matusita distance criterion. To test the experimental accuracy of current proposal, we employ three hyperspectral images justifying its performance against other state-of-the-art methods using Principal Components Analysis (PCA) feature extraction algorithm in combination with the Jeffries-Matusita distance criterion for its components selection and employing a Support Vector Machine (SVM) for classification.

Keywords: DFT · Feature extraction · Hyperspectral images · Jeffries-Matusita distance · PCA · Support vector machine

1 Introduction

Classification is a widely studied problem in remote sensing applications, especially in hyperspectral imagery (HSI). HSI data can be represented as a cube data structure where two dimensions (2D) represent spatial information and the third one represents information obtained by sensors that record the spectral radiance, normally, in more than a hundred contiguous spectral bands. Then, each pixel formed by the 2D can be viewed as a vector, which is composed by the radiance value at each spectral band. This spectrum is used to identify different materials present in a pixel [1,2].

© Springer International Publishing Switzerland 2015
O. Pichardo Lagunas et al. (Eds.): MICAI 2015, Part II, LNAI 9414, pp. 337–348, 2015.
DOI: 10.1007/978-3-319-27101-9_25

For the classification problem, each band can be considered as a feature. Therefore, the data size grows according to the number of features, so this turns classification into a more complex problem. Moreover, data can be redundant and irrelevant causing lower accuracy rates. As a result, a feature extraction stage should be performed in order to reduce dimensionality and redundancy in training data.

PCA is a popular method for feature extraction in remote sensing imagery. It is used previously to a classification stage because of the linear transformation that it can perform reducing data dimension, whereas the output data conserve the most information of the input data [3,4].

The DFT is a linear transformation, which can be used to feature extraction considering spatial characteristics of the image such as textures [5]. Besides, DFT is used in data mining as a time series dimension reduction method that decreases redundancy [6].

The feature extraction stage's goal is to obtain biased information related to each class so, that every class could obtain linear separability between each other. Several interclass distances are used as criterion functions to measure feature extraction algorithms performance, in particular Bhattacharyya, Jeffries-Matusita or Kullback-Leibler divergence [7]. Nevertheless, Bhattacharyya distance can be used as a basis of a texture feature selector in grey-scaled imagery [8].

In this paper, we propose a novel feature extraction method for HSI employing the magnitude of the DFT coefficients and selecting the number of magnitudes by applying Jeffries-Matusita distance in order to obtain the maximum separability between classes with the decreased number of features. We compare the proposed method performace using PCA feature extraction algorithm and the Jeffries-Matusita distance criterion over two Airborne Visible InfraRed Imaging Spectrometer (AVIRIS) images, and a Reflective Optics System Imaging Spectrometer (ROSIS) image. As the performance of a SVM with a Radial Basis Function (RBF) kernel has leaded to good accuracy rates for HSI [9], we use the same kind of SVM with one-against-all (OAA) strategy for the comparison.

2   Methodology

A hyperspectral image is denoted as $X = \{x_i \in \mathbb{R}^N, i = 1, 2, ..., h\}$, where N represents the number of bands and h is the number of pixels in an image X. It is considered that the image may contain a set $W = \{w_1, w_2, ..., w_m\}$ of classes, so there are m labels $L = \{l \in \mathbb{Z}, l = 1, 2, ..., m\}$ for each one of the classes identification.

The proposal involves calculating the DFT of the values from the image pixels bands, subsequently obtaining the magnitude of the coefficients of the exponential Fourier series and posteriorly selecting a number of features according to Jeffries-Matusita distance criterion. Finally, we employ a SVM with RBF kernel for classification.

2.1   Feature Extraction

The Fourier transform is the frequency domain representation of a temporal function in time domain:

$$F(\omega) = \int_{-\infty}^{\infty} f(t) e^{-j\omega t} dt. \tag{1}$$

This function values are repeated after a regular period of NT, where N is the number of samples in $f(t)$. According to this, Eq. (1) can be expressed as:

$$F(k) = \sum_{n=0}^{N-1} f(n) e^{-j\frac{2\pi}{N} kn}. \tag{2}$$

Any function $f(t)$ can be represented in form of exponential Fourier series every $t_0 < t < t_0 + T$ interval:

$$f(t) = \sum_{n=-\infty}^{\infty} C_n e^{jn\omega_0 t};$$

$$C_n = \frac{1}{T} \int_{t_0}^{t_0+T} f(t) e^{-jn\omega t} dt. \tag{3}$$

Taking into consideration that the signal $f(t)$ has N samples in the interval $0 < t < N - 1$, the Eq. (3) can be presented as follows:

$$f(t) = \sum_{k=0}^{N-1} C_k e^{jk\omega_0 t};$$

$$C_k = \frac{1}{T} F(k) = \frac{1}{T} \sum_{n=0}^{N-1} f(n) e^{-j\frac{2\pi}{N} kn}, \tag{4}$$

where complex coefficients C_k are expresed in such a form:

$$C_k = A_k + jB_k. \tag{5}$$

According to the previous nomenclature, if x_i is a pixel with N band values, let x_i be a band function $x_i(n)$ with N samples. Then, the Eq. (2) is represented as

$$X_i(k) = \sum_{n=0}^{N-1} x_i(n) e^{-j\frac{2\pi}{N} kn}. \tag{6}$$

Thus, Eq. (4) can be written as

$$x_i(t) = \sum_{k=0}^{N-1} C_k e^{jk\omega_0 t};$$

$$C_k = \frac{1}{T} X_i(k). \tag{7}$$

The spectral data of a pixel can be represented by Eq. (7). We take the C_k magnitudes as features of a pixel as follows:

$$F_k = |C_k| = \sqrt{A_k^2 + B_k^2} \tag{8}$$

as a pixel x_i has N samples, it has N features.

A flowchart of explained above feature extraction algorithm is shown in Fig. 1.

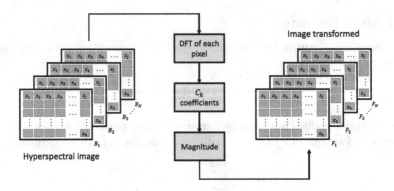

Fig. 1. Flowchart of the feature extraction algorithm.

2.2   Feature Selection

Once the features are extracted from an image, it is necessary to perform their selection, so the data dimension might be reduced. However, if there are a less number of features than it is necessary to obtain linear separability between the classes, the classifier may result in lower recognition rates. For this reason, the number of features that should be taken into consideration for the classifier should be controlled by a separability distance criterion.

The probability density function of each class can be approximated as a multivariate Gaussian distribution:

$$G\left(x; \mu, \Sigma\right) = \frac{1}{\sqrt{\left(2\pi\right)^k |\Sigma|}} \exp\left[\frac{1}{2}\left(x - \mu\right)^T \Sigma^{-1}\left(x - \mu\right)\right], \qquad (9)$$

where μ is the mean and Σ is the covariance matrix. For these parameters estimation, we use the labels of true position provided by the ground truth information for separating into classes the x_i pixels data from the hyperspectral image. The x_i pixels corresponding to the w_j class are denoted as $O_{i_{w_j}}$ observations. If each of the classes has h_{w_j} number of observations, then the maximum-likelihood estimators for parameters μ and Σ can be computed as:

$$\hat{\mu}_j = \frac{1}{h_{w_j}} \sum_{i=0}^{h_{w_j}} O_{i_{w_j}},$$

$$\hat{\Sigma}_j = \frac{1}{h_{w_j}} \sum_{i=0}^{h_{w_j}} \left(O_{i_{w_j}} - \hat{\mu}\right)\left(O_{i_{w_j}} - \hat{\mu}\right)^T. \qquad (10)$$

In order to measure the separability between the Gaussian functions of the classes, Bhattacharyya distance is employed. The Bhattacharyya distance between w_i and w_j classes is given by:

$$B_{ij} = \frac{1}{8}\left(\mu_i - \mu_j\right)^T \left[\frac{\Sigma_i + \Sigma_j}{2}\right]^{-1}\left(\mu_i - \mu_j\right) + \frac{1}{2}\log\left(\frac{|\Sigma_i + \Sigma_j|}{2\sqrt{|\Sigma_i||\Sigma_j|}}\right). \qquad (11)$$

Equation (11) uses a covariance weighting Euclidean distance called Mahalanobis distance (first term), which measures the dissimilarity between the means taking into consideration the variances of the variables and their level of correlation. The second term of Eq. (11) determines the similarity between the covariance matrices and it vanishes when the covariance matrices are equal.

Bhattacharyya distance does not have an upper limit. For this reason, it is difficult to know when the Gaussian functions are sufficiently separated in order to consider them linearly separable. The Jeffries-Matussita distance uses Eq. (11), where distance between w_i and w_j classes is given by:

$$D\left(w_i, w_j\right) = 2\left(1 - e^{-B_{ij}}\right).$$ (12)

For the feature selection algorithm, the Jeffries-Matusita distance between all pair of classes is computed as follows:

$$Z_k = \frac{1}{m}\sum_{i=0}^{m} J_{w_i},$$ (13)

$$J_{w_i} = \frac{1}{m-1}\sum_{j=1;j\neq i}^{m} D\left(w_i, w_j\right).$$ (14)

In Fig. 2, it is seen how the average distance between classes is computed. For making the classes linearly separable with the least number of features, the average distances Z_k are calculated using the features F_1 to F_k; where k is iterated from 1 to N. Let N be the total number of features resulted from the feature extraction algorithm. This results in N average distances calculation. Finally, the number of characteristics employed for the classification's stage is the lowest which leads to the maximum averaged distance. A point worth mentioning is that we approximate the exponential term $e^{-B_{ij}}$ to zero when its value is smaller than 1×10^{-16}.

2.3   Classification Scheme

The goal of a feature selection algorithm is to reduce dimensionality maintaining the separability between classes in such a way that a classifier can obtain a better accuracy. In order to test if the goal of the proposed algorithm is achieved, we use a SVM classifier with RBF kernel with a parameter $\sigma = \frac{1}{S}$, where S is the number of features.

Since each of the classes has a different number of observations, we propose a random selection with a v percentage of each class during training. The training set employed for the classifier consist of:

$$R = \left\{R_{1_{w_1}}, R_{2_{w_1}}, ..., R_{q_{w_1}}, R_{1_{w_2}}, R_{2_{w_2}}, ..., R_{q_{w_2}}, R_{1_{w_m}}, R_{2_{w_m}}, ..., R_{q_{w_m}}\right\},$$ (15)

where $R_{i_{w_j}}$ is an observation, belonging to the class w_j, selected for training and q_{w_j} is the number of selected observations of each class:

$$q_{w_j} = v h_{w_j}.$$ (16)

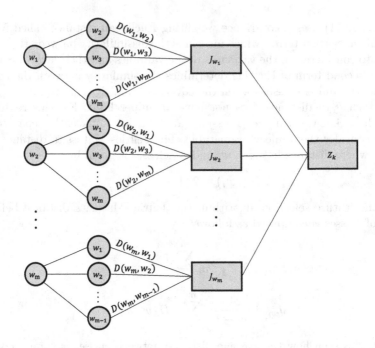

Fig. 2. Computing of the average distance between classes.

The other part of data set is used for testing, so the test set U is given by

$$U = \{X \neq R\}. \tag{17}$$

The flowchart of the proposed algorithm and the classification scheme are presented in Fig. 3.

3   Simulation Results

Three hyperspectral images were employed to evaluate the accuracy of the proposed method: two landscapes taken from the AVIRIS data set (Salinas and Salinas Subscene, which is a subscene of a certain region of Salinas image), and other one taken from ROSIS: Pavia University. The ground truths (GT) of these images can be observed in Fig. 4.

Salinas image contains 16 classes, it has a size of 512×217 pixels, where each pixel is composed by 224 bands. Bands 108 to 112, 154 to 167 and 224 are discarded because they express water absorption and do not give sufficient discriminant information; finally, the image employed contains only 204 bands. Salinas Subscene image contains only 6 classes and it has the size of 86×83 pixels. Pavia University data contain 610×340 pixels with 103 spectral bands representing 9 classes.

The proposed method is compared with PCA feature extraction algorithm [3]. The number of PCA components to use in the classifier is calculated by

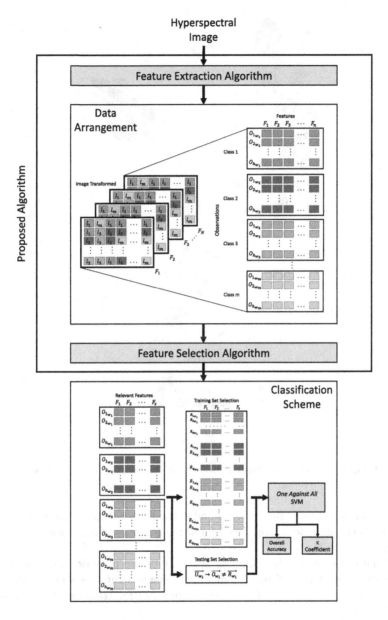

Fig. 3. Flowchart of the proposed algorithm and classification scheme.

the Jeffries-Matusita distance criterion. Figure 5 shows the variation of the distance error $\epsilon = 2 - Z_k$ as a function of the number of PCA components taken. Figure 6 exposes the distance error according the number of Fourier coefficient magnitudes taken into account.

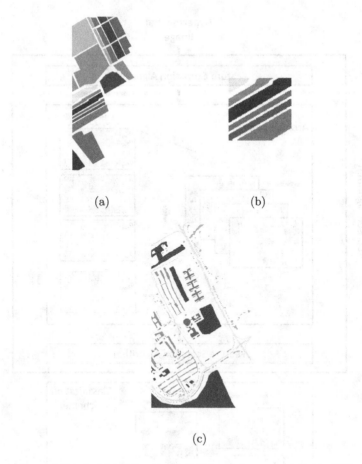

(a)   (b)

(c)

Fig. 4. Ground Truths: (a) Salinas. (b) Salinas Subscene. (c) Pavia University.

As it can be observed from Figs. 5 and 6, the higher is the number of features, the lower is the distance error. The number of features selected for each scheme is shown in Table 1.

For the purpose of validating the accuracy of the proposed method against PCA feature extraction, four classification scheme strategies were used: where 40 %, 50 %, 60 % and 70 % of data were employed for training. These schemes

Table 1. Number of features employed

Image	Fourier Coefficient Magnitudes	Principal Components Analysis
Salinas	3	2
Salinas Subscene	4	5
Pavia University	2	2

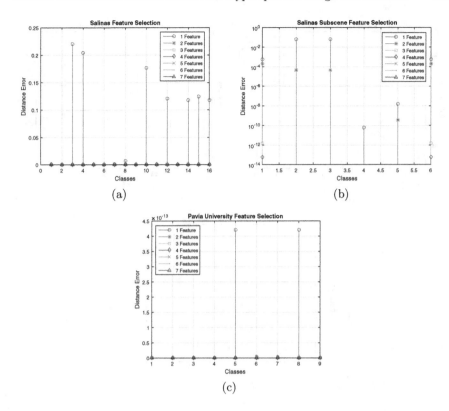

Fig. 5. Error of averaged distances depending on the number of PCA selected. (a) Salinas. (b) Salinas Subscene. (c) Pavia University.

were performed 10 times over each image with a different selection of the training set. Classification accuracies (training and test) and κ coefficients were calculated.

The κ coefficient represents the difference between the agreement, which is actually present in the classification, and the proportion of agreement that would be corrected by chance, where the last one is known as expected agreement. Classification results with κ coefficient in the range from 0.61 to 0.80 can be defined as a substantial agreement, and in a range from 0.81 to 1.00 is considered as almost perfect agreement [10].

The average accuracy rates and average κ coefficients resulted from the experiments using the proposed method can be observed in Table 2, as well as the results of another method that uses PCA procedure are presented in Table 3. In these tables, Tr. oa. is training overall accuracy, Tr. κ is training κ coefficient, Te. oa. is test overall accuracy and Te. κ is test κ coefficient.

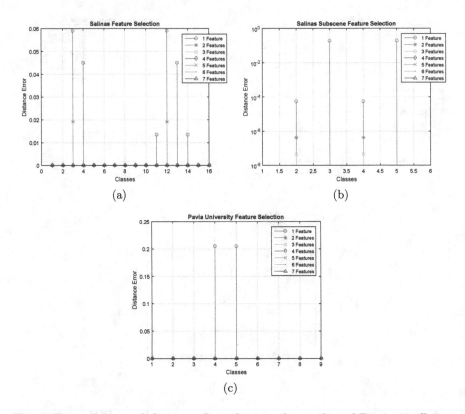

(a)

(b)

(c)

Fig. 6. Error of averaged distances depending on the number of Fourier coefficients magnitudes selected. (a) Salinas. (b) Salinas Subscene. (c) Pavia University.

Table 2. Average classification accuracy and average κ coefficients of each classification scheme obtained with the proposed method.

		40 %	50 %	60 %	70 %
Salinas	Tr. oa	0.9835	0.9812	0.9791	0.9771
	Tr. κ	0.9816	0.9790	0.9767	0.9744
	Te. oa	0.8039	0.8231	0.8375	0.8515
	Te. κ	0.7831	0.8039	0.8199	0.8353
Salinas Subscene	Tr. oa	0.9999	0.9997	0.9999	0.9998
	Tr. κ	0.9998	0.9997	0.9998	0.9998
	Te. oa	0.8581	0.8849	0.9077	0.9196
	Te. κ	0.8195	0.8540	0.8832	0.8985
Pavia University	Tr. oa	0.9352	0.9304	0.9263	0.9385
	Tr. κ	0.9115	0.9048	0.8991	0.9167
	Te. oa	0.5891	0.6040	0.6141	0.6228
	Te. κ	0.3560	0.3873	0.4074	0.4254

Table 3. Average classification accuracy and average κ coefficients of each classification scheme obtained using PCA feature extraction method.

		40%	50%	60%	70%
Salinas	Tr. oa	0.9999	1.0000	0.9999	0.9999
	Tr. κ	0.9999	1.0000	0.9999	0.9999
	Te. oa	0.3557	0.3899	0.4245	0.4576
	Te. κ	0.2066	0.2528	0.2993	0.3432
Salinas Subscene	Tr. oa	1.0000	1.0000	1.0000	1.0000
	Tr. κ	1.0000	1.0000	1.0000	1.0000
	Te. oa	0.4675	0.5106	0.5541	0.5913
	Te. κ	0.2774	0.3402	0.4028	0.4560
Pavia University	Tr. oa	0.6037	0.6647	0.6183	0.6602
	Tr. κ	0.3757	0.4761	0.4334	0.4669
	Te. oa	0.4363	0.4366	0.4364	0.4369
	Te. κ	0.0009	0.0014	0.0013	0.0023

4 Conclusions

In this work, we have developed a novel feature extraction-selection scheme for hyperspectral image classification. The experiments have demonstrated that the proposed method can obtain better classification accuracy rates than other one based on PCA feature extraction algorithm.

According to the proposed feature selection algorithm, the Gaussian functions of the classes contained in Pavia University image should be sufficiently separated in order to obtain a good classification accuracy that results in κ coefficients range between 0.61 and 1.00. However, as it can be observed, this image has a test overall accuracy near of 60% with κ coefficients between 0.35 and 0.42 in contrast to the AVIRIS images, where it can be obtained a test overall accuracy over 80% with κ coefficients over 0.78. Under these circumstances, we think that the usage of the Jeffries-Matusita distance criterion should be employed in combination with another criteria that uses diverse statistical distances to obtain an efficient feature selection, which can result in better classification accuracy rates. In addition, we think that this accuracy may be increased with the employment of spatial characteristics.

In future, a combination between spectral and spatial feature extraction algorithms should be performed employing the criteria mentioned before.

Acknowledgments. The authors would like to thank Consejo Nacional de Ciencias y Tecnologia (CONACyT, grant 220347), and Instituto Politecnico Nacional (IPN) for their economic support.

References

1. Shaw, G., Manolakis, D.: Signal processing for hyperspectral image exploitation. Sig. Process. Mag. **19**(1), 12–16 (2002)
2. Zhang, L., Zhang, L., Tao, D., Huang, X.: Sparse transfer manifold embedding for hyperspectral target detection. IEEE Trans. Geosci. Remote Sens. **52**(2), 1030–1043 (2014)
3. Cao, L.J., Chua, K.S., Chong, W.K., Lee, H.P., Gu, Q.M.: A comparison of PCA, KPCA and ICA for dimensionality reduction in support vector machine. J. Neurocomput. **55**, 321–336 (2003)
4. Slavkovic, M., Reljin, B., Gavrovska, A., Milivojevic, M.: Face recognition using Gabor filters, PCA and neural networks. In: 20th International Conference on Systems, Signals and Image Processing, pp. 35–38. IEEE Press, Bucharest (2013)
5. Tao, Y., Muthukkumarasamy, V., Verma, B., Blumenstein, M.: A texture feature extraction technique using 2D-DFT and hamming distance. In: 5th International Conference on Computational Intelligence and Multimedia Applications, pp. 120–125. IEEE Press (2003)
6. Morchen, F.: Time series feature extraction for data mining using DWT and DFT. Technical Report No. 33, Philipps-University Marburg (2003)
7. Serpico, S.B., DInc, M., Melgani, F., Moser, G.: A comparison of feature reduction techniques for classification of hyperspectral remote-sensing data. In: Proceedings of the SPIE, Image and Signal Processing for Remote Sensing VIII, vol. 4885, pp. 347–358. SPIE (2003)
8. Reyes-Aldasoro, C.C., Bhalerao, A.: The Bhattacharyya space for feature selection and its application te texture segmentation. J. Pattern Recogn. **39**, 812–826 (2006)
9. Melgani, F., Bruzzone, L.: Classification of hyperspectral remote sensing images with support vector machines. IEEE Trans. Geosci. and Remote Sens. **42**(8), 1778–1790 (2004)
10. Landis, J.R., Koch, G.G.: The measurement of observer agreement for categorical data. Biometrics **33**(1), 159–174 (1977)

Unconstrained Facial Images: Database for Face Recognition Under Real-World Conditions

Ladislav Lenc[1,2](✉) and Pavel Král[1,2]

[1] Department of Computer Science and Engineering,
University of West Bohemia, Plzeň, Czech Republic
[2] NTIS - New Technologies for the Information Society,
University of West Bohemia, Plzeň, Czech Republic
{llenc,pkral}@kiv.zcu.cz

Abstract. The objective of this paper is to introduce a novel face database. It is composed of face images taken in real-world conditions and is freely available for research purposes at http://ufi.kiv.zcu.cz. We have created this dataset in order to facilitate to researchers a straightforward comparison and evaluation of their face recognition approaches under "very difficult" conditions. It is composed of two partitions. The first one, called *Cropped images*, contains automatically detected faces from photographs. The number of individuals is 605. These images are cropped and resized to have approximately the same face size. Images in the second partition, called *Large images*, contain not only faces, however some background objects are also present. Therefore, it is necessary to include the face detection task before the face recognition itself. This partition contains images of 530 individuals. Another contribution of this paper is to show the recognition accuracy of several state-of-the-art face recognition approaches on this dataset to provide a baseline score for further research.

Keywords: Unconstrained Facial Images · UFI · Face database · Face recognition · Unconstrained conditions

1 Introduction

Face recognition has become a mature research field and the amount of approaches published every year is very high. We could state that the problem is already well solved but it is always not true. It holds only for the cases when the images are sufficiently well aligned and have limited amount of variations. Face recognition under general *unconstrained* conditions still remains a very challenging task.

Since the beginning of the era of computerized face recognition there have existed an important issue with a straightforward comparison and interpretation

---

This work has been partly supported by the project LO1506 of the Czech Ministry of Education, Youth and Sports. We would like also to thank Czech New Agency (ČTK) for support and for providing the data.

O. Pichardo Lagunas et al. (Eds.): MICAI 2015, Part II, LNAI 9414, pp. 349–361, 2015.
DOI: 10.1007/978-3-319-27101-9_26

of the results. Evaluation of the developed methods was often done on different databases. This issue was fortunately recognized very early. The FERET [1] database and a clearly defined testing protocol was designed in 1993. The FERET program motivated by the Defense Advanced Research Projects Agency (DARPA) brought a significant progress in the face recognition field.

It may seem straightforward to compare the methods on such a dataset but there may also emerge problems with the comparison of the results. The authors usually crop the faces according to the eye positions and the size of the resulting image can thus differ. This may cause differences in the recognition accuracy. An interesting comparison is available in [2] where three well known techniques (PCA, LDA and ICA) are compared on exactly the same data and the results are sometimes in contradiction with the previously reported ones of other authors.

There was much work done since the origin of the FERET database and some new datasets have been created since then. An important issue is that the majority of them was created in more or less controlled environment. There are only few datasets, such as Labeled Faces in the Wild (LFW) [3], Labeled Wikipedia Faces (LWF) [4], Surveillance Cameras Face Database (SCface) [5] and FaceScrub [6] that are acquired in real conditions. Therefore, we believe there is still room for another challenging face database.

Therefore, we would like to introduce a novel real-world database that contains images extracted from real photographs acquired by reporters of a news agency. It is further reported as Unconstrained Facial Images (UFI) database and is mainly intended to be used for benchmarking of the face identification methods, however it is possible to use this corpus in many related tasks (e.g. face detection, verification, etc.).

We prepared two different partitions. The first one contains the cropped faces that were automatically extracted from the photographs using the Viola-Jones algorithm [7]. The face size is thus almost uniform and the images contain just a small portion of background. The images in the second partition have more background, the face size also significantly differs and the faces are not localized. The purpose of this set is to evaluate and compare complete face recognition systems where the face detection and extraction is included.

Together with the dataset description we provide a set of experiments realized on this corpus. We use several state-of-the-art feature based methods that perform well on the other databases and that give particularly good accuracy on real-world data. The results should serve as a baseline and we would like to encourage researchers to surpass these results.

The structure of this paper is as follows. Section 2 describes the most important databases used for face recognition. The following section introduces the created database and the testing protocol. Section 4 shows the baseline recognition results on this dataset. Finally, Sect. 5 concludes the paper and proposes some further possible improvements of this dataset.

2   Summary of the Main Face Databases

FERET. Creation of this dataset [1] is connected with the FERET program that started in 1993. It was designed to allow a straightforward comparison of newly developed face recognition techniques under the same conditions. This database was acquired during 15 sessions within 3 years and contains 14,051 face images belonging to 1,199 individuals. The images are divided into the following categories according to the face pose: frontal, quarter-left, quarter-right, half-left, half-right, full-left and full-right. The images are also grouped into several probe sets. The main probe sets of the frontal images are summarized in Table 1.

Table 1. Image numbers in the main frontal probe sets of the FERET dataset.

Type	Description	Images no
fa	face gallery (for training)	1,196
fb	different facial expressions	1,195
fc	different illuminations	194
dup1	obtained over a three year period	722
dup2	sub-set of the *dup1*	234

CMU PIE. CMU PIE database [8] was created at the Carnegie Mellon University (CMU). It contains images of 68 people and the total number of images is 41,368. All the images were recorded in a single session. There are variations in pose (13 poses) and lighting conditions (43 different illumination conditions). The differences in facial expression are limited and can be categorized to 4 expressions.

Multi-PIE. This database [9] builds on the success of the CMU PIE database. Its goal is to remove the shortcomings that the PIE database has. The number of individuals is 337 and the total number of images is 755,370. The images were taken under 15 different viewpoints and 19 lighting conditions. There were 4 recording sessions compared to just one in the case of the CMU PIE.

Yale Face Databases. The original Yale Face Database [10] contains images of only 15 subjects, 11 images are available for each person. They differ in lighting conditions and in the details as for instance wearing glasses or not. This dataset was extended to the Yale Face Database B [11] which contains 16,128 face images of 28 individuals under 9 poses and 64 lighting conditions.

AT&T "The Database of Faces". AT&T database [12] (formerly known as "The ORL Database of Faces") was created at the AT&T Laboratories[1]. It contains facial images of 40 people that were captured between the years 1992

---

[1] http://www.cl.cam.ac.uk/research/dtg/attarchive/facedatabase.html.

and 1994. 10 pictures for each person are available. The images have a black homogeneous background. They may vary due to three following factors: (1) time of acquisition; (2) head size and pose; (3) lighting conditions.

AR Face Database. The AR Face Database[2] was created at the Universitat Autònoma de Barcelona. This database contains more than 4,000 colour images of 126 individuals. The individuals are captured under significantly different lighting conditions and with varying expressions. Another characteristic is a possible presence of glasses or scarf.

CAS-PEAL. The creation of CAS-PEAL face database [13] was sponsored by the National Hi-Tech Program and ISVISION. It contains the faces of 1,040 Chinese people which represents in total 99,594 face images. The images differ in pose, expression, accessories (glasses and caps) and lighting. One part of this database called CAS-PEAL-R1 containing 30,900 images is available for the researchers.

Banca. This database [14] was designed for testing of multi-modal verification systems. It consists of image and audio data and contains the images of 208 people. The images were captured under three different conditions: controlled, degraded and adverse.

Labeled Faces in the Wild. Labeled Faces in the Wild (LFW) [3] is a database collected from the web. It contains the images of 5,749 people and the total number of images is more than 13,000. 1,680 people has two or more images. Its purpose is to test the face verification scenario under unconstrained conditions. There are four available sets. The first one is the original and the others are aligned using three different methods.

PubFig. PubFig [15] database comprises also the images collected from the Internet. Compared to LFW, it has lower number of individuals (200). The total number of images is 58,797 and thus the number of images per person is much higher. There are significant differences in lighting, pose, expression, camera quality and other factors. This dataset is also used for the face verification.

Labeled Wikipedia Faces. Labeled Wikipedia Faces (LWF) [4] is a large collection of images from Wikipedia biographic entries. It contains 1,500 individuals which represents 8,500 images in total. There are available the original raw images as well as the aligned ones. Compared to LFW, it contains also historical images of a particular person and the time span is thus very large.

SCface. Surveillance Cameras Face Database (SCface) [5] was captured in indoor environment using 5 surveillance cameras of different qualities. It contains 4,160 images of 130 individuals. Some of the images are in the infrared spectrum.

---

[2] http://www2.ece.ohio-state.edu/~aleix/ARdatabase.html.

FaceScrub. FaceScrub [6] dataset was collected from the images available on the Internet. There is an automatic procedure that verifies that the image belongs to the right person. It contains the images of 530 people which is 107,818 in total. The images are provided together with the name and gender annotations.

The other thorough summaries of face databases can be found in [3] or in [16].

3   Unconstrained Facial Images Database

The Unconstrained Facial Images (UFI) database is composed of real photographs chosen from a large set of photos owned by the Czech News Agency(ČTK)[3]. Each photograph is annotated with the name of a person. However, some background objects and also other persons are often available. Due to (a) financial/time constraints; (b) necessity to be able to create quickly another face dataset on demand, we would like to create the database as automatic as possible (with minimal human efforts). We are inspired by [17] and we do thus a similar series of tasks in order to build the UFI database. As already mentioned, we created two different partitions.

3.1   Cropped Images: Creation and Dataset

The first step is face detection in the input images. We utilized the widely used Viola-Jones detector [7]. It is possible that the given photograph contains more than one person. In this case, we do not know which of the detected faces belongs to the correct person in annotation. In this step, we do not solve this problem and choose the first detected one. Another important issue is a presence of false detections (e.g. background objects instead of the faces) among the results. This issue will be addressed in the following steps.

Next, we detect the eyes in the detected faces. This step has two reasons: (a) to remove a significant number of non-face images (false detections); (b) to remove some face images that have significant out-of-plain rotation. The images with both eyes detected are then rotated to have the eyes on a horizontal line and resized to a specified size.

The resulting set of images is used as an input to the cleaning algorithm. The algorithm tries to chose the most similar images in the set of images for one person. Its aim is to remove the faces belonging to the other people and the possible non-face images that were not excluded in the previous step.

From the remaining images of each person we randomly choose one example for the test set. The remaining ones will be used for training. Finally, the database is manually checked to correct the possible errors.

The resulting set contains images of 605 people with an average of 7.1 images per person in the training set and one in the test set. The distribution of training examples per person is depicted in Fig. 1. The images are cropped to a size of 128×128 pixels. Figure 2 shows the images of two individuals from the *Cropped images* partition.

---

[3] http://www.ctk.eu/.

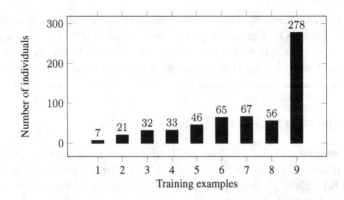

Fig. 1. Distribution of the training image numbers in the *Cropped images* partition.

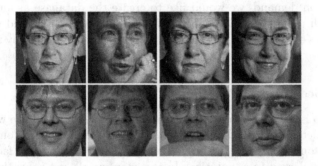

Fig. 2. Example images of two individuals from the *Cropped images* partition.

3.2   Large Images: Creation and Dataset

First, we apply the three similar tasks as in the previous case (i.e. face detection, eye detection and rotation according to the eyes and cleaning algorithm).

Then, we randomly choose the image portion that the face should fill in the image and random shifts in both horizontal and vertical axis are made. The random values define the maximal size of the freely available images for research purposes (the size of all images in this partition is 384 × 384 pixels). After applying this step, the face can be located in any part of the resulting image. Moreover, the face size is not specified and can occupy the whole image as well as only a small part.

This procedure is followed by a manual checking and no additional alignment or rotation is performed. The total number of the subjects in this partition is 530 and an average number/person of training images is 8.2. The distribution of the numbers of training examples is depicted in Fig. 3. Figure 4 shows some example images from the *Large images* partition.

The main goal of this partition is to evaluate and compare complete face recognition systems. Therefore, additional steps before recognition itself are expected (face detection, background removal, etc.).

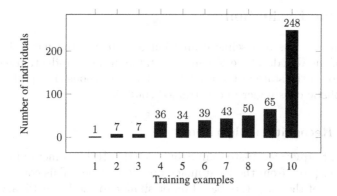

Fig. 3. Distribution of the training image numbers in the *Large images* partition.

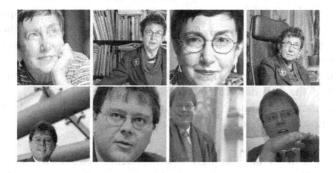

Fig. 4. Example images of two individuals from the *Large images* partition.

3.3   Testing Protocol

We would like to keep the testing protocol as straightforward and simple as possible. Therefore, both partitions are divided into training and testing sets. All images from the training sets are available as a gallery for training. The test sets are used as test images.

The images in the *Cropped images* partition should be used in its original size. Additional cropping or resizing is undesirable because of the comparability of the results. The images may be preprocessed and the preprocessing procedure must be described together with the reported results.

On the other hand we allow any preprocessing or cropping in the case of *Large images* partition. However, the whole procedure must be reported and thoroughly described. The recognition results should be reported as an accuracy (i.e. ratio between correctly recognized faces and all the faces).

Database Structure. The database is distributed in a directory structure. Each partition contains *train* and *test* directories which are composed of the sub-directories for each person named *sxxx* (*xxx* is the number of the subject).

4   Baseline Evaluation

This section provides a baseline evaluation of four selected methods on both partitions of the UFI database. As already stated in the introduction section, we concentrated on the state of the art feature based methods that perform better than the holistic ones under unconstrained conditions.

4.1   Face Recognition Algorithms

Histogram Sequence. Histogram Sequence (HS) [18] is a method of creating the face descriptors from the local image operator values. This concept is common for most of the operators based on or similar to the Local Binary Pattern (LBP) and therefore it is briefly described in this section.

The image is first divided into rectangular regions according to a regular grid. In each of these regions a histogram of operator values is computed. The histograms are then concatenated into a vector called *histogram sequence* that is used as a descriptor. This method ensures that the corresponding image parts are correctly compared.

Although there are a lot of sophisticated classifiers that can be employed for classification of the face descriptors created using the HS, we chose the simple nearest neighbour algorithm for classification in this baseline evaluation. It is used in all following methods.

Local Binary Patterns. The LBP operator [19] is based on a simple procedure that encodes a small neighbourhood of a pixel as follows: 8 neighbouring pixels are compared against the central one. The pixels with higher intensity are assigned to 1 and those with lower intensity are assigned to 0. The result is an eight bit binary number which corresponds to the decimal value in the interval $[0; 255]$.

The LBP operator was extended to use the points on a circle of given radius R that are compared to the central pixel. The number of the points is not fixed and is marked P. LBP operator in this form is referred to as $LBP_{P,R}$.

The LBP Histogram Sequences (LBPHS) were first used for face recognition by Ahonen in [20] and we use this method as the first baseline.

Local Derivative Patterns. Local Derivative Patterns (LDP) operator was proposed in [21]. Its main difference against LBP is that it uses the features of higher order than the LBP operator. It thus should capture more information than LBP. We will refer next the face recognition method as LDP Histogram Sequences (LDPHS).

Patterns of Oriented Edge Magnitudes (POEM). This operator [22] uses gradient magnitudes instead of the intensity values in LBP. The magnitudes of pixels within a *cell* (square region around the central pixel) are accumulated in a histogram of gradient orientations. The values for each orientation are then encoded using a circular LBP operator with a radius $L/2$. The circular neighbourhood of a pixel with a diameter L is called *block* in this method. The operator value is thus d-times longer (d is the number of discrete orientations). We will next refer to this method used for face recognition as POEM Histogram Sequences (POEMHS).

Face Specific LBP. This method [23] differs from the previous ones in the way of the computing the image representation. First, the representative face points are detected automatically using Gabor wavelets (instead of the regularly defined grid). Then, the LBP histograms are created in the regions around these points in the same way as in the other three previous approaches. However, the face is not represented by a single descriptor but by a set of the features (histograms). No HS is used in this case because the features are compared individually. We will further refer to this method as Face Specific LBP (FS-LBP).

4.2 Results on the Cropped Images Partition

This section presents results of the four selected methods on the *Cropped images* partition. The images are used in their original form as defined in the testing protocol (see Sect. 3.3). The Histogram Intersection (HI) metric is used for descriptor comparison in all cases. The grid size is set to 13 for LBPHS, LDPHS and POEMHS. It means that the histograms are computed within the square regions of size the 13×13 pixels. The similar value is used also in the FS-LBP method where it cannot be referred as a grid but it has similar interpretation that the histograms are computed within 13×13 square region. We use the circular $LBP_{8,2}$ in the FS-LBP method. POEM descriptors are calculated using three gradient directions. The cell size is set to 7 and the block size to 10. The results reported for the LDP method use LDP of first order because it surprisingly reaches better accuracy than the higher ones.

Table 2 shows the results of the four selected baseline methods on this partition. This table shows that the best performing method is POEMHS. Surprisingly, LDPHS has the worst results on this partition.

Table 2. Recognition results of the baseline methods on the *Cropped images* partition.

Method	Accuracy in %
LBPHS	55.04
LDPHS	50.25
POEMHS	**67.11**
FS-LBP	63.31

Then, we have done some error analysis. Two incorrectly recognized face examples/method are depicted in Fig. 5. This examples shows the complexity of

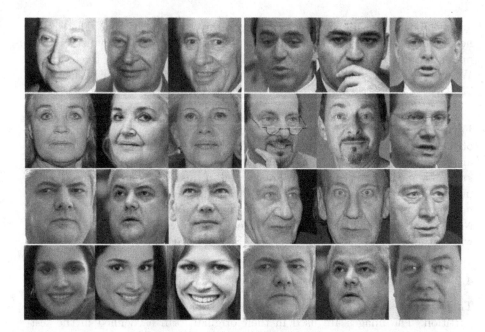

Fig. 5. Examples of the incorrectly recognized face images from the *Cropped images* partition using LBPHS, LDPHS, POEMHS and FS-LBP methods (from top to bottom). Each triplet contains a probe image, corresponding gallery image, incorrectly recognized image (from left to right).

this dataset where some examples are difficult to be correctly recognized even by humans.

4.3   Results on the Large Images Partition

As already stated, the recognition methods cannot be applied directly on the images in this partition. We therefore first applied the Viola-Jones algorithm to detect the faces. Additionally, we tried to detect the eyes and if both eyes were detected the faces were rotated and aligned according to the ayes. All resulting images were resized to the size 128 × 128 pixels. For the face recognition itself, we use the same configuration of the baseline methods as in the *Cropped images* case (see Sect. 4.2).

Table 3 summarizes the face recognition results on this partition. In this case, the best performing method is FS-LBP with score nearly 10 % higher than the remaining methods. The other methods perform comparably.

Then, we have also realized some error analysis. Two incorrectly recognized face examples/method are depicted in Fig. 6. This examples shows the complexity of this dataset even more clearly than the ones in the previous experiment.

Table 3. Recognition results of the baseline methods on the *Large images* partition.

Method	Accuracy in %
LBPHS	31.89
LDPHS	29.43
POEMHS	33.96
FS-LBP	**43.21**

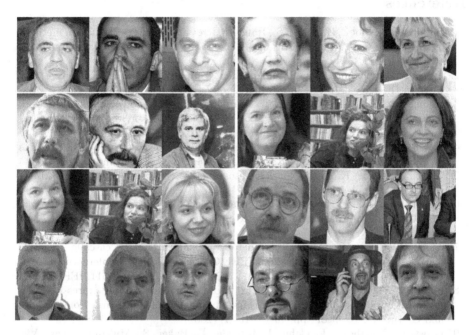

Fig. 6. Examples of the incorrectly recognized face images from the *Large images* partition using LBPHS, LDPHS, POEMHS and FS-LBP methods (from top to bottom). Each triplet contains a probe image, corresponding gallery image, incorrectly recognized image (from left to right).

5 Conclusions

In this work, we presented a novel face database intended primarily for testing of the face recognition algorithms. It represents a challenging dataset that addresses the main issues of the current face recognition approaches, the performance on low quality real-world images. We provide a simple testing scenario that must be kept so that the results are directly comparable. Together with the dataset we provide a set of experiments that evaluate some state-of-the-art face recognition approaches on this dataset. The best obtained accuracy on *Cropped images* partition is 67.1 % using the POEMHS method. The highest score on

Large images partition is 43.2 % obtained by the FS-LBP method. The database is freely available for research purposes[4].

One possible future work consists in adding the coordinates of the faces in the *Large images* partition and the coordinates of the important facial features. The dataset could then be used also for face detection and facial landmark detection algorithms.

References

1. Phillips, P.J., Moon, H., Rizvi, S., Rauss, P.J., et al.: The feret evaluation methodology for face-recognition algorithms. IEEE Trans. Pattern Anal. Mach. Intell. **22**, 1090–1104 (2000)
2. Delac, K., Grgic, M., Grgic, S.: Independent comparative study of PCA, ICA, and LDA on the feret data set. Int. J. Imaging Syst. Technol. **15**, 252 (2005)
3. Huang, G.B., Ramesh, M., Berg, T., Learned-Miller, E.: Labeled faces in the wild: a database for studying face recognition in unconstrained environments. Technical report, Technical report 07–49, University of Massachusetts, Amherst (2007)
4. Hasan, M.K., Pal, C.: Experiments on visual information extraction with the faces of wikipedia. In: Twenty-Eighth AAAI Conference on Artificial Intelligence (2014)
5. Grgic, M., Delac, K., Grgic, S.: Scface-surveillance cameras face database. Multimedia Tools Appl. **51**, 863–879 (2011)
6. Ng, H.W., Winkler, S.: A data-driven approach to cleaning large face datasets. In: 2014 IEEE International Conference on Image Processing (ICIP), pp. 343–347. IEEE (2014)
7. Viola, P., Jones, M.: Rapid object detection using a boosted cascade of simple features. In: Proceedings of the 2001 IEEE Computer Society Conference on Computer Vision and Pattern Recognition, CVPR 2001. vol. 1. pp. I-511. IEEE (2001)
8. Sim, T., Baker, S., Bsat, M.: The CMU pose, illumination, and expression (pie) database. In: Proceedings Fifth IEEE International Conference on Automatic Face and Gesture Recognition, pp. 46–51. IEEE (2002)
9. Gross, R., Matthews, I., Cohn, J., Kanade, T., Baker, S.: Multi-pie. Image Vis. Comput. **28**, 807–813 (2010)
10. Georghiades, A., et al.: Yale face database. Center for computational Vision and Control at Yale University (1997). http://cvc.yale.edu/projects/yalefaces/yalefa
11. Georghiades, A.S., Belhumeur, P.N., Kriegman, D.J.: From few to many: illumination cone models for face recognition under variable lighting and pose. IEEE Trans. Pattern Anal. Mach. Intell. **23**, 643–660 (2001)
12. Jain, A.K., Li, S.Z. (eds.): Handbook of Face Recognition, vol. 1. Springer, London (2005)
13. Gao, W., Cao, B., Shan, S., Chen, X., Zhou, D., Zhang, X., Zhao, D.: The cas-peal large-scale chinese face database and baseline evaluations. IEEE Trans. Syst. Man Cybernetics Part A Syst. Hum. **38**, 149–161 (2008)
14. Bailly-Bailliére, E., et al.: The banca database and evaluation protocol. In: Kittler, J., Nixon, M.S. (eds.) AVBPA 2003. LNCS, vol. 2688, pp. 625–638. Springer, Heidelberg (2003)
15. Kumar, N., Berg, A.C., Belhumeur, P.N., Nayar, S.K.: Attribute and simile classifiers for face verification. In: 2009 IEEE 12th International Conference on Computer Vision, pp. 365–372. IEEE (2009)

---

[4] http://ufi.kiv.zcu.cz.

16. Gross, R.: Face databases. In: Handbook of Face Recognition, pp. 301–327. Springer (2005)
17. Lenc, L., Král, P.: Automatic face recognition system based on the SIFT features. Comput. Electr. Eng. (2015)
18. Ahonen, T., Hadid, A., Pietikäinen, M.: Face recognition with local binary patterns. In: Pajdla, T., Matas, J.G. (eds.) ECCV 2004. LNCS, vol. 3021, pp. 469–481. Springer, Heidelberg (2004)
19. Ojala, T., Pietikäinen, M., Harwood, D.: A comparative study of texture measures with classification based on featured distributions. Pattern Recogn. **29**, 51–59 (1996)
20. Ahonen, T., Hadid, A., Pietikainen, M.: Face description with local binary patterns: application to face recognition. IEEE Trans. Pattern Anal. Mach. Intell. **28**, 2037–2041 (2006)
21. Zhang, B., Gao, Y., Zhao, S., Liu, J.: Local derivative pattern versus local binary pattern: face recognition with high-order local pattern descriptor. IEEE Trans. Image Process. **19**, 533–544 (2010)
22. Vu, N.S., Dee, H.M., Caplier, A.: Face recognition using the poem descriptor. Pattern Recogn. **45**, 2478–2488 (2012)
23. Lenc, L., Král, P.: Automatically detected feature positions for LBP based face recognition. In: Iliadis, L. (ed.) AIAI 2014. IFIP AICT, vol. 436, pp. 246–255. Springer, Heidelberg (2014)

Application of a Face Recognition System Based on LBP on Android OS

Marco Calderon-Lopez, Tadeo Torres-Gonzalez, Jesus Olivares-Mercado[✉],
Karina Toscano-Medina, Gabriel Sanchez-Perez,
Hector Perez-Meana, and Silvestre Garcia-Sanchez

National Polytechnic Institute of Mexico,
Av. Santa Ana 1000 San Francisco Culhuacan Coyoacan, Mexico City, Mexico
jolivares@ipn.mx

Abstract. This paper presents the application of the algorithm of Local Binary Pattern (LBP) for face feature extraction and its implementation on Android operating system. The algorithm LBP is used for texture characterization and based on good performance was used to face characterization showing a good effectiveness, due to this is chosen to apply in a mobile device. To perform system testing on a mobile device was used a standard database (AR Facedatabase) to simulate the capture of images, which has 120 people and 21 images each, the average of 3 images was used for obtaining a template by person and using Euclidean distance it was obtained a 70 % correct classification, showing that the LBP obtains good results using a simple classification algorithm with a limited processing power as have a mobile device, further tests were performed with 10 people where up to 94 % recognition was obtained.

Keywords: Mobile device · Face recognition · Local Binary Pattern · Euclidean distance

1 Introduction

Face recognition is one of the most widely used biometric technologies because the data acquisition approach is non-intrusive. Face recognition is performed by taking a picture and can be performed with or without the cooperation of the person under analysis. Thus, face recognition is a biometric technology that has obtained high acceptance among users [2,3]. A face recognition system can be used for either identity verification or person identification. In the identity verification task, the system is asked to determine whether the person is who he/she claims to be, whereas during the person identification task, the system is asked to determine, among a set of persons whose facial characteristics are stored in a database, the person who most closely resembles the image under analysis [1].

The Local Binary Pattern (LBP) [4] algorithm is one of the best texture descriptor methods. The acceptance and popularity level of this feature extraction method has propitiate its implementation even in facial expression recognition systems, achieving good results. Therefore, This texture descriptor method

© Springer International Publishing Switzerland 2015
O. Pichardo Lagunas et al. (Eds.): MICAI 2015, Part II, LNAI 9414, pp. 362–370, 2015.
DOI: 10.1007/978-3-319-27101-9_27

is chosen to be applied, because have a lot of benefits like a low complexity to develop on a mobile device. The LBP algorithm has been implemented only in simulation environments, where it has responded satisfactorily, as is shown in [5], but has not yet been implemented in a biometric system that works in an uncontrolled environment, to prove if it responds acceptably in situations that are not presented in a simulation environment.

LBP will be implemented as feature extractors as part of a facial recognition system for the Android operating system, in order to assess the effectiveness and efficiency of this algorithm.

2   Theoretical Framework

Biometric systems are a set of automated methods for recognizing people using physiological or personal behavior characteristics [2,3]. A biometric system is, essentially, a pattern recognition system and, generally, can be divided into four main modules: a capture module, a feature extraction module, a comparison and decision (classification) module and a database module. In capture module is taken the picture to analyze; in the feature extraction module, biometric data are processed, and a set of outstanding discriminatory features is extracted to represent the most important features of the identity of the person under analysis, in this work are used the LBP for feature extraction. In the decision module is use the Euclidean distance to determine the winner class, and finally in the database module are storage all de models of each person to identify.

2.1   Android OS

The importance of mobile devices called "smart phones" has been increasing in recent years, thanks to technological development in this area. Then the percentage of use of smartphones by brand is show in the Fig. 1.

Android is an operating system based on Linux kernel, and was developed by Android Inc., which was acquired by Google in 2005. Android was introduced

Worldwide Smartphone Sales to End Users by Vendor in 2014 (Thousands of Units)

Company	2014 Units	2014 Market Share (%)	2013 Units	2013 Market Share (%)
Samsung	307,597	24.7	299,795	30.9
Apple	191,426	15.4	150,786	15.5
Lenovo*	81,416	6.5	57,424	5.9
Huawei	68,081	5.5	46,609	4.8
LG Electronics	57,661	4.6	46,432	4.8
Others	538,710	43.3	368,675	38.0
Total	1,244,890	100.0	969,721	100.0

Source: Gartner (March 2015)

*The results for Lenovo include sales of mobile phones by Lenovo and Motorola.

Fig. 1. Worldwide Smartphones sales until 2014.

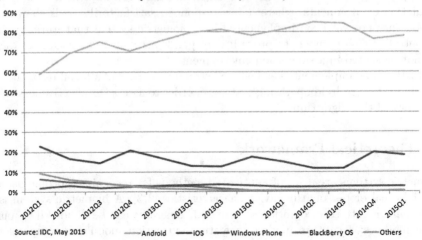

Fig. 2. Worldwide Smartphones OS Market until 2015.

in 2007 and is currently the most widely used mobile operating system in the world, as is reported by IDC and is shown in Fig. 2.

2.2 LBP Algorithm

The original Local Binary Pattern (LBP) method uses windows of 3×3 pixels of an image representing a neighborhood around the central pixel, as shown in Fig. 3(a), where the central pixel is used as a threshold to compare values of its 8 neighbors. The pixels whose values are less than the threshold must be labeled with 0 and those that are greater than the threshold are labeled by with 1, as shown in Fig. 3(b). Then, the labels of pixels are multiplied by 2^P, where $0 \le P \le 7$ represents the position of each pixel in the neighborhood, as shown in Fig. 3(c). Finally, the resulting values are added to obtain the label of the central pixel of that neighborhood, as shown in Fig. 3(d). This method produces 256 possible values for the label of the central pixel. This process is repeated for the entire image and produces a LBP label matrix (LBP image).

2.3 Proposed System

In order to apply the LBP algorithm, it will be used in a face recognition system; this system will be implemented on the Android operating system. In Fig. 4, the block diagram of the face recognition system is shown, which blocks will be explained below.

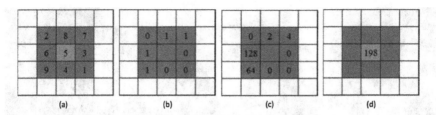

Fig. 3. LBP Algorithm: (a) Values of neighbors around the central pixel. (b) Comparison of each neighbor with the central pixel. (c) Substitution of each value of the comparison by the corresponding 2^P value. (d) Adding and replacing of the central pixel with the resultant value.

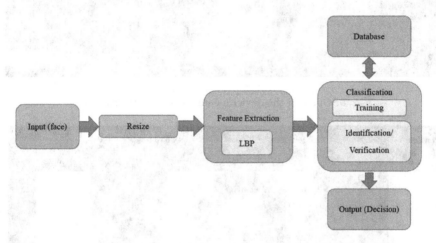

Fig. 4. Block diagram of proposed face recognition system.

Input (face). Through the device's camera, a picture will be taken, as shown in Figs. 5 and 6. The system will identify the face of the person and will discriminate all parts of the image that does not correspond to it. The resulting image will be the test sample.

Resize. In order to standardizing the images, each of these were converts to grayscale and resize it, having the same picture size, regardless of the resolution of the camera device or distance of person with respect to device.

Feature Extraction. In this block, the LBP algorithm will be implemented, to obtain the feature vector of the sample. Figure 7 shows the result of this block in the application on the mobile device. After apply the LBP to the image, this is converted to row vector concatenating each row one after another. Finally the average of 3 different images of the same person is used like model to the classification stage.

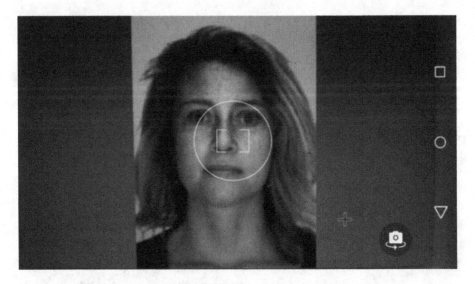

Fig. 5. Opening the device's camera to take the sample.

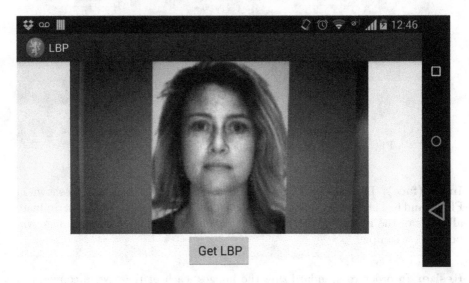

Fig. 6. Taking the test sample.

Classification. This block is divided into two parts:

Training: It will take place when individuals are entered to the database. The feature vectors of each person will be marked with the ID of the person to which they belong, and then, will be stored in the database.

Identification: It will happen when it is desired to identify a person. By euclidean distance, the feature vector of the sample will be compared against all existing models in the database, the winner will be that which possess a less

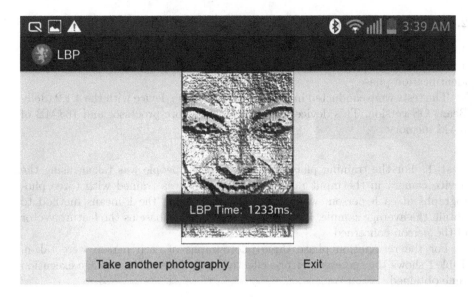

Fig. 7. Sample after application of the LBP, the execution time of the algorithm is shown.

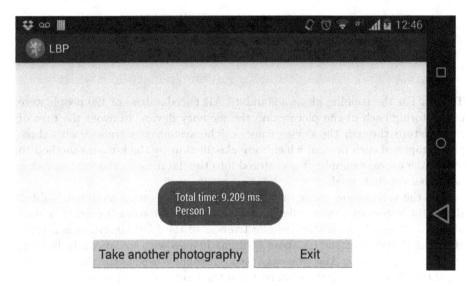

Fig. 8. The system identifies the person that has been entered. The ID and the execution time of the algorithm are shown.

euclidean distance. The winner will be shown on the screen, where a decision will be made on, as shown in Fig. 8.

2.4 Experimental Results

Three tests were performed in order to measure the performance of the LBP on a mobile device, which consist in a previous training phase and in a subsequent identification phase.

The tests were conducted in an Android midrange device with the 4.1.2 (Jelly Bean) OS version. This device has a 1 GHz dual-core processor and 768 MB of RAM memory.

Test 1. For the training phase a database of 10 people was taken, using the device camera in the input module. The system was trained with three photographs of each person, which were classified using the k-means method to obtain the average sample. It was stored into the database as the feature vector of the person concerned.

For the recognition phase three photographs of each person were taken. Table 1 shows the successes, errors, effectiveness rate and the average execution time obtained.

Table 1. Results obtained with the LBP algorithm in the test 1, with a database of 10 people and a training of 3 images per person.

Algorithm	Successes	Failures	Effectiveness	Execution time
LBP	28	2	93.33 %	9.2 seg

Test 2. For the training phase a standard AR Facedatabase of 120 people were used, storing each of the pictures on the memory device, to avoid the take of each picture through the device camera. The system was trained with three photographs of each person, which were classified using the k-means method to obtain the average sample. It was stored into the database as the feature vector of the person concerned.

For the recognition phase, a total of 2458 pictures were analyzed. Table 2 shows the successes, errors, effectiveness rate and the average execution time obtained. It can be seen that the effectiveness of the LBP algorithm is acceptable considering that the database contains images with variations in lighting and facial expressions. Also whereas a basic classifier is used as the Euclidean distance that has low computational cost and the model of each person is obtained from a non-supervised method, as is the K-means, the results are considered satisfactory.

Also is remarkable that the time of execution for all images is considerably short, considering that the application is on a mobile device.

Table 2. Comparison of results obtained with LBP in the test 2, with a database of 120 people and a training of 3 images per person. A total of 2458 photographs were analyzed.

Algorithm	Successes	Failures	Effectiveness	Execution time
LBP	1508	950	61.35 %	73 seg

Test 3. It was determined that with a higher level of training, it could be possible to achieve better performance results, so, for this training phase, the same database, used in the previous test, were charged, but the system was trained with five photographs of each person. For the recognition phase, the same 2458 photographs of the Test 2 were analyzed. The percentage of effectiveness obtained by the LBP algorithm is shown in Table 3.

Table 3. Comparison of results obtained with LBP in the test 3, with a database of 120 people and a training of 5 images per person. A total of 2458 photographs were analyzed.

Algorithm	Successes	Failures	Effectiveness	Execution time
LBP	1745	713	71 %	73 seg

3   Conclusions

The application on a mobile device a method such as LBP for feature extraction of face shows it have a good performance in addition to the computational cost is low, since the tests were done with a standard database with 120 people having a recognition rate of up to 70 % when models with 5 images per person are obtained. It notes that the implementation of a method of facial recognition on a mobile device has many applications, besides that, the count database within the device does not limit its use only with an Internet connection allowing the user to make an identification in real time. One possible application may be for police department in the pursuit of suspects. Another advantage of this application is that the runtime for identification is very short which makes the application even more attractive. Using a mobile device using the Android operating system is because it is the most currently used in the market. When the test 1 was developed shown that with a short real database (only 10 persons) the identification rate is until 93 %, obviously when the database increase the number of individuals the identification rate decrease and the confusion in the application increase because of the possible similarity between individuals.

Acknowledgement. We thanks the National Science and Technology Council of Mexico and to the National Polytechnic Institute for the financial support during the realization of this work.

References

1. Chellappa, R., Sinha, P., Phillips, P.J.: Face recognition by computers and humans. Computer **43**(2), 46–55 (2010)
2. El-Bakry, H.M., Mastorakis, N.: Personal identification through biometric technology. In: 9th WSEAS International Conference on Applied Informatics and Communications (AIC09), Moscow, Russia, pp. 325–340 (2009)
3. Kung, S.Y., Mak, M.W., Lin, S.H.: Biometric authentication: a machine learning approach. Prentice Hall Professional Technical Reference (2005)
4. Ojala, T., Pietikainen, M., Harwood, D.: Performance evaluation of texture measures with classification based on kullback discrimination of distributions. In: Proceedings of the 12th IAPR International Conference on Pattern Recognition, vol. 1 - Conference A: Computer Vision AMP; Image Processing, vol. 1, pp. 582–585, October 1994
5. Yuan, B., Cao, H., Chu, J.: Combining local binary pattern and local phase quantization for face recognition. In: 2012 International Symposium on Biometrics and Security Technologies (ISBAST), pp. 51–53. IEEE (2012)

Feature to Feature Matching
for LBP Based Face Recognition

Ladislav Lenc[1,2] and Pavel Král[1,2]($\boxtimes$)

[1] Department of Computer Science and Engineering, Faculty of Applied Sciences,
University of West Bohemia, Plzeň, Czech Republic
[2] NTIS - New Technologies for the Information Society, Faculty of Applied Sciences,
University of West Bohemia, Plzeň, Czech Republic
{llenc,pkral}@kiv.zcu.cz

Abstract. This paper presents a novel face recognition method called
Local Binary Patterns with Feature to Feature Matching (LBP-FF).
Contrary to other LBP approaches, we do not focus on the operator itself,
however we would like to improve the matching procedure. The current
LBP based approaches concatenate all feature vectors into one vector and
then compare these large vectors. By contrast, our method compares the
features separately. A sophisticated distance measure composed from two
parts is used for face comparison. Chi square distance and histogram
intersection metrics are utilized for vector distance computation. The
proposed approach is evaluated on four face corpora: AT&T, FERET,
AR and ČTK database. We experimentally show that our method significantly outperforms all compared state-of-the-art methods on all the
databases. It is also worth of noting that the ČTK corpus is a novel
face dataset composed of the images taken in real-world conditions and
is freely available for research purposes at http://ufi.kiv.zcu.cz or upon
request to the authors.

Keywords: Automatic face recognition · Czech News Agency · LBP
with Feature to Feature Matching · LBP-FF · Local Binary Patterns

1 Introduction

Face recognition became one of the most popular biometric identification methods. It has a very broad spectrum of applications: access control, surveillance of
people, automatic annotation of photographs and so on. The most of currently
emerging approaches can be categorized as feature based because these methods
proved to be more accurate than the holistic ones especially in case of images
with significant variations in pose, lighting, etc.

One of the most popular methods for feature extraction are Local Binary Patterns (LBP). It was originally proposed for texture classification in [1]. Lately,
it is frequently used also for other tasks such as facial expression recognition,
content based image retrieval, face recognition or medical applications. The
first method utilizing LBP for face recognition was proposed by Ahonen in [2].

© Springer International Publishing Switzerland 2015
O. Pichardo Lagunas et al. (Eds.): MICAI 2015, Part II, LNAI 9414, pp. 371–381, 2015.
DOI: 10.1007/978-3-319-27101-9_28

The image is divided into a set of non-overlapping rectangular regions and a histogram of LBP values is computed in each one. One feature corresponds to one region. All features are finally concatenated and treated as one large vector that represents the face.

The LBP algorithm inspired many other, more sophisticated, image descriptors but the principle of creating the face representation remains usually the same. Histograms are created from the values obtained from the particular algorithm and are concatenated to one vector that creates the face representation. In our work, we concentrate rather on the comparison procedure than the descriptor itself.

We use the features individually and compare them one to another. A similar method was already presented in [3]. It showed significantly better performance than the method that uses one concatenated vector.

The main goal of this work is to improve the matching scheme and to show its impact on several face corpora. We use features equally distributed on a grid as in the original method to allow a direct comparison. For the face matching step we propose a novel method that combines two distance measures.

The rest of the paper is organized as follows. Section 2 describes the fundamental face recognition methods based on LBP. Section 3 describes the LBP algorithm and the proposed face recognition method. Section 4 first describes the databases we used for evaluation and then presents the results of experiments performed on these datasets. In the last section, we discuss the results and propose some ideas for future research.

2   Related Work

As already stated, the first method using LBP for face recognition was proposed by Ahonen in [2]. The authors also proposed a weighted LBP modification which gives more importance to the regions around central parts of the face.

An important idea proposed already by Ojala in [1] are Uniform Local Binary Patterns. The pattern is called uniform if it contains at most two transitions from 0 to 1 or from 1 to 0. The histogram is then shortened from 256 intervals (bins) to 59.

Li et al. propose in [4] Dynamic Threshold Local Binary Pattern (DTLBP). They consider the mean value of the neighbouring pixels and also the maximum contrast between the neighbouring points. The authors claim that this variation is less sensitive to the noise than the original LBP method.

Another LBP extension are Local Ternary Patterns (LTP) [5]. LTP uses three states to capture the differences between the central pixel and the neighbouring ones. Similarly to the DTLBP this method is less sensitive to the noise.

Local Derivative Patterns (LDP) are proposed in [6]. The difference from the original LBP is that it uses features of higher order. It thus can represent more information than the original approach.

Local Tetra Patterns (LTrPs) are proposed in [7]. The standard LBP and LTP encode the relationship between the reference pixel and its surrounding neighbours by computing gray-level difference. The proposed method encodes the relationship between the reference pixel and its neighbours by the directions calculated using the first-order derivatives in vertical and horizontal directions. The results on several benchmark datasets show that the performance of this method is better than the LBP, LTP and LDP.

Yang et al. propose in [8] an interesting method which uses uniform patterns. The authors state that the histogram bin containing non-uniform patterns dominates among the other bins and gives thus too much importance to this bin. Therefore they propose to assign such patterns to the closest uniform pattern.

A novel LBP based approach, patch based descriptor is proposed in [9]. The authors show that this approach improves the accuracy of the original LBP method in both multi-option identification and same/not-same classification on the LFW corpus [10]. Three-patch LBP (TPLBP) and Four-patch LBP (FPLBP) are proposed.

Zhang et al. propose in [11] Multiblock LBP (MB-LBP) which captures not only the microstructures but also the macrostructures. The main difference of this method from the original LBP is that it compares average intensities of neighbouring subregions instead of comparing individual pixels.

Mawloud et al. propose in [12] a novel alternative to the original LBP, Modied Local Binary Pattern (MLBP). This method exploits the sparsity of the representative set of MLBPs for recognition of different faces. Compressive sensing theory was employed to construct a so-called sparse representation classifier. Experimental results on three popular face databases show the superiority of the proposed method over other state-of-the-art techniques.

He et al. present in [13] a modified LBP operator with a pyramid model. In this approach, a separate output label for each uniform pattern and all non-uniform patterns is reclassified. The experiments on the AT&T and Honda/UCSD video databases show that this novel approach outperforms other related methods.

Davarzani et al. propose in [14] a weighted and adaptive LBP-based texture descriptor. This approach successfully handles some issues in the previously proposed LBP-based approaches such as invariance to scaling, rotation, viewpoint variations and non-rigid deformations. In this method, both the radius of the circular neighbourhood and the orientation of sampling in LBP descriptor are defined in adaptive manner. The authors experimentally show that this approach achieves significantly better results over other LBP-based methods.

Local Gabor Binary Pattern Histogram (LGBPH) [15,16] combines Gabor wavelets with LBP. It first filters the image with a set of Gabor filters and obtains a set of magnitude images. Then the LBP operator is applied to each of the magnitude images.

For additional information about the LBP based methods, please see the surveys [17,18].

It is worth of mentioning that in all above described LBP methods, the images are divided into rectangular regions and histograms are computed in each region. All histograms from one image are then concatenated to create the face representation.

A method that differs from the above described ones is proposed in [3]. The features are not placed on a rectangular grid. The method instead detects the feature points automatically using the Gabor wavelets. The points thus differ for each image. The dynamically determined points proved to be more suitable for images with higher amount of variations. One important part of the method is the matching scheme that compares the features individually. Chi square distance is used for vector comparison.

3   LBP with Feature to Feature Matching (LBP-FF)

Our method extends the LBP based face recognition method proposed by Ahonen [2]. The first step in the face representation creation is applying the LBP operator to the facial image. We use the $LBP_{8,2}$ operator that proved to be superior in [3]. The resulting LBP image is then divided into a set of square cells lying on a regular grid. The feature vector is composed of two parts. The first one are the coordinates of the feature point and the second one is the histogram of LBP values computed in a given cell. The coordinates of the feature point are set to the center of the cell. The resulting feature vector is thus composed of $2 + 256$ values.

3.1   Local Binary Patterns

The original LBP operator uses a 3×3 square neighbourhood centred at the given pixel. The algorithm assigns either 0 or 1 value to the 8 neighbouring pixels by Eq. 1.

$$N = \begin{cases} 0 \text{ if } g_N < g_C \\ 1 \text{ if } g_N \geq g_C \end{cases} \tag{1}$$

where N is the binary value assigned to the neighbouring pixel, g_N denotes the gray-level value of the neighbouring pixel and g_C is the gray-level value of the central pixel. The resulting values are then concatenated into an 8 bit binary number. Its decimal representation is used for further computation.

Currently, LBP is mostly used with a circular neighbourhood which is formed by a certain number of points P placed on a circle with a given diameter R. Values in the points that are not placed exactly in the centre of a pixel are interpolated from the values of neighbouring pixels. The points are compared to the central pixel in the same way as in the original descriptor. The operator is then denoted as $LBP_{P,R}$.

The value of the operator is computed by Eq. 2.

$$LBP_{P,R} = \sum_{p=1}^{P-1} s(g_p - g_c)2^p, S(x) = \begin{cases} 0 \text{ if } x < 0 \\ 1 \text{ if } x \geq 0 \end{cases} \tag{2}$$

where g_p denotes the points on the circle and g_c is the central point. The computation is illustrated by Fig. 1.

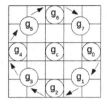

Fig. 1. Computation of LBP operator with a circular neighbourhood, P = 8, R = 2

3.2   Face Comparison

Face comparison is the main contribution of the proposed method. As stated previously, we compare the features individually instead of concatenating them into one large vector. Let T be a test image and G a gallery one. The distance of the two faces $dist_{T,G}$ is defined as:

$$dist_{T,G} = \alpha D_{T,G} + (1 - \alpha)V_G \tag{3}$$

where α is a weighting coefficient and its optimal value will be found experimentally. The first variable $D_{T,G}$ represents an average vector similarity in a given region and is defined as:

$$D_{T,G} = mean\,\{d(t,g), t \in T, g \in G(N_t)\} \tag{4}$$

where $G(N_t)$ is the neighbourhood of feature t defined by a distance threshold DT (see Eq. 5) and $d(t,g)$ is the (distance) metric used for histogram comparison. We evaluate two different metrics: Chi square distance and histogram intersection.

$$\sqrt{(x_t - x_g)^2 + (y_t - y_g)^2} \leq DT \tag{5}$$

The second variable V_G determines the face with the most similar vector to the test vector t as follows.

$$V_G = C_G/N_G \tag{6}$$

The variable C_G defines how many times the gallery face G was the closest to some of the vectors of the test face T and N_G is the number of features in the face G. Same as for the variable $D_{T,G}$, only the vectors within a neighbourhood defined by the distance threshold DT are considered.

The recognized face $\hat{G}$ is then defined as:

$$\hat{G} = \arg\min_{G}(dist(T, G)) \tag{7}$$

4   Experimental Setup

4.1   Corpora

This section briefly summarizes the face databases used for evaluation of our approach.

AT&T Database of Faces. This database [19] was formerly known as the ORL database. It was created at the AT&T Laboratories[1]. The pictures were captured between years 1992 and 1994. The database contains the faces of 40 people, 10 pictures for each person are available. Each image contains one face with a black homogeneous background. They may vary due to the different time of acquisition, head size and pose and lighting conditions. The size of pictures is 92×112 pixels. We used these images without any modification of size.

FERET Dataset. FERET dataset [20] contains 14,051 images of 1,199 individuals. The images were collected between December 1993 and August 1996. The resolution of the images is 256×384 pixels. The images are divided into the following categories according to the face pose: frontal, quarter-left, quarter-right, half-left, half-right, full-left and full-right, and they are stored in the *.tiff* format. The images are also grouped into several probe sets. The main probe sets of the frontal images are summarized in Table 1. Note that only one image per person/set is available. We used images cropped to 130×150 pixels in our experiments.

Table 1. Image numbers in the main frontal probe sets of the FERET dataset

Type	Images no.
fa	1,196
fb	1,195
fc	194
dup1	722
dup2	234

AR Face Database. AR Face Database[2] [21] was created at the Univerzitat Autonòma de Barcelona. This database contains more than 4,000 colour images of 126 individuals. The images are stored in a *raw* format and their size is 768×576 pixels. The individuals are captured under significantly different lighting conditions and with varying expressions. Another characteristic is a possible presence of glasses or scarf. In our experiments, we used images cropped to 120×165 pixels.

---

[1] http://www.cl.cam.ac.uk/research/dtg/attarchive/facedatabase.html.
[2] http://www2.ece.ohio-state.edu/~aleix/ARdatabase.html.

Czech News Agency (ČTK) Database. This database was created automatically from real-world photographs owned by the Czech News Agency and contains gray-scale images of 638 people of the size 128 × 128 pixels. All images were taken over a long time period (20 years or more) and have significant variations in pose and lighting conditions. Up to 10 images for each person are available. The testing part contains one image for each person whereas the remaining part is used for training. Note that only the testing part was checked manually. No additional cropping was performed on these images.

Figure 2 shows three example images from this corpus. The corpus is available freely for research purposes at http://ufi.kiv.zcu.cz or upon request to the authors.

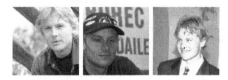

Fig. 2. Three example images from the ČTK face database

4.2 Experiments

The first series of experiments was realized on the AT&T database of faces. We used the scenario where only one image is used for training and the remaining 9 for testing. As baselines, we used the algorithm designed by Ahonen [2] and an approach based on automatically detected feature points [3]. The recognition accuracies of these two baseline approaches are 56.17 % and 68.8 % respectively. The experiments on this small dataset were performed in order to choose the best performing distance metric and to set up optimal values for the parameters of the method.

Distance Metric Determination. In the first experiment, we compare the results when Chi square distance and histogram intersection are used as distance metrics. The coefficient α is set to 0.5 and the distance threshold DT is set to 0 (only features at the same positions are compared) in this experiment. Table 2 shows the results of these two metrics for cell sizes set to 11, 13 and 15.

The table shows clearly that the histogram intersection outperforms the Chi square distance in all cases. Therefore, we use this metric in all following experiments.

Optimal Value of the α Coefficient Determination. In the second experiment, we determine an optimal value of the coefficient α (see Eq. 3). The results of this experiment are depicted in Fig. 3. We also compare the results with the distance threshold DT set to 0 and with a value that allows comparison of neighbouring cells. AT&T database is utilized in this experiment.

Table 2. Recognition accuracies in % of the Chi square distance and histogram intersection metrics on the AT&T database.

Distance	Cell size		
	11	13	15
Chi square	36.81	54.81	61.86
Histogram intersection	69.61	71.00	72.28

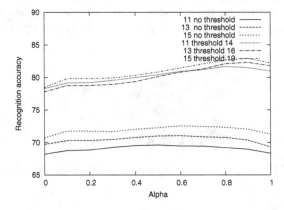

Fig. 3. Dependency of recognition accuracy on the coefficient α on the AT&T database. Histogram intersection distance is used and no distance threshold. Three values of cell size are tested.

Based on this experiment, we can conclude that:

- It is beneficial to use the distance threshold DT;
- The optimal value of the coefficient α is around 0.9.

The best obtained recognition accuracy in this experiment reached 82.92 %.

Optimal Cell Size Determination. The following experiment is realized in order to set an optimal value of the cell size. These tests are also done on the AT&T database. Figure 4 shows the dependency of recognition accuracy on the cell size. The results show that the suitable values of the cell size are $cellSize \in \langle 15; 18 \rangle$. The rapid changes at some values are caused by placing the grid on the image. In case of larger cell the cells may not correspond to the image features.

Experimental Evaluation on Three Face Datasets. In the last and the most important experiment, we would like to evaluate and compare our method with the other state-of-the-art (SoTa) approaches (see Table 3). We use two standard datasets: AR and FERET and our ČTK corpus. For the AR database, we use a scenario with 7 training and 7 testing examples for each person. The reported FERET experiments use fa set for training and fb set for testing.

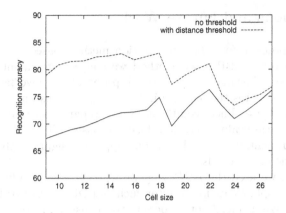

Fig. 4. Dependency of recognition accuracy on the cell size

For the ČTK dataset, we use one image for testing and the remaining ones for training. According to the previous experiments was the cell size set to 18 in all cases.

This table shows that the proposed FBP-FF method outperforms the Ahonen's baseline in all cases. Moreover, the results on AR and FERET datasets are significantly better than the method reported in [3] as well as the other reported SoTa methods.

In the case of the ČTK dataset, the scores are slightly lower. This is probably caused by the real-world character of images in this dataset where it is more important to detect the most representative feature points. It must be also mentioned that the novel method has lower computational costs than the method [3] which is an important factor for practical applications.

Table 3. Recognition accuracy in % on AR, FERET and ČTK datasets

Method	Database		
	AR	FERET	ČTK
Orig. LBP (Ahonen) [2]	87.71	93.89	39.81
DP-LBP (Lenc) [3]	97.00	98.24	59.10
Scale adaptive features [22]	92.78	98.16	-
Direct LGBPHS [15]	98.00	94.00	-
LBP + SRC [14]	96.00	-	-
LBP-FF (proposed)	99.57	99.16	57.37

5   Conclusions and Future Work

This paper proposes a novel face recognition method based on LBP features. Compared with other LBP-based method we concentrate mainly on the face comparison process. The main contribution is proposal of a novel face comparison algorithm that compares the features individually. The distance of two faces is computed as a weighted linear combination of two partial distance metrics. The proposed method was evaluated on four face databases: AT&T, AR, FERET and ČTK. We experimentally showed that our approach significantly outperforms other state of the art methods.

In this work, we used the $LBP_{8,2}$ operator. Therefore, the first perspective is to use a more sophisticated descriptor such as LDP, POEM or LQP together with our matching scheme. Another perspective consists in using other distance metrics or use weighting of the features according to its position in the face.

Acknowledgements. This work has been partly supported by the project LO1506 of the Czech Ministry of Education, Youth and Sports. We also would like to thank Czech New Agency (ČTK) for support and for providing the photographic data.

References

1. Ojala, T., Pietikäinen, M., Harwood, D.: A comparative study of texture measures with classification based on featured distributions. Pattern Recogn. **29**, 51–59 (1996)
2. Ahonen, T., Hadid, A., Pietikäinen, M.: Face recognition with local binary patterns. In: Pajdla, T., Matas, J.G. (eds.) ECCV 2004. LNCS, vol. 3021, pp. 469–481. Springer, Heidelberg (2004)
3. Lenc, L., Král, P.: Automatically detected feature positions for LBP based face recognition. In: Iliadis, L., Maglogiannis, I., Papadopoulos, H. (eds.) AIAI 2014. IFIP AICT, vol. 436, pp. 246–255. Springer, Heidelberg (2014)
4. Li, W., Fu, P., Zhou, L.: Face recognition method based on dynamic threshold local binary pattern. In: Proceedings of the 4th International Conference on Internet Multimedia Computing and Service, pp. 20–24. ACM (2012)
5. Tan, X., Triggs, B.: Enhanced local texture feature sets for face recognition under difficult lighting conditions. IEEE Trans. Image Process. **19**, 1635–1650 (2010)
6. Zhang, B., Gao, Y., Zhao, S., Liu, J.: Local derivative pattern versus local binary pattern: face recognition with high-order local pattern descriptor. IEEE Trans. Image Process. **19**, 533–544 (2010)
7. Murala, S., Maheshwari, R., Balasubramanian, R.: Local tetra patterns: a new feature descriptor for content-based image retrieval. IEEE Trans. Image Process. **21**, 2874–2886 (2012)
8. Yang, H., Wang, Y.: A lbp-based face recognition method with hamming distance constraint. In: Fourth International Conference on Image and Graphics, ICIG 2007, pp. 645–649. IEEE (2007)
9. Wolf, L., Hassner, T., Taigman, Y., et al.: Descriptor based methods in the wild. In: Workshop on Faces in 'Real-Life' Images: Detection, Alignment, and Recognition (2008)

10. Huang, G.B., Ramesh, M., Berg, T., Learned-Miller, E.: Labeled faces in the wild: a database for studying face recognition in unconstrained environments. Technical report 07–49, University of Massachusetts, Amherst (2007)
11. Zhang, L., Chu, R.F., Xiang, S., Liao, S.C., Li, S.Z.: Face detection based on multi-block LBP representation. In: Lee, S.-W., Li, S.Z. (eds.) ICB 2007. LNCS, vol. 4642, pp. 11–18. Springer, Heidelberg (2007)
12. Mawloud, G., Djamel, M.: Modified local binary pattern for human face recognition based on sparse representation. Int. J. Comput. Appl. **36**, 64–71 (2014)
13. He, W.: Improved local binary pattern with pyramid model and its application in face recognition. Int. J. Commun. Netw. Distrib. Sys. **13**, 380–390 (2014)
14. Davarzani, R., Mozaffari, S.: Robust image description with weighted and adaptive local binary pattern features. In: 2014 22nd International Conference on Pattern Recognition (ICPR), pp. 1097–1102. IEEE (2014)
15. Zhang, W., Shan, S., Gao, W., Chen, X., Zhang, H.: Local gabor binary pattern histogram sequence (lgbphs): a novel non-statistical model for face representation and recognition. In: Tenth IEEE International Conference on Computer Vision, ICCV 2005, vol. 1, pp. 786–791. IEEE (2005)
16. Xie, Z.: Single sample face recognition based on DCT and local gabor binary pattern histogram. In: Huang, D.-S., Bevilacqua, V., Figueroa, J.C., Premaratne, P. (eds.) ICIC 2013. LNCS, vol. 7995, pp. 435–442. Springer, Heidelberg (2013)
17. Huang, D., Shan, C., Ardabilian, M., Wang, Y., Chen, L.: Local binary patterns and its application to facial image analysis: a survey. IEEE Trans. Syst. Man Cybern. Part C Appl. Rev. **41**, 765–781 (2011)
18. Nanni, L., Lumini, A., Brahnam, S.: Survey on lbp based texture descriptors for image classification. Expert Syst. Appl. **39**, 3634–3641 (2012)
19. Jain, A.K., Li, S.Z. (eds.): Handbook of Face Recognition. Springer, New York (2005)
20. Phillips, P.J., Wechsler, H., Huang, J., Rauss, P.: The FERET database and evaluation procedure for face recognition algorithms. Image Vis. Comput. **16**, 295–306 (1998)
21. Martinez, A., Benavente, R.: The AR face database. Technical report, Univerzitat Autonòma de Barcelona (1998)
22. Mehta, R., Yuan, J., Egiazarian, K.: Face recognition using scale-adaptive directional and textural features. Pattern Recogn. **47**, 1846–1858 (2014)

Classification of Different Vegetation Types Combining Two Information Sources Through a Probabilistic Segmentation Approach

Francisco E. Oliva[1]([✉]), Oscar S. Dalmau[2], Teresa E. Alarcón[1],
and Miguel De-La-Torre[1]

[1] Centro Universitario de los Valles, Universidad de Guadalajara,
Ameca, Jalisco, Mexico
{francisco.oliva,teresa.alarcon,
miguel.delatorre}@profesores.valles.udg.mx
[2] Centro de Investigación en Matemáticas, Guanajuato, Mexico
dalmau@cimat.mx

Abstract. In this work we propose a new probabilistic segmentation model that allows us to combine more than one likelihood. The algorithm is applied to identify vegetation types in images from Landsat 5 satellite. Firstly, we obtain histograms from two information sources: spectral bands and principal components obtained from vegetation indices. Then, given an image, we compute two likelihoods of pixels to belong to each class (vegetation type), one for each source of information. The computed likelihoods are the inputs of the proposed probabilistic segmentation algorithm. This algorithm gives an estimation of the probability of a pixel of belonging to a class. The final segmentation is easily obtained by maximizing the estimated discrete probability for each pixel of the image. Experiments with real data show that the proposed algorithm obtains competitive results compared with state of the art algorithms.

Keywords: Probabilistic segmentation · Remote sensing · Vegetation indices · Histogram

1 Introduction

There are different approaches for extracting and classifying vegetation in remotely sensed imagery, some of them are: Artificial Neural Networks (ANNs) [32], Maximum Likelihood Classifier (ML) [22], Particle Swarm Optimization (PSO), Minimum Euclidean Distance (MED) [28], ECHO (Extraction and Classification of Homogeneous Objects) Spectral Spatial classifier (ESS) [15, 16], Fisher Linear Likelihood (FLL) [13] and probabilistic approach [21] among others. On the other hand, vegetation indices (VI) are one of the methods employed to enhance the vegetation information. These indices are a result of algebraic operations in which two or more spectral bands are combined [8]. The design of vegetation indices is based on the spectral signature of the vegetation

© Springer International Publishing Switzerland 2015
O. Pichardo Lagunas et al. (Eds.): MICAI 2015, Part II, LNAI 9414, pp. 382–392, 2015.
DOI: 10.1007/978-3-319-27101-9_29

and they are widely used to analyze and monitor temporal and spatial variations of crop patterns [30]. VIs that are computed through visible and near-infrared spectral regions such as: Normalized Difference Vegetation Index (NDVI) [26], Green Normalized Difference Vegetation Index (GNDVI) [29], Renormalized Difference Vegetation Index (RDVI) [11], Modified Simple Ratio (MSR) [11], Green Chlorophyll Index (CI) [5], Enhanced Vegetation Index (EVI) [7], Wide-Dynamic Range Vegetation Index (WDRVI) [6], Soil-Adjusted Vegetation Index (SAVI) [12], Modified SAVI (MSAVI) [2] and Atmospherically Resistant Vegetation Index (SARVI) [14] among others are indices reported to examine the different spectral responses of the crop and for assessing the influence of background soil. In [23] several vegetation indices are explored and together with textural features derived from visible, near-infrared and short-wave infrared bands of ASTER satellite, a Decision Tree [19] is constructed to classify 13 types of crops. In [30] NDVI, GNDVI and Normalized Difference Red Edge Index (NDRE) [1,33] derived from Rapid Eye imagery, are investigated and the effect of each one is studied for classification accuracy by means of a Support Vector Machine [31].

The similarity of spectral characteristic of some agricultural classes, the spectral variability of the canopy reflectance, and the bare soil background together with the presence of mixed pixels at the boundary between classes, lead to a complex process of crops classification [4,23]. For that reason the conventional pixel based methodology is not enough to discriminate different crops, and it is necessary to incorporate the contextual information to diminish the misclassification rate. The work described in [23] is an example of the technique based on objects, in order to include contextual information around the pixel. In [21] an algorithm was elaborated in which pixel information is combined with local information through a Gaussian Markov Measure Fields (GMMF) [18]. The works proposed in [21,23,30] lead to improve the discrimination of crops, however the classification accuracy could be improved. In [21], an algorithm that combines the use spectral bands with a probabilistic segmentation algorithm was presented, this approach proved to be successful in comparison with other algorithms. Based on the previous approaches and by taking into consideration the advantages of vegetation indices to examine vegetation, we propose an algorithm that combines information from different sources: spectral bands and principal components obtained from vegetation indices. For the final segmentation we propose a new probabilistic segmentation model, which is based on GMMF [18]. This new approach results in a *fusion probabilistic segmentation algorithm*. Although we apply this algorithm to detect vegetation types in remote sensing images, the formulation is more general and could be applied to other types of segmentation problems in which the feature space comes from different sources.

The structure of this work is as follows. Section 2 describes in detail of the proposed algorithm. Section 3 presents experiments along with the discussion of the results and finally, Sect. 4 presents the conclusions.

2 Classification Algorithm

The segmentation approach has three stages. In the first stage we obtained histograms from two information sources: spectral bands and principal components obtained from vegetation indices. Then, given an image, we compute two likelihoods of pixels to belong to each class (vegetation type), one for each source of information. For the final segmentation we propose a new probabilistic segmentation model, which is based on a modification to the GMMF model, that allows us to combine more than one likelihood. We explain the details in next subsections.

2.1 Histogram Computation

We propose to compute two likelihood sources. As histograms give information about the likelihood of a pixel to belong to different classes, we first compute the corresponding histogram. For that, one needs to identify the features on which to build the histogram. In particular, we use the spectral bands [21], and principal components based on vegetation indices [2,11,12,14,26,29]. On the other hand, we also use information about the classes provided by an expert, which allows us to obtain the histograms, i.e., using a supervised learning. Let us denote the normalized histogram as:

$$h(x_1, x_2, x_3; k) \propto N(x_1, x_2, x_3; k), \tag{1}$$

$$\sum_{x_1, x_2, x_3} h(x_1, x_2, x_3; k) = 1, \ \forall k \in \mathcal{K}, \tag{2}$$

where K is the number of classes, $\mathcal{K} = \{1, 2, \cdots, K\}$, (x_1, x_2, x_3) corresponds to a 3D feature vector, for example, three spectral bands; and $N(x_1, x_2, x_3; k)$ denotes the number of times the feature vector (x_1, x_2, x_3) is in class k.

Spectral-Band Histogram. In this work, we use satellite images from LANSAT-5 Thematic Mapper. Therefore, and similar to [21], we use the color scheme TM432, i.e., spectral bands TM2, TM3 and TM4; to compute the histogram based on spectral bands. This, because it is well-known that the infrared (TM4), red (TM3) and green (TM2) bands provide information related to crops and are commonly used in vegetation studies. The Spectral-Band histogram is denoted as $h_{SB}(\cdots ; \cdot)$, see Eq. (1).

PCA-Vegetation Index Histogram. To compute the histogram based on vegetation indices, denoted here as $h_{PV}(\cdots ; \cdot)$ Eq. (1)., we obtain the first 3 principal components computed on 10 vegetation indices. The vegetation indices are computed from reflectance values, ρ, of the acquired images. The reflectance values are calculated according to the algorithm in [3,9,10,25,34]. Table 1 shows the mathematical expressions for each examined spectral vegetation index where

Table 1. Explored vegetation indices. ρ_r, ρ_g, ρ_b and ρ_{NIR} denote the reflectance values for the red, blue, green and infrared bands respectively

Spectral vegetation index	Equation
MSR [11]	$\dfrac{\frac{\rho_{NIR}}{\rho_r}-1}{\sqrt{\frac{\rho_{NIR}}{\rho_r}+1}}$
CI [5]	$\dfrac{\rho_{NIR}}{\rho_g} - 1$
NDVI [30]	$\dfrac{\rho_{NIR}-\rho_r}{\rho_{NIR}+\rho_r}$
GNDVI [29]	$\dfrac{\rho_{NIR}-\rho_g}{\rho_{NIR}+\rho_g}$
EVI [7]	$2.5\left[\dfrac{\rho_{NIR}-\rho_r}{1+\rho_{NIR}+6\rho_r-7.5(\rho_b)}\right]$
SARVI [14]	$\dfrac{(1+L)(\rho_{NIR}-\rho_{rb})}{(\rho_{NIR}+R_{rb}+L)}$ $\rho_{rb}=\rho_r-\gamma(\rho_b-\rho_r)$
RDVI [11]	$\dfrac{\rho_{NIR}-\rho_r}{\sqrt{\rho_{NIR}+\rho_r}}$
SAVI [12]	$\dfrac{(1+L)(\rho_{NIR}-\rho_r)}{\rho_{NIR}+\rho_r+L}$
MSAVI [2]	$\frac{1}{2}\left[(2\rho_{NIR}+1-\sqrt{(2\rho_{NIR}+1)^2-8(\rho_{NIR}-\rho_r)})\right]$
WDRVI [6]	$\dfrac{\alpha\times\rho_{NIR}-\rho_r}{\alpha\times\rho_{NIR}+\rho_r}$

ρ_r, ρ_g, ρ_b and ρ_{NIR} denote the reflectance values for the red, blue, green and infrared bands respectively. According to [12] we considered $L = 0.5$ to compute the SAVI and SARVI expressions. The authors of SARVI [14], recommended $\gamma = 1$. The images corresponding to the computed indices are shown in Fig. 1. Observe that in the obtained images the vegetation information is enhanced. Although the first four indices provide more details about vegetation regions, all the 10 indices were considered for the PCA.

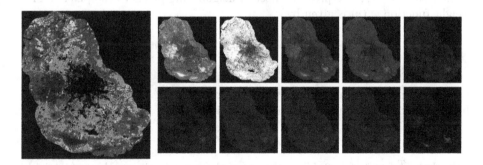

Fig. 1. Images of the calculated vegetation indices. First column contains the ground truth. The remainder columns represent: in the first row from left to right MSR, CI, NDVI, GNDVI and EVI image indices; in the second row from left to right SARVI, RDVI, SAVI, MSAVI and WDRVI image indices.

2.2 Likelihood Computation

In order to compute the likelihood of a pixel $r \in \mathcal{L}$ to belong to a class k, where $\mathcal{L}$ is the lattice of the image, one first obtains the corresponding feature vector $(x_1(r), x_2(r), x_3(r))$ and then assigns

$$v_k(r) \propto h(x_1(r), x_2(r), x_3(r); k), \tag{3}$$

such that $\sum_{k \in \mathcal{K}} v_k(r) = 1$. Note that, we need to compute the likelihood for both information sources, i.e., based on *Spectral-Band Histogram* and *PCA-Vegetation Index Histogram*.

2.3 Segmentation Approach

In the previous section, we provided two ways to compute the likelihood of pixels to belong to a class. The challenge is how to combine both information sources in order to get a good segmentation result. Here, we present a segmentation model for probabilistic segmentation, that allows us to compute the discreet probability of each pixel to belong to a class (vegetation type). This model is based on the GMMF algorithm [17] and allows us to combine two likelihoods that come from two information sources.

$$\boldsymbol{p}^* = \arg\min_{\boldsymbol{p}} \sum_{r \in \mathcal{L}} \sum_{k \in \mathcal{K}} \sum_{i=1}^{2} \omega_i(r)(p_k(r) - v_k^i(r))^2 + \lambda \sum_{s \in \mathcal{N}_r} (p_k(r) - p_k(s))^2, \tag{4}$$

where $v^i(r)$ is the likelihood that comes from the i-th source, $\lambda > 0$ is a regularization parameter, $\mathcal{N}_r$ represents a set of neighboring pixels to the pixel r. The weight function $\omega_i(r)$ is given by

$$\omega_i(r) = \begin{cases} 1 & \text{if } \mathcal{E}(v^i(r)) < \mathcal{E}(v^{3-i}(r)) \\ 0 & \text{otherwise}, \end{cases} \tag{5}$$

$i \in \{1, 2\}$ and $\mathcal{E}(\cdot)$ is an entropy measure, for example, Shanon's entropy [27]. In the experiment we use the Gini impurity index, i.e.,

$$\mathcal{E}(\boldsymbol{f}) = 1 - \boldsymbol{f}^T \boldsymbol{f}, \tag{6}$$

such that $\mathbf{1}^T \boldsymbol{f} = 1, \boldsymbol{f} \succeq 0$. The solution of the optimization problem (4) yields the following Gauss-Seidel scheme

$$p_k(r) = \frac{\sum_{i=1}^{2} \omega_i(r) v_k^i(r) + \lambda \sum_{s \in \mathcal{N}_r} p_k(s)}{1 + \lambda |\mathcal{N}_r|}. \tag{7}$$

According to Eq. (7) the weight function basically selects one likelihood for each pixel. The final segmentation is obtained by using 'the winner takes it all' strategy, i.e., given the vector field $\boldsymbol{p}^*$, Eq. (4), the segmentation is computed with the following equation:

$$s(r) = \arg\max_{k \in \mathcal{K}} p_k(r), \ \forall r \in \mathcal{L}. \tag{8}$$

In the experiment we use

$$v_k^1(r) \propto h_{SB}(x_1(r), x_2(r), x_3(r); k), \tag{9}$$
$$v_k^2(r) \propto h_{PV}(y_1(r), y_2(r), y_3(r); k), \tag{10}$$

where $(x_1(r), x_2(r), x_3(r))$, $(y_1(r), y_2(r), y_3(r))$ are 3D feature vectors obtained from the selected spectral bands and the first 3 principal components computed on 10 vegetation indices.

3   Experiments and Discussion

3.1   Study Area

The study area is located in western México at coordinates Lat. 20° 39′ 58″ N, Long. 103° 21′ 7″ W, an altitude of 1550 m above sea level, in the geographical area known as Valle de Atemajac [24]. The examined vegetation species are: irrigation agriculture (C1), seasonal agriculture (C2), forest (C3), scrub (C4), pastureland (C5), green area (C6), aquatic vegetation (C7) and riparian vegetation (C8), Fig. 2.

3.2   Data Sources

Data sources are from Landsat 5 TM satellite imagery. The images have resolution of 30 m and 2^8 radiometric resolution. The studied images correspond to March 1st 2011. Data was delivered in level 1T, in which geometric correction was applied [20]. These multispectral images were obtained from the

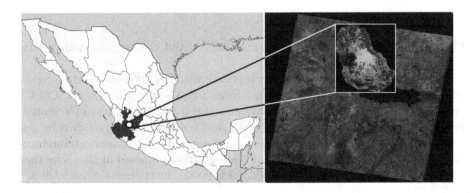

Fig. 2. Study area: Lansat-5 TM satellite image from Guadalajara Jalisco, México.

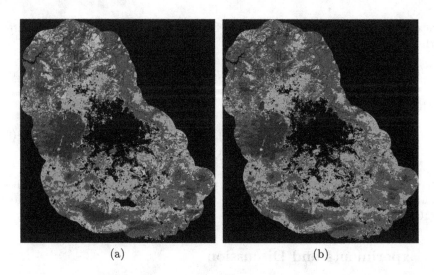

(a)   (b)

Fig. 3. (a) Ground truth, (b) segmentation result by the new proposal

Table 2. Numerical results of different classification methods

Method	C1	C2	C3	C4	C5	C6	C7	C8	Overall accuracy	Kappa
ESS	0.80	0.41	0.31	0.75	0.56	0.09	0.18	0.09	0.7773	0.6880
FLL	0.43	0.35	0.39	0.74	0.79	0.10	0.36	0.16	0.7770	0.6867
ML	0.54	0.40	0.30	0.73	0.61	0.11	0.29	0.29	0.7676	0.6751
MED	0.15	0.22	0.53	0.77	0.89	0.11	0.24	0.13	0.7721	0.6768
Proposal in [21]	0.75	0.90	0.65	0.90	0.45	0.003	0.03	0.0003	0.8962	0.8499
Our Proposal	**0.69**	**0.84**	**0.87**	**0.92**	**0.54**	**0.04**	**0.06**	**0.02**	**0.9120**	**0.8731**

USGS Global Visualization Viewer site (http://glovis.usgs.gov/). For comparison purposes and error analysis, the explored image was manually segmented by experts[1], see Fig. 3(a).

3.3 Experimental Work

Figure 3 shows the labeled image by an expert and the segmentation results obtained by our new approach.

Table 2 shows a comparison of our approach with five different reported methods, whose numerical results are taken from [21]. C1, C2, C3, C4, C5, C6, C7 and C8 denote the study classes mentioned in Sect. 3.1. According to the numerical result in Table 2, the overall accuracy and the kappa index reached by our proposal are competitive with state of the art algorithms, obtaining an improvement in both measures, with respect to the algorithm proposed in [21]. Note that the classification of classes C2, C3 and C4 is good. Nevertheless, classes C6, C7

---

[1] The experts work at Land Information Institute of Jalisco (IITEJ).

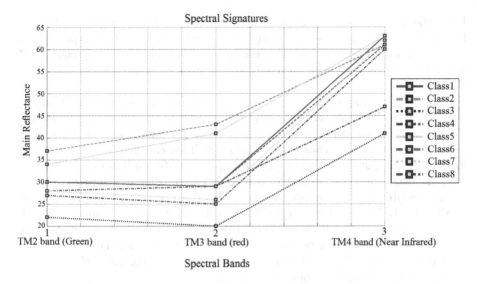

Fig. 4. Mean reflectance values for the TM432 bands for each vegetation type under study (Color figure online).

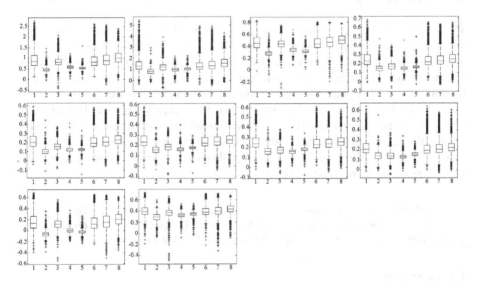

Fig. 5. Boxplot vegetation index per classes. First row (from left to right): boxplot for MSR, CI, NDVI and GNDVI indices. Second row (from left to right): EVI, SARVI, RDVI and SAVI indices. Third row (from left to right): boxplot for MSAVI and WDRVI indices.

and C8 present a poor classification. On the other hand, the algorithm presented in [21] and our approach present the worse results for classes C6, C7 and C8. In order to understand the misclassification of the proposed algorithm, we show in

Fig. 4 the mean reflectance values in the color scheme TM432 under study. The Figure depicts the spectral signatures of the eight classes for all experiments. As we can see, classes C1 and C6 overlap in some bands; similarly classes C7 and C8 appear very close in all bands, which leads to misclassification of these classes.

Furthermore, Fig. 5 depicts the boxplot by class for each vegetation index. Observe that, the mean value of class C1 is similar to the mean value of classes C6, C7 and C8; and the variance of class C1 is, for almost all indices, greater than the variance of classes C6, C7 and C8. This can help to comprise the misclassification of these classes when using the vegetation indices.

This insight allows us to take into account two possible strategies in order to tackle this problem. One alternative is a hierarchical solution, in which, for the first level only 5 classes C0 = {C1, C6, C7, C8}, C2, C3, C4, C5 are considered; and in a second level, a refinement could be carried out with the estimated C0, by classifying C0 in 4 classes. Another strategy is to improve the feature space or to propose new indices or features that discriminate better these classes. Both strategies are beyond the scope of this work.

4   Conclusions

We proposed a new probabilistic segmentation model that combines more than one likelihood. This new approach results in a *fusion probabilistic segmentation algorithm*. In this work, the algorithm was applied to detect vegetation types in remote sensing images, however, our formulation is more general and can be applied on other types of segmentation problems in which the feature space comes from different sources. In particular, for solving the segmentation of vegetation types, here we proposed to combine the information of spectral bands and principal components obtained from vegetation indices. Experiments with real images show that the proposed algorithm obtains competitive results compared with algorithms found in the literature.

Acknowledgments. We thank Maximiliano Bautista Andalón and Ana Teresa Ortega Minakata, members of Land Information Institute of Jalisco (IITEJ), for providing the ground truth images and the required information for this research.

References

1. Barnes, E.M., Clarke, T.R.: Coincident detection of crop water stress, nitrogen status and canopy density using ground based multispectral data. In: Proceedings of the Fifth International Conference on Precision Agriculture (2000)
2. Broge, N.H., Leblanc, E.: Comparing prediction power and stability of broadband and hyperspectral vegetation indices for estimation of green leaf area index and canopy chlorophyll density. Remote Sens. Environ. **76**(2), 156–172 (2001)
3. Chen, D., Huan, J., Jackson, T.J.: Vegetation water content estimation for corn and soybeans using spectral indices derived from modis near- and short-wave infrared bands. Remote Sens. Environ. **98**, 225–236 (2005)

4. De Wit, A.J.W., Clevers, J.G.P.W.: Efficiency and accuracy of per-field classification for operational crop mapping. Int. J. Remote Sens. **25**(20), 4091–4112 (2004)
5. Gitelson, A.A., Merzlyak, M.N.: Relationships between leaf chlorophyll content and spectral reflectance and algorithms for non-destructive chlorophyll assessment in higher plant leaves. J. Plant Physiol. **160**(3), 271–282 (2003)
6. Gitelson, A.A.: Wide dynamic range vegetation index for remote quantification of biophysical characteristics of vegetation. J. Plant Physiol. **161**(2), 165–173 (2004)
7. Huete, A.R., Liu, H., Batchily, K., Van Leeuwen, W.: A comparison of vegetation indices over a global set of TM images for EOS-MODIS. Elsevier **59**, 440–451 (1997)
8. Jackson, R.D., Huete, A.R.: Interpreting vegetation indices. Remote Sens. Environ. **8**(2), 185–200 (1979)
9. Ji, L., Zhang, L., Bruce, W.: Analysis of dynamic thresholds for the normalized difference water index. Photogram. Eng. Remote Sens. **75**(11), 1307–1317 (2009)
10. Jiang, H., Feng, M., Zhu, Y., Lu, N., Huang, J., Xiao, T.: An automated method for extracting rivers and lakes from landsat imagery. Remote Sens. **6**(6), 5067–5089 (2014)
11. Jordan, C.: Derivation of leaf area index from quality of light on the forest floor. Ecology **50**(4), 663–666 (1969)
12. Jordan, C.: A soil-adjusted vegetation index (SAVI). Remote Sens. Environ. **25**(3), 295–309 (1988)
13. Karakahya, H., Yazgan, B., Ersoy, O.K.: A spectral-spatial classification algorithm for multispectral remote sensing data. In: Kaynak, O., Alpaydın, E., Oja, E., Xu, L. (eds.) ICANN 2003 and ICONIP 2003. LNCS, vol. 2714, pp. 1011–1017. Springer, Heidelberg (2003)
14. Kaufman, Y., Tanre, D.: Atmospherically resistant vegetation index (ARVI) for EOS-MODIS. Geosci. Remote Sens. **30**(2), 261–270 (1992)
15. Kettig, R.L., Landgrebe, D.A.: Computer classification of remotely sensed multispectral image data by extraction and classification of homogeneous objects. IEEE Trans. Geosci. Electron. **14**(1), 19–26 (1976)
16. Landgrebe, D.: The development of a spectral-spatial classifier for earth observational data. Pattern Recogn. **12**(3), 165–175 (1980)
17. Marroquín, J.L., Botello, S., Calderón, F., Vemuri, B.C.: The MPM-MAP algorithm for image segmentation. Pattern Recogn. **1**, 303–308 (2000)
18. Marroquin, J.L., Velasco, F.A., Rivera, M., Nakamura, M.: Gauss-markov measure field models for low-level vision. IEEE Trans. Pattern Anal. Mach. Intell. **23**(4), 337–348 (2001)
19. Moore, D.M., Lees, B.G., Davey, S.M.: A new method for predicting vegetation distributions using decision tree analysis in a geographic information system. Environ. Manage. **15**(1), 59–71 (1991)
20. Northrop, A., Team, L.S.: Ideas-lansat products description document. Technical report, Telespazio VEGA UK Ltd. (2015)
21. Oliva, F.E., Dalmau, O.S., Alarcón, T.E.: A supervised segmentation algorithm for crop classification based on histograms using satellite images. In: Gelbukh, A., Espinoza, F.C., Galicia-Haro, S.N. (eds.) MICAI 2014, Part I. LNCS, vol. 8856, pp. 327–335. Springer, Heidelberg (2014)
22. Omkar, S.N., Senthilnath, J., Mudigere, D., Kumar, M.M.: Crop classification using biologically-inspired techniques with high resolution satellite image. J. Indian Soc. Remote Sens. **36**(2), 175–182 (2008)

23. Pena-Barragán, J., Ngugi, M., Plant, R., Six, J.: Object-based crop identification using multiple vegetation indices, textural features and crop phenology. Remote Sens. Environ. **115**, 1301–1316 (2011)

24. Pulido, H.G., Bautista, A.M., Guevara, R.M.: Jalisco territorio y problemas de desarrollo. iterritorial (2013)

25. Rokni, K., Ahmad, A., Selamat, A., Hazini, S.: Water feature extraction and change detection using multitemporal landsat imagery. Remote Sens. **6**(5), 4173–4189 (2014)

26. Rouse, J.W., Haas, R.H., Schell, J.A., Deering, D.W., Harlan, J.C.: Monitoring the vernal advancements and retrogradation of natural vegetation. Technical report, NASA/GSFC (1974)

27. Shannon, C.E.: A mathematical theory of communication. Bell Syst. Tech. J. **27**, 379–423 (1948)

28. Su, B., Noguchi, N.: Agricultural land use information extraction in miyajimanuma wetland area based on remote sensing imagery. Environ. Control. Biol. **50**(3), 277–287 (2012)

29. Tucker, C.J.: Red and photographic infrared linear combinations for monitoring vegetation. Remote Sens. Environ. **8**(2), 127–150 (1979)

30. Ustuner, M., Sanli, F., Abdikan, S., Esetlili, M., Kurucu, Y.: Crop type classification using vegetation indices of rapideye imagery. In: The International Archives of the Photogrammetry, Remote Sensing and Spatial Information Sciences, pp. 195–198 (2014)

31. Vapnik, V.N.: The Nature of Statistical Learning Theory. Springer, New York (2001)

32. Wang, H., Zhang, J., Xiang, K., Liu, Y.: Classification of remote sensing agricultural image by using artificial neural network. In: International Workshop on Intelligent Systems and Applications, pp. 1–4, May 2009

33. Weichelt, H., Rosso, P., Marx, A., Reigber, S., Douglass, K., Heynen, M.: The rapideye red edge band. Technical report, BlackBridge (2012)

34. Yashon, O., Tateishi, R.: A water index for rapid mapping of shoreline changes of five east african rift valley lakes: an empirical analysis using landsat TM and ETM+ data. Int. J. Remote Sens. **27**(15), 3153–3181 (2006)

Place Recognition Based Visual Localization Using LBP Feature and SVM

Yongliang Qiao$^{(\boxtimes)}$, Cindy Cappelle, and Yassine Ruichek

IRTES-SET, UTBM, 90010 Belfort Cedex, France
{yongliang.qiao,cindy.cappelle,yassine.ruichek}@utbm.fr

Abstract. This paper presents a visual localization method based on HOG-LBP and disparity information using stereo images. The method supposes the availability of a database composed with geo-referenced images of the traveling environment. Given an image, the method consists in searching the similar image in the geo-referenced database using SVM (support vector machine) image recognition model. To perform that, a global descriptor obtained by concatenating LBP (Local Binary Pattern) descriptors and HOG features built from the gray-scale image and its disparity map is constructed. Then, a SVM recognition model built on the global descriptors was used to identify the top best similar images. The matched image (from the reference database) to the given image is finally determined using a probability threshold. If no candidate can be selected, the current position is estimated by extrapolating the previous known positions. The integration of disparity information into HOG-LBP is valuable to decrease perceptual aliasing problems in case of bidirectional trajectory situation. To show its effectiveness, the proposed method is tested and evaluated using real data sets acquired in outdoor environments.

Keywords: Visual localization · SVM · Place recogntion · LBP · HOG · Disparity map

1 Introduction

Visual localization is a challenging problem for developing ADAS (Advanced Driver Assistance Systems) and/or unmanned driving cars. In this context, each location is represent by an image, localization can be achieved through visual (place) recognition. One of the typical approaches is adopting image matching (retrieval) method [4,5,8] to recognize geo-referenced places of the traveling environment. Some works like FAB-MAP [4] and SeqSLAM [9] have been proposed in the past years. However, most of these works exhibit a high computation cost and large storage due to complex feature extraction or image matching.

During the last several years, local binary patterns (LBP) [10], as one of the widely used binary descriptors, which is invariant to monotonic changes in grayscale and fast to calculate, has achieved good performance in image description and visual recognition [1]. Using binary codes, the computation and storage are

© Springer International Publishing Switzerland 2015
O. Pichardo Lagunas et al. (Eds.): MICAI 2015, Part II, LNAI 9414, pp. 393–404, 2015.
DOI: 10.1007/978-3-319-27101-9_30

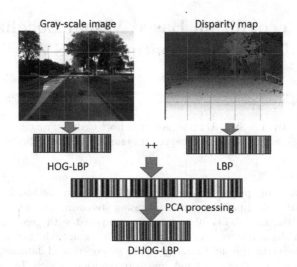

Fig. 1. Block based D-HOG-LBP descriptor built from gray-scale image and its disparity map.

more efficient and effective than non binary descriptors like SIFT or SURF. This makes them applicable in mobile devices or small smart agents with low processing and storage capacities [1].

In this paper, a novel visual localization approach is proposed based on stereo images using an augmented descriptor D-HOG-LBP as illustrated in Fig. 1. D-HOG-LBP feature, which is built from gray-scale image and its disparity map, incorporates texture, shape and disparity information that help to reduce some typical problems related to visual place recognition, such as perceptual aliasing. The descriptor extraction process is based on image blocks. Principal Component Analysis (PCA) is used to further reduce data dimension. Basing on the constructed descriptor, visual place recognition is achieved by SVM recognition modeling.

2   Related Works

Due to cheap and easy-use, visual sensor can be a complementary or alternative option for localization with respect to other sensing techniques such as LiDAR-based or GPS-based. Vehicle localization based on vision approaches enable to recover vehicle current position from a reference database.

FAB-MAP [4] can be considered as the milestone in visual topological localization methods for detecting loop closures. It employs Bag-of-Words (BOW) and Chow-Liu trees algorithm to measure the co-occurring visual words to achieve robust image matching.

Some related image retrieval works use binary descriptors. Local binary patterns (LBP) has been popularized in texture classification, face recognition and image retrieval [12]. LBP is invariant to monotonic changes in gray-scale and fast to calculate. Its efficiency originates from the detection of different micro patterns (edges, points, constant areas etc.). HOG as one of the best features to capture edge or local shape information also has been widely used. HOG-LBP feature resulting from the combination of HOG feature and LBP feature is also used in the literature to take simultaneously into account texture and shape information.

Apart from texture and shape information provided by HOG-LBP, disparity information from scene is also interesting for place recognition. Some works use 3D information to improve performance of vision-based navigation methods, such as [2,3]. In [2], the author proposed a SLAM system that combines both appearance and 3-D geometric information. However, the calculation and matching 3D information is associated with a high computational cost. For this reason, an augmented feature vector (D-HOG-LBP), proposed in our work, is a promising approach, since 3D information is efficiently integrated in the binary descriptor, improving place recognition performance.

3   Proposed Vehicle Localization Approach

The proposed localization approach uses pairs of images acquired by a stereo camera. Given a current query image, the objective is to find the matching image from a reference database containing geo-referenced images. The whole system proposed in this paper is outlined in Fig. 2.

Our proposed system is composed of two phases: training and testing. Training consists of constructing a reference database composed of geo-referenced images acquired by the stereo set-up when the vehicle traversed a path at the first time. Both in training and testing phases, each image is characterized by a global descriptor D-HOG-LBP (HOG-LBP extracted from the gray-scale image, and LBP descriptor extracted from its disparity map). Given a current query image in the testing phase, we start by searching from the reference database a set of potential matching images using an image retrieval circle, calculated from the previous vehicle position. This set of reference images is then used to

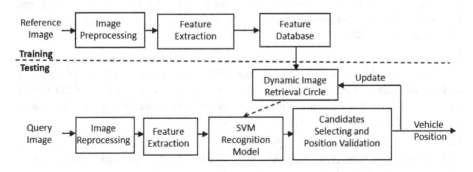

Fig. 2. Architecture of the proposed system

train a SVM model. This allows to reduce learning/searching processing time and matching ambiguities.

When the query image is applied to the SVM model, we obtain a confidence value for each potential candidate. A thresholding validation procedure is finally applied to select the best candidate image.

3.1   Image Preprocessing and Feature Extraction

For decreasing computation time, the original color images are converted into 640×480 gray-scale images. At each acquisition time, we have stereo images. HOG-LBP extraction is applied to the left gray-scale image and LBP feature is extracted from its disparity map. Here disparity map is calculated using the SGBM (Semi-Global Block Matching) algorithm [7]. In order to describe large scale structure (macro-structure), D-HOG-LBP feature is computed using blocks.

LBP: The generalized LBP definition is used with N sample points evenly distributed on a radius R around a center pixel located at (x_c, y_c). The position (x_p, y_p) of the neighbor points, where $p \in \{0, ..., N-1\}$, is given by:

$$(x_p, y_p) = (x_c + Rcos(2\pi/N), y_c - Rsin(2\pi/N)) \tag{1}$$

The local binary code for the pixel (x_c, y_c) can be computed by comparing its gray-scale value g_c and its neighbor pixel gray-scale values g_p. The value of the LBP at the pixel (x_c, y_c) is given by:

$$LBP_{N,R}(x_c, y_c) = \sum_{p=0}^{N-1} s(g_p - g_c)2^p \tag{2}$$

where

$$s(x) = \begin{cases} 1, & x \geq 0 \\ 0, & otherwise \end{cases} \tag{3}$$

In our work, we set N to 8 sampling points and radius R to 3 pixels around the center pixel to get the LBP feature. The computed LBP pattern is uniform patterns "U2" (U refers to the measure of uniformity, 2 is the number of 0/1 and 1/0 transitions in the circular binary code pattern) which decreases the original 256 dimension to 59.

HOG: For HOG feature computation, the size of the cell is 8×8 pixels and the size of the block is the same as for LBP, the direction of the gradient at each pixel is discretized into 9 bins. For each pixel, the gradient is a 2D vector with a real-valued magnitude and a discretized direction (9 possible directions uniformly distributed in $[0, \pi]$).

D-HOG-LBP: Each image can be represented using a single vector v (D-HOG-LBP feature) by concatenating the block features from gray-scale image and its disparity map, as the following equation shows:

$$v = P_1 ++ P_2 ++ ... ++ P_s ++ Q_1 ++ Q_2 ++ ... ++ Q_k \tag{4}$$

where $++$ means concatenation, P_i is HOG-LBP feature of the ith block and s is the block number in the gray-scale image. Q_i is LBP feature of the ith block obtained from disparity map and k is the block number in the disparity map. Here, due to removing the "black area" in the disparity map, s and k are not identical.

Since the vector v is a high dimension data, principal component analysis (PCA) is also performed to reduce the data dimension (as shown in Fig. 1).

3.2   Image Recognition Model Based on SVM

Support Vector Machine: SVM are state-of-the-art discriminative classifiers which have recently gained popularity within visual pattern recognition [11]. Consider separating positive and negative place matches (x_1, y_1), (x_2, y_2), $\cdots$ (x_m, y_m) into two classes, where $x_i \in R^N$ is a feature vector and $y_i \in \{-1, 1\}$ is its class label.

If we assume that the two classes can be separated by a hyperplane in Hilbert space H, search for the optimal hyperplane that maximizes the margin (distance) to the closest points in the training data, can be regarded as a constrained minimization problem, using Lagrange multipliers $\alpha_i (i = 1, ...m)$:

$$f(x) = \sum_{i=1}^{m} \alpha_i y_i K(x_i, x) + b \tag{5}$$

The sign of $f(x)$ indicates the classification result, α_i and b are found by using sequential minimal optimization (SMO) algorithm. The x_i with nonzero α_i are the "support vectors".

The Kernel $K(x_i, x)$ maps the input data into a high dimension space H where the non-linearly separable data may be separated linearly. In our work, sigmoid kernel was selected after comparing four different kernel types (RBF, polynomial, linear and sigmoid).

Dynamic Image Retrieval Circle: In order to improve recognition accuracy and time searching, SVM recognition models were built on a subset of reference images from the training database rather than on the whole database. For that, a searching circle centered at the last known vehicle position is used. If the chosen radius of searching circle is too wide, it will lead to time-consuming and if it is to small, it will be hard to guarantee that the target reference image is included in. In this paper, we set the searching circle radius to 10 m according to our experiment. Given a query image, we consider that its corresponding reference image is in the defined local searching circle. As Fig. 3 shows, the reference images in the searching circle were selected according to the tagged GPS information and the last estimated vehicle position (at time t-1). The searching circle is dynamic since the vehicle moves.

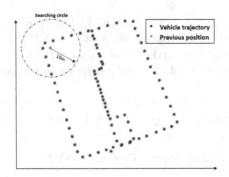

Fig. 3. Example of an image searching circle

Dynamic SVM Recognition Model: For a given query image (from test-ing database), suppose that there are M reference images (potential matching images) from training database in the searching circle. Then M SVM models are constructed for these reference images. For each reference image, the SVM recog-nition model is constructed by labeling the current reference image as $Y=+1$ and the remaining reference images as $Y=-1$, as shown in Fig. 4. For each SVM model, the input predictor matrix X is composed of D-HOG-LBP features of the reference images.

After the training step, the D-HOG-LBP feature of the query image is used as the input predictor matrix for the M SVM models, and M probability values are obtained, each one representing a matching confidence measure between the query image and a reference one. The best candidate for matching is the reference image with highest confidence value.

Best Candidate Validation: To accept the best matching candidate defi-nitely, we set a reliable threshold to guarantee precise results. The confidence value, which is originally in the range [-1 1], is converted to the range [0 1]. If the confidence value is larger than a threshold T, then the matching candidate is validated; otherwise it is rejected. The threshold T is set experimentally to 0.28. It is noted that the value 0.28 is a strict threshold that guarantees the validated candidates are true positives. Then the vehicle position can be get according to the GPS measurements of the matched reference image. If no candidate is validated, the position is estimated according to the last known positions using extrapolation technique.

4   Experimental Results

The proposed method is tested with real data acquired by our experimental GEM vehicle equipped with a stereoscopic Bumblebee XB3 system (16 Hz, image size is 1280×960), a RTK-GPS receiver (10 Hz) and two SICK LMS221 laser range

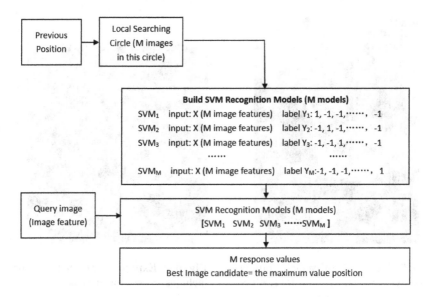

Fig. 4. SVM recognition method

finders, as shown in Fig. 5. In this paper, we just use the left and right cameras of the stereoscopic Bumblebee XB3 system. The camera field of view (FOV) is 66°. For fast computation, the original images are converted into 640×480 gray-scale images.

During the training database acquisition, the experimental vehicle traversed about 4 Km in a typical outdoor environment, which is surrounded by lake, trees, factories and buildings. As shown in Fig. 6, in the traveled trajectory, three typical areas are traversed: urban city road (area A), lots of factories building (area B) and a nature scene surrounding a lake (area C). Data for training and testing were acquired and stored at different times.

The training and testing data were collected respectively in 2014/9/11 and 2014/9/5 independently. The training database is composed of 849 images while the testing database is composed of 819 images. The average distance interval between two successive frames was around 3.5 m. To tag the reference images (training database), GPS position of each image is obtained by RTK-GPS.

Place recognition experiment was conducted in unidirectional and bidirectional driving situations. Our proposed method is also compared with the FAB-MAP method [4]. Here, we use the OpenFABMAP code [6] and focus on its recognition performance at 100 % precision.

4.1   Place Recognition in Unidirectional Driving Situation

In this part, we firstly focus on the unidirectional driving situation (areas A and C in Fig. 6). The visual localization results are shown in Fig. 7 (area A) and Fig. 8 (area C).

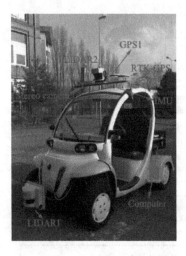

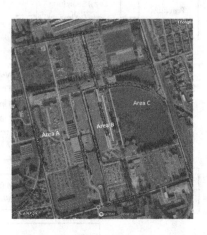

Fig. 5. Experimental vehicle equipped with sensors (camera and RTK-GPS)

Fig. 6. Experimental field which includes three typical areas

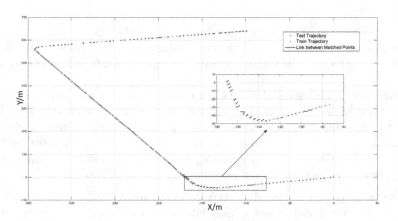

Fig. 7. Appearance-based matching results within the area A. Training and testing locations are marked by black "." and green "+" respectively. Two correct image matches coming from the same location are joined with a red line (Color figure online).

In Table 1, image recognition rates of our approach and FAB-MAP method were compared. It can be seen that with 32×32 block size our approach achieves 64.22 % in area A and 68.36 % in area C. More smaller block sizes can obtain more better performance. This is easy to understand because more blocks can bring more image local spatial information. One can see that the result of our approach outperforms FAB-MAP method.

Table 1. Image recognition results in unidirectional driving situation

Method	Recognition rate in area A (%)	Recognition rate in area C (%)
D-HOG-LBP (Block size:16×16)	156/232 (67.24)	183/256 (71.48)
D-HOG-LBP (Block size:24×24)	154/232 (66.38)	181/256 (70.70)
D-HOG-LBP (Block size:32×32)	149/232 (64.22)	175/256 (68.36)
FAB-MAP	120/232 (52.16)	137/256 (53.52)

Also it can be noted that the D-HOG-LBP feature with the SVM classification method has good recognition rate in the area C when compared to the results in the area A. This is due to the nature of scenes within the area C which contain more local texture information than in the area A. We can see that when the block size increases the place recognition rate decreases. However, by decreasing the block size, the number of blocks increases and thus the computation time increases also.

4.2 Place Recognition in Bidirectional Driving Situation

In the most place recognition methods, bidirectional driving situation, which may lead to ambiguous matching, is not considered. In this part, we test our proposed method in the area B (see Fig. 6) which includes a bidirectional driving trajectory. The visual localization results are shown in Fig. 9 and the image matching rates are reported in Table 2.

As can be seen, in bidirectional environment, the average recognition rate is lower for the unidirectional situation. However, our method improves place recognition compared to the state-of-art FAB-MAP method. This is due to the fact that FAB-MAP method uses SURF descriptor which can not distinguish the same scene image taken from two directions as shown in the example of Fig. 10.

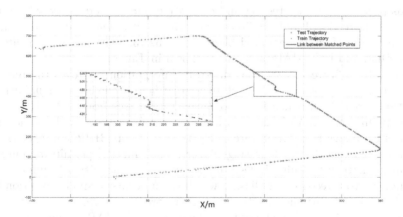

Fig. 8. Appearance-based matching results within the area C. Training and testing locations are marked by black "." and green "+" respectively. Two correct image matches coming from the same location are joined with a red line (Color figure online).

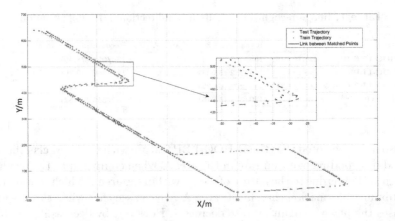

Fig. 9. Appearance-based matching results within the area B. Training and testing locations are marked by black "." and green "+" respectively. Two correct image matches coming from the same location are joined with a red line (Color figure online).

Table 2. Image recognition results in bidirectional driving situation

Method	Recognition rate in area B (%)
D-HOG-LBP (Block size:16×16)	202/331 (61.03)
D-HOG-LBP (Block size:24×24)	184/331 (55.59)
D-HOG-LBP (Block size:32×32)	183/331 (55.29)
FAB-MAP	103/331 (31.12)

4.3   Place Recognition Results in Whole Field

In this part, we focus on testing and evaluating our method in the whole field with the bidirectional and unidirectional driving situations, with and without disparity map. Here, the adopted block size is 32×32. The recognition rates of our method and FAB-MAP method are shown in Table 3.

From Table 3, we can see that disparity information improves the recognition rates in each area. Especially, it gives great help in the bidirectional driving situation (area B) in which the recognition rate passes from 30.82 %, without disparity information, to 55.29 % with disparity information. At the same time, the average image recognition rate of FAB-MAP is only 31.12 % in area B. We can thus conclude that integrating disparity information permits to improve the image matching results. Indeed, image matching with disparity information permits to avoid recognition aliasing which often occurs in similar position but from two opposite driving directions. Furthermore, the average recognition rate of our method (61.90 %) is higher than the one of FAB-MAP method (43.96 %). Hence, the proposed method outperforms the FAB-MAP method and demonstrates more robust results in different typical areas and situations.

Table 3. Image recognition rates with and without disparity map in three different areas

Method	Area A (%)	Area B (%)	Area C (%)	Average (%)
With disparity map (D-HOG-LBP)	149/232 (64.22)	183/331 (55.29)	175/256 (68.36)	507/819 (61.90)
Without disparity map (HOG-LBP)	138/232 (59.48)	102/331 (30.82)	163/256 (63.67)	403/819 (49.21)
FAB-MAP	120/232 (52.16)	103/331 (31.12)	137/256 (53.52)	360/819 (43.96)

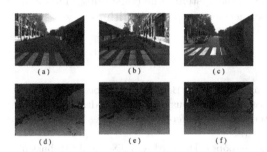

Fig. 10. Disparity map in the bidirectional driving situation. Image (a), (b), (c) are the camera acquired images and (d), (e), (f) are their corresponding disparity maps. It is noted that image (a) and (c) are taken from the same driving direction while the image (b) taken from the opposite direction

As Fig. 10 shows, image (a) and image (c) are taken from the same direction while the image (b) is taken from the opposite direction. When using traditional features like SIFT or SURF, these three images may be matched, because their visual content represents almost the same image context and then their SIFT or SURF descriptors will be very close.

Although disparity information based improvement, the recognition rate is still low due to two main reasons. The first is that the distance interval between two successive images is little small, overlapping parts make the image distinguishing more difficult. The second reason is that the view of our camera is not wide enough and the images are taken with front view, so there are not enough discriminating information.

5 Conclusion

In this paper, we presented a vehicle localization based on place recognition using stereo vision. The proposed method consists in matching reference (geo-referenced) and testing images thanks to a SVM recognition model using D-HOG-LBP features built from gray-scale images and their disparity maps. The experimental tests conducted in different typical outdoor areas showed that our method is effective and the integration of disparity information is very useful especial in bidirectional situation where it is more difficult to discriminate between scenes acquired in opposite directions. The proposed place recognition method was also compared to the state-of-the-art FAB-MAP method. The evaluation demonstrated that our method outperforms the FAB-MAP method.

In our method, the image searching is performed in a fixed local range with the assumption that vehicle is moving at a constant speed. The dynamic of searching range can be improved in future work by adjusting it according to the vehicle speed. Furthermore, our method builds SVM model at each given query image, making the whole system time-consuming. This issue can be solved by using GPU or other accelerate speed algorithms.

References

1. Arroyo, R., Alcantarilla, P.F., Bergasa, L., Yebes, J.J., Bronte, S.: Fast and effective visual place recognition using binary codes and disparity information. In: IEEE/RSJ International Conference on Intelligent Robots and Systems (IROS), pp. 3089–3094 (2014)
2. Cadena, C., Gálvez-López, D., Tardós, J., Neira, J.: Robust place recognition with stereo sequences. IEEE Trans. Robot. 28(4), 871–885 (2012)
3. Chong, Z., Qin, B., Bandyopadhyay, T., Ang, M., Frazzoli, E., Rus, D.: Synthetic 2D LIDAR for precise vehicle localization in 3D urban environment. In: IEEE International Conference on Robotics and Automation (ICRA), pp. 1554–1559 (2013)
4. Cummins, M., Newman, P.: Fab-map: probabilistic localization and mapping in the space of appearance. Int. J. Robot. Res. 27(6), 647–665 (2008)
5. Glover, A., Maddern, W., Milford, M.J., Wyeth, G.: FAB-MAP+ RatSLAM: appearance-based SLAM for multiple times of day. In: IEEE International Conference on Robotics and Automation (ICRA), pp. 3507–3512 (2010)
6. Glover, A., Maddern, W., Warren, M., Reid, S., Milford, M., Wyeth, G.: Openfabmap: an open source toolbox for appearance-based loop closure detection. In: 2012 IEEE International Conference on Robotics and Automation (ICRA), pp. 4730–4735, May 2012
7. Hirschmuller, H.: Stereo processing by semiglobal matching and mutual information. IEEE Trans. Pattern Anal. Mach. Intell. 30(2), 328–341 (2008)
8. Johns, E., Yang, G.: Dynamic scene models for incremental, long-term, appearance-based localisation. In: IEEE International Conference on Robotics and Automation (ICRA), pp. 2731–2736 (2013)
9. Milford, M., Wyeth, G.: SeqSLAM: visual route-based navigation for sunny summer days and stormy winter nights. In: IEEE International Conference on Robotics and Automation (ICRA), pp. 1643–1649 (2012)
10. Ojala, T., Pietikäinen, M., Harwood, D.: A comparative study of texture measures with classification based on featured distributions. Pattern Recogn. 29(1), 51–59 (1996)
11. Schuldt, C., Laptev, I., Caputo, B.: Recognizing human actions: a local SVM approach. In: 2004 Proceedings of the 17th International Conference on Pattern Recognition, ICPR 2004, vol. 3, pp. 32–36. IEEE (2004)
12. Yuan, X., Yu, J., Qin, Z., Wan, T.: A SIFT-LBP image retrieval model based on bag of features. In: IEEE International Conference on Image Processing (2011)

Search and Optimization

TSP in Partitioning with Tabu Search

María Beatríz Bernábe-Loranca[1(✉)], Rogelio González Velázquez[1],
Martín Estrada Analco[1], Alejandro Fuentes Penna[1,2],
Ocotlan Díaz Parra[2], and Abraham Sánchez López[1]

[1] Facultad de Ciencias de la Computación,
Benemérita Universidad Autónoma de Puebla, Puebla, Mexico
beatriz.bernabe@gmail.com
[2] Universidad Autónoma del Estado de Hidalgo, Pachuca, Hidalgo, Mexico

Abstract. Solving Territorial Design problems implies grouping territorial units into k of groups with compactness and/or contiguity restrictions. However each group formed is often treated in accordance to a conflict of interest; one of them is the routing problem. In this work grouping geographical units is also known as classification by partitions, which is a well-known high complexity problem. This complexity requires reaching approximated partitioning solutions of the territory in a reasonable computing time; therefore we have chosen the tabu search metaheuristic because it has achieved very efficient results in several optimization problems. Once tabu search has returned a solution, we apply an exact algorithm to the elements of the partition, which solves a routing problem.

Keywords: Tabu search · Territorial design · Traveling salesman problem

1 Introduction

Zone design occurs when small areas or geographical units must be grouped into acceptable zones according to the requirements imposed by the problem under study. Depending on the context, these requirements can include the generation of connected zones with the same amount of habitants, clients, communication means, public services, etc. Zone design appears in diverse applications such as the creation of school zones, zones with appropriate characteristics for socio-economic analysis, sales territories design, services or maintenance and geographic design for censuses. In general, zone design or Territorial Design (TD) is a problem present in geographical tasks and requires taking into account multiple objectives and/or restrictions, which implies that this problem is particularly hard due to the size of the solutions space. Even for a small number of geographical units and zones, the amount of possible configurations can be considerably high. On the other hand, when the zones have been designed with a clustering method, they must be analyzed in accordance to a specific objective, such as routing, and this implies the need to apply a routing algorithm adequate to the problem.

One of the most common applications of the routing problem is attaining an efficient minimum cost route in the supply chain. For example, the classic Vehicle Routing Problem (VRP), one of the most demanded problems, has classic restrictions such as satisfying customers' demand where the vehicles can visit several clients in one

© Springer International Publishing Switzerland 2015
O. Pichardo Lagunas et al. (Eds.): MICAI 2015, Part II, LNAI 9414, pp. 407–421, 2015.
DOI: 10.1007/978-3-319-27101-9_31

trip. The VRP can be reduced to finding the shortest way possible traveled by the vehicles while employing the minimum amount of these. In the classic interpretation of the (VRP), connections between clients are allowed, providing a complete graph, but it has been given little attention to the problem of an incomplete network or when there aren't connections between all the nodes or customers. VRP is an NP-Complete problem [1], and only small instances can be solved in a reasonable amount of time by exact methods. Our work is focused on this point considering two phases to solve a routing problem: First the territorial design is solved under geometric compactness restrictions using a partitioning algorithm. Considering that this is an NP-Complete problem, employing a heuristic is necessary, and after analyzing several proposals we have chosen tabu search (TS) because of its capability to attain good solutions in a reasonable amount of time for several problems [2]. The second phase consist of applying a routing procedure to every partition, using the traveling salesman problem (TSP) model while omitting sub-tours to optimize the best one, this was solved with an optimization software in an exact way. To test our methodology we chose a map with 469 objects; Toluca city, Mexico.

The following work is organized as follows: this introduction is Sect. 1. In Sect. 2 the territorial partitioning problem is exposed. Section 3 explains the tabu search methodology and Sect. 4 presents a TS approximation method to find a partition of a territory. Finally, Sect. 5 shows the application of the routing with TSP and conclusions are discussed in Sect. 6.

2 The Territorial Design Problem and Partitioning of Geographical Units

TD problems are generally presented from different points of view due to the multiple applications it can have, however common and essential factors exist to solve this kind of problems. Among the most common factors, two are essential: the definitions and the mathematical models, the ones that have been important in this area and they're usually employed as a support. Furthermore, it can be observed in the TD literature that authors propose terms that can originate diverse interpretations: regionalization, zonification, territorial distribution, zone categorization, territorial aggregation, territorial ordering, regional design and even territorial lining. Nonetheless, the terminology doesn't make any noticeable conceptual differences between each other. The territory design also known as zone design problem (ZD), may be viewed as the problem of grouping small geographic coverage units into larger geographic clusters called territories such that the territories are acceptable according to managerially relevant alignment criteria. Depending on the context, these criteria can have economical motive (potential sales average, workload or number of salespeople) or they can have a demo-graphic background (number of habitants, people that can vote). At this stage, concepts like spatial restrictions, contiguity and compactness are formalized and required [3, 4]. Zone design is a complex geographic problem present in several geographic tasks. The geographic zones design occurs when n area units are aggregated into k zones such that the value of a function is optimized, depending on the restrictions over the topology of the zones (for example internal connectivity). The ZD solution requires a process that classifies zones based on restrictions, where the grouping generally forces the comparison of several configurations, and then the problem becomes NP-hard [5]; therefore an optimization model supported on a metaheuristic is needed to obtain a good grouping/solution.

To deal with the zone design problem, we must analyze diverse algorithms al-ready proposed to solve it. There are two important problems in the application of the automatic algorithms for zone design. First, most of the algorithms described in the literature aren't available due to the fact that most of them are a product of research efforts and most of these weren't released as software packages. Secondly, most of the algorithms are based on a regional perspective of the zone design problem; this means that they use entire areas whereas the basic units aren't well determined for the zone they design. However, currently some algorithmic proposals more or less clear are available for zone design and they employ several optimization strategies, including simulated annealing, tabu search, and lineal programming associated to branch and bound [6, 7]. The genetic algorithms (GA) [5, 8] still are pretty much unexplored in this field, a good reference is [5], but it doesn't provide details about how the GA was applied to this particular problem. Still, GA has been extensively used as search procedure in related fields such as the P-Median problem [9]. The design of districts for electoral processes is one of the most demanded applications of TD and consist in partitioning area units (usually administrative units), into a predetermined number of zones (districts) such that the units in every zone are contiguous, geographically compact and the sum of the population of the area units in every district is as homogeneous as possible or with a certain tolerance within a predetermined range [6]. We assume the importance of this definition resides in its simplicity and flexibility that allows it to be adjusted to other similar problems, for example, commercial or sales territories design. On this stage we locate our work: we propose an algorithm that solves geometric compactness while it partitions a territory with TS. The territory under study is formed by geographic units called Agebs (an acronym in Spanish which means basic geo-statistical areas). This Agebs partitioning algorithm minimizes the interclass distance in the objective function, which guarantees that the elements of the partition formed are very close to its distribution center. However, once the Agebs clusters have been obtained, it is important to treat these groups in accordance with a routing problem. It is assumed that from the distribution centers, the most optimal route must be given to the salespeople to optimize costs, at this stage, a routing algorithm is necessary. This routing is solved employing a TSP algorithm without subtours, implemented in Lingo, which ensures it provides an optimal route.

2.1 Modeling in Geographic Partitioning

Partitioning as an optimization method produces a unique partition of the objects into a particular number (k) of non-overlapping clusters, as a result of minimizing or maximizing an objective function. Usually, these methods start with an initial partition of the set of objects into k clusters, for each cluster a centroid (representative) is defined, and then each object is allocated into the cluster that has the nearest centroid, afterwards a new set of centroids is generated (randomly or strategically, one or more new centroids) and each object is reallocated accordingly. This recalculation continues until there aren't any changes in the clusters or no further improvement is made.

Generally, the objects are represented by D descriptive attributes in the form of vectors in the R^D space, and by a similarity comparison measure, such as distance to create clusters formed by similar objects. In the clustering of the information, a series of variables for every object is used and in accordance with them, the similarity between the objects is measured. Once the similarity has been determined, the objects are gathered into internally homogeneous groups but different to one another. The similarity measures depend on the assumptions and the use that is given to the data; different results from the same data can obtained due to the use of different similarity measures, where each one of them can be equally valid for a particular goal.

In the classification by partitions we have $\Omega = \{X_1, X_2, \ldots, X_n\}$ as the set of n objects to classify and $k \in \mathbb{N}$, the number of classes, in which the objects will be classified and $k < n$. One partition $P = \{C_1, C_2, \ldots, C_k\}$ of Ω into k classes is characterized by the following two conditions, the first $\Omega = \bigcap_{i=1}^{k} C_i$, and the second $C_i \cap C_j, \forall i \neq j$. For our partitioning problem, let Ω be a set of n geographical objects named Agebs in the form of $X_i = (x_{i1}, x_{i2}, \ldots x_{iD})$, are vectors with D components, and let k be an integer number known beforehand. The clustering problem consists in finding a partition P of Ω such that $|P| = k$ and that minimices the Euclidean distance between objetos, defined as similarity function between the Agebs and denoted by

$d(X_i, X_j) = \sqrt{\sum_{l=1}^{D} (x_{il}, x_{jl})^2}$, therefore the objective function of the combinatory optimization problem to form compact groups is:

$$\sum_{C_i \in P} \sum_{X_i \in C_i} d(X_i, X_{C_i})$$

Where X_{C_i} is the representative Ageb of C_i.

The previous formulation can be implemented with diverse programming languages using heuristic methods. In previous works we have incorporated simulated annealing (SA) and variable neighborhood search (VNS) where several statistical tests proved that VNS obtains better results, considering time and quality [10]. In this work we have propose tabu search as approximation method and with some random tests we have observed that it obtains better approximations for TD partitioning than the heuristics previously implemented.

3   Tabu Search

The origins of tabu search can be traced back to several works published in the late 1970's. Officially, the name and the methodology were introduced by Fred Glover and Manuel Laguna in 1989 in the book tabu search [2, 11]. The philosophy behind TS is to derive and exploit a collection of intelligent principles to solve problems. On this sense, it can be said that TS is based on select concepts that unite the artificial intelligence and optimization fields.

TS is a metaheuristic that guides a local search heuristic to explore the solution space beyond local optima. The local procedure is a search that uses an operation named "move" to define the neighborhood of any given solution. One of its main elements is the use of adaptive memory, which creates a more flexible search behavior. This memory based strategy is a distinctive point of tabu search approaches. Furthermore TS imposes restrictions to guide the search process to reach regions that would be hard to access otherwise. The restrictions are imposed or created by making reference to memory structures designed for this specific purpose. The restrictions work over the local searches (LS), which have a tendency to become stuck in suboptimal regions or on plateaus, to break out of these difficult areas. TS translates the restrictions into memory structures that describe the visited solutions or attributes of it in order to get stuck in the same areas of the solution space [2]. If a latent solution has been previously visited within a certain short period of time or if it has violated a rule, it is marked as "tabu" (forbidden) so it isn't considered repeatedly. TS uses LS or a neighborhood search procedure to move iteratively from one potential solution x to an improved solution x' within the neighborhood of x, until a stopping criterion has been fulfilled. The memory structures form what is known as the tabu list, a set of rules, attributes and/or banned solutions used to filter which solutions will be explored in the neighborhood $N*(x)$. In its simplest form, a tabu list is a short-term set of the solutions that have been visited in the recent past (less than l iterations ago).

Different memory structures can be used in TS: (a) Short-term: The list of solutions recently considered. If a potential solution appears on this list, it cannot be revisited until it reaches an expiration point, (b) Intermediate-term: A list of rules intended to bias the search towards promising areas of the search space and (c) Long-term: Rules that promote diversity in the search process (i.e. regarding restarts when the search becomes stuck in a plateau or a suboptimal area).

On the other hand, TS has weaknesses as well, a major issue is that it is only effective in discrete spaces. Another problem with TS is that if the search space is very large or of high dimensionality, it can be easy to get stuck in a small area of the search space. To work around this pitfall, is important to create a tabu list consisting of the attributes of a solution, rather than complete candidate solutions [2]. The tabu lists containing attributes (rather than entire solutions) can be more effective for some domains, although they raise a new problem; when a single attribute is marked as tabu, this typically results in more solutions becoming tabu as well. Some of these solutions that must be avoided could be of excellent quality and might not be visited. Nonetheless, there's a solution to mitigate this problem, the "aspiration criteria", which override the tabu state of a solution, thereby including the otherwise-excluded solutions in the allowed set. A common aspiration criterion used is allowing solutions which are better than the current best solution to be accepted despite being tabu.

4 A Tabu Search Partitioning Algorithm in TD

The model presented in Sect. 2, has been implemented and adapted to a tabu search scheme. For this TS algorithm we have a main data structure, which is an array of initial size equal to k (number of clusters to form) in which the centroids are stored, and its associated tabu list that stores the "tabu centroids". A centroid that recently replaced another centroid from the solution array is considered tabu-active for a certain number of iterations to forbid the early replacement of this new centroid. The size of this list is dynamic; however, the sum of the size of the solution array and the size of the list of tabu centroids is always equal to k, this means that the centroids are split into two sections; the replaceable ones and the irreplaceable ones. In the following Fig. 1, we can see a graphic representation of the structures:

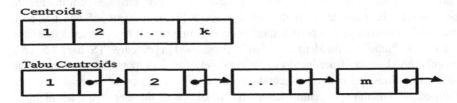

Fig. 1. Array of centroids (m < k)

On the other hand Agebs are stored analogously into two structures, an array of size n and its associated tabu list. A centroid recently replaced by a new one, becomes a tabu Ageb (non-centroid), and will under a tabu-active state for a certain number of iterations to forbid its early reinsertion into the solution array.

These four structures diversify the search avoiding revisiting the same solutions. The Fig. 2 shows the Agebs structures:

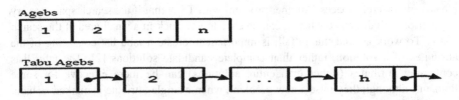

Fig. 2. Array of Agebs (h < n)

4.1   Tabu Search Algorithm Pseudocode

```
Input:
Number of groups k
Array C of centroids
Number of iterations nit
Number of iterations for the second phase nit2
Number of no-improvement iterations before perturbation ip
Tabu Add Tenure tat
Tabu Drop Tenure tdt
pc ← 0;
ic ← 1;
x ← InitialSolution();
x'← S;
While ic < nit do
 costp ← CostOf(S);
 MoveToAnotherSolution(x);
 If CostOf(x) > costp then
     pc ← pc+1;
 end if
 If CostOf(x) < CostOf(x') then
     x' ← x;
 end if
 If pc > ip then
     PerturbSolution(x);
     pc ← 0;
 end if
 UpdateTabuLists();
 ic ← ic+1;
end while
x ← x';
ClearTabuStates();
For i←0 to nit2 do
 MoveToAnotherSolution(x);
 If CostOf(x) < CostOf(x') then
     x' = x;
 end if
 UpdateTabuLists();
 ic ← ic+1;
end for
return x'

MoveToAnotherSolution Function (Neighborhood)
Input:
Solution x
Neighborhood size ns
localS ← x;
index ← RandomIndex();
first ← FisrtAgebFrom(index);
Swap(localS[index], first);
local_cost = CostOf(localS);
xn ← localx;
For i←1 to ns do
    Rand ← RandomAgebFrom(index);
    Swap(xn[index], rand);
    cost_n ← CostOf(xn);
    If cost_n < local_cost then
        localx ← xn;
        local_cost ← costo_n;
    end if
end for
x ← localx;
cost ← local_cost;
StartTabuStates();
UpdateMemory();
```

Parameters description:

nit: Determines the number of iterations for the first phase (stopping criteria).

nit2: Determines the number of moves or iterations that will be made over the best solution found in the first phase.

ip: Determines the maximum number of worse solutions that will be accepted before perturbing the current solution (only during phase one).

tat: The tabu-add tenure determines for how many iterations a new centroid added to the current solution won't be replaced.

tdt: The tabu-drop tenure determines for how many iterations a centroid dropped from the current solution won't be added to the solution array again.

ns: Determines the number of neighbors to evaluate in the local search process (size of candidate list).

The algorithm works in the following way: A random initial solution is generated, which is considered up to this point the best solution found (x'). This happens at the beginning of the search, then the first search phase starts. Within this phase the cost of the current solution is stored in costp to continue with a move over this solution (x). This move is a local search that returns the best neighbor in the neighborhood defined. If the cost of the new solution (x) is worse than the cost of the previous solution (costp) the perturbation counter is increased (pc) and when it reaches the limit (ip), the current solution will be perturbed generating a new one from where the search will be restarted, that is, the search will move to another place of the solution space with the expectative to find even better solutions. On the other hand, if the cost of S is better than the cost of the best solution found so far (x'), then x becomes the new best solution.

At the last step the tabu lists are updated, this consists in transferring Agebs or centroids from the tabu lists to their respective arrays if the maximum number of iteration given by tat and tdt has been reached. When this phase finishes, a new search over the best solution found begins, which is stored back into the array S. The tabu lists are emptied to restart a completely new search without previous information. In this second phase the perturbation strategy is removed in order to intensify the search over the best solution of the previous phase, therefore, only if the move made over x finds a better solution than x', this new solution is stored and otherwise discarded. Finally the tabu list are updated before increasing the global iteration counter (ic).

On the other hand, in the move function, according to the value of ns, a limited amount of neighbors will be explored. We have defined a neighbor as the action of replacing one of the centroids from the current solution (randomly chosen) by a new one, which is chosen from the Agebs assigned to the centroid being replaced. Finally the tabu-active states are initialized, that is, the dropped centroid is now tabu-active and so is the new centroid. Implicitly the algorithm has an internal memory to determine when the tabu states begin and end, also a frequency memory to keep control of the centroids that appear more often in the evaluated solutions, these structures are updated in the last step of the move function.

The map we treat in this article is of the Toluca city formed by 469 geographic objects (basic units) Agebs. The following Fig. 3 shows the Toluca map divided into Agebs when it hasn't been partitioned.

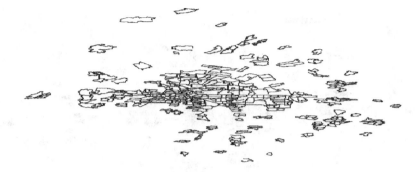

Fig. 3. The territory (Toluca)

Table 1. Cost and time for 6 algorithms (24 groups)

Method	Cost	Time (s)
Hybrid SA-VNS	11.838	3
SA	11.893	9
VNS	11.855	1
GAMS	9.2	936
PAM	9.1986	89
TS	9.3	28

In accordance with the empirical comparison made with other heuristics: simulated annealing (SA) [13], variable neighborhood search (VNS) [14], general algebraic modeling system GAMS [15], partitioning around the medoids (PAM) [16] and VNS-SA hybrid [17]; tabu search has reached good results close to the optimum for small instances of the problem. These results are presented in the following Table 1.

We can see that the cost achieved by TS for a partition of 469 Agebs is good, however for bigger territories; the quality of the solutions is questionable. Recently we made an evaluation of SA, VNS, GAMS, PAM and a SA-VNS hybrid with the goal of analyzing the behavior of the computing cost and of the quality function [17]. These results have been reported and are currently being reviewed.

Given that TS returns better results for this TD problem than the other meta-heuristics, it has been employed to cluster 469 geographic objects from Toluca city, Mexico achieving a compactness cost of 9.357 for 24 groups in 28 s. From the 24 groups formed, we chose cluster 1 as study case to apply TSP. This group (circled in red) contains 26 Agebs with centroid in the Ageb 378 and the elements that belong to it are: 301, 307, 309, 77, 375, 383, 302, 299, 377, 300, 298, 376, 389, 303, 379, 304, 65, 382, 381, 405, 390, 66, 380, 384 and 288.

The Fig. 4 shows the partition of the Toluca territory into 24 groups and in the following section we present the TSP application over this cluster. The map has been generated with a geographic information system (GIS) application [18].

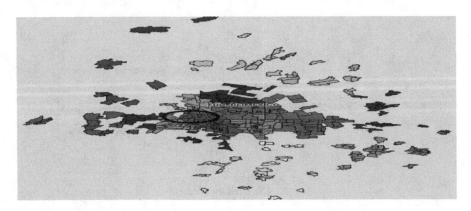

Fig. 4. Partition of the territory into 24 groups with TS (Color figure online)

5 TSP Applied in Territorial Partitioning

The commercial distribution has the goal of putting manufacturers or producers in contact with the consumers, that is, the enterprises that distribute their products directly need to divide a geographic area into commercial territories, each one of them administrated as a business unit.

In general, optimization gives answer to the commercial territory design problem regarding one or more criteria of interest, for example the workload and the turnover or distance minimization between the distribution center and the salespeople. When the territory is divided into zones (partitioned) with a heuristic method and because each element of the territory is considered a business unit, it is necessary to organize the workload of each salesperson in the best way possible. For this, once the territory has been partitioned, it is convenient to employ a routing technique to every element of the partition to determine optimal visiting sequences. This will ensure the decrement of the unproductive times in the territorial groups formed allowing bigger attention spans to every sales point, and to the transportation expenses between them looking to improve the team of salespeople's performance, with the lowest investment possible. Considering that it is common to have many sales points to look over, this is a factor that increases the difficulty of the optimization algorithms to solve this kind of problems. With the purpose of decreasing the complexity of the feasible region, the sales points are grouped into basic units called groups or partitions that will be considered as one entity. The restrictions of the model must be defined based on geographic criteria. For our problem, in Sects. 2 and 3, we have already designed the territory with a partitioning algorithm that optimizes the distance minimization between the distribution centers and the salespeople. Now the challenge is to determine an optimal sequence for every zone formed. Considering each Ageb as a basic unit, implies that the distance between its distribution points and salespeople has the lowest cost in an optimal route without omitting that from every basic unit it must be possible to reach any other basic unit within the same territory. Such characteristic will allow us to apply a routing optimization method based on TSP to travel between the units of the same territory without exiting it. The territories must be as compact as possible, which has been achieved with a TS partitioning algorithm.

Let $G = (V, A)$ be a graph where V is a set of n vertices and A is a set of arcs that connect the vertices in V, let $C = (C_{ij})$ be a distance matrix between the vertices in V associated with A. We associate a variable X_{ij} to every arc (i, j) equal to 1 if and only if the arc (i, j) is used in the optimal solution and 0 otherwise. The linear integer programming model for TSP is credited to Miller, Tucker and Zemlin and modified by Desrochers and Laporte [19].

$$\text{Minimize} \sum_{i \neq j} c_{ij} x_{ij} \tag{1}$$

$$\text{Subject to} \sum_{j=1}^{n} x_{ij} = 1 \quad i = 1, \ldots, n, \tag{2}$$

$$\sum_{i=1}^{n} x_{ij} = 1 \quad j = 1, \ldots, n, \tag{3}$$

$$u_i - u_j + (n-1)x_{ij} + (n-3)x_{ji} \leq \\ n - 2, i, j = 1, \ldots, n, i \neq j \tag{4}$$

$$1 \leq u_i \leq n - 1, \quad i = 2, \ldots, n, \tag{5}$$

$$x_{ij} \in \{0, 1\}, \quad i, j = 1, \ldots, n, i \neq j \tag{6}$$

The objective function (1) describes the cost of an optimal tour, the restrictions (2), (3) are the restrictions to ensure a single assignation of each arc, the restrictions (4) prevent the generation of subtours in the optimal solution and the variables u_j describe the optimal tour. In this article this model has been implemented in LINGO 10.0 [20] and as representative example we have chosen cluster 1 of the partition obtained in this work. The model presented in this section is known as the TSP and is one of the most widely studied combinatorial optimization problems. Its modeling is deceptively simple, and yet it remains one of the most challenging problems in operational research [21].

One of the most common practical applications of the TSP is the vehicle routing problem (VRP). The TSP is used to solve the VRP and both are NP-hard, in both cases several approximation methodologies have been employed to solve them.

Another interesting application related to TSP and that is possible to incorporate it to this work is the Inventory-Routing Problem (IRP), which combines the critical routing logistic activities and the handling of the inventories at the lowest cost possible, where the demand of a set of customers most be attended, employing a fleet of vehicles that travel from a central storage to the distribution routes [22]. Without losing generality, in this article we solve the integration of a territorial design problem with a routing problem for every cluster of the territorial design such that a vehicle can travel through every geographic unit and go back to the departing point. Although the TSP is an NP-hard problem and using a metaheuristic is necessary for big instances, in the application that is presented it isn't needed because the cardinality of the clusters is adequate to use available software such a LINGO.

Laporte defines the TSP in terms of graphs and Hamilton circuits [21]. The TSP consists of determining a minimum distance circuit passing through each vertex once and only once. Such a circuit is known as a tour or Hamiltonian circuit (or cycle). In several applications, C can also be interpreted as a cost or traveling time matrix. It will be useful to distinguish between the cases where C is symmetrical, that is, when $C_{ji} = C_{ij}$, $\forall i,j \in V$, and the case when it is asymmetrical.

In this article we partitioned the territory of Toluca to get 24 groups and we chose randomly the cluster 1 of the partition which centroid is Ageb 378. Let's suppose that this cluster 1 of the partition of Toluca must attend the shipment of merchandise from a distribution center to the customers without capacity restrictions in one trip and in only one vehicle. In this way, we calculate the vehicle route from Ageb 378 and finishes at the same spot, by means of a TSP model. Ageb 378 is the centroid of the cluster where a distribution center can be established and the rest of the Agebs are the customers. In congruence with the mathematical model presented in this section and discussed by Desrochers and Laporte [19], we included restrictions that avoid the generation of subtours in the optimal solution. The implementation used was executed in LINGO 10.0 producing the optimal sequence shown in Table 2.

Table 2. Optimal Tour with 26 Agebs (Group 1)

Ordinal	1	2	3	4	5	6	7	8	9	10	11	12	13
AGEB	378	65	66	77	288	298	299	300	301	302	303	304	307
TSP route	0	15	16	19	3	9	4	8	7	6	5	10	11
Ordinal	14	15	16	17	18	19	20	21	22	23	24	25	26
AGEB	309	375	376	377	379	380	381	382	383	384	389	390	405
TSP route	13	14	12	25	24	23	21	22	1	2	20	18	17

Figure 5 shows this group with 26 Agebs which has been obtained with a geographic information system.

The version of Lingo available that we used for this instance of 26 nodes, is efficient for a maximum of 26 customers, with 676 integer variables. However, with more than 26 customers this version of Lingo (10.0) doesn't respond well regarding the computing time or the feasibility of the solutions. At this stage we decided to test TSP in a new version of Lingo (13.0) and after 38 h for 80, 90 and 100 customers, finding a feasible solution wasn't possible. The optimization software called Lingo 13 was installed and used on a workstation with 4.00 GB RAM, a 1397 GB hard drive and CPU Intel (R) Core (TM) i7-3770 at 3.40 GHz.

According to these results, incorporating a metaheuristic to solve the TSP in this work is necessary.

On the other hand, in an effort to compare the efficiency and optimality of the solution, we processed it with a TSP implementation that consists of a genetic algorithm in Java [23] where we obtained the tour shown on Table 3.

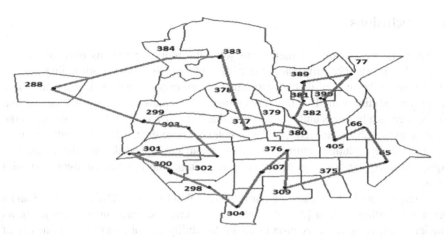

Fig. 5. Cluster 1 with its Agebs: 301, 307, 309, 77, 375, 383, 302, 299, 377, 300, 298, 376, 389, 303, 379, 304, 65, 382, 381, 405, 390, 66, 380, 384, 288. TSP Lingo 10.0.

Table 3. SUB-Optimal Tour with 26 Agebs (Group 1) WITH JAVA ANG GENETIC

Ordinal	1	2	3	4	5	6	7	8	9	10	11	12	13
Ageb Tour	77	405	376	298	65	381	379	382	288	299	303	384	377
Ordinal	14	15	16	17	18	19	20	21	22	23	24	25	26
Ageb Tour	380	66	389	390	375	309	302	378	383	300	304	307	301

Despite the response time of 6 s for this solution [23], it isn't good; it doesn't keep the same starting centroid (Ageb 378) that represents the optimal solution (Fig. 6).

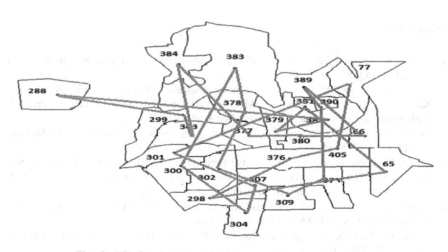

Fig. 6. TSP for cluster 1 solved by a genetic algorithm in java

6 Conclusions

In this work we proposed a method to solve the routing problems over an already designed territory. The proposal consists of 2 phases: the first is partitioning the territory with TS because of its high efficiency in territorial clustering. The second phase is applying routing with TSP to every element of the partition, which is a cluster that can be seen as a business unit. Considering that TD and TSP are NP-hard problems, the solution in two phases has reduced the complexity: once the territory is partitioned with TS, the routing solution returns an optimum tour cost given the smaller amount of Agebs in every cluster, which makes easier getting the optimal configuration with Lingo.

Without a doubt, by measuring our results, TSP in Lingo 10, TSP in Lingo 13 and a genetic algorithm in Java [23], the solution we have presented in this article shows efficiency regarding the execution time, the feasibility and of course the optimality of the solution.

We have developed a graphic interface with a GIS in order to have a graphic representation of the territory [18] and with some modifications; this interface can show each cluster separately, such that a graphic analysis of every cluster can be done within the GIS or with other tools. This contribution helps us to express the routing over an element of the partition graphically.

Another evident application of our methodology can be within the context of location-allocation, because we solve the partitioning and also define the location of facilities in the centroid of every group, from which a route can be established to visit each customer with a minimum transportation cost considering all the distances.

Finally, an additional demanded restriction is the satisfaction of the homogeneity in regard with the number of customers, and currently we are solving this restriction under a multi-objective context including the characteristics required in territorial design: geometric compactness and homogeneous cluster sizes [24, 25].

References

1. Lenstra, K., Rinnooy Kan, A.H.: Complexity of vehicle routing and scheduling problems. **11** (2), 221–227 (1981)
2. Glover, F., Laguna, M.: Tabu Search. Kluwer Academic Publishers, Boston (1997)
3. Kalcsics, J., Nickel, S., Schröder, M.: Toward a unified territorial design approach: applications, algorithms, and GIS integration. TOP **13**(1), 1–56 (2005)
4. Zoltners, A., Sinha, P.: Towards a unified territory alignment: a review and model. Manage. Sci. **29**, 1237–1256 (1983)
5. Bação, F., Lobo, F., Painho, V.: Applying genetic algorithms to zone design. In: Soft Computing - A Fusion of Foundations, Methodologies and Applications vol. 9, no. 5, pp. 341–348. Springer, Berlin, Heidelberg (2005). ISSN 1432-7643
6. Mehrotra, A., Johnson, A., Nemhause, E.: An optimization based heuristic for political districting. Manage. Sci. **44**(8), 1100–1114 (1998)
7. Openshaw, S., Rao, L.: Algorithms for reengineering 1991 Census geography. Environ. Plann. A **27**, 425–446 (1995)

8. Altman, M.: The computational complexity of automated redistricting: is automation the answer? Rutgers Comput. Technol. Law J. **23**(1), 81–142 (1997)
9. Correa, E.S., Steiner, M.T., Freitas, A.A., Carnieri, C.: A genetic algorithm for the P-median problem. In: Proceeding Genetic and Evolutionary Computation Conference, pp. 1268–1275 (2001)
10. Bernábe, B., Osorio, L., Espinosa, R., Ramirez, R., Aceves, R.: A comparative study of simulated annealing and variable neighborhood search for the geographic clustering problem. In: The 2009 International Conference on Data Mining, pp. 595–599 (2009)
11. Martí, R.: Procedimientos metaheurísticos en optimización combinatoria. Tech. rep., Departamento de Estadística e Investigación Operativa, Facultad de Matematicas, Universidad de Valencia (2002)
12. Edleston, O.S., Bartlett, L.M.: A tabu search algorithm applied to the staffing roster problem of Leicestershire police force. J. Oper. Res. Soc. **63**(1), 489–496 (2012)
13. Kirkpatrick, S., Gelatt, C.D., Vecchi, M.P.: Optimization by simulated annealing. Science **220**, 671–680 (1983)
14. Hansen, P., Mladenovic, N., Pérez, M.: Variable Neighbourhood Search. Inteligencia Artificial, Revista Iberoamericana de Inteligencia Artificial. Number 19, pp. 77–92 (2003). ISSN 1137-3601
15. http://www.gams.com/
16. Kaufman, L., Rousseeuw, P.: Clustering by means of medoids. Statistical Data Analysis based on the L1 Norm, North-Holland, Amsterdam, pp. 405–416 (1987)
17. Bernábe-Loranca, B., Pinto, D., Olivares-Benitez, E., Ramirez Rodríguez, J., Martínez-Flores, J.: Simulated annealing and variable neighborhood search hybrid metaheuristic for the geographic clustering. In: Fourth International Workshop of Knowledge Discovery, Knowledge Management and Decision Making, EUREKA 2013, vol. 5, pp. 140–147 (2013). ISSN 1951-6851
18. Loranca, M.B.B., Velázquez, R.G.: Integración de un sistema de información geográfica para algoritmos de particionamiento. In: Research in Computing Science Avances en la Ingeniería del Lenguaje y Conocimiento, vol. 88, pp. 31–44 (2014). ISSN 1870-4069
19. Desrochers, M., Laporte, G.: Improvements and extensions to the Miller-Tucker-Zemlin subtour elimination constraints. Oper. Res. Lett. **10**, 27–36 (1991)
20. http://www.lindo.com/
21. Laporte, G.: The traveling salesman problem: an overview of exact and approximate algorithms. Eur. J. Oper. Res. **59**, 231–247 (1992)
22. Elizondo, M., Aceves, R.: Strategy of solution for the inventory routing problem based on separable cross decomposition. J. Appl. Res. Technol. **3**(2), 139–149 (2005)
23. http://jclec.sourceforge.net/
24. Rincón-García, E.A., Gutiérrez-Andrade, M.A., de-los-Cobos-Silva, S.G., Lara-Velázquez, P., Mora-Gutiérrez, R.A., Ponsich, A.S.: A multiobjective algorithm for redistricting. J. Appl. Res. Technol. 324–330 (2012)
25. Bernábe, B., Guillén, C.: Búsqueda de entorno variable multiobjetivo para resolver el problema de particionamiento de datos espaciales con características poblacionales. Computación y Sistemas **16**(3), 335–347 (2012)

On a Relative MaxSAT Encoding for the Steiner Tree Problem in Graphs

Ricardo Tavares de Oliveira[✉] and Fabiano Silva

Departamento de Informática, Universidade Federal Do Paraná, POBox 19081,
Curitiba 81531-980, Brazil
{rtoliveira,fabiano}@inf.ufpr.br
http://www.inf.ufpr.br

Abstract. In [1] it was presented some MaxSAT encodings for trees
in graphs which can be used to solve the Steiner Tree Problem. In this
paper we focus exclusively on the relative encoding which was called
Parental-based. We review this encoding and improve it by applying two
techniques. One of them is a known improvement to encode transitivity,
previously used for other relative encodings. The other one consists on
deducing unit clauses from the dominance relation of the given graph.
Finally, we use the improved encodings to solve relevant instances, and
present experimental results.

Keywords: Boolean satisfiability · SAT encodings · MaxSAT encodings · Relative encoding · Steiner Tree

1 Introduction

The efficiency of SAT and MaxSAT solvers has grown in the last decades. This
motivates solving relevant problems by encoding them to (Max)SAT and providing the resulting formulae as input to state-of-art (Max)SAT solvers.

Many encodings of relevant problems are known [1–4]. In this paper, we focus
on an encoding for the *Steiner Tree Problem*. This problem is known to be NP-
Hard [5], and has applications, for instance, in Computational Geometry and
Circuit Design [6].

Previously, it was presented different MaxSAT encodings for the Steiner Tree
Problem [1], which were classified as *absolute*, *relative* or *counting-based*. In this
paper, we review and improve the relative *Parental-based* encoding, the most
efficient encoding among the relative ones presented previously.

We apply two improvements on this encoding. One of the procedures we use
to improve the encoding was previously used by Bryant & Velev [3] and Velev
& Gao [4] to encode transitivity for other problems. The other one consists on
using the dependence relation of the given graph to deduce unit clauses.

This paper is organized as follows: Section 2 provides preliminary definitions and notations. Section 3 provides a brief background on SAT and MaxSAT
encodings for problems in graphs. Section 4 reviews the *Parental-based* encoding.

© Springer International Publishing Switzerland 2015
O. Pichardo Lagunas et al. (Eds.): MICAI 2015, Part II, LNAI 9414, pp. 422–434, 2015.
DOI: 10.1007/978-3-319-27101-9_32

Section 5 presents the first improvement on the encoding, while Sect. 6 presents the second one. Finally, Sect. 7 shows experimental results, while Sect. 8 concludes and present future works.

2   Preliminaries

In this section we present some preliminaries notions and definitions. First, the *Steiner Tree Problem* consists in, given a weighted graph $G = (V, E, w : E \rightarrow \mathbb{N}^+)$ and a set of vertices $S \subseteq V$ (the *terminal* vertices), find a connected subgraph of G containing all terminal vertices whose sum of the weight of its edges is minimized. Such subgraph is clearly a tree.

A *(Boolean) variable* can assume either 0 (false) or 1 (true). A *literal* is a variable x_i or its negation $\neg x_i$. A *clause* is a disjunction ($\vee$) of literals. The expression $A \rightarrow B$ denotes $(\neg A) \vee B$, which always results in a clause in this text. An *unit* clause is a clause containing exactly one literal, and an *empty* clause is a clause containing no literals, which is always evaluated to 0 (false). A *Conjective Normal Form (CNF)* formula is a conjunction ($\wedge$) of clauses.

An *assignment* is a set of literals where a variable and its negation do not occur simultaneously in it. Given a CNF formula, an assignment A is *total* if $x_i \in A$ or $\neg x_i \in A$ for all variable x_i occurring in the formula, and *partial* otherwise. An assignment A is an *extension* of a partial assignment A' (or, equivalently, A' can be *extended to* A) if $A' \subset A$. An assignment A *satisfies* a clause C if there is a literal in both the assignment A and the clause C. An assignment satisfies a CNF formula if it satisfies all its clauses. A total assignment that satisfies a CNF formula is a *model* of it. The *Boolean Satisfiability Problem* (SAT) consists in, given a CNF formula, decide whether it has a model.

Unit Propagation is a procedure used by most state-of-the-art SAT solvers to simplify a CNF formula [7,8]. If a given CNF formula contains an unit clause (x_i) (resp. $(\neg x_i)$), then the procedure *propagates* the literal x_i (resp. $\neg x_i$) in the formula, i.e., it replaces each occurrence of the variable x_i by 1 (true) (resp. 0 (false)). The procedure is repeated until the formula does not contain any unit clause or contains an empty clause.

Let A be a partial assignment (possibly empty) which can be extended to a model of a given CNF formula, and consider that all literals in A are propagated in such formula. The resulting formula is *Generalized Arc-Consistent (GAC)* if there is not a variable x_i such that: (i) $A \cup \{\neg x_i\}$ can be extended to a model of the formula; (ii) $A \cup \{x_i\}$ can *not* be extended to a model of the formula; (iii) $\neg x_i \notin A$. Informally, the formula is GAC if all variables that must be set to 0 (false) to make the formula satisfiable are present in the current partial assignment, and thus are not present in the resulting formula at all. Also, the given formula is *maintained GAC by Unit Propagation* if the literal $\neg x_i$ is propagated by such procedure, for all variable x_i such that $A \cup \{\neg x_i\}$ can be extended to a model of the formula, but $A \cup \{x_i\}$ can not, for all such partial assignments A during the search.

The *Partial Weighted Maximum Boolean Satisfiability Problem* ((PW)MaxSAT) consists in, given a CNF formula F_h (the *hard* formula), a set of clauses F_s (the *soft* clauses), and a function $W : F_s \rightarrow \mathbb{N}^+$ (the *weight* or *cost* of each *soft* clause), find a model of the *hard* formula whose sum of the weight of the satisfied *soft* clauses is maximized. Unit Propagation can also be used by MaxSAT solvers to simplify the *hard* formula [9].

Finally, given a graph $G = (V, E)$, we denote by $N(v_i) = \{v_j \in V | \{v_i, v_j\} \in E\}$ the set of neighbors of a given vertex v_i.

3   Background

In this section we give a brief background about SAT and MaxSAT encodings for problems in graphs.

There is more than one way to reduce a given problem to SAT or MaxSAT. A possible way to do so is by describing the problem as a Constraint Satisfiability Problem (CSP) and then encode its constraints into CNF formulae. These encodings are referred as *absolute* encodings. This notation was used by Prestwich [2] to describe an encoding for the Hamiltonian Cycle Problem. In his encodings, a permutation of the vertices in the given graph, which described the path, is encoded. In the absolute encoding, there is a boolean variable for each vertex in the given graph and each position of the permutation. Many distinct absolute encodings can be used, such as the *direct*, *muldirect*, and *log* encodings. For a review of these encodings, the reader may referrer to Velev [10].

For some problems, one can describe the problem as a binary relation instead of a CSP. The encodings that describe a binary relation are referred as *relative* encodings. This notation was also used by Prestwich [2] to describe another encoding for the Hamiltonian Cycle Problem. In this encoding, each boolean variable states the relative positions, in the described permutation, between vertices in the given graph.

In relative encodings, it is usually necessary to describe a *transitive* relation. The transitivity property can naturally be encoded by a cubic number of clauses in the form $(r_{a,b} \wedge r_{b,c}) \rightarrow r_{a,c}$, where $r_{a,b}$ states the relation between elements a and b. Bryant & Velev [3] suggested an improvement for this property in particular. Velev & Gao [4] then improved Prestwich's encoding. This improvement is shown in Sect. 5 applied to the *Parental-based* encoding.

Previously [1], it was presented, among others, two relative encodings for the Steiner Tree Problem to (PW)MaxSAT. In this work, we focus on the *Parental-based* encoding. The encoding describes the partial (binary) relation induced by a tree in the given graph. This encoding is reviewed in the next section.

4   The *Parental-based* encoding

In this section we review the *Parental-based* encoding. Given a graph $G = (V, E)$ and a set of its vertices $S \subseteq V$, the *Parental-based* encoding creates a *hard* formula $F_{PrB}(G, S)$ which is satisfiable if and only if all vertices in S are in the same connected component of G [1]. Also, each model of $F_{PrB}(G, S)$ describes a tree in G containing all vertices in S. To solve the Steiner Tree Problem, *soft* clauses are then created to minimize such tree [1].

The encoded tree is rooted in an arbitrary terminal vertex $v_r \in S$. The root of the tree is chosen among the terminal vertices during a pre-processing step. We suggest seven heuristics to select such vertex: (1) Select the first terminal vertex in the input file; (2) Select a terminal vertex with maximum degree. Break ties by selecting the first such vertex in the input file; (3) Select a terminal vertex with maximum degree. Break ties by randomly selecting one such vertex; (4) Select a terminal vertex with minimum degree. Break ties by selecting the first such vertex in the input file; (5) Select a terminal vertex with minimum degree. Break ties by randomly selecting one such vertex; (6) Select a terminal vertex whose average distance to all others terminal vertices is minimum. Break ties by randomly selecting one such vertex; (7) Select a terminal vertex whose average distance to all others terminal vertices is maximum. Break ties by randomly selecting one such vertex. One can use the Floyd-Warshall algorithm [11] to compute the distances used by heuristics 6 and 7.

The formula $F_{PrB}(G, S)$ is built as follows [1]: for each edge $\{v_i, v_j\} \in E$, two boolean variables $p_{i,j}$ and $p_{j,i}$ are created. The variable $p_{i,j}$ (resp. $p_{j,i}$) states that v_j (resp. v_i) is the *parent* of v_i (resp. v_j) in the described tree.

Also, two other boolean variables $a_{i,j}$ and $a_{j,i}$ are created for each pair of distinct vertices $v_i, v_j \in V$. The variable $a_{i,j}$ (resp. $a_{j,i}$) states that v_j (resp. v_i) is an *ancestor* of v_i (resp. v_j) in the described tree. It is worth noticing that variables $p_{i,j}$ encode a *binary relation* P over the vertices of the given graph, while variables $a_{i,j}$ encode its *transitive closure* P^+.

Finally, another boolean variable $y_{i,j}$ is created for each edge $\{v_i, v_j\} \in E$. The variable $y_{i,j}$ states that the edge $\{v_i, v_j\}$ is present in the described tree.

The *hard* formula $F_{PrB}(G, S)$ contains eight types of clauses:

(*terminal-presence*) $(\bigvee_{v_j \in N(v_s)} p_{s,j})$ for each $v_s \in S, v_s \neq v_r$. These clauses ensure that all terminal vertices, except for the root, must have a parent in the tree, and thus are present in the described subgraph;

(*at-most-one-parent*) $(p_{i,j} \rightarrow \neg p_{i,k})$ for each $v_i \in V, v_i \neq v_r$ and for each pair of distinct vertices $v_j, v_k \in N(v_i)$. These clauses ensure that no vertex has more than one parent in the tree;

(*connectedness*) $(p_{j,i} \rightarrow \bigvee_{v_k \in N(v_i)} p_{i,k})$, for each $v_i \in V, v_i \neq v_r$ and for each $v_j \in N(v_i), v_j \neq v_r$. These clauses ensure that, if a given vertex has a parent in the tree, then its parent also has a parent in such tree, except for the root;

(*subset*) $(p_{i,j} \rightarrow a_{i,j})$ for each $v_i \in V, v_i \neq v_r$ and for each $v_j \in N(v_i)$. These clauses state that if a vertex is the parent of another vertex in the tree, then it is also one of its ancestors. This encodes $P \subseteq P^+$;

(*transitivity*) $((a_{i,j} \wedge a_{j,k}) \rightarrow a_{i,k})$ for each triple of distinct vertices $v_i, v_j, v_k \in V$. These clauses encode the transitivity of the ancestor relation P^+;

(*asymmetry*) $(a_{i,j} \rightarrow \neg a_{j,i})$ for each pair of distinct vertices $v_i, v_j \in V$. These clauses state that the ancestor relation P^+, and thus also the parental relation P, is asymmetric;

(*root-path*) $(a_{s,r})$ for all $v_s \overset{*}{\in} S, v_s \neq v_r$. These unit clauses state that the root of the tree is an ancestor of all other terminal vertices;

(*edge-vertex-relation*) $(y_{i,j} \leftrightarrow (p_{i,j} \vee p_{j,i})) = (y_{i,j} \rightarrow (p_{i,j} \vee p_{j,i})), (p_{i,j} \rightarrow y_{i,j})$ and $(p_{j,i} \rightarrow y_{i,j})$, for each edge $\{v_i, v_j\} \in E$. These clauses state that an edge is present in the tree iff one of its vertices is the parent of its other one.

Finally, an unit *soft* clause $(\neg y_{i,j})$ with weight $w(\{v_i, v_j\})$ is created for each edge $\{v_i, v_j\} \in E$, stating that the sum of the weights of the edges in the tree must be minimized.

This encoding creates $O(|V|^2)$ boolean variables, $O(|V|^3)$ *hard* clauses and $|E|$ *soft* clauses. The total number of literals in both the *hard* and *soft* clauses is also in $O(|V|^3)$. Asymptotically, this encoding creates the smaller number of variables, clauses and literals among the Path-based encodings presented in [1]. Also, it is worth noticing that the largest portion of the instance is due the encoding of the *transitivity* property, which requires a cubic number in $|V|$ of *hard* clauses. In the next section we present an improvement on this part of the formula in particu lar.

It is also worth observing that a model A of the *hard* formula may describe a subgraph $G'(A)$ containing more vertices and edges than the ones presented in the described tree. These elements are removed from the solution exclusively via MaxSAT optimization.

5   An Improvement on the Transitivity Relation

As previously stated, this encoding creates a *hard* formula with $O(|V|^2)$ variables, $O(|V|^3)$ clauses and $O(|V|^3)$ literals in total, and $|E|$ unit *soft* clauses.

The number of variables and clauses in the *hard* formula can be reduced using a method described by Bryant & Velev [3] and applied to the Hamiltonian Cycle Problem by Velev & Gao [4]. Their method is based on the fact that the transitive relation between some pairs of vertices is not directly relevant to the solution, and thus some variables may be omitted from the formula.

Let us define the *relational graph* as the graph $G_R = (V, E \cup \{\{v_r, v_s\}|v_s \in S, v_s \neq v_r\})$, i.e., G_R is the graph G with additional edges connecting the root v_r and all other terminal vertices in S (if not present already). Instead of defining variables $a_{i,j}$ and $a_{j,i}$ for each pair of distinct vertices $v_i, v_j \in V$, we define these variables only for each pair of vertices where $\{v_i, v_j\} \in E(G_R)$. In practice, we remove from the encoding the variables that originally occur in the *transitivity* and *asymmetry* clauses *only*. These variables are not directly relevant to the encoding and their values could be inferred from other variables in the solution.

Transitivity can then be encoded by enumerating all chord-free cycles in G_R, as suggested by Bryant & Velev [3]. For each chord-free cycle with k vertices, k clauses are added to the formula. Each clause states the relation between the vertices in one edge and the vertices in all the other edges in the cycle.

As also suggested by Bryant & Velev [3], the transitivity property can be encoded efficiently if every chord-free cycle in G_R is a triangle with 3 vertices, i.e., if G_R is *chordal*. If G_R is not chordal, it is possible to add a set of edges (called a *fill*) to the graph to make it chordal. It is NP-Hard to obtain a fill with the smallest possible number of edges [12]. However, some heuristics can be used to obtain a "good" set of edges.

Velev & Gao [4] presented the following procedure to obtain such a set: Let G^+ be a graph initially equal to G_R, and let F be an initially empty set. Select a vertex $v_i \in G^+$ and, for each pair of distinct vertices v_j, v_k such that $\{v_i, v_j\} \in E(G^+)$ and $\{v_i, v_k\} \in E(G^+)$, add the edge $\{v_j, v_k\}$ to both the set F and the graph G^+, if not present already. Then, remove the vertex v_i and all its incident edges from G^+. Repeat the procedure until G^+ is empty. At the end, include all edges in F to G_R to make it chordal [4].

Twelve heuristics to choose a vertex at each step are known [4]: (1) Select a vertex in G^+ with minimum degree. Break ties by selecting the vertex whose sum of the degrees of its neighbors is minimum; (2) Select a vertex in G^+ with minimum degree. Break ties by selecting the vertex whose sum of the degrees of its neighbors is maximum; (3) Select a vertex in G^+ with minimum degree. Break ties by selecting the vertex whose number of edges to be added at that step of the procedure, if that vertex is selected, is minimum; (4) Select a vertex in G^+ with minimum degree. Break ties by selecting the vertex whose number of edges to be added at that step of the procedure, if that vertex is selected, is maximum; (5) Select a vertex in G^+ with minimum degree. Break ties by selecting one such vertex whose degree in G_R is minimum; (6) Select a vertex in G^+ with minimum degree. Break ties by selecting one such vertex whose degree in G_R is maximum; (7) Select a vertex in G^+ with minimum degree. Break ties by selecting the vertex that, if selected, minimizes the number of triangles, in the graph given by the union of G_R with the edges currently in F, containing the selected vertex and some edge in F; (8) Select a vertex in G^+ with minimum degree. Break ties by selecting the vertex that, if selected, maximizes the number of triangles, in the graph given by the union of G_R with the edges currently in F, containing the selected vertex and some edge in F; (9) Select a vertex in G^+ that, if selected, minimizes the number of edges to be added to G^+ at that step of the procedure. Break ties by selecting the first such vertex in the input file; (10) Select a vertex in G^+ that, if selected, minimizes the number of edges to be added to G^+ at that step of the procedure. Break ties by randomly selecting one such vertex; (11) Select a vertex to G^+ that, if selected, minimizes the number of triangles, in the graph given by the union of G_R with the edges currently in F, containing the selected vertex and some edge in F. Break ties by selecting the first such vertex in the input file; (12) Select a vertex to G^+ that, if selected, minimizes the number of triangles, in the graph given by the union of G_R with the edges currently in F, containing the selected vertex and some edge in F. Break ties by randomly selecting one such vertex. For all heuristics, if not stated otherwise, if there are still ties, break it by selecting the first vertex in the input that matches the given criteria.

We define variables $a_{i,j}$ and $a_{j,i}$ only for pairs of vertices $v_i, v_j \in V$ that are adjacent in G_R. Also, a *transitivity* clause $((a_{i,j} \wedge a_{j,k}) \to a_{i,k})$ is added only when all variables $a_{i,j}, a_{j,k}$ and $a_{i,k}$ are defined. Since G_R is chordal, a *transitivity* clause is created for each triangle in this graph. The number of triangles in G_R

may be way smaller than the number of *transitivity* clauses created in the original encoding, which is near to $|V|^3$.

Finally, a *asymmetry* clause $(a_{i,j} \rightarrow \neg a_{j,i})$ is also added only when the variables $a_{i,j}$ and $a_{j,i}$ are defined. The number of *asymmetry* clauses created is equal to the number of edges in G_R, which is in $O(|E| + |S| + |F|)$, the sum of the number of edges in the original graph, the number of edges connecting the root to all terminal vertices, and the number of edges in F.

As stated by Bryant & Velev [3], this improvement can be applied without invalidating the correctness of the transitivity encoding. Indeed, the solutions found during our experiments are all optimal according to benchmark descriptions and previous experiments.

6   On Deducing Unit Clauses from the Dominance Relation

In this section we suggest another improvement on the *Parental-based* encoding.

It is possible to anticipate a truth value for some variables before starting the MaxSAT solver by analyzing the input graph. Informally, this improvement consists on *deducing unit clauses* based on the original problem and the meaning of the variables in the encoding.

Let $G' = (V, E')$ be the directed graph obtained by replacing each edge in the original graph G by two directed arcs, i.e., $E' = \{(v_i, v_j), (v_j, v_i)|\{v_i, v_j\} \in E\}$. Also, let v_r be the terminal vertex selected to be root of the encoded tree, as defined in Sect. 4.

The *dominator tree* D of G' w.r.t. v_r is a tree rooted at v_r such that, if a vertex v_i is an ancestor of a vertex v_j in D, then every path from v_r to v_j in G contains the vertex v_i [13]. Hence, if v_i is an ancestor of v_j in D, then it *not* possible to obtain a tree in G such that v_j occurs *before* v_i in a path starting in v_r. Thus, v_j cannot be an ancestor of v_i in the described tree, so we can deduce that the variable $a_{i,j}$, if defined, must be set to 0 (false). In this case, we create the unit clause $(\neg a_{i,j})$ and add it to the *hard* formula.

If the vertex v_j is present in the tree described by a model of the *hard* formula, then the literal $a_{j,i}$ is certainly present in such model. However, there is a model containing $a_{j,i}$ even if the vertex v_j is not present in the encoded tree. Notice that the *subset* clause $(p_{j,i} \rightarrow a_{j,i})$ is satisfied in this case even if $p_{j,i}$ is set to 0 (false). Hence, it is also possible to add the unit clause $(a_{j,i})$ to the formula.

We use the Lengauer-Tarjan algorithm [13] to build the dominator tree. Then, for each pair of vertex v_i, v_j such that v_i is an ancestor of v_j in the dominator tree and the variables $a_{i,j}$ and $a_{j,i}$ are defined, we add the unit clauses $(\neg a_{i,j})$ and $(a_{j,i})$ to the *hard* formula. These literals will be propagated by the Unit Propagation procedure as the solver starts.

It is worth mentioning that the addition of the unit clause $(\neg a_{i,j})$ makes Unit Propagation propagate the literal $\neg p_{i,j}$ (if defined), due to the *subset* clause $(p_{i,j} \rightarrow a_{i,j})$. In fact, we conjecture that, with this improvement, Unit Propagation makes the *hard* formula *Generalized Arc-Consistent* (GAC), i.e., if there is any variable that must be set to 0 (false) in order to make the formula satisfied, then Unit Propagation will propagate such assignment. However, this fact may be valid only for the formula given as input to the solver – GAC is not *maintained* by Unit Propagation during the search. This maintenance is discussed as a future work in Sect. 8.

It is also worth noticing that, although we applied this technique on the *Parental-based* encoding in particular, this improvement may actually be applied on any relative encoding that encodes the transitivity property.

7   Experimental Results

In this section we present some experimental results obtained by solving relevant instances of the Steiner Tree Problem using the presented encoding.

We used the encoding to reduce some random instances of the Steiner Tree Problem and instances from the SteinLib benchmark [6]. The random instances used in our experiments, namely *20_45_13, 25_54_15, 30_70_17* and *35_98_19*, as well as all source codes of all tools used in this paper, can be downloaded at http://www.inf.ufpr.br/rtoliveira/.

To efficiently encode a given instance of the problem, it is needed to determine (i) the root v_r of the encoded tree and (ii) the vertex to be selected at each step of the procedure used to make G_R chordal, presented in Sect. 5. We consider seven heuristics for the selection of the root and twelve for the selection of such vertex, as presented in Sects. 4 and 5.

First, we encoded the instances with the improvement on the transitivity property using all combinations of both heuristics. We then compared the size of the resulting formulae against the size of the formulae obtained by the *Parental-based* encoding *as-is*, i.e., as presented in [1].

Table 1 shows the results. The column *PrB* stands for the *Parental-based* encoding *as-is*, while *IPrB* stands for the improved version of the encoding, with the improvement on the transitivity property. Columns *Vars* indicate the number of variables in the formulae, while columns *Claus* indicate the number of clauses in them. The columns *h(i)* and *h(ii)* indicate which heuristic to (i) select

Table 1. Size of the formulae generated by the encodings

Encoding	PrB		IPrB				Encoding	PrB		IPrB			
Instance	Vars	Claus	Vars	Claus	h(i)	h(ii)	Instance	Vars	Claus	Vars	Claus	h(i)	h(ii)
20_45_13	511	7750	**279**	**1543**	3	1	es30fst01	6505	479011	**879**	**3897**	3	3
25_54_15	758	14920	**382**	**2371**	7	2	es30fst02	5259	346623	**712**	**2828**	7	3
30_70_17	1076	25937	**507**	**3670**	2	2	es30fst03	7162	556189	**904**	**3994**	3	10
35_98_19	1480	41663	**743**	**7035**	7	2	es30fst04	6664	497572	**872**	**3767**	7	3
i080-001	6673	497740	**817**	**4246**	1	2	es30fst05	3517	187649	**531**	**1957**	2	3
i080-002	6676	497772	**860**	**4766**	3	2	es30fst07	2946	142714	**464**	**1638**	2	2
i080-003	6672	497736	**840**	**4368**	1	2	es30fst08	4968	317846	**676**	**2584**	7	10
i080-004	6674	497768	**858**	**4870**	1	10	es30fst09	1937	75471	**310**	**936**	2	1
i080-005	6677	497732	**904**	**5487**	2	2	es30fst10	2411	105526	**355**	**1081**	3	2
							es30fst11	6496	478955	**858**	**3739**	3	10
							es30fst12	2213	92691	**321**	**928**	2	1
							es30fst13	4410	265192	**630**	**2471**	2	10
							es30fst14	2929	142638	**389**	**1177**	2	2

the root and (ii) select the vertex at each step of the procedure resulted in the smaller number of variables and clauses in the formulae.

As expected, this improvement on the encoding reduced the size of the resulting formulae. For the instance *i080-001*, the number of variables was reduced by aprox. 8 times, while the number of clauses was reduced by aprox. 117 times. It is also worth noticing that the selections 2, 3 and 7 showed to be the best heuristics overall to choose the root of the tree.

We then encoded all instances: with the improvement on the transitivity property only; with the improvement on deducing unit clauses only; and with both improvements. In the cases where the first improvement applies, we considered all 12 heuristics to choose the vertex to be selected at each step of the procedure, and the heuristics 2, 3 and 7 to select the root of the tree. In the case where only the second improvement applies, we used the heuristic 1 to select the root of the encoded tree, as implemented by [1]. The resulting formulae were given as input to MaxSAT solvers MiniMaxSAT (`minimaxsat1.0`) [9] and EvaSolver (`eva500a_`) [14]. We then ran the solvers on an *AMD Opteron(tm) Processor 6136, 2.4 Ghz, 120 Gb RAM, Linux 3.16.7.*

Table 2 shows the best obtained results. *PrB* stands for the *Parental-based* encoding *as-is*; *IPrB* stands for the improved version of the encoding, with the improvement on the transitivity property only; *UPrB* stands for the improved version with deduced unit clauses only; *UIPrB* stands for the encoding improved by both improvements. In the cases where the first improvement applies, each

Table 2. Best results for both solvers with the first improvement, with the second one and with both

Encoding	PrB	IPrB				UPrB	UIPrB			
	CPU	CPU	σ	h(i)	h(ii)	CPU	CPU	σ	h(i)	h(ii)
Solver	MiniMaxSAT [9]									
20_45_13	4.77	**0.64**	0.00	7	2	6.97	0.78	0.00	7	3
25_54_15	1.19	0.68	0.00	3	5	6.06	**0.56**	0.00	2	2
30_70_17	265.48	18.28	0.00	2	1	273.88	**12.92**	0.00	7	1
35_98_19	TLE	TLE	-	-	-	TLE	TLE	-	-	-
es30fst01	TLE	TLE	-	-	-	TLE	TLE	-	-	-
es30fst02	TLE	TLE	-	-	-	TLE	TLE	-	-	-
es30fst03	TLE	TLE	-	-	-	TLE	TLE	-	-	-
es30fst04	TLE	TLE	-	-	-	TLE	TLE	-	-	-
es30fst05	TLE	35.71	0.00	7	2	TLE	**23.01**	0.00	7	2
es30fst07	TLE	1.20	0.00	2	3	TLE	**0.95**	0.00	2	4,5
es30fst08	TLE	TLE	-	-	-	TLE	TLE	-	-	-
es30fst09	0.82	**0.01**	0.00	*	*	0.33	**0.01**	0.00	*	*
es30fst10	0.52	**0.01**	0.00	*	*	0.32	**0.01**	0.00	*	*

(Continued)

Table 2. (Continued)

Encoding	PrB	IPrB				UPrB	UIPrB			
	CPU	CPU	σ	h(i)	h(ii)	CPU	CPU	σ	h(i)	h(ii)
es30fst11	TLE	TLE	-	-	-	TLE	TLE	-	-	-
es30fst12	0.20	**0.00**	0.00	*	*	0.33	**0.00**	0.00	*	*
es30fst13	TLE	502.12	1.03	2	2	TLE	**17.77**	0.00	2	6
es30fst14	0.75	**0.00**	0.00	*	*	0.47	**0.00**	0.00	*	*
i080-001	TLE	765.94	1.5	2	1	1292.42	**272.99**	0.45	2	6
i080-002	TLE	281.10	0.55	2	9	920.36	**250.42**	1.33	2	6
i080-003	TLE	**90.97**	0.17	2	5	TLE	205.42	0.46	2	7
i080-004	TLE	197.70	0.46	2	2	TLE	**101.05**	0.20	2	6
i080-005	TLE	1146.93	5.08	2	9	TLE	**304.91**	0.38	3	2
Solver	EvaSolver [14]									
20_45_13	87.74	**2.55**	0.00	7	9	150.01	5.77	1.20	7	10
25_54_15	13.81	**0.22**	0.00	*	*	1.27	0.24	0.00	7	6
30_70_17	TLE	TLE	-	-	-	TLE	TLE	-	-	-
35_98_19	1128.26	**135.55**	3.63	7	4	955.81	236.30	17.34	7	4
es30fst01	TLE	**1698.69**	31.18	2	5	TLE	TLE	-	-	-
es30fst02	172.47	**10.33**	0.00	7	5	160.05	13.05	0.33	7	5
es30fst03	1392.26	23.06	0.14	7	2	896.13	**20.34**	0.20	7	4
es30fst04	TLE	**662.33**	6.30	2	5	TLE	1275.68	44.45	2	6
es30fst05	TLE	TLE	-	-	-	TLE	TLE	-	-	-
es30fst07	9.22	**0.28**	0.00	*	*	10.31	0.30	0.00	*	*
es30fst08	93.14	**8.15**	0.00	3	4	94.66	8.89	0.22	2	4
es30fst09	3.91	**0.24**	0.00	7	10	8.99	0.33	0.00	7	9
es30fst10	2.54	**0.08**	0.00	3	2	3.45	**0.08**	0.00	3	7
es30fst11	TLE	**460.37**	8.57	7	4	TLE	523.47	12.52	7	4
es30fst12	0.70	**0.01**	0.00	*	*	0.80	**0.01**	0.00	*	*
es30fst13	46.22	**2.18**	0.00	*	*	61.22	2.39	0.00	2	4
es30fst14	1.13	**0.01**	0.00	*	*	0.99	**0.01**	0.00	*	*
i080-001	**245.63**	313.09	54.94	7	12	377.24	294.36	9.99	7	1
i080-002	1100.40	**242.45**	4.24	7	9	1169.88	259.70	9.27	7	9
i080-003	119.52	**115.31**	2.94	2	9	143.96	138.22	8.93	3	2
i080-004	**724.11**	954.66	16.33	7	6	753.81	887.64	53.00	2	6
i080-005	688.35	**531.31**	9.92	7	7	887.96	833.94	46.88	7	3

instance was encoded 10 times for each combination of heuristics. Column *CPU* indicates the average CPU time took by the solver in seconds, while column σ indicates its standard deviation. TLE (*Time Limit Exceeded*) indicates that the given formula was not solved within 1800 s. The symbol * indicates that there was not an unique best combination of heuristics for that instance.

Let us first analyze the results obtained by the improvement on the transitivity property only (*IPrB*). As it can be observed, except for isolated cases, this improvement on the encoding impacted significantly on the run time taken by solvers to solve the obtained formulae. Indeed, some instances previously unsolved by MiniMaxSAT with the *Parental-based* encoding, such as the ones in the class *I080*, can be solved with the improved encoding by the same solver.

It is also worth observing that the combination of heuristics that generates the smaller formulae is not necessarily the combination that generates the easier formulae. It is also interesting noticing that there is not an overall best MaxSAT solver to solve these instances. EvaSolver performed better than MiniMaxSAT for some instances, mainly for the class *ES30FST*, while MiniMaxSAT performed better than EvaSolver in others. This may indicate there is a relation between the instances' characteristics and the internal algorithms and heuristics used by the solvers.

Let us then analyze the results obtained by the improvement by deducing unit clauses only (*UPrB*). We expected this improvement to make the formulae easier to solve. Surprisingly, although this improvement did make the solvers solve specific instances faster, it did *not* improved their overall run time. In fact, this improvement made some instances actually *harder* to be solved.

To help us to investigate this fact, we combined the second improvement with the $12 \times 3 = 36$ combinations of heuristics used for the experiments for the first improvement, and analyzed the cases where the second improvement made the resulting formulae easier or harder to solve.

Table 3 shows the results. Column *UIPrB* indicates the number of combinations of heuristics for which the formula obtained by using *both* improvements were solved faster, while column *IPrB* indicates the number of combinations of heuristics for which the formula obtained by using the first improvement only were solved faster. It is worth mentioning that the sum of both values may not add to 36 due to formulae that were not solved within the time limit.

Table 3. Number of combinations that performed better for each instance

Solver	MiniMaxSAT [9]		EvaSolver [14]		Solver	MiniMaxSAT [9]		EvaSolver [14]	
Encoding	UIPrB	IPrB	UIPrB	IPrB	Encoding	UIPrB	IPrB	UIPrB	IPrB
20_45_13	29	7	6	30	es30fst01	0	0	0	1
25_54_15	22	14	11	20	es30fst02	0	0	16	20
30_70_17	22	6	0	0	es30fst03	0	0	21	13
35_98_19	0	0	16	20	es30fst04	0	0	3	8
i080-001	4	4	10	26	es30fst05	30	0	0	0
i080-002	10	2	8	20	es30fst07	22	11	3	32
i080-003	16	15	6	30	es30fst08	0	0	2	34
i080-004	21	6	9	3	es30fst09	22	1	2	31
i080-005	4	3	4	17	es30fst10	13	3	7	29
					es30fst11	0	0	0	11
					es30fst12	0	4	1	4
					es30fst13	1	2	7	29
					es30fst14	6	12	1	6

By analyzing Table 3, we can notice that, overall, the formulae obtained by using both improvements are better solved by MiniMaxSAT, while the formula obtained by not using the second improvement are better solved by EvaSolver. This seems particularity true for the random instances and the class *ES30FST*, where the differences between the respective number of easier instances are larger.

We suspect that the performance obtained with and without the improvement may be related to the base algorithm and to the internal heuristics used by the solvers. MiniMaxSAT is based on a *Branch and Bound* DPLL-like algorithm [9], while EvaSolver is based on successive eliminations of *unsatisfiable cores* [14]. Since the base algorithm used by each solver is different, it may be expected that the deduced unit clauses may impact them differently.

Also, the deduced unit clauses may interfere in the internal heuristics used by the solvers. After unit propagation, the resulting formulae may be such that the solver decides to use "worse" heuristics and hence explore the search space poorly, which may not be the case if the formula remains unchanged, without the deduced unit clauses. Further investigation on the solver' internal algorithms and instances' characteristics is needed to confirm this conjecture.

As stated in Sect. 6, we conjecture that the second improvement makes the (initial) formula GAC, but unit propagation does not maintains it during the search. We also conjecture that, if the formula is *maintained* GAC by unit propagation during the search, then the solvers will perform better with the second improvement for *all* instances. We suggest studying such maintenance as a future work, as discussed in Sect. 8.

Finally, let us briefly analyze the results obtained by both improvements (*UIPrB*). Again, it is possible to notice that the second improvement did not make all instances easier as expected, as previous discussed. However, for some particular instances, such as *30_70_17*, *es30fst03*, *es30fst05* and *i080-004*, the combination of both improvements did make the instance easier to be solved.

8   Conclusion and Future Work

In this paper we review the *Parental-based* relative encoding which is used to solve the Steiner Tree Problem in graphs and improve it by using a method described and used previously by Bryant & Velev [3] and Velev & Gao [4], and another one that explore the dominance relation in the given graph.

As shown in Sect. 7, the first method reduced the size of the resulting formulae and the run time taken by MaxSAT solvers to solve them, as expected. The second method made some instances easier to solve, but did not improved the run times overall.

As mentioned in Sect. 6, we conjecture that the second improvement makes the *hard* formula GAC, but unit propagation does not maintains this property during the search. As mentioned in Sect. 7, we also conjecture that maintaining GAC during search may make the second method always improve the solvers.

Since it is polynomial to decide whether all terminal vertices are in the same connected component, we suspect that it may be possible to build the *hard* formula in such a way that GAC is maintained by unit propagation. As a future work, we suggest studying some encoding for which the *hard* formula is maintained GAC by unit propagation, or prove that such encoding does not exist.

References

1. Oliveira, R.T.D., Silva, F.: Sat and maxsat encodings for trees applied to the steiner tree problem. In: 2014 Brazilian Conference on Intelligent Systems (BRACIS), pp. 192–197, October 2014
2. Prestwich, S.: Sat problems with chains of dependent variables. Disc. Appl. Math. **130**(2), 329–350 (2003)
3. Bryant, R.E., Velev, M.N.: Boolean satisfiability with transitivity constraints. ACM Trans. Comput. Logic **3**(4), 604–627 (2002)
4. Velev, M.N., Gao, P.: Design of parallel portfolios for sat-based solving of hamiltonian cycle problems. In: International Symposium on Artificial Intelligence and Mathematics (ISAIM 2010), Fort Lauderdale, Florida, USA, January 6–8, 2010 (2010)
5. Karp, R.: Reducibility among combinatorial problems. In: Miller, R., Thatcher, J., Bohlinger, J. (eds.) Complexity of Computer Computations. The IBM Research Symposia Series, pp. 85–103. Springer, US (1972)
6. Koch, T., Martin, A., Voß, S.: Steinlib: an updated library on steiner tree problems in graphs. Technical Report 00–37, Zuse-Institut Berlin (ZIB), November 2000
7. Davis, M., Logemann, G., Loveland, D.: A machine program for theorem-proving. Commun. ACM **5**, 394–397 (1962)
8. Biere, A.: Lingeling, plingeling and treengeling entering the sat competition 2013. In: Proceedings of SAT Competition 2013. Volume B-2013-1, University of Helsinki (2013)
9. Heras, F., Larrosa, J., Oliveras, A.: Minimaxsat: an efficient weighted max-sat solver. J. Artif. Intell. Res. **31**, 1–32 (2008)
10. Velev, M.N.: Exploiting hierarchy and structure to efficiently solve graph coloring as sat. In: IEEE/ACM International Conference on Computer-Aided Design, ICCAD 2007, pp. 135–142, November 2007
11. Floyd, R.W.: Algorithm 97: shortest path. Commun. ACM **5**(6), 345 (1962)
12. Yannakakis, M.: Computing the minimum fill-in is np-complete. SIAM J. Algebraic Discrete Methods **2**(1), 77–79 (1981)
13. Lengauer, T., Tarjan, R.E.: A fast algorithm for finding dominators in a flowgraph. ACM Trans. Program. Lang. Syst. **1**(1), 121–141 (1979)
14. Narodytska, N., Bacchus, F.: Maximum satisfiability using core-guided maxsat resolution. In: Proceedings of the Twenty-Eighth AAAI Conference on Artificial Intelligence, July 27–31, 2014, Québec City, pp. 2717–2723 (2014)

Left-Right Relations for Qualitative Representation and Alignment of Planar Spatial Networks

Malumbo Chipofya[✉], Angela Schwering, Carl Schultz, Emily Harason, and Sahib Jan

Institut Für Geoinformatik, Universität Münster,
48149 Heisenbergstraße 2, Münster, Germany
{mchipofya,schwering,schultzc,e_hara01,s_jan001}@uni-muenster.de

Abstract. The spatial relations "left-of" and "right-of" are important for distinguishing relative positions of objects within and with respect to elements of plane embedded networks such as networks of streets. We present a representation of the "left/right" relations that is suitable for use in sketch-to-metric map alignment. The new representation is based on a new family of qualitative spatial calculi called $\mathcal{ULSTRA}$. Although left/right relations have already been formalized for line segments in the Dipole Relation Algebra ($\mathcal{DRA}$) family of qualitative spatial calculi, the distinctions made by those calculi are too strong for applications such as sketch-to-metric map alignment. We show in an empirical evaluation that performing sketch-to-metric map alignment with the new representation is more effective than using the original $\mathcal{DRA}$ calculi.

Keywords: Left-right relations · Qualitative spatial representation · Sketch-metric map alignment

1 Introduction

Qualitative matching algorithms [4,13,19] have applications in sketch-to-metric map alignment [5,17] as well as other areas such as image retrieval [18] and object recognition [6]. These algorithms take qualitative descriptions of two spatial scenes and search for a correspondence between objects in one scene with objects in the other such that the similarity of spatial relations between corresponding pairs is maximized. The qualitative descriptions are fundamental to these algorithms because the measure of similarity depends on the representation [13].

Representations can be constrained to differing degrees. For line segments the undirected graph representation is one of the simplest, distinguishing only whether two line segments share an end point or not. The $\mathcal{DRA}_{80}$ calculus [11] may be considered to be at the other end of this spectrum. It is so expressive that it distinguishes between parallel, anti-parallel, and non-aligned configurations of line segments. However, this great expressive power comes at the expense of flexibility. That is, the distinctions made by the calculus may be finer than the

© Springer International Publishing Switzerland 2015
O. Pichardo Lagunas et al. (Eds.): MICAI 2015, Part II, LNAI 9414, pp. 435–450, 2015.
DOI: 10.1007/978-3-319-27101-9_33

distinctions required by an application. Therefore, to use a representation for qualitative matching problems involving line segments, it may first have to be adapted to make only as many distinctions as necessary to preserve relations between matched segments.

In this paper we present a family of spatial calculi for qualitative representation and reasoning about undirected line segments called the *Undirected Line Segment Ternary Relation Algebra* ($\mathcal{ULSTRA}$). The target application for which we developed these calculi is sketch-metric map alignment but their generality makes them useful for representing and reasoning about connectivity and left-right relations between adjacent segments in spatial networks in general. The main goal of this representation is to be able to capture information about the connectivity of the segments and at the same time allow one to distinguish the cyclic order of segments that meet at a three way or higher order junction. The design choices made in the development of the new calculus are justified by results from experiments in sketch-metric map alignment [5] that showed that the cyclic order of streets around a junction was preserved with high accuracy in sketch maps. In the experiments reported in [5] it was found that the connectivity relations or network topology of street segments drawn in sketch maps was mostly correct with respect to the same relations for the corresponding street segments in the metric map. It was also found that the ordering of street segments at junctions was always correct whenever the connectivity relations were correct [2]. On the other hand precise relations such as metric lengths and angles are not necessarily correlated due to typical schematization and distortion effects [20].

Based on $\mathcal{ULSTRA}_{119}$, a version of the $\mathcal{ULSTRA}$ calculus and the qualitative spatial calculus $\mathcal{DRA}_7$ [2,19], we devise a binary representation of $\mathcal{ULSTRA}$ relations called $\mathcal{DRA}_{7-lr}$. This allows us to apply $\mathcal{ULSTRA}$ constraints directly using existing sketch-metric map alignment algorithms that only accept binary constraints.

We will begin our presentation with an overview of the state of the art in qualitative spatial representation of left/right relations for directed line segments and highlight some difficulties that arise when representing spatial networks (Sect. 2). The $\mathcal{ULSTRA}$ calculus is introduced in Sect. 3. Section 4 contains evaluations of the two new representations with sketch maps from the SketchMapia database[1]. In Sect. 4.2 we evaluate the robustness of $\mathcal{ULSTRA}$ against typical distortions of sketch maps. The results of Sect. 4.2 partly motivate development of the $\mathcal{DRA}_{7-lr}$ representation. The relations $\mathcal{DRA}_{7-lr}$ are introduced in Sect. 4.3 with details of their application to a sketch-metric map alignment algorithm [3]. We close the paper with a conclusion in Sect. 5.

2   Qualitative Representation with Left/Right Relations

Relative direction relations can be defined many ways depending on the application and the domain of spatial objects involved. The common aspect to relative direction relations that can be interpreted as representing "being left of" and

---

[1] www.sketchmapia.de.

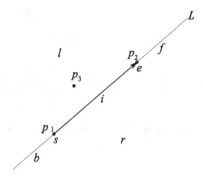

Fig. 1. Any two points p_1 and p_2 induce a planar partition into sectors $l,b,s,i,e,$ $f,$ and r. Any other point in the plane, e.g. p_3, must be located in exactly one of these sectors.

"being right of" is that the referent set of objects have an intrinsic front. At any point in time, an object will have an orientation determined by the bearing of its front. "Left" can thus be taken to be a region contained in the left half-plane determined by the line through the front of the object that has the same bearing as the front. The choice of which region is considered is one of the main differences between models of left and right relations.

2.1 The $\mathcal{LR}$ calculus

One of the simplest relative orientation calculi is the ternary $\mathcal{LR}$ calculus which distinguishes several configurations that three points can be in. Given an ordered list of three points, (p_1, p_2, p_3), consider the planar partition $P(p_1, p_2)$ induced by the points p_1 and p_2 with the following classes: the open left (l) and right (r) half-planes bounded by the directed line L incident with p_1 and p_2 and oriented with bearing p_1 to p_2; the points of L lying before p_1 (b), coincident with p_1 (s), between p_1 and p_2 (i), after p_2 (f), and coincident with p_2 (e).

The triple (p_1, p_2, p_3) are in a relation R if the point p_3 is the region with the label R. For example if p_3 is in the left half-plane bounded by L then the corresponding relation is l (Fig. 1).

For the sake of clarity, we will use the symbols l, b, s, i, e, f, r to refer to the relations. When referring to the regions of the partition, we will annotate the relation symbol with a subscript containing the point pair defining the partition. That is, $l_{(p,q)}$ refers to the left two dimensional region of $P(p,q)$. If $A = (p,q)$ is the line segment determined by the point pair (p,q) we may equivalently use l_A to refer to the same two dimensional region.

2.2 The $\mathcal{DRA}$ Calculi

In $\mathcal{DRA}$ the relative positions of directed line segments, also called dipoles in [11], are based on the relations of their vertices. Formally, a dipole is an ordered pair of points in $\mathbb{R}^2$ which can be written as $\mathbf{A} = (A_s, A_e)$, where A_s and A_e

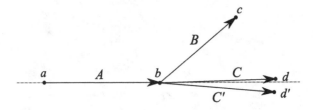

Fig. 2. The qualitative spatial calculi $\mathcal{DRA}_{72}$ and $\mathcal{DRA}_{80}$ are over constrained as tools for representing spatial networks

are, respectively, the start- and end-point of **A**. We refer to A_s and A_e as nodes of **A**.

A basic $\mathcal{DRA}$ relation between two dipoles **A** and **B** is given by the 4-tuple of $\mathcal{LR}$ relations $s_B e_B s_A e_A$ of the respective triples (A_s, A_e, B_s), (A_s, A_e, B_e), (B_s, B_e, A_s), and (B_s, B_e, A_e). The resulting system of 72 relations is called $\mathcal{DRA}_f$ [11]. $\mathcal{DRA}_{80}$ refines $\mathcal{DRA}_{72}$ by introducing orientation descriptors '+', '-', 'A', and 'P' that describe the orientation of **B** with respect to **A** where the orientation is '+' if **B** is oriented towards the left of **A**, '-' if it is oriented towards the right, 'P' if **A** and **B** are parallel and 'A' if they are anti-parallel. The descriptors are defined only for the four relations $rrrr, rrll, llll, llrr$ [11]. The "coarsened" $\mathcal{DRA}_c$ [11] demands that points be in general position (i.e. no three points can be collinear). This means that only the values l, r, s, e are allowed. The resulting calculus has 24 relations (see [11] for details). The coarsest version of $\mathcal{DRA}$ described so far is $\mathcal{DRA}_7$, so called because only 7 relations can be realised between any pair of dipoles [2,19]. For $\mathcal{DRA}_7$, $\mathcal{P}(\mathbf{A})$ is a partition of the plane into only three parts, namely, A_s (s_A), A_e (e_A), and the rest of plane (x_A). The resulting seven relations are $sese$ (coincidence), $sxsx$ (share same start point), $xsex$ (start point of first dipole coincident with end point of second dipole), $xxxx$ (disjoint), $exxs$ (start point of second dipole is coincident with end point of first dipole), $xexe$ (share same end point), and $eses$ (reverse of each dipole is coincident with the other). The $\mathcal{DRA}_7$ relations give the information captured by a directed graph without loops.

2.3 Representing Spatial Networks

Representing relative directions between segments in spatial networks can be performed at least two levels. At the finest level, relative directions between nodes of the network can be used to describe all relative direction relations in the network. Using $\mathcal{LR}$ this would mean recording the $\mathcal{LR}$ relation for every three nodes. But for many applications such constraints would be too strict. For example, it is not disagreeable that the configurations (a, b, d) and (a, b, d') of points in Fig. 2 are more similar than the configurations (a, b, d) and (a, b, c). Yet, to the contrary, $\mathcal{LR}$ would consider the former pair to be different and the latter indistinguishable. Another example of this strictness can be seen when considering the constraint between nodes where one is not adjacent to any of the other two. In many applications (e.g. Sketch-metric map alignment [5]) such constraints are not given in strict form, often remaining completely undetermined.

A solution might be to coarsen constraints to allow for expressing uncertainty but this would introduce more problems than not, because even for small $\mathcal{LR}$ constraint networks of four to five nodes using only the base relations l and r it is impossible to detect inconsistencies using algebraic closure [10]. A solution may instead lie in using $\mathcal{DRA}_{72}$ to directly represent relative directions between the segments of the network. This approach, however, has the same shortfalls. Again the configurations (A, B) and (A, D) would be considered indistinguishable while the configurations (A, D) and (A, D') would be seen as being significantly different. The problem here is that the semantics of the left and right relations as captured here are different from the expected semantics for the given domain of spatial networks.

In [19], Wallgrün et al. did away with these problems by disregarding all relative direction information, instead introducing $\mathcal{DRA}_7$ relations between street segments and using cardinal direction relations between street intersections to constrain orientations of the street segments relative to the entire spatial scene. This of course applies only to situations where the correspondence between the two input networks is expected to preserve orientations globally.

The $\mathcal{ULSTRA}$ calculi which we present below support alternative representations that do not share some of the aforementioned shortfalls. $\mathcal{ULSTRA}$ builds upon our previous work [2] and on the work of Moratz et al. [11,12] on the $\mathcal{DRA}$ calculus.

3 $\mathcal{ULSTRA}$ Calculi

The $\mathcal{ULSTRA}$ calculi are defined by ternary relations over the set of undirected line segments in $\mathbb{R}^2$. However, our characterization of them derives from the $\mathcal{DRA}$ relations, i.e. we first consider relations on directed line segments and collapse these relations to relations on undirected line segments. In this section we will present the $\mathcal{ULSTRA}$ calculi. Subsection 3.1 introduces a few terms and concept the we will refer to in the sequel. In Subsect. 3.2 we define four members of the $\mathcal{ULSTRA}$ family and in Subsect. 3.3 we how reasoning can be done using $\mathcal{ULSTRA}$ relations in the spatial solver CLP(QS).

3.1 Preliminaries

We denote the set of undirected line segments by *USegs* and denote the set directed line segments by *Segs*. Thus all $\mathcal{ULSTRA}$ relations are subsets of *USegs* × *USegs* × *USegs* and all $\mathcal{DRA}$ relations are subsets of *Segs* × *Segs*. For a directed line segment $A \in Segs$ we will write $rev(A)$ to denote the directed line segment covering the same set of points as A but having the opposite orientation. In the sequel we shall treat rev as an equivalence relation on *Segs* so that we shall be also able to use the fact that

$$USegs = Segs/rev = \{\{A, B\} \mid A, B \in Segs \land B = rev(A)\}.$$

Where the division represents taking the quotient of *Segs* by identifying line segments that cover the same set of points. Let R be a binary relation on *Segs*. Then there is a relation R' on *USegs* satisfying $(A', B') \in R'$ if and only if there exists a pair $(A, B) \in R$ such that A and A' cover the same points, and B and B' cover the same points. Thus with some abuse of notation we will also write $R/rev \subseteq R'$ to describe the relationship between R and R'. This notation is extended to three and higher arity relations.

In the next Subsection below we will refer to ternary incarnations of $\mathcal{DRA}_7$ and $\mathcal{DRA}_{72}$. These will be denoted $\mathcal{DRA}_{7t}$ and $\mathcal{DRA}_{72t}$ respectively, and are what we call Induced Ternary Calculi [2]. A ternary calculus, $\mathcal{C}$, is said to be an induced ternary calculus if every relation of $\mathcal{C}$ has a decomposition into binary relations of some binary calculus, say $\mathcal{B}$, such that if R is a base relation of $\mathcal{C}$ then there are base relations R_1, R_2, R_3 of $\mathcal{B}$ with $R = \{(A, B, C) \mid (A, B) \in R_1, (B, C) \in R_2, (A, C) \in R_3\}$.

3.2   Defining $\mathcal{ULSTRA}$ Relations

Any simple undirected graph with three or less edges such that each node is incident with at least one edge can have no more than six nodes and there are exactly eight such graphs up to isomorphism (which can be enumerated exhaustively - see Sloane's sequence number A000088 [9]). In [2] we introduced the notion of the shape of a triple of line segments which in fact refers to these eight graphs (See Fig. 3). The set of classes of line segment triples belonging to the same shape is a JEPD set of relations (by isomorphism). The closure of these eight relations under permutations comprises 16 JEPD relations. The 16 shape relations together with the standard relation algebraic operations form the coarsest member of the $\mathcal{ULSTRA}$ family of qualitative spatial calculi which we call $\mathcal{ULSTRA}_{16}$.

For a further refinement consider the the system of induced ternary relations, $\mathcal{S}$, comprising the components S_0, S_1, S_2 where

$$S_1 = \{(A, B) \in Segs \times Segs \mid (A, B) \in eifs \cup iebe \cup sisf \cup iseb\}\}$$
$$S_2 = \{(A, B) \in Segs \times Segs \mid (A, B) \in ebis \cup beie \cup sfsi \cup fsei\}\}$$
$$S_0 = (Segs \times Segs) - (S_1 \cup S_2).$$

The symbols $eifs$, $iebe$, $sisf$, $iseb$, $ebis$, $beie$, $sfsi$, $fsei$ in the definitions of S_1, S_2, and S_3 represent $\mathcal{DRA}_{72}$ the relations. S_1 identifies pairs of line segments that share an end point and the first contains the second, while S_2 identifies pairs of line segments that share an end point where the second contains the first. The 27 relations in $\mathcal{S}$ have the form

$$S_{ijk} = \{(A, B, C) \in Segs \times Segs \times Segs \mid (A, B) \in S_i \land (B, C) \in S_j \land (A, C) \in S_k\},$$

$0 \le i, j, k \le 2$, some of which are empty.

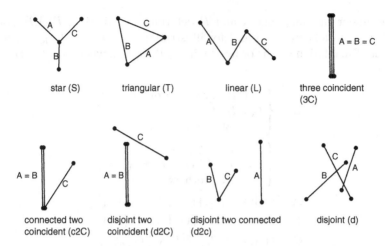

star (S)   triangular (T)   linear (L)   three coincident (3C)

connected two   disjoint two   disjoint two connected   disjoint (d)
coincident (c2C)   coincident (d2C)   (d2c)

Fig. 3. The eight basic shapes describing possible configurations of three line segments in the plane based on shared end points.

We now introduce the mechanisms for distinguishing between left and right in the $\mathcal{ULSTRA}$ calculus. Let $A = (A_s, A_e)$ and $B = (B_s, B_e)$ be two directed line segments with $\mathcal{DRA}_7$ relation R_{AB}. We can alter the orientations of A and B by the following mapping

$$\text{if } R_{AB} \in \{sese, exxs\}(A, B) \longmapsto (A, B)$$
$$\text{if } R_{AB} \in \{xexe, eses\}(A, B) \longmapsto (A, rev(B))$$
$$\text{if } R_{AB} = sxsx(A, B) \longmapsto (rev(A), B)$$
$$\text{if } R_{AB} = xesx(A, B) \longmapsto (rev(A), rev(B))$$

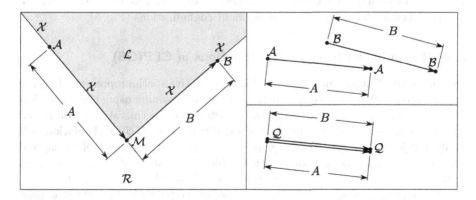

Fig. 4. The $\mathcal{ULSTRA}$ zones determined by a configuration of directed line segments.

Then under this mapping A and B determine a partition, $P(A,B)$, of the plane defined as follows (see Fig. 4 for illustration). Let $t_{AB} = R_{\mathcal{LR}}(A_s, p, B_e)$ denote the $\mathcal{LR}$ relation on the ordered triple (A_s, p, B_e), where $p \in \{A_e\} \cap \{B_s\}$, and let

$$\mathcal{L} = \begin{cases} l_A \cap l_B & \text{if } t_{AB} = l \text{ or } t_{AB} = f \\ l_A \cup l_B & \text{if } t_{AB} = r \\ \emptyset & \text{otherwise} \end{cases} \tag{1}$$

$$\mathcal{R} = \begin{cases} r_A \cap r_B & \text{if } t_{AB} = r \\ r_A \cup r_B & \text{if } t_{AB} = l \text{ or } t_{AB} = f \\ \emptyset & \text{otherwise} \end{cases} \tag{2}$$

$$\mathcal{A} = (\{A_s\} - \{B_e\}) \cup (\{A_e\} - \{B_s\}) \tag{3}$$

$$\mathcal{B} = (\{B_s\} - \{A_e\}) \cup (\{B_e\} - \{A_s\}) \tag{4}$$

$$\mathcal{Q} = (\{A_s\} \cap \{B_s\}) \cup (\{A_e\} \cap \{B_e\}) \tag{5}$$

$$\mathcal{M} = (\{A_s\} \cap \{B_e\}) \cup (\{A_e\} \cap \{B_s\}) \tag{6}$$

$$\mathcal{X} = \mathbb{R}^2 - (\mathcal{L} \cup \mathcal{A} \cup \mathcal{Q} \cup \mathcal{M} \cup \mathcal{B} \cup \mathcal{R}) \tag{7}$$

We call the parts of the partition $P(A,B)$ the $\mathcal{ULSTRA}$ zones of the pair (A, B). Then any triple (A, B, C) of line segments can be placed into a relation $\{s_C, e_C\} \wedge \{s_B, e_B\} \wedge \{s_A, e_A\}$ where the values s_I and e_I, $I \in \{A, B, C\}$, specify the respective sectors of the partition determined by the remaining *ordered* pair in which I_s and I_e lie (à la $\mathcal{DRA}$). We assume $\mathcal{L} = \mathcal{R} = \emptyset$ whenever $\mathcal{M} = \emptyset$.

Note that this set of relations has the property that changing the orientations of any line segments in a triple will not change the relation computed. That is, forgetting the orientations of the line segments does not add or reduce the amount of information at our disposal. So we can in fact treat these relations as if they were relations on *USegs*. We denote by $\mathcal{ULSTRA}_{65}$ the closure of the resulting relations under permutations.

The base relations of $\mathcal{ULSTRA}_{119}$ are those obtained as intersections of the set $\mathcal{S}/rev$ of relations on *USegs* and $\mathcal{ULSTRA}_{65}$ base relations. $\mathcal{ULSTRA}_{119}$ distinguishes 33 disjoint sets of line segment configurations (Fig. 5).

3.3   Reasoning with $\mathcal{ULSTRA}$ Relations in CLP(QS)

One of the most important tasks to which qualitative spatial representations are applied is reasoning. We are currently working on reasoning using the $\mathcal{ULSTRA}$ representation, specifically in order to (1) determine the consistency of a mixed qualitative-numerical descriptions of a scene using the $\mathcal{ULSTRA}$ relations (2) verify the jointly-exhaustive, pairwise disjoint properties of the relations, and (3) automatically generate composition tables for relation algebraic reasoning. Importantly, these tasks require both sound and complete spatial reasoning.

One approach to achieve this is by encoding the $\mathcal{ULSTRA}$ relations as *polynomial constraints*; determining spatial consistency of a scenario is then equivalent to determining satisfiability of the corresponding polynomial constraint

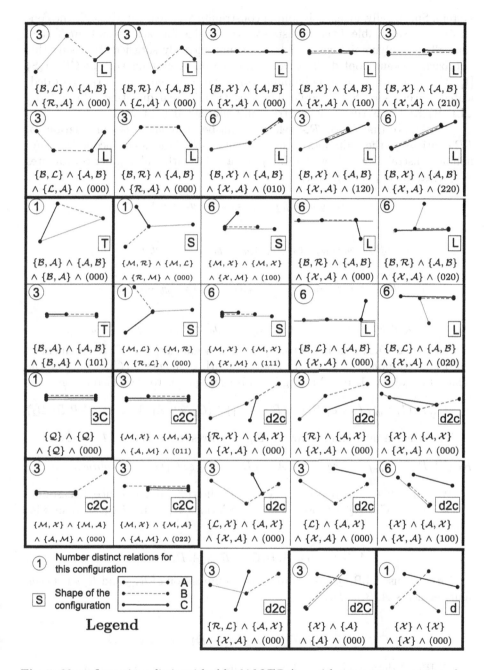

Fig. 5. 33 configurations distinguished by $\mathcal{ULSTRA}_{119}$ with some representative relation labels. The first three conjuncts of each label correspond to the underlying $\mathcal{ULSTRA}_{65}$ relation while the last conjunct corresponds to the underlying member of the set $\mathcal{S}/rev$.

system. Specifically, given polynomial constraints over real variables X, the constraints are satisfiable if there exists some real value for each variable in X such that all the polynomial constraints are simultaneously satisfied. By using this approach we can adopt declarative spatial reasoning systems such as CLP(QS) [1]; within such reasoners, polynomial solving is achieved using a range of dedicated solvers such Sat Modulo Theories (SMT), real quantifier elimination, CLP(R), and constructive geometric constraint solving [14–16].

We observe that $\mathcal{ULSTRA}$ relations can be formulated as combinations of LR relations on the endpoints of the segments. LR relations are encoded as polynomial constraints as follows [1]. Let p_i be a point with real number coordinates $x_i, y_i \in \mathbb{R}$; given points p_a, p_b, p_c:

$$p_a \ eq \ p_b \equiv_{def} (x_a = x_b) \wedge (y_a = y_b)$$

$$p_c \ left \ p_a \ p_b \equiv_{def} (x_b - x_a)(y_c - y_a) > (y_b - y_a)(x_c - x_a)$$

$$p_c \ collinear \ p_a \ p_b \equiv_{def} (x_b - x_a)(y_c - y_a) = (y_b - y_a)(x_c - x_a)$$

$$p_c \ right \ p_a \ p_b \equiv_{def} (x_b - x_a)(y_c - y_a) < (y_b - y_a)(x_c - x_a)$$

Each $\mathcal{ULSTRA}$ relation consists of three segments A, B, C; let segment A consist of endpoints A_1 and A_2 (likewise with segments B, C). Consider the relation in column 1, row 2 in Fig. 5. This corresponds to the LR relations:

$$R_{1,2}(A, B, C) \equiv_{def} (A_2 \ eq \ B_1) \wedge (B_2 \ eq \ C_1) \wedge (C_2 \ left \ A_1 \ A_2) \wedge (C_2 \ left \ B_1 \ B_2)$$

The relation in column 1, row 3 (Fig. 5) corresponds to the LR relations:

$$R_{1,3}(A, B, C) \equiv_{def} (A_1 \ eq \ C_2) \wedge (A_2 \ eq \ B_1) \wedge (B_2 \ eq \ C_1) \wedge \neg (C_1 \ collinear \ A_1 \ A_2)$$

We similarly encode relation $R_{2,4}$ for the following proof of concept reasoning tasks. Firstly, CLP(QS) proves that the relations $R_{1,2}$ and $R_{1,3}$ are pair-wise disjoint:

$$\exists A, B, C \big(R_{1,2}(A, B, C) \wedge R_{1,3}(A, B, C) \big) \equiv \bot$$

Next, we use CLP(QS) to compute the composition of $R_{1,2}$ and $R_{1,3}$ between four segments A, B, C, D:

$$\exists A, B, C, D \big(R_{1,2}(A, B, C) \wedge R_{1,3}(B, C, D) \wedge R_{i,j}(A, B, D) \big) \equiv \top$$

CLP(QS) determines that this is satisfiable when $R_{i,j}$ is the relation in column 2 row 4 (Fig. 5).

Given a partially numerically defined scene, CLP(QS) can determine which $\mathcal{ULSTRA}$ relations are possible; e.g. let $A_1 = (0, 0)$, $A_2 = (10, 0)$ and $B_1 = (10, 0)$, then CLP(QS) determines that $R_{1,2}$ and $R_{2,4}$ can hold between A, B, C

(restricted to the subset of relations that we have defined for this proof of concept):

$$\exists A, B, C\big(A_1 = (0,0) \wedge A_2 = (10,0) \wedge B_1 = (10,0) \wedge R_{i,j}(A,B,C)\big) \equiv \top$$

... for $i = 1, j = 2$ or $i = 2, j = 4$.

Finally, given the following incomplete qualitative LR description of a scenario, CLP(QS) determines which $\mathcal{ULSTRA}$ relations are possible:

$$\exists A, B, C\big((C_2 \ collinear \ A_1 \ A_2) \wedge R_{i,j}(A,B,C)\big) \equiv \top$$

... for $i = 1, j = 3$ or $i = 2, j = 4$.

We are in the process of completing this polynomial formalisation of all $\mathcal{ULSTRA}$ relations.

4   Representation of Networks for Sketch Map Alignment

Spatial representation with $\mathcal{ULSTRA}$ can be done directly for plane embedded networks. We performed experiments to compare $\mathcal{ULSTRA}$ representations with those of $\mathcal{DRA}_7$ and $\mathcal{DRA}_{72}$ for efficacy in sketch-metric map alignment. In past experiments with sketch-metric map alignment [7] we explored using $\mathcal{DRA}_7$ and $\mathcal{DRA}_{72}$ for representing spatial relations between street segments. Results from those experiments showed that $\mathcal{DRA}_{72}$ relations were over constrained for this task. The results from our first experiment presented in Subsect. 4.2 below support the hypothesis that the $\mathcal{ULSTRA}$ calculi are at least as robust against typical distortions in sketch maps as are the $\mathcal{DRA}$ calculi. In addition, the results of Subsect. 4.3 show that representations based on $\mathcal{ULSTRA}$ are competitive in terms of their impact on algorithm performance when compared with pure $\mathcal{DRA}$ representations.

4.1   The Sketch Map Alignment Problem

For the sake of clarity, we will introduce a formal characterization of the sketch map alignment problem as the problem involving matching sets of constraints. Given a domain of objects such as line segments, one can describe the spatial configuration of these objects by labelling each pair of objects with the relation that holds between them. We call such labels constraints.

Suppose the relations that we use as constraints in our description are given by a qualitative spatial calculus with base relations $\mathfrak{B}$. If N is a set representing the set of objects in our description then the function $C : N \times N \rightarrow 2^{\mathfrak{B}}$ is called the constraint function for our description and the pair (N, C) called a Qualitative Constraint Network (QCN). Thus a set of spatial constraints can equivalently be expressed as a QCN. In order to say what it means to match two QCNs we require the following definition.

Definition 1 (Disjoint Union of QCNs [4]). *Let $\mathcal{N} = (N, C)$ and $\mathcal{N}' = (N', C')$ be QCNs with $N \cap N' = \emptyset$. The disjoint union of $\mathcal{N}$ and $\mathcal{N}'$ is the QCN $\mathcal{N} \uplus \mathcal{N}' = (N \cup N', C'')$ where*

$$
C''(i,j) = \begin{cases} C(i,j) & if \ i,j \in N \\ C'(i,j) & if \ i,j \in N' \\ 1 & otherwise \end{cases}
$$

The set of arcs connecting nodes from N to N' are called the joining arcs. A QCN matching problem is the problem of finding refinements of the joining arcs that maximize the number of those arcs labelled with relations under $1'$, the identity relation. Formally, let $\mathbf{Id}_\mathcal{N} = \{(i,j) \in \mathcal{N} \mid C(i,j) \leq 1'\}$ denote the arcs of QCN $\mathcal{N}$ labelled with relations under $1'$. The QCN matching problem is stated as follows.

Definition 2 (QCN Matching Problem [4,19]). $P(\mathcal{N}, \mathcal{N}')$: *find $\mathcal{M} \leq \mathcal{N} \uplus \mathcal{N}'$ such that*

1. *$\mathcal{M}$ is closed, and*
2. *for any closed $\mathcal{M}' \leq \mathcal{N} \uplus \mathcal{N}'$, $|\mathbf{Id}_{\mathcal{M}'}| \leq |\mathbf{Id}_{\mathcal{M}}|$.*

The sketch map alignment algorithms that we presented in [3,4] all perform the alignment by solving this QCN matching problem. In Subsect. 4.3 below we claim that solving the QCN matching problem with $\mathcal{ULSTRA}_{119}$ constraints is equivalent to maximizing a certain sum.

4.2 Robustness Against Typical Distortions: A Comparitive Evaluation

For evaluating the efficacy of $\mathcal{ULSTRA}$ representations for alignment we compared how robust the representations were to the distortions inherent in sketch maps. The data used were extracted from 10 sketch maps taken from the Sketch Mapia database[2]. The sketch maps were produced by participants in a study on information contained in sketch maps. One general location in the city Münster, Germany, was selected and participants were asked to draw a sketch map of this location indicating all features that they considered important for describing the location. In the original study, participants were asked to draw a sketch map of the designated region from a survey perspective. Other than landmarks used to mark the maximum extents of the regions to be drawn no other information was provided to the participants. At the end of the drawing exercise each participant georeferenced their sketch map by ground truthing as many sketched objects as they could. The ground truthing involved assigning an object in the metric map to the sketch object that is being georeferenced.

---

[2] http://www.uni-muenster.de/Geoinformatics/en/sketchmapia/
sketch-map-database.php.

In our evaluation we used the ground truthing data provided in the original experiment to determine the number of constraint violations the sketch map data contained when compared with the metric map data. The results of our comparison are summarized in Table 1. Each row in the table represents data for a single sketch map. For each calculus we computed the number of spatial constraints on which the sketch map and the metric map agreed. The columns titled 'Actual' contain the actual numbers counted while the '%age' column contains the same count as a proportion of the total number of constraints in the sketch map ($^nC_3$ for a map of size n). $\mathcal{DRA}_{7t}$ and $\mathcal{ULSTRA}_{16}$ had almost the same performance both overall and for the individual maps with an average gain in robustness of 1.2 % from $\mathcal{DRA}_{7t}$ to $\mathcal{ULSTRA}_{16}$. They both resulted in fewer constraint violations when compared with $\mathcal{DRA}_{72t}$ and $\mathcal{ULSTRA}_{119}$. The performance of $\mathcal{ULSTRA}_{119}$ was surprisingly much better than that of $\mathcal{DRA}_{72t}$. In fact the average reduction in robustness of 52.2 % from $\mathcal{ULSTRA}_{119}$ to $\mathcal{DRA}_{72t}$ is by far much higher than that observed between $\mathcal{ULSTRA}_{16}$ and $\mathcal{ULSTRA}_{119}$ (4.5 %).

The results reported here suggest that for the given data either $\mathcal{DRA}_{7t}$ or $\mathcal{ULSTRA}_{16}$ may be the best suited models for representing them. However, previous experience [4,19] has shown that these calculi are considerably under-constrained for the matching task. $\mathcal{DRA}_{72t}$, and therefore the binary $\mathcal{DRA}_{72}$, on the other hand, are most unsuitable for this task. In addition the cubic size of ternary representations present a bottleneck when large amounts of data are involved. In the next section, we therefore explore a binary representation of $\mathcal{ULSTRA}_{119}$ relations for this task.

4.3 $\mathcal{DRA}_{7-lr}$: Binary Re-representation of $\mathcal{ULSTRA}_{119}$ constraints

We have found that performing sketch-metric alignment using model/graph matching algorithms is orders of magnitude faster using $\mathcal{DRA}_{72}$ than using $\mathcal{DRA}_7$ [3,4]. We therefore sought to find an alternative representation for line segments spatial relations that could be used in place of $\mathcal{DRA}_{72}$ to increase the robustness against typical distortions in sketch maps with a smaller penalty on performance. Because the graph matching algorithm that we have developed for sketch-metric map alignment [3], requires binary rather than ternary constraints, we present here $\mathcal{DRA}_{7-lr}$, an alternative, binary, representation of $\mathcal{ULSTRA}_{119}$ constraints.

An atomic $\mathcal{DRA}_{7-lr}$ constraint between two line segments A and B is specified by a 4-tuple of two-part constraints of the form

$$R_{\mathcal{DRA}_{7-lr}}(A,B) = \bigwedge_{i,j \in \{1,2\}} \left(R_{\mathcal{DRA}_7}(A_i, B_j) \wedge \left(\bigwedge_{\tau,\kappa \in \{\mathcal{L},\mathcal{A},\mathcal{Q},\mathcal{X},\mathcal{M},\mathcal{B},\mathcal{R}\}} \#\{\tau,\kappa\} \right) \right),$$

(8)

where $i, j \in \{1, 2\}$ each indicate one of the two possible orientations of the respective line segments A and B, τ and κ are any two compatible $\mathcal{ULSTRA}$ zone symbols, and $\#$, when applied to $\{\tau, \kappa\}$ returns the number of line segments with one end-point in τ and the other end-point in κ. The first term of the

Table 1. Robustness of different calculi against distortions inherent in sketch maps measured as the proportion of constraints on sketched objects that are consistent with constraints on corresponding metric map objects.

Sketch map	# of line segments	$\mathcal{DRA}_{7t}$		$\mathcal{ULSTRA}_{16}$		$\mathcal{ULSTRA}_{119}$		$\mathcal{DRA}_{72t}$	
		Actual	%age	Actual	%age	Actual	%age	Actual	%age
SM1	43	11354	92.0	11943	96.8	11564	93.7	2562	20.8
SM2	24	1882	93.0	1981	97.9	1855	91.7	514	25.4
SM3	17	574	84.4	584	85.9	559	82.2	275	40.4
SM4	10	120	100.0	120	100.0	114	95.0	59	49.2
SM5	20	1140	100.0	1140	100.0	1095	96.1	564	49.5
SM6	18	816	100.0	816	100.0	749	91.8	272	33.3
SM7	29	3499	95.8	3524	96.4	3347	91.6	1251	34.2
SM8	31	4060	90.3	4060	90.3	3887	86.5	1556	34.6
SM9	37	7073	91.0	7073	91.0	6830	87.9	3275	42.1
SM10	28	2925	89.3	2925	89.3	2836	86.6	1691	51.6

conjunct is the $\mathcal{DRA}_7$ constraint between A_i and B_j. The four constraints in Subsect. 4.3 can be treated independently of each other.

To match two sets of $\mathcal{DRA}_{7-lr}$ constraints one simply compares pairs of constraints one from each set for equality. This means that the input sets are restricted to have the same cardinality. There are at least two simple variations on this approach that can be used to overcome this restriction. First, one can digitize the count values into binary values setting all non-zero values to 1. Then a pair of constraints match provided they agree on the $\mathcal{DRA}_7$ part and preference is given to the constraint pair that has the most matching positions in the binary string.

The second variation involves comparing the actual counts and still accepting the constraints if they agree on the $\mathcal{DRA}_7$ portion but preferring instead the pair that has the greatest sum of the pairwise minima over all counts. That is, preference is given to the pair $(R_{\mathcal{DRA}_{7-lr}}(A, B), R_{\mathcal{DRA}_{7-lr}}(A', B'))$ of constraints maximizing the sum

$$\sum_{\{\mathcal{L},\mathcal{A},\mathcal{Q},\mathcal{X},\mathcal{M},\mathcal{B},\mathcal{R}\}} \min\left(\#\{\tau, \kappa\}, \#\{\tau', \kappa'\}\right) \tag{9}$$

This last variation is the most robust for sketch-to-metric alignment because it does not penalize differences in the sizes of the input data and does not throw away as much detail as does the digitized version. In fact we obtain the following:

Statement 1. *Let $\mathcal{U}$ and $\mathcal{V}$ be two $\mathcal{DRA}_{7-lr}$ QCNs and let $\mathcal{U}'$ and $\mathcal{V}'$ be their respective underlying $\mathcal{ULSTRA}_{119}$ QCNs. Then every solution to the QCN matching problem for $\mathcal{U}'$ and $\mathcal{V}'$ is optimal if and only if it is a solution to the matching for $\mathcal{U}$ and $\mathcal{V}$ that maximizes the sum of counts over all mutually consistent pairs of constraints in $\mathcal{U} \times \mathcal{V}$.*

5   Conclusions and Outlook

We have presented the $\mathcal{ULSTRA}$ calculus and discussed how it improves the performance of our sketch-metric map alignment algorithm. $\mathcal{ULSTRA}_{119}$ is less constrained than $\mathcal{DRA}_{72}$ and more constrained than $\mathcal{DRA}_7$. The way that $\mathcal{ULSTRA}_{119}$ brings advantage to the matching process is by distinguishing fewer configuration per pair of line segments while maintaining distinctions induced planar partitions corresponding to simple circuits (sequences of line segments forming closed polygons).

$\mathcal{ULSTRA}_{119}$ leads to better solutions during alignment as it is robust against some typical distortions inherent in sketch maps. However, it is not robust to all distortion effects encountered during sketch processing. In particular, when the third line segment is disconnected from the other two, then the relation in the sketch map may differ from the corresponding relation in the metric map. In addition, constraints involving one dimensional sectors are unlikely to remain stable across hand draw sketch maps. The same applies for other applications where such relations are directly observed and reported (e.g. robotics).

Another problem that we have not been able to address yet with $\mathcal{ULSTRA}_{119}$ is that of maintaining spatial consistency under spatial aggregation. When a string of segments is aggregated, the resulting configuration may change the relation of the aggregate to one that significantly deviates from the majority of the original constraints involving the component line segments.

Our future work will focus on the two shortfalls outlined above. In addition we will address the question of deciding consistency of networks of $\mathcal{ULSTRA}$ constraints. By the curious and strong result of Lee [8], we believe that $\mathcal{ULSTRA}_{119}$ is $\exists\mathbb{R}$–complete. We also believe that the $\exists\mathbb{R}$–completeness result can be, alternatively, shown by reduction from the rectilinear crossing number problem. We will write about this next.

Acknowledgements. This work was partially funded by Universität Münster and the German Research Foundation (DFG) under grant Grant SCHW 1372/7-1:SketchMapia.

References

1. Bhatt, M., Lee, J.H., Schultz, C.: CLP(QS): a declarative spatial reasoning framework. In: Egenhofer, M., Giudice, N., Moratz, R., Worboys, M. (eds.) COSIT 2011. LNCS, vol. 6899, pp. 210–230. Springer, Heidelberg (2011)
2. Chipofya, M.: Combining DRA and CYC into a network friendly calculus. In: Raedt, L.D., Bessière, C., Dubois, D., Doherty, P., Frasconi, P., Heintz, F., Lucas, P.J.F. (eds.) ECAI, vol. 242 of Frontiers in Artificial Intelligence and Applications, pp. 234–239. IOS Press (2012)
3. Chipofya, M., Schultz, C., Schwering, A.: A metaheuristic approach for efficient and effective sketch-to-metric map alignment. Int. J. Geogr. Inf. Sci. 29 (2015)
4. Chipofya, M., Schwering, A., Binor, T.: Matching qualitative spatial scene descriptions á la tabu. In: Castro, F., Gelbukh, A., González, M. (eds.) MICAI 2013, Part II. LNCS, vol. 8266, pp. 388–402. Springer, Heidelberg (2013)

5. Chipofya, M., Wang, J., Schwering, A.: Towards cognitively plausible spatial representations for sketch map alignment. In: Egenhofer, M., Giudice, N., Moratz, R., Worboys, M. (eds.) COSIT 2011. LNCS, vol. 6899, pp. 20–39. Springer, Heidelberg (2011)
6. Grimson, W.E.L.: Object Recognition by Computer - The Role of Geometric Constraints. MIT Press, Cambridge (1990)
7. Jan, S., Schwering, A., Chipofya, M., Wang, J.: Qualitative representations of schematized and distorted street segments in sketch maps. In: Freksa, C., Nebel, B., Hegarty, M., Barkowsky, T. (eds.) Spatial Cognition 2014. LNCS, vol. 8684, pp. 253–267. Springer, Heidelberg (2014)
8. Lee, J.H.: The complexity of reasoning with relative directions. In: Schaub, T., Friedrich, G., O'Sullivan, B. (eds.) Frontiers in Artificial Intelligence and Applications, ECAI 2014, vol. 263, pp. 507–512 (2014)
9. T.O. line Encyclopedia of Integer Sequences. Number of graphs on n unlabeled nodes: Accessed 14 July 2015
10. Lücke, D.: Qualitative Spatial Reasoning about Relative Orientation: A Question of Consistency. Ph.D. thesis, University of Bremen (2012)
11. Moratz, R., Lücke, D., Mossakowski, T.: Oriented straight line segment algebra: Qualitative spatial reasoning about oriented objects. CoRR, abs/0912.5533 (2009)
12. Moratz, R., Renz, J., Wolter, D.: Qualitative spatial reasoning about line segments. In: ECAI, pp. 234–238. Citeseer (2000)
13. Nedas, K., Egenhofer, M.: Spatial-scene similarity queries. Trans. GIS **12**(6), 661–681 (2008)
14. Schultz, C., Bhatt, M.: Spatial symmetry driven pruning strategies for efficient declarative spatial reasoning. In: Proceedings of the 12th International Conference on Spatial Information Theory, COSIT 2015, Santa Fe, New Mexico, USA (2011)
15. Schultz, C., Bhatt, M.: Declarative spatial reasoning with boolean combinations of axis-aligned rectangular polytopes. In 21st European Conference on Artificial Intelligence (ECAI 2014), Prague, Czech Republic (2014)
16. Schultz, C., Bhatt, M.: Encoding relative orientation and mereotopology relations with geometric constraints in clp(qs). In: 1st Workshop on Logics for Qualitative Modelling and Reasoning (LQMR 2015), Lodz, Poland, September 2015
17. Schwering, A., Wang, J., Chipofya, M., Jan, S., Li, R., Broelemann, K.: Sketchmapia: qualitative representations for the alignment of sketch and metric maps. Spati. Cognit. Comput. **14**(3), 220–254 (2014)
18. Sciascio, E.D., Donini, F., Mongiello, M.: Spatial layout representation for query-by-sketch content-based image retrieval. Pattern Recogn. Lett. **23**(13), 1599–1612 (2002)
19. Wallgrün, J.O., Wolter, D., Richter, K.-F.: Qualitative matching of spatial information. In: Proceedings of the 18th SIGSPATIAL International Conference on Advances in Geographic Information Systems, GIS 2010, pp. 300–309, New York, USA. ACM (2010)
20. Wang, J., Mülligann, C., Schwering, A.: An empirical study on relevant aspects for sketch map alignment. In: Geertman, S., Reinhardt, W., Toppen, F. (eds.) Advancing Geoinformation Science for a Changing World. Lecture Notes in Geoinformation and Cartography, vol. 1, pp. 497–518. Springer, Heidelberg (2011)

Multiobjective Optimization Approach for Preference-Disaggregation Analysis Under Effects of Intensity

Nelson Rangel-Valdez[1]($\boxtimes$), Eduardo Fernández[2], Laura Cruz-Reyes[1], Claudia Gómez Santillán[1], and Rodolfo Iván Hernández-López[1]

[1] Postgraduate and Research Division, National Mexican Institute of Technology/Madero Institute of Technology, 89440 Tamaulipas, Mexico
nelson.rangel@itcm.edu.mx, cruzreyeslaura@gmail.com, cggs71@hotmail.com, rodolfo_hdezlopez@yahoo.com
[2] Faculty of Civil Engineering, Autonomous University of Sinaloa, 80040 Sinaloa, Mexico
eddyf@uas.edu.mx

Abstract. A widely used approach in Multicriteria Decision Aid is the Preference Disaggregation Analysis (or PDA). This is an indirect approach used to characterize the decision process of a Decision Maker (or DM). By means of a limited set of examples (called a reference set) provided by the DM, the PDA approach estimates the parameter values of a preference model that is characterized by the DM. This paper proposes a new optimization model for PDA, and its solution through an evolutionary algorithm. The novel features in the definition of the model include the use of the effect of the intensity (i.e. the variations among the criteria values used to evaluate decision alternatives), and new ways to combine the number of consistencies and inconsistencies with respect to the reference set. Through an experimental design performed to evaluate the fitness of the new model, it was corroborated its effectiveness to fit the DM preferences, and also it showed comparable results with that provided by an state-of-the-art strategy.

1 Introduction

In Multi-Criteria Decision Aid (MCDA) the decisions made by a Decision Maker (DM) can be expressed through a prespecified mathematical structure. A multi-criteria decision model that is made in this way relies commonly in a set of preferential parameters that are meant to reflect the preference information of a DM, which in turn becomes a crucial aspect in building the decision models ([1]). The development of these models is based on direct or indirect methods. In the first case, the DM is involved in the process of specifying the preferential parameters ([2]), a process that presents difficulties for the DM when assigning values to parameters, commonly because it is hard for a DM to know the exact values required by the parameters, and because it is a time consuming task. On the other hand, the indirect methods, which include the preference-disaggregation

© Springer International Publishing Switzerland 2015
O. Pichardo Lagunas et al. (Eds.): MICAI 2015, Part II, LNAI 9414, pp. 451–462, 2015.
DOI: 10.1007/978-3-319-27101-9_34

analysis (PDA), use a reference set provided by a DM to infer the values for the preferential parameters.

According to Greco et al., in [3], the relatively less effort from the DM implied by disaggregation paradigms is becoming more attractive among the MCDA approaches. The scientific literature relates several works to the PDA paradigm (e.g., [4–6]), ([7]). Of particular interest for this research is the PDA in ELEC-TRE methods (see [8]), which are one of the most popular multi-criteria decision tools; they are commonly used to model the preferences of a DM in different type of problems as sorting, choosing, and ranking. However, due to the ELECTRE-based models requires solving a difficult non-linear programming problem (cf. [9,10]), the use of evolutionary techniques has become an important tool to solve them. Doumpos et al., in [2], use a differential evolution algorithm for inferring parameter values in the ELECTRE TRI method. In [5,6], the authors present evolutionary multi-objective algorithms for inferring parameters of a fuzzy indifference relation model for multi-criteria sorting purposes, these works use the ELECTRE III method. In [7], Covantes et al. present a robustness analysis over a PDA in ELECTRE III, through the use of an artificial DM and multi-objective evolutionary algorithm.

Because of the importance of the ELECTRE-based methods in MCDA, and the relatively small number of works devoted to their solution, the research presented in this paper is focused to extend the state of the art of existing PDA in ELECTRE methods, through the development of a new optimization model. In particular, the model is developed for the PDA in the ELECTRE III method, such that it can contribute in the solution of decision problems e.g., as in the portfolio selection problem(cf. [11,12]). The results derived from the experimental design provide additional evidence that it is competitive against a state-of-the-art strategy; they also reveal, as expected, that the existing models could be improved to fit better a model for the DM's preferences. In order to be consistent with the decision policy, embedded in the chosen reference set, the model explores a novel feature based on the effect of the intensity, and the type of inconsistencies derived from the preference system.

The paper is organized as follows. Section 2 describes the outranking model based on ELECTRE III, and the basic concepts. Section 3 presents the new parameter optimization model based on the PDA paradigm. Section 4 details the experimental design performed to evaluate the performance of the optimization models in the characterization of the DM's preferences. Section 5 presents the results derived from the experiment performed. Finally, Sect. 6 presents the conclusions derived from the research.

2   Assumptions and Notations

The proposed model is based on the Relational System of Preferences presented by Roy [8], and extended by Fernandez et al., in [6], to include fuzzy preference relations. This section describes the elements of the Relational System of Preferences, which will be used in the following section to define the proposed model.

In order to define the optimization model in this paper, it is necessary to define a preference relation A_P over pair of alternatives for which a DM must take a decision. The preference relation A_P is defined according to the fuzzy preference relations proposed by Fernandez et al., in [6]; there, each alternative has a set of objective values g_i associated to it, where $1 \le i \le n$, and n is the number of criteria. The relations over each pair of alternatives x, y are described as follows:

1. *Strict preference*: Denoted as xPy, corresponds to the existence of clear and positive reasons that justify significant preference in favor of one of the two alternatives.
2. *Indifference*: It corresponds to the existence of clear and positive reasons to support the idea that two alternatives have high degree of equivalence between both. This relationship is denoted as xIy.
3. *Weak preference*: Represented as xQy, it corresponds to the existence of clear and positive reasons in favor of x over y, but that are not sufficient to justify strict preference. Indifference and strict preference cannot be distinguished appropriately.
4. *Incomparability*: None of the preceding situations predominates, since there is high heterogeneity between the alternatives. That is, absence of clear and positive reasons that justify any of the above relations, so he/she cannot set a preference relation. This is denoted as xRy.
5. *k-Preference*: It corresponds to the existence of clear and positive reasons that justify strict preference in favor of one of the two alternatives, or incomparability between the two alternatives, but with no significant division established between the situations of strict preference and incomparability. It is denoted as xKy.

In order to formally define the relations previously described, the methodology uses the outranking method ELECTRE III to calculate the value of $\sigma(x, y, \rho)$, which expresses the degree of truth of the predicate x *is at least as good as* y in terms of a set of preferential parameters ρ, and the value of the parameter λ. The parameter λ is commonly known as the outrank threshold, and it is assigned accordingly to the preferences of the DM. Table 1 shows the formal definition for each of the relations previously described.

3   Method for Inferring Parameters of a Decision Model

The closest related work to the model proposed in this paper, is the one presented by Fernandez et al., in [6]; there, the authors present an optimization model based on the PDA paradigm for estimating the values of the parameters of ELECTRE III, where the degree of differences among criteria are not taken into account. Our approach deals with that degree of difference, which is referred as *effect of intensity*, and it tries to fit the DM's preferences by leaving out those cases where it occurs. The remaining of this section is meant to describe the proposed model. It is important to point out that in this work the set of criteria that defines an

Table 1. Preference relations used to define the optimization model proposed.

Preference	Definition
$x\mathbf{P}y$-Strict Preference	$(x$ dominates $y) \vee$ $([\sigma(x,y,\rho) \geq \lambda] \wedge [\sigma(y,x,\rho) < 0.5]) \vee$ $([\sigma(x,y,\rho) \geq \lambda] \wedge [0.5 \leq \sigma(y,x,\rho)] \wedge [\sigma(y,x,\rho) < \lambda] \wedge [\sigma(x,y,\rho) - \sigma(y,x,\rho) \geq \beta])$
$x\mathbf{I}y$-Indifference	$([\sigma(x,y,\rho) \geq \lambda] \wedge [\sigma(y,x,\rho) \geq \lambda]) \wedge$ $(\sigma(x,y,\rho) - \sigma(y,x,\rho) \leq \epsilon)$
$x\mathbf{Q}y$-Weak Preference	$(\neg x\mathbf{P}y) \wedge$ $(\neg x\mathbf{I}y) \wedge$ $([\sigma(x,y,\rho) \geq \lambda] \wedge [\sigma(x,y,\rho) > \sigma(y,x,\rho)])$
$x\mathbf{K}y$-K-Preference	$([0.5 \leq \sigma(x,y,\rho)] \wedge [\sigma(x,y,\rho) < \lambda]) \wedge$ $(\sigma(y,x,\rho) < 0.5) \wedge$ $(\sigma(x,y,\rho) - \sigma(y,x,\rho) > \epsilon)$
$x\mathbf{R}y$-Incomparability	$(\sigma(x,y,\rho) < 0.5) \wedge$ $(\sigma(y,x,\rho) < 0.5)$

alternative are considered as objectives that are wished to be improved in the decision process; and for that reason, objectives and criteria are related terms, and are considered the same.

The section is organized in two parts. Firstly, the main feature of the model is introduced, the effects of intensity. After that, the new optimization model is presented.

3.1   Effects of Intensity

To define the optimization model proposed in this paper, let us introduce the concept of *Effects of Intensity*, or EI, as follows. Let x, y be two alternatives among which a DM should choose one. Let $\{g_1, g_2, ..., g_n\}$ be the set of n criteria, and w.l.o.g. in the form of maximization functions, that characterizes the alternatives. Then, $EI(x, y)$, or the EI among x and y, is defined according to Eq. 1, where α denotes a threshold established according to the DM preferences.

$$EI(x,y) = \begin{cases} true & \text{If there is at least a criterion } i \text{ such that } |g_i(x) - g_i(y)| > \alpha \\ false & \textbf{otherwise} \end{cases}$$

(1)

The function $EI(x, y)$ triggers an indicator of relative importance of a certain criterion to define the overall importance of an alternative x over another one y, i.e. whenever one alternative x outranks another alternative y in the presence of EI, it means that with a high probability it is due to only one criterion. Equation 2 gives an example of EI. This is an example of the existence of the EI among two alternatives x, y with three criteria. Note that the threshold α is set to 2, such that the EI exists only due to the first criterion, where the difference is 9 and surpasses this value. The latter situation can be deceivable, because it could provoke in a DM to choose an alternative like x, only because of the intensity of one criterion, before realizing that in the remaining criteria it is worst; this represents the main reason to exclude such cases from the decision model proposed.

$$x = (10, 5, 9)$$
$$y = (1, 6, 10)$$
(2)

3.2 New Parameter Optimization Model for ELECTRE III

The model proposed in this paper considers the definition of ELECTRE III as described in [6], which involves the use of the parameters λ, and $\rho = \{w, q, p, v, u\}$, to compute $\sigma(x, y, \rho)$. The parameters are described in Table 2.

The new optimization model is based on a reference set T provided by a DM. The reference set T is formed by related pairs $x \succeq y$, where x, y are a couple of alternatives, and the relation $\succeq$ specifies a preference of x over y defined by the DM. The implication defined in Eq. 3 indicates that if the proposed model specifies preference of x over y, then the DM must also have specified the same, i.e. $x \succeq y \in T$. On the other hand, the implication in Eq. 4 indicates the opposite, i.e. if the DM specifies a preference, then the model should have predicted the same. The model predicts a preference based on the relation established according to ELECTRE III, i.e. if $\sigma(x, y, \rho) \geq \lambda$ then the preference holds.

$$\sigma(x, y, \rho) \geq \lambda \rightarrow x \succeq y$$
(3)

$$x \succeq y \bigwedge \sim EI(x, y) \rightarrow \sigma(x, y, \rho) \geq 0.51$$
(4)

3.3 Solution for the Proposed Optimization Model

Based on the previously defined implications in Eqs. 3 and 4, the functions N_1, N_2 are defined to count the inconsistencies derived from them. The functions N_1 and N_2 count the inconsistencies derived from Eqs. 3 and 4, respectively, i.e. when the implications are false. Note that N_2 incorporates the use of EI in its definition, which means that only those relations provided by the DM without effects of intensity (denoted $\sim EI$) will be considered. These functions are used to define the proposed optimization model as shown in Eq. 5, where $R.F.$ stands for a

Table 2. Parameters of the proposed model.

Parameter	Purpose
λ	Outrank threshold
$w = \{w_1, w_2, ..., w_n\}$	Vector of weight for each objective i
$q = \{q_1, q_2, ..., q_n\}$	Vector of indifference thresholds for each objective i
$p = \{p_1, p_2, ..., p_n\}$	Vector of preference thresholds for each objective i
$u = \{u_1, u_2, ..., u_n\}$	Vector of pre-veto thresholds for each objective i
$v = \{v_1, v_2, ..., v_n\}$	Vector of veto thresholds for each objective i

feasible region of solutions defined by the set of parameters ρ. This optimization model does not consider the value of λ, because it is fixed during its solution.

$$\begin{aligned} & \min N_1, N2 \\ & \text{s.t.} \qquad \rho \in \textbf{R.F.} \end{aligned} \tag{5}$$

The minimization of the functions N_1, N_2 allows a better fit of the parameters to the DM preferences, represented by the reference set T. Given that founding an exact solution for this new model might be hard, an evolutionary approach is used instead. Both functions N_1, N_2 are used as objectives, and the chromosome is formed by the set of parameters ρ that define ELECTRE III. The following section presents the integration of the model presented in this section, the relational system of preferences described in Sect. 2, and a multi-objective metaheuristic.

4   Experimental Design

This sections presents details on the experiment conducted to test the performance of the new optimization model for PDA in ELECTRE III. The experiment is divided in five parts. The first part refers to the use of an artificial DM to generate the instances to test the performance of the model, i.e. a reference set T was generated using the artificial DM. The second part describes the constraints that can be considered when solving the instances. The third part involves the implementation of the solution for the proposed model using the multi-objective metaheuristic NSGAII. The fourth part involves the performance indicators to evaluate the solutions for the proposed model found through the metaheuristic. And finally, the fifth part describes with detailed the methodology followed in the experiment to integrate all the other parts. The results were compared against one of the best results reported by the state-of-the-art approach proposed in [6].

4.1   Generation of Instances: Building Reference Sets

In order to test the model, it was necessary to emulate a DM, and with it to generate a set of instances as cases of study. For this purpose, the function V described in [6] was used. This function considers a universe U formed by objects x with four criteria $(F_1, F_2, F_3, F_4) \in \Re^4$, where each F_i can take random real values in the range of $[1, 7]$, and the model shown in Eq. 6. The preference over the criteria is incremental, i.e. they are maximizing functions.

$$V = \frac{F_1 + F_2 + F_3 + F_4 + \sqrt[4]{F_1 \cdot F_2 \cdot F_3 \cdot F_4}}{5} \tag{6}$$

Each element (x, y) of the reference set T is formed by four criteria generated at random, then its preference relation is established according to the expression shown in Eq. 7, where the value 0.25 emulates certain preference threshold.

$$\forall (x, y) \in T, \, x \succeq y \rightarrow V(x) \geq V(y) - 0.25 \tag{7}$$

Table 3. Configuration of the parameters for the algorithm NSGAII implemented in jMetal, and used to solve the proposed model defined in Sect. 3.2.

Feature	Meaning
Objective	Minimization of the values $N1, N2$ defined in Sect. 3.2
Crossover operator	$SBXCrossover$, defined in jMetal, with a probability set to 0.9
Mutation operator	$PolynomialMutation$, with a probability set to $\frac{1}{5*N}$
Selection operator	$BinaryTournament2$
Maximum Evaluations	25000
Population size	100

4.2 Constraints

The parameter values of the preference model were described in Table 2. Some of the parameter values of the preference model were fixed, in order to compare with the state-of-the-art approach reported in [6]. For this experiment we fixed $\lambda = \{0.67, 0.70, 0.75\}$, and $\alpha = 2$ (note that the values of λ were taken from values reported in related work derived from the scientific literature [5,6]). Additionally, some constraints used in the literature, as in [6], were considered over the values of the parameters ρ; these constraints are depicted as follows:

– $w_i > 0$;
– $\lambda > 0.51$;
– $0 \leq q_i \leq p_i < u_i < v_i (i = 1, \cdots, n)$;
– $|w_m - w_j| < 0.125$, for $m = \{1, 2, 3\}$ y $j > m$;
– For each criterion j, $0 < q_j \leq 0.34$, $0.5 \leq p_j \leq 0.9$, $1.0 \leq u_j \leq 2.4$, $2.5 \leq v_j \leq 6$;
– $|(v_j + p_j)/2 - u_j| \leq 0.1(v_j - p_j)$;

4.3 The Evolutionary Multi-objective Approach

The *framework* jMetal[1] is developed for multi-objective optimization with meta-heuristics. The algorithm NSGAII implemented in this framework was used to solve the optimization model proposed in Eq. 5. The parameters of the algorithm were configured as indicated in Table 3.

The proposed model searches for an adequate configuration of parameter values for the preference model based on ELECTRE III, such that they fit the DM's preferences. For this purpose, the NSGAII algorithm represents the set of parameters as individuals of a population, each chromosome of the individual represents one the parameters that define ELECTRE III, i.e. the parameters $\{w, p, q, v, u\}$ for each objective are the chromosomes of an individual in the algorithm.

---

[1] http://jmetal.sourceforge.net/.

4.4   Performance Indicators

Once that the parameters of a generic decision model have been estimated using an optimization model, a sorting decision over new objects has to be performed in order to determine the quality of a set of parameter values. For this purpose, it can be used the outranking relations defined in Sect. 2, and the implications shown in Eqs. 8 and 9.

$$xS(\lambda, \rho)y \rightarrow x \succeq y \tag{8}$$

$$x \succeq y \rightarrow xS(\lambda, \rho)y \tag{9}$$

Based on the previous information, the following indicators are defined to measure the performance of the optimization model:

- **Correct Decisions** DC_1. This indicator corresponds to a decision taken properly in the sense of the DM preference. It counts the times that both, the antecedent and the consequent in implications in Eqs. 8 and 9 were true, and must be maximized.
- F_1. This indicator counts the inconsistencies from implication in Eq. 8, and must be minimized. It relates assertions of the model on preferences of x over y when the DM indicates the contrary.
- F_2. This indicator counts the inconsistencies derived from implication in Eq. 9, and must be minimized. It relates assertions of the DM on preferences of x over y when the model indicates the contrary.
- AC_F. This indicator corresponds to vague decisions derived from the model, and must be minimized. It counts the times that both, the antecedent and the consequent in implications in Eqs. 8 and 9 were false.
- A_1. This indicator counts the times that both, the antecedent and the consequent in implications in Eq. 4 were true, without EI among pairs (x, y), and must be maximized.
- A_2. This indicator counts the times that both, the antecedent and the consequent in implications in Eq. 9 were true, only considering pairs (x, y) with EI, and must be maximized.
- G^1. It counts the inconsistencies from implication in Eq. 4, without EI, and must be minimized.
- G^2. It counts the inconsistencies from implication in Eq. 9, with EI, under the constraints $\sigma(x, y, \rho) \geq 0.51$ and $\sigma(x, y) < \lambda$, and must be minimized.
- G^3. It counts the inconsistencies from implication in Eq. 9, with EI, under the constraints $\sigma(x, y, \rho) \geq 0.51$, and must be minimized.

The previous performance indicators were used to compare each set of parameter values ρ derived from our optimization model, against the solution $P_{best^*}(2)$ reported in [6] (see Table 4).

Table 4. Set of parameter values $P_{best*}(2)$ reported in [6], using $\lambda = 0.70$.

Solution	λ	w_1	w_2	w_3	w_4	q_1	q_2	q_3	q_4	p_1	p_2	p_3	p_4	u_1	u_2	u_3	u_4	v_1	v_2	v_3	v_4
$P_{best*}(2)$	0.70	0.250	0.250	0.25	0.25	0.15	0.154	0.147	0.149	0.693	0.694	0.695	0.694	2.036	2.043	2.040	2.036	3.461	3.464	3.461	3.483

4.5   Detailed Experiment

The methodology followed to test the algorithm NSGAII on the solution of the proposed model was based in the following steps:

1. Initially, 8 alternatives were created, each having 4 objectives with values generated at random in the range $[1, 7]$.
2. Using the set of 8 alternatives of the previous step, 28 instances were generated. Each instance is one of the possible subsets of size 6 that can be constructed from the initial 8 alternatives. Hence, there are 30 possible pairs of relations, defined through the model described in Sect. 4.1, per instance.
3. The optimization model derived from each instance was solved 10 times by NSGAII, and the parameter values generated were used to determine $\overline{\rho}^*$, the central solution from the generated Pareto front. The value of $\overline{\rho}^*$ was taken as the best solution for the instance, regarding that it also belong to the Pareto

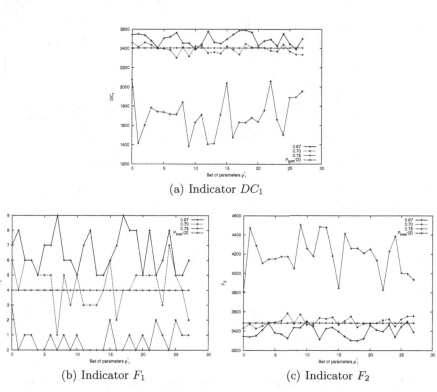

(a) Indicator DC_1

(b) Indicator F_1

(c) Indicator F_2

Fig. 1. Graph of results of the performance indicators DC_1, F_1, and F_2.

front. The value $\overline{\rho}^*$ of an instance is computed as the mean value of each
parameter value obtained from a solution in the Pareto front.
4. The fitness of the set of parameter values $\overline{\rho}^*$ was evaluated. For this purpose,
$\overline{\rho}^*$ was used to establish the preference relations over the pairs of alternatives
derived from an entire new set of 100 random alternatives. Then, the rela-
tion between each pair (x, y) in the new set of alternatives was determined

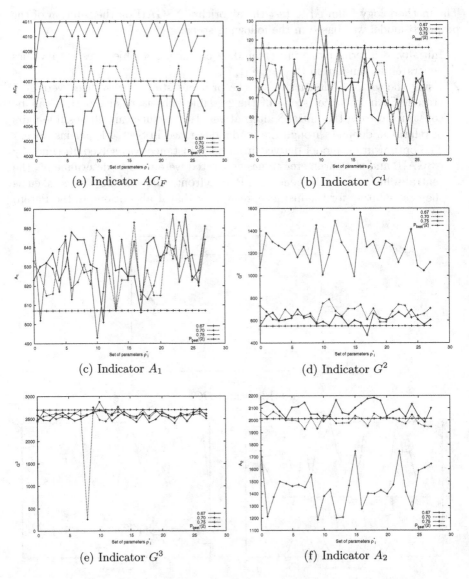

(a) Indicator AC_F (b) Indicator G^1

(c) Indicator A_1 (d) Indicator G^2

(e) Indicator G^3 (f) Indicator A_2

Fig. 2. Graph of results of the performance indicators AC_F, G^1, A_1, G^2, G^3, and A_2.

using $\sigma(x, y, \overline{\rho}^*)$ in the model described in Sect. 2. The performance indicators presented in Sect. 4.4 were used.

5. The results were compared against one of the best values reported in [6].

Note that the considered values of the outrank threshold where fixed to $\lambda = \{0.67, 0.70, 0.75\}$. The following section presents the results derived from the present experiment.

5   Results

Figures 1 and 2 show graphs that summarizes the results obtained from the experiment described in Sect. 4. There is a graph per performance indicator, and each of these graph contains the value obtained by each of the 28 set of parameter values $\overline{\rho}^*$ considered. Additionally, each graph shows a different line per distinct value of $\lambda = \{0.65, 0.70, 0.75\}$, and it is compared against the state-of-the-art value $P_{best*}(2)$ taken from [6]; this value is represented as a straight line.

Finally, note that in all the indicators, the performance in the prediction of preferences of the proposed model over 100 random alternatives is competitive, since it improves the solution $P_{best*}(2)$, in at least one set of parameter values $\overline{\rho}^*$. This information provide evidence that the preference models can still be improved in PDA.

6   Conclusions

This paper presents a new optimization model for PDA in ELECTRE III. The model incorporated the effects of the intensity derived from the extreme variations in the differences between same criteria among pairs of alternatives. The model minimized two objectives, derived from the inconsistencies found in the model with respect to a reference set provided by the DM. For small instances, the optimization model solved by NSGAII obtained zero inconsistency in both objectives. For prediction purposes in new randomly sets, the central value from the Pareto front generated previously showed competitive results against an state-of-the-art approach, by improving it in some of the performance indicators defined in this work.

Finally, it is open the question whether or not exists a better optimization model that yields values which support better the predictions given by a preference model, in comparison to the real preferences provided by a DM.

Acknowledgments. This research was partially funded by the following projects: the project 3058-Optimización de Problemas Complejos of the *Programa de Cátedras CONACyT*.

References

1. Dias, L., Mousseau, V., Figueira, J., Climaco, J.: An aggregation/disaggregation approach to obtain robust conclusions with electre-tri. EJOR **138**, 332–348 (2002)
2. Doumpos, M., Marinakis, Y., Marimaki, M., Zopounidis, C.: An evolutionary approach to construction of outranking models for multicriteria classification: The case of electre tri method. EJOR **199**, 496–505 (2009)
3. Greco, S., Mousseau, V., Slowinski, R.: Ordinal regression revisited: Multiple criteria ranking with a set of additive value functions. EJOR **191**, 415–435 (2008)
4. Mangasarian, O.: Multisurface method for pattrn separation. IEEE Trans. Inf. Theor. **14**, 801–807 (1968)
5. Fernandez, E., Navarro, J., Bernal, S.: Multicriteria sorting using a valued indifference relation under a preference disaggregation paradigm. EJOR **198**, 602–609 (2009)
6. Fernandez, E., Navarro, J., Mazcorro, G.: Evolutionary multi-objective optimization for inferring outranking model's parameters under scarce reference information and effects of reinforced preference. Found. Comput. Decis. Sci. **37**, 163–197 (2012)
7. Covantes, E., Fernández, E., Navarro, J.: Robustness analysis of a moea-based elicitation method for outranking model parameters. In: CCE, pp. 209–214 (2013)
8. Roy, B.: The outranking approach and the foundations of electre methods. Theor. Decis. **31**, 49–73 (1991)
9. Dias, L., Mousseau, V.: Inferring electre's veto-related parameters from outranking examples. EJOR **170**, 172–191 (2006)
10. Mousseau, V., Slowinski, R.: Inferring an electre-tri model from assignment examples. J. Global Optim. **12**, 157–174 (1998)
11. Cruz, L., Fernandez, E., Gomez, C., Rivera, G., Perez, F.: Many-objective portfolio optimization of interdependent projects with a priori incorporation of decision-maker preferences. Appl. Math, (8)
12. Bastiani Medina, S., Cruz Reyes, L., Fernandez, E., Gómez Santillán, C., Rivera Zarate, G.: An ant colony algorithm for solving the selection portfolio problem, using a quality-assessment model for portfolios of projects expressed by a priority ranking. In: Design of Intelligent Systems Based on Fuzzy Logic, Neural Networks and Nature-Inspired Optimization, pp. 357–373 (2015)

TwoPILP: An Integer Programming Method for HCSP in Parallel Computing Centers

José Carlos Soto-Monterrubio, Héctor Joaquín Fraire-Huacuja,
Juan Frausto-Solís[✉], Laura Cruz-Reyes, Rodolfo Pazos R.,
and J. Javier González-Barbosa

Instituto Tecnológico de Cd. Madero, Ciudad Madero, Mexico
{soto190,juan.frausto}@gmail.com, {automatas2002,
r_pazos_r,jjgonzalezbarbosa}@yahoo.com.mx,
lauracruzreyes@itcm.edu.mx

Abstract. Scheduling is a problem in computer science with a wide range of applicability in industry. The Heterogeneous Computing Scheduling Problem (HCSP) belongs to the parallel computing area and is applicable to scheduling in clusters and high performance data centers. HCSP has been solved traditionally as a mono-objective problem that aims at minimizing the makespan (termination time of the last task) and has been solved by Branch and Bound (B&B) algorithms. HCSP with energy is a multi-objective optimization problem with two objectives: minimize the makespan and the energy consumption by the machines. In this paper, an integer linear programming model for HCSP is presented. In addition, a multi-objective method called TwoPILP (Two-Phase Integer Linear Programming) is proposed for this model. TwoPILP consists of two phases. The first minimizes the makespan using a classic branch and bound method. The second phase minimizes the energy consumption by selecting adequate voltage levels. The proposed model provides advantages over mono-objective models which are discussed in the paper sections. The experimentation presented compares TwoPILP versus B&B and NSGA-II, showing that TwoPILP achieves better results than B&B and NSGA-II. This method offers the advantage of providing only one solution to the user, which is particularly useful for applications where there is no decision maker for choosing from a set of solutions delivered by multi-objective optimization methods.

Keywords: Scheduling · Branch and bound · Modeling · Planning

1 Introduction

Scheduling is among the most difficult NP-hard problems in combinatorial optimization [1]. The classic scheduling problem consists of a set of jobs which should be executed in a set of machines. The objective of this problem is to minimize the makespan, which is the time when all the tasks are completed. A multi-objective scheduling problem (MSP) consists of minimizing two or more objectives such as the makespan, energy, cost, and tardiness. In a MSP the goal is to find the Pareto Frontier which contains all the non-dominated solutions. The non-dominated solutions are equally good or none of them is worse than any other. The main issue in multi-objective optimization is that the

© Springer International Publishing Switzerland 2015
O. Pichardo Lagunas et al. (Eds.): MICAI 2015, Part II, LNAI 9414, pp. 463–474, 2015.
DOI: 10.1007/978-3-319-27101-9_35

objectives are usually in conflict, because the optimization of one of the objectives debases the optimization of the others.

The scheduling problem HCSP with energy consists not only in the minimization of the makespan but also deals with the minimization of the energy consumption of the machines. To achieve these objectives, DVFS (Dynamic Voltage and Frequency Scaling) capable machines are used. These machines are capable to work at different speeds, allowing to manage the energy consumption during the execution of allocated tasks. DVFS is an energy management technique in computer architectures, which allows to increase or decrease the voltage applied. DVFS is normally used in laptops and other mobile devices as energy saver.

In 1992, the Energy Star program was created [2] and the efficient energy-aware consumption was started. Nowadays, this approach is applied in data centers and distributed systems due to the concern for environmental care in the last years.

The consumption by data centers has increased in the last years. For instance in the United States the energy consumption in millions of kilowatt-hours was 61000 in 2006, which was equivalent to around 1.5 % of the total energy consumption in this country [3]. Nowadays to save energy by datacenters is more important, because the costs are higher due to energy awareness and environmental care. In November 2008 there were a total of 14 High Performance Computing Centers (HPCC) with an energy consumption higher than 1 MW. The number of HPPC in June 2013 was 43. The total of super-computers for USA and Europe was almost 363 in 2014. The National University of Defense Technology (NUDT) in China developed a super-computer with 3,120,000 cores with a performance of 33.9 Pflops and energy consumption of 17.9 MW [3]. Although more cores provide more computing power, this has strong implications in energy consumption and thermal conditions. The more energy used to compute an application, the larger the economic costs and heat problems.

HCSP (Heterogeneous Computing Scheduling Problem) with DVFS is a problem where the goal is to find the best allocation of tasks to machines, which produces the lowest makespan and also generates the lowest energy consumption. HCSP is in fact a two-objective optimization problem which deals with both, minimize the energy consumption and the makespan, and it was solved by a Genetic Algorithm, mainly by NSGA-II [4]. In this paper, an integer linear programming model for HCSP is presented. Besides, a multi-objective method called TwoPILP (Two-Phase Integer Linear Programming) is proposed for this model. TwoPILP consists of two phases. The first minimizes the makespan using a classic branch and bound method. The second phase minimizes the energy consumption by selecting adequate voltage levels. The proposed model provides advantages over mono-objective models which are discussed in the paper sections. In addition TwoPILP is compared versus a classic B&B and NSGA-II algorithms for mono-objective and two-objective formulations respectively.

This paper is organized as follows. Section 2 contains the multi-objective methods for scheduling. HCSP and its mathematical formulation are described in Sect. 3. Section 4 details the phases of the TwoPILP method for solving HCSP, which aims at minimizing the energy and the makespan. The experimentation and results are discussed in Sect. 5. Section 6 presents the conclusions.

2   Multi-objective Methods for Scheduling

The multi-objective scheduling problem is currently solved by metaheuristics [5–10]. Also to solve it several heuristics are used, some of them are genetic and evolutionary algorithms like NSGA-II [11], MOEA/D [12], and ant colonies [13]. Some methods work over populations or individuals which improve simultaneously all the objectives. Other methods use aggregative functions which combine all the objectives in only one. Usually these methods work to find the Pareto frontier which includes all the non-dominated solutions found by the algorithm.

In the Job Shop Scheduling Problem (JSSP) a set of jobs needs to be executed in a set of machines subject to some constraints. These tasks and machines have some characteristics, which are used for classifying JSSP problems [14]. Specifically, each problem can be classified by three fields $\alpha|\beta|\gamma$:

- α : Represents the type of machine in the system.
- β : Represents the type of task.
- γ : Represents the criteria on which the schedule is evaluated.

Some JSSP variants are the following:

- Related independent and equal machines.
- Machines require some time to wait between tasks.
- Objective function optimizes makespan, costs, lateness, and tardiness. The problems can be multi-objective optimization.
- Tasks can have some constraints; for example, to start a job i needs to finish a job j.
- Tasks and machines have mutual constraints, for example, certain tasks can be allocated only to specific machines.
- Processing times can be fixed or probabilistic.

The most common multi-objective version of JSSP is the Flexible JSSP. In this problem the tasks can only be allocated to specific machines. JSSP normally minimizes the makespan combined with one of the other criteria: energy, cost, tardiness, idle time, and work load.

The scheduling problem has been solved by metaheuristics like NSGA-II, MOEAD/D, Simulated Annealing, Tabu Search and also exact models for makespan minimization. To explore the solution space among metaheuristics, there are some heuristic rules. The most common rules are min-min, max-min, largest job on fastest resource-shortest job on fastest resource, and suffrage [7, 15, 16].

2.1   NSGA-II and HCSP

NSGA-II has been used to solve a wide variety of scheduling problems [4, 9, 17, 18]. NSGA-II is a multi-objective algorithm based on dominance [11]. This algorithm has two principal methods which improve the lack of elitism, the front sorting complexity, and the diversity of NSGA. These methods are the fast_nondominated_sorting and the crowding_distance_assignment. The former sorts the population in a set of fronts with non-dominated solutions. The later assigns to each solution a crowding distance value, which measures the density of solutions around it. The crowding distance is the size of the largest cuboid enclosing one solution without including any other population.

3 HCSP

In recent years the fast growth of computing power in low cost equipment and the technology development of networks with high speed have accelerated the spread of distributed systems to solve complex problems. Heterogeneous computing systems are composed by computer equipment with different characteristics and computing power. These characteristics allows to create an infrastructure that provides a high computing capacity with good relation between cost and effectiveness to solve very large and complex problems.

Normally heterogeneous computing systems provide high performance machines in parallel and/or distributed systems, which work cooperatively to solve problems that require an intensive computer power and have diverse computational requirements. Heterogeneous computing systems have been used to solve a wide variety of problems that require high power consumption [15].

The main issue in heterogeneous computing consists in finding the best schedule of tasks on machines such that it satisfies some requirements related to efficiency, work load, economic benefits, costs, and others. This is a scheduling problem where JSSP considers diverse operations per job and dependencies between jobs. Typically, dependency is modeled by a disjunctive graph [19, 20]. HCSP not only minimizes the makespan but also minimizes the energy. This problem is called HCSP with energy and is described in the next subsection.

3.1 HCSP Description

The formal definition of HCSP is the following [21]: Given an HC system that has a set of computer resources (machines) $M = \{m_1, m_2, \ldots, m_L\}$ and a set of jobs $J = \{j_1, j_2, \ldots, j_N\}$ to be executed in the HC system. Given a function with execution times $P : \{1, \ldots, N\} \times \{1, \ldots, L\} \to R^+$, where $P(i,j)$ is the required time to execute the job j in the machine M_i. The purpose of HCSP is to find an allocation of tasks in machines which minimizes the makespan, more specifically, the function $(f : J^N \to M^L)$ such that:

$$\max_{i \in \{m_1, \ldots, m_L\}} \sum_{j \in J, f(i)=j} P(i,j) \qquad (1)$$

HCSP with energy is defined as follows [22]: Given a set of n jobs, m processors and a constraint of time T. Find the processors configurations $e_1, e_2, \ldots, e_L$ for the N jobs and a schedule with N jobs in L processors, such that the energy consumption is minimized and the makespan does not exceed T. Notice that this problem is two-objective since it minimizes makespan and energy consumption.

Exact models with two phases for HCSP with energy have not been found in the literature. Most methods use a non-deterministic approach. The few integer linear programming (ILP) methods in the state of the art focus on minimizing makespan or minimizing energy consumption [23]. In this work the problem addressed is HCSP with energy, which aims at minimizing the two objectives (makespan and energy consumption) considering the following conditions: (a) every job that has been allocated and started, cannot be interrupted; (b) each job is an atomic unit and cannot be split, and it can only be executed in one processor at a time; (c) the execution time for a job may vary from one machine to another; (d) all the tasks are independent; (e) idle time is not considered. The two objectives of HCSP with energy are described in the following subsections.

3.2 Makespan

Let $\{J_1,\ldots,J_N\}$ a set of jobs and $\{M,\ldots,M_L\}$ a set of machines. Each job j has associated a computation cost $P_{i,j}$ in machine M_i at a maximal speed and voltage. The relative cost in terms of execution time $P'_{i,j}$ is given by the next equation [19, 20]:

$$P'_{ij} = \frac{P_{i,j}}{speed} \tag{2}$$

where $P_{i,j}$ represents the time that requires j to be executed in the machine M_i, and *speed* is associated to each level of processor configuration. Makespan is the time in which the last job is finished and is given by the following equation:

$$makespan = MAX_{j=1}^{k}\left(\sum P'_{i,j} \forall j \text{ allocated to } M_i\right) \tag{3}$$

3.3 Energy

The energy model used in this work is derived from the consumption energy model CMOS (Complementary Metal-Oxide Semiconductor) [26], where V_i is the voltage supplied to the processor in which job j is processed, and $P'_{i,j}$ is the relative computational cost for job j with the voltage configuration and machine scheduled. The energy consumption is given by

$$E_c = \sum_{i=0}^{n} V_{l,i}^2 P'_{i,j} \forall j \text{ allocated to } M_i \tag{4}$$

where l is the configuration index in selected processor with a voltage V_i. Since machines are DVFS capable, the makespan objective function is modified as follows:

$$\min MAX_{i=1}^{k}(\sum P'_{i,j} \forall j \text{ allocated to } M_i) \tag{5}$$

4 TwoPILP Method for HCSP with Energy

TwoPILP (Two-Phase Integer Linear Programming) is an integer linear programming model which works in two phases. The first phase of this method consists in optimizing the makespan, and then the objective value found is passed to the second phase to optimize the energy function [9]. These phases are sequenced this way because in HPCC the priority is execution time, and then the energy consumption. In In other words, the problem focuses on optimizing only one objective at a time. Furthermore, this is an exact method that guarantees great quality in both objectives.

Figure 1 shows the process representation of the TwoPILP method. The first phase uses a B&B with the classical simplex method to solve the model and to obtain the makespan, which is provided to the second phase. The second phase also applies a B&B and the simplex method to minimize the energy consumption.

The formal descriptions for the integer linear programming models for HCSP with energy are presented in the next section. First, the model of phase I is described which was taken from [27]. Then the proposed model for phase II is presented.

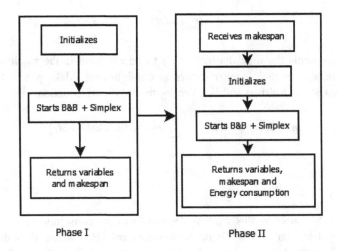

Fig. 1. Phases of TwoPILP.

4.1 TwoPILP: Phase I

In the first phase a binary variable x_{ij} is defined. This variable takes the value of 1 if job j is allocated to machine M_i. Variable y stores the makespan. Constant $P_{i,j}$ is the execution time of job j in machine M_i.

$$min\ y \tag{6}$$

subject to:

$$\sum_{i=1}^{m} x_{i,j} = 1, \quad j = 1, \ldots, n. \tag{7}$$

$$\sum_{j=1}^{n} P_{i,j} x_{i,j} \leq y, \quad i = 1, \ldots, m. \tag{8}$$

$$x_{i,j} \in \{0, 1\} \tag{9}$$

$$y \in \{\mathbb{R}^{+}\} \tag{10}$$

In this formulation (6) represents the objective function to minimize. Constraint (7) is related to the allocation, which allows a job to be executed only in one machine. Constraint (8) associates the maximum of the total execution times from each machine Mi to the makespan. The allowed variable values are defined by constraints (9) and (10).

4.2   TwoPILP: Phase II

The purpose of this model is to find a processing level configuration in machines that minimizes the energy consumption. The makespan obtained in phase I is established as a bound in phase II constraint (14). This phase uses Eq. (6) to avoid exceeding the makespan established from phase I. This model defines a binary variable $x_{i,j,k}$, which takes the value 1 if job j is allocated to machine M_i with the configuration k. Constants v_{kj} and V_{kj} represent speed and voltage respectively. These constants are associated with the configuration k selected in machine M_i where job j is executed. Constant *makespan* represents the optimal makespan from the first phase.

$$\min \sum_{i=1}^{m} \sum_{j=1}^{n} \sum_{k=1}^{K} \frac{P_{ij}}{v_{kj}} V_{kj}^2 x_{i,j,k} \tag{11}$$

subject to:

$$\sum_{i=1}^{m} \sum_{k=1}^{K} x_{i,j,k} = 1, \quad j = 1, \ldots, n. \tag{12}$$

$$\sum_{j=1}^{n} \sum_{k=1}^{K} \frac{P_{ij}}{v_{kj}} x_{i,j,k} \leq y, \quad i = 1, \ldots, m. \tag{13}$$

$$y \leq makespan \tag{14}$$

$$x_{i,j,k} \in \{0, 1\} \tag{15}$$

$$y \in \{\mathbb{R}^+\} \tag{16}$$

The objective function is defined by (11) and Eq. (5) is used to compute energy consumption. Constraint (12) allows to select one processor speed configuration in a machine when a job is executed, this is an allocation constraint. Constraint (13) calculates the total execution time of machine M_i. Constraint (14) is used to avoid exceeding the makespan from phase I. The allowed variable values are defined by constraints (15) and (16).

5 Branch and Bound for TwoPILP

A classic B&B was implemented to solve HCSP. This B&B works in two phases. In the first phase each tree level represents a job and each tree node represents the machine in which a job will be executed. Thus, the first tree level corresponds to the first job, the second tree level to the second job, and so forth. In the second phase each tree level represents one job and each tree node represents the processor configuration of the machine in which the job will be executed.

The first phase explores job allocations to the machines. The process starts setting as upper bound the objective value obtained when all the jobs are executed in the first machine. Then a depth-first tree exploration is performed and a machine is chosen for each level; next the makespan is partially computed with the solution built. If the solution value is better than the upper bound, then the exploration continues on the current branch until the last level is reached. If the value of any partial solution is equal or worse than the upper bound, this branch is cut off. When the last level is reached, the solution is stored and the upper bound is updated. Afterwards a backtracking process is started. In this process the exploration moves one level back on the tree to visit unexplored branches. The first phase ends when all the branches are explored or cut off. The solution found and its makespan will be the input for the second phase. The second phase explores processor speed configurations for machines in order to minimize energy consumption. This phase carries out the same procedure as that of phase one; however, in phase two, the process searches voltage configurations (related to processor speed) of the machines for each job to be executed. In this phase, if a current branch decreases the energy consumption but the makespan is increased, then the branch is cut off. Branches are explored only when the energy consumption is decreased, and the makespan remains equal or becomes lower than the makespan found in phase one. At the end of phase two, the makespan and energy consumptions are retrieved.

6 Experiment and Results

In this experiment the performance of the TwoPILP and classic B&B methods are compared. Although the HCSP with energy problem has drawn a great attention, there does not exist a benchmark set of instances with optimal solutions. For this experimentation a reference set of instances is used, which have been developed by different authors. These instances are defined for dependent jobs and are identified by a character string with the following pattern: A_m_j_M where A stands for the author name, m the number of machines, j the number of jobs, and M the makespan. In this paper the M value is deprecated. These instances are shown in Table 1; for example, the instance Ahmad_3_9_28 has m = 3 machines, j = 9 jobs, and a makespan M = 28.

Table 1. Comparative results from TwoPILP, B&B, and NSGA-II.

Instance	TwoPILP			B&B			NSGA-II		
	M	E	TT	M	E	TT	M	E	TT
Ahmad_3_9_28	13.00	79.58	0.34	13.00	123.71	0.03	29.28	87.75	0.142
Bittencourt_3_9_184	89.00	454.78	0.06	89.00	806.75	0.02	213.36	511.67	0.126
Cao_3_10_536	379.00	1952.10	0.09	379.00	3768.31	0.00	1245.67	2169.37	0.129
Hsu_3_10_84	36.00	218.84	0.06	36.00	334.71	0.03	84.29	236.67	0.127
Eswari_2_11_61	55.50	186.30	0.04	55.50	293.31	0.02	150.49	214.40	0.123
Ilavarasan_3_15_114	79.00	771.75	0.08	79.00	802.05	0.36	237.89	480.18	0.143
Kang_3_10_84	36.00	388.94	0.08	36.00	337.80	0.02	71.86	216.04	0.134
Kuan_3_10_28	11.00	134.75	0.09	11.00	103.87	0.00	21.21	71.20	0.139
Liang_3_10_80	36.00	388.94	0.07	36.00	337.80	0.00	75.59	215.18	0.135
Mohammad_2_11_64	55.50	186.30	0.03	55.50	293.31	0.02	150.66	214.33	0.120
Rahmani_3_7	912.00	5179.04	0.07	912.00	9096.63	0.00	2035.13	5269.82	0.128
SahB_3_6_76	22.00	136.08	0.04	22.00	180.18	0.00	46.32	137.64	0.138
Xu_3_8_66	23.31	130.44	0.05	23.31	201.15	0.02	61.18	144.86	0.131
YCLee_3_8_80	29.00	161.84	0.05	29.00	247.36	0.00	88.94	178.23	0.121
Average	**126.88**	**740.69**	**0.08**	**126.88**	**1209.07**	**0.04**	**322.28**	**724.81**	**0.131**

In this paper NSGA-II was implemented using a uniform crossover and a mutation where 10 % of the chromosome is modified. The initial population is randomly generated. The parents are selected from the population by binary tournament based on the rank front and crowding distance. For the NSGA-II experimentation, the mutation and crossover rates were set to 100 %. The population size was 200 individuals and the number of generations was 300. A total of 50 independent runs were performed for every instance. The averages of the makespan and energy from the solutions in the Pareto frontier were calculated. The experiment was executed on a computer with an Intel Core i7 64-bit processor at 2.40 GHz, 6 GB in RAM, and Operating System Windows 8. The experimentation consisted of solving every instance with the proposed method.

Table 1 shows the experiment results. The first column indicates the instance name. The makespan (M) achieved by TwoPILP is in the second column. The third column presents the energy obtained (E) by TwoPILP. The total time (TT) that TwoPILP spent to solve the instance is shown in the fourth column. The fifth, sixth and seventh columns present the same values obtained by the classic B&B. The eighth, ninth, and tenth columns show the averages of the makespan, the energy, and the execution time respectively from NSGA-II.

Notice in Table 1 that the NSGA-II and B&B methods do not always achieve the same energy. Classic B&B usually obtains an energy higher than TwoPILP. This occurs because B&B sometimes cuts off a branch that reduces makespan but increases energy. Observe that TwoPILP produces the same makespan quality but with lower energy consumption on average than the classic B&B. TwoPILP requires more execution time than B&B. In addition, observe that NSGA-II does not achieve the solution quality obtained by TwoPILP; however, NSGA-II found a diversity of solutions in the Pareto frontier.

7 Conclusions

In this work a model for the two-objective HCSP with energy is presented. This is a novel model, since for this problem an exact two-objective version combining makespan minimization and energy minimization was not previously published. The Two-PILP method is applied to an integer linear programming model, which is presented in this work. HCSP is approached by TwoPILP as a hierarchical method, where makespan minimization was given priority over energy minimization. Tested on a set of instances, Two PILP was able to obtain the optimal makespan and energy. The TwoPILP method obtained an energy consumption lower than a classic B&B. Experiment results show that TwoPILP achieves better results than B&B and NSGA-II, and the TwoPILP results are applicable in real cases. This method offers the advantage of achieving a great quality solution in both objectives and retrieves only one solution to the user, which is particularly useful for applications where there is no decision maker for choosing from a set of solutions delivered by multi-objective optimization methods. Additionally, the second phase can be implemented independently to carry out only the energy minimization, in the case that a schedule is given and just energy minimization is required. The experimentation results show that for this set of instances an exact method is better.

References

1. Garey, A.M., Johnson, D.S.: Computers and Intractability: A Guide to the Theory of NP-completeness. Freeman, San Francisco (1979)
2. ENERGY, S.: Energy Star. History: ENERGY STAR (2011)
3. TOP500.org: The 43rd top500 list published during isc14 in Leipzig, Germany. ISC (2014)
4. Friese, R., Brinks, T., Oliver, C., Siegel, H.J., Maciejewski, A.A.: Analyzing the trade-offs between minimizing makespan and minimizing energy consumption in a heterogeneous resource allocation problem. In: INFOCOMP, The Second International Conference on Advanced Communications and Computation (2012)
5. Pooranian, Z., Harounabadi, A., Shojafar, M., Hedayat, N.: New hybrid algorithm for task scheduling in grid computing to decrease missed task. World Acad. Sci. Eng. Technol. **55**, 924–928 (2011)
6. Pooranian, Z., Shojafar, M., Javadi, B.: Independent task scheduling in grid computing based on queen bee algorithm. IAES Int. J. Artif. Intell. (IJ-AI) **1**(4), 171–181 (2012)
7. Chaturvedi, A.K., Sahu, R.: New heuristic for scheduling of independent tasks in computational grid. Int. J. Grid Distrib. Comput. **4**(3), 25–36 (2011)
8. Raj, R.J.S., Vasudevan, V.: Beyond simulated annealing in grid scheduling. Int. J. Comput. Sci. Eng. (IJCSE) **3**(3), 1312–1318 (2011)

9. Huacuja, H.J.F., Santiago, A., Pecero, J.E., Dorronsoro, B., Bouvry, P., Monterrubio, J.C.S., Barbosa, J.J.G., Santillan, C.G.: A comparison between memetic algorithm and seeded genetic algorithm for multi-objective independent task scheduling on heterogeneous machines. Design of Intelligent Systems Based on Fuzzy Logic, pp. 377–389. Neural Networks and Nature-Inspired Optimization. Springer International Publishing, Berlin (2015)

10. Guzek, M., Pecero, J.E., Dorronsoro, B., Bouvry, P., Khan, S.U.: A cellular genetic algorithm for scheduling applications and energy-aware communication optimization. In: 2010 International Conference on High Performance Computing and Simulation (HPCS), pp. 241–248. IEEE (2010)

11. Deb K., A. S., P. A. and M. T.: A fast elitist non-dominated sorting genetic algorithm for multi-objective optimization: Nsga-ii. In: Proceedings of the 6th International Conference on Parallel Problem Solving from Nature, vol. 1917 (2000)

12. Chang, P.C., Chen, S.H., Zhang, Q., Lin, J.L.: MOEA/D for flowshop scheduling problems. In: IEEE Congress on Evolutionary Computation. CEC 2008 (IEEE World Congress on Computational Intelligence), pp. 1433–1438 (2008)

13. Yagmahan, B., Yenisey, M.M.: A multi-objective ant colony system algorithm for flow shop scheduling problem. Expert Syst. Appl. 37(2), 1361–1368 (2010)

14. Graham, R., Lawler, E., Lenstra, J., Kan, A.R.: Optimization and Approximation in Deterministic Sequencing and Scheduling: a Survey. North-Holland Publishing Company, Amsterdam (1979)

15. Braunt, T.D., Siegel, H.J., Beck, N., Boloni, L.L., Maheswarans, M.: A comparison study of eleven static heuristics for mapping a class of independent tasks onto heterogeneous distributed computing systems. J. Parallel Distrib. Comput. 61, 810–837 (2001)

16. Diaz, C.O., Guzek, M., Pecero, J.E., Danoy, G., Bouvry, P., Khan, S.U.: Energy-aware fast scheduling heuristics in heterogeneous computing systems. In: 2011 International Conference on High Performance Computing and Simulation (HPCS), pp. 478–484. IEEE (2011)

17. Guzek, M., Diaz, C.O., Pecero, J.E., Bouvry, P., Zomaya, A.Y.: Impact of voltage levels number for energy-aware bi-objective dag scheduling for multi-processors systems. In: Papasratorn, B., Charoenkitkarn, N., Lavangnananda, K., Chutimaskul, W., Vanijja, V. (eds.) IAIT 2012. CCIS, vol. 344, pp. 70–80. Springer, Heidelberg (2012)

18. Ishibuchi, H., Yoshida, T., Murata, T.: Balance between genetic search and local search in memetic algorithms for multiobjective permutation flowshop scheduling. IEEE Trans. Evol. Comput. 7(2), 204–223 (2003)

19. Conway, R.W., Maxwell, W.L., Miller, L.W.: Theory of Scheduling. Courier Corporation, New York (2012)

20. Jones, A., Rabelo, L.C., Sharawi, A.T.: Survey of job shop scheduling techniques. Wiley Encyclopedia of Electrical and Electronics Engineering. Wiley, New York (1999)

21. CECAL: HCSP - Heterogeneous Computing Scheduling Problem. CECAL, 1993. http://www.fing.edu.uy/inco/grupos/cecal/hpc/HCSP/index.html. Accessed 1 September 2013

22. Lee, Y.C., Zomaya, A.Y.: Energy efficient distributed computing systems. Wiley Series on Parallel and Distributed Computing, vol. 88, pp. 1–34. Wiley, New York (2012)

23. Emami, M., Ghiasi, Y., Jaberi, N.: Energy-aware scheduling using dynamic voltage-frequency scaling. CoRR, vol. abs/1206.1984 (2012)

24. Pecero, J.E., Bouvry, P., Fraire Huacuja, H.J., Khan, S.U.: A multi-objective grasp algorithm for joint optimization of energy consumption and schedule length of precedence-constrained applications. In: Cloud and Green Computing (CGC 2011) (2011)

25. Pecero, J.E., Bouvry, P., Barrios, C.J.: Low energy and high performance scheduling on scalable computing systems. In: Latin-American Conference on High Performance Computing, pp. 1–8 (2010)

26. Lee, Y.C., Zomaya, A.Y.: Energy conscious scheduling for distributed computing systems under different operating conditions. IEEE Trans. Parallel Distrib. Syst. **22**, 1374–1381 (2011)
27. Mokotoff, E., Jimeno, J.: Heuristics based on partial enumeration for the unrelated parallel processor scheduling problem. Annals of Operations Research, pp. 133–150. Kluwer Academic Publishers, Netherlands (2002)

Building Optimal Operation Policies for Dam Management Using Factored Markov Decision Processes

Alberto Reyes[✉], Pablo H. Ibargüengoytia, Inés Romero, David Pech, and Mónica Borunda

Instituto de Investigaciones Eléctricas, Cuernavaca, Morelos, México
{areyes,pibar,monica.borunda}@iie.org.mx,
{senileon,davidpech_01}@hotmail.com

Abstract. In this paper, we present the conceptual model of a real-world application of factored Markov Decision Processes to dam management. The idea is to demonstrate that it is possible to efficiently automate the construction of operation policies by modelling compactly the problem as a sequential decision problem that can be easily solved using stochastic dynamic programming. We will explain the problem domain and provide an analysis of the resulting value and policy functions. We will also present a useful discussion about the issues that will appear when the conceptual model to be extended into a real-world application.

1 Introduction

The construction of operation policies for dam management is a complex and time-consuming task that requires multi-disciplinary expert knowledge. Usually, a group conformed of specialists such as meteorologists, hydrologists, civil engineers, and others are encouraged of performing this task. However, one of the main challenges is how to represent the uncertainty of the rainfall behavior to change the water level of the big storage container and the significance of keeping the dam safe. A reservoir used solely for hydropower or water supply is better able to meet its objectives when it is full of water, rather than when it is empty. On the other hand, a reservoir used solely for downstream flood control is best left empty, until the flood comes of course. A single reservoir serving all three purposes introduces conflicts over how much water to store in it and how it should be operated. In basins where diversion demands exceed the available supplies, conflicts will exist over water allocations. Finding the best way to manage, if not resolve, these conflicts that occur over time and space are other reasons for planning. In general, water resources planning and management activities are usually motivated by the realization that there are both problems to solve and opportunities to obtain increased benefits from the use of water and related land resources. However, the uncertain and intermittent nature of this resources make them hard to solve.

© Springer International Publishing Switzerland 2015
O. Pichardo Lagunas et al. (Eds.): MICAI 2015, Part II, LNAI 9414, pp. 475–484, 2015.
DOI: 10.1007/978-3-319-27101-9_36

Among the most traditional artificial intelligence (AI) techniques to deal with a planning and decision making problems under uncertainty, the decision trees approach [14] can be found. A decision tree represents a problem in such a way that all the options and consequences can be reviewed. They allow quantifying the costs of all possible results before making a decision. They also quantify the probability of occurrence of each event. The problem with this technique is that it only can be applicable when the number of actions is small and not all combinations of them are not possible. Other approaches such as influence diagrams or decision networks [8,12] allow representing a situation with many variables involved, identifying the source of the information required to make a decision, and modelling dynamic decisions in time. A limitation with this technique is that it exploits spatial and temporally as the problem grows up. The approaches based on classical planners like DRIPS [7], WEAVER [10] or MAXPLAN [11] introduce a non-deterministic representation of actions, represent conditional planning to estimate the maximum utility of a plan, explicitly represent exogenous events, or profit the main concepts under decision-theory and constraint logic programming. The problem with this techniques is that given that each planner solves different parts of the planning problem and that each one visualizes the problem from a different perspective, their integration results hard to implement. The framework of Markov Decision Processes (MDP) [2] meets in one single approach many of the main features of the traditional AI tools to deal with a planning and decision making problems under uncertainty.

From the point of view of water resources management and planning problems, some related work can also be found. In [6] for instance, a deep review about different applications of MDPs is presented. Among them, the water reservoir optimization problem is well described. In others such as [9], non linear optimization models, linear programming, fuzzy optimization, dynamic programming, Markov processes, stochastic optimization, and data-base approaches are also presented. The problem with the MDP approach has been the "curse of dimensionality" implicit on its own nature. This lack results in a big difficulty to solve a decision problem with a few variables. Due to its compactness, ability to exploit the domain structure, and feasibility to integrate the features of other logic-based planners, the factored MDP approach [3] is used in this work. This approach introduces a series of methods under the concept of intentional (or factored) representations through which a combinational problem can be solved to make tractable a planning under uncertainty problem computationally speaking. Another feature is that it concentrates the main features of other planners in just one.

This paper is organized as follows: Sect. 2 presents a formalization of a simplified dam management problem. Section 3 provides a brief background about factored MDPs. Section 4 formalizes the dam problem in terms of a sequential decision problem represented as a factored MDP. Section 5 provides an analysis of the resulting value and policy functions for to test scenarios. Finally, conclusion and future directions are established in Sect. 6.

2   Problem Domain

Consider the problem of creating the best operation policies for the hydroelectric system described in Fig. 1.

The system consists of: a reservoir; an inflow conduit, regulated by V0, which can either be a river or a spillway from another dam; and two spillways for outflow: the first penstock, V1, which is connected to the turbine and thus generates electricity, and the second penstock, V2, allowing direct water evacuation without electricity generation. In this way the reservoir has two inflow sources coming either from the inflow conduit or the rainfall and two outflow sources namely the two spillways. We quantize all flows to a unit of flow, L, and consider them as multiples of this unit. We consider the four reservoir levels MinOperL, MaxOperL, MaxExtL and Top and consider the transition from one level to the other above the bottom of the reservoir.

The unit L is the required amount of displaced water required to move from one level in the reservoir to another one and it is defined by

$$L = \frac{Q}{S}\Delta t,\tag{1}$$

where $Q = [m^3/s]$ is a unit of flow, $S = [m^2]$ is the surface of the reservoir and $\Delta t = [s]$ is a unit of time. Therefore the rainfall, LL, and the inflow and outflows are multiples of L,

$$LL = n_{LL}L,\tag{2}$$
$$Q_i = n_iL,\tag{3}$$

where the subindex $i = 0, 1, 2$ and Q_0 is the inflow at V_0 and Q_1 and Q_2 are the outflows at V_1 and V_2 and $n_{LL}, n_i \in (0, N)$. Given this, we classify the rainfall as follows

$$LL = \begin{cases} \text{No rain;} & LL = 0, \\ \text{Moderate rain;} & LL = L, \\ \text{Heavy rain;} & LL \geq L. \end{cases}\tag{4}$$

The aim of the optimization process is to control V_0, V_1 and V_2 such that the water volume in the reservoir is as much as possible in the optimum level,

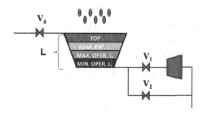

Fig. 1. Simplified hydroelectric system.

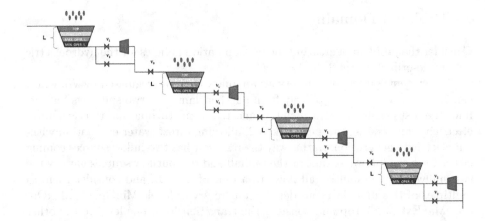

Fig. 2. Multiple dam system.

namely the MaxOperL level, given the rainfall conditions. This optimization process creates the optimal operation conditions of the dam and becomes a decision maker depending on the meteorological and hydrological conditions of the site.

With the idea of having four interconnected dams, now the system is modeled by the interconnection of the previous set-up and three more copies as shown in Fig. 2.

This process is more complex since the decision maker takes into account the inflows and outflows of each dam, the rainfall conditions, which may be different from one dam to another because they are located at different sites, in addition to keep consulting the operation policies of each of them to maintain the four dams as close as possible to the MaxOperL levels.

3   Factored Markov Decision Processes

A Markov decision process (MDP) [13] models a sequential decision problem, in which a system evolves over time and is controlled by an agent. At discrete time intervals the agent observes the state of the system and chooses an action. The system dynamics are governed by a probabilistic transition function Φ that maps states $\mathbf{S}$ and actions $\mathbf{A}$ (both at time t) to new states $\mathbf{S}'$ (at time $t+1$). At each time, an agent receives a scalar reward signal R that depends on the current state s and the applied action a. The performance criterion that the agent should maximize considers the discounted sum of expected future rewards, or value V: $E[\sum_{t=0}^{\infty} \gamma^t R(s_t)]$, where $0 \leq \gamma < 1$ is a discount rate. The main problem is to find a control strategy or *policy* π that maximizes the expected reward V over time.

For the discounted infinite-horizon case with any given discount factor γ, there is a policy π^* that is optimal regardless of the starting state and that satisfies the *Bellman* equation [2]:

Table 1. State space for a single-dam system. The description is in terms of the values for the Level and Rain variables.

State ID	Description	State ID	Description	State ID	Description
1	MinOperL1, Null	9	MinOperL1, Moderate	17	MinOperL1, Intense
2	MinOperL2, Null	10	MinOperL2, Moderate	18	MinOperL2, Intense
3	MaxOperL1, Null	11	MaxOperL1, Moderate	19	MaxOperL1, Intense
4	MaxOperL2, Null	12	MaxOperL2, Moderate	20	MaxOperL2, Intense
5	MaxExtL1, Null	13	MaxExtL1, Moderate	21	MaxExtL1, Intense
6	MaxExtL2, Null	14	MaxExtL2, Moderate	22	MaxExtL2, Intense
7	Top1, Null	15	Top1, Moderate	23	Top1, Intense
8	Top2, Null	16	Top2, Moderate	24	Top2, Intense

$$V^*(s) = max_a\{R(s,a) + \gamma \sum_{s\in \mathbf{S}} \Phi(a,s,s')V^*(s')\} \tag{5}$$

Two methods for solving this equation and finding an optimal policy for an MDP are: (a) dynamic programming [13] and (b) linear programming.

In a factored MDP, the set of states is described via a set of random variables $\mathbf{S} = \{X_1, ..., X_n\}$, where each X_i takes on values in some finite domain $Dom(X_i)$. A state $\mathbf{x}$ defines a value $x_i \in Dom(X_i)$ for each variable X_i. Thus, as the set of states $\mathbf{S} = Dom(X_i)$ is exponentially large, it results impractical to represent the transition model explicitly as matrices. Fortunately, the framework of dynamic Bayesian networks (DBN) [4,5] gives us the tools to describe the transition model concisely. In these representations, the post-action nodes (at the time $t + 1$) contain smaller matrices with the probabilities of their values given their parents' values under the effects of an action. For a more detailed description of factored MDPs see [3].

4   Factored MDP Problem Specification

The MDP problem specification consists in establishing the set of states, set of actions, immediate reward function, and an state transition function. A simplified space state is composed of the possible values for the variables rain intensity (Rain) and dam level (Level). The variable Rain can take three different nominal values: Null, Moderate and Intense, and Level can take eight values MinOperL1, MinOperL2, MaxOperL1, MaxOperL2, MaxExtL1, MaxExtL2, Top1 and Top2. As a consequence, the state space dimension will be 24 (31 * 81) with the values combination shown in Table 1.

The possible actions are given in terms of the operations permitted on the control elements (valves or gates) V0, V1 and V2. V0 is the inflow conduit valve, V1 is the spillway to the hydraulic turbine, and V2 is the direct evacuation gate or turbine bypass valve (see Sect. 2 for details.). For this simple example, the actions could be close or open a control element. The possible actions combination are shown in Table 2.

Table 2. Action space. The recommended actions are open or close the valves V0, V1 or V2.

Action ID	V0	V1	V2
A1	Close_Valve	Close_Valve	Close_Valve
A2	Close_Valve	Close_Valve	Open_Valve
A3	Close_Valve	Open_Valve	Close_Valve
A4	Close_Valve	Open_Valve	Open_Valve
A5	Open_Valve	Close_Valve	Close_Valve
A6	Open_Valve	Close_Valve	Open_Valve
A7	Open_Valve	Open_Valve	Close_Valve
A8	Open_Valve	Open_Valve	Open_Valve

In order to set a reward function for this problem, consider that keeping a dam level of MaxOperL1 or MaxOperL2 represents 100 economic units (best case). If the level is MaxExtL1 or MaxExtL2 the immediate reward value is -0 (irrelevant), if the level is Top1 or Top2 the reward value is -100 (worst case), and finally if the level is MinOperL the reward received is -50 (bad). In general terms, the dam levels around the MaxOperL value are awared while the levels nearby the top limits are penalized significantly. Notice that the reward rate is independent of the rainfall intensity. The decision tree of Fig. 3 shows graphically the reward distribution as a function of the dam levels.

The transition model is represented using a two steps dynamic bayesian network for each action. Figure 4 shows the action A1 in three different scenarios. In all three scanarios the level of the dam is established in the **MaxOperL level** (red mark on interval 3-4). In the left case, Rain is instantiated in **Null** value (blue mark in interval 1). In this scenario, the level of tha dam has no change. Level_1 is maintained in interval 3-4 (orange mark). In the center scenario, Rain is **Moderate** (interval 1-2) and the dam level increments to reach interval 4-5 with 80 % probability. Finally, in the rigth scenario, the Rain is intense (interval 2-3) and the dam level is incremented to interval 5-6 with 80 % probability. The model and the inferences are visualized using the Hugin package [1].

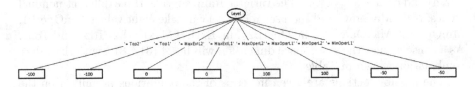

Fig. 3. Reward function

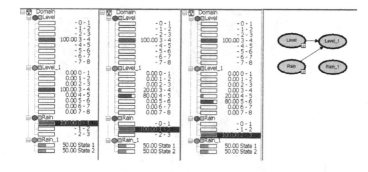

Fig. 4. Transition model (Color figure online).

5   Experimental Results

Given the reward and transition functions, we solved the factored MDP to obtain the policy and expected utility functions. As factored MDP solver we used the SPI (Planning under Uncertainty System in spanish) tool which managed to estimate 14 different values with a value iteration implementation. The minimum value obtained for this MDP model was 136.5961 and the maximum value was 771.2321. These values are represented with labels and colors in Fig. 5 (left). The utility values for each state are shaded with light green color when the value is optimal and with darker colors as the value decreases. In the same figure, we show the resulting policy (recommended action) using labels with the action id. In all cases we used a discount value $= 1$.

For example, the effect of the action A1, framed with red in Fig. 5 (left) and represented by the symbol $\oplus$ (pointed with a red asterisk) in Fig. 5 (right), means that the policy effect on the level is null due that the recommended action will keep the level. This is because the rain has no influence on the system. In the case of having a low level of the dam, independently of the rain condition, the policy function will recommend action A5 with the effect of increasing the level $\uparrow$. In this case, the influence of the rain could increase the level in one step or two depending on the rain intensity. In the opposite case when the dam has a high level the action effect of A4 will decrease $\downarrow\downarrow$ the level of the dam according to the rain intensity. The policy effects on the dam level are shown in Table 3.

In order to show the system behavior, we followed the recommended actions from an random initial state until achieving the goal state under two different scenarios: 1-dam process and 4-dam process. In this demonstration we obtained each next state from the transition state function with the maximum probability of occurrence.

In the first case, one dam was set up under the minimum operation level (level = MinOperL) and with no rain (rain = Null). The policy was applied for a time horizon of twenty steps to observe the utility trend through the states transited. Figure 6 (left) shows how the dam starts with a minimum operation level with an expected utility $= 427.68$ units, in the next step the system reaches

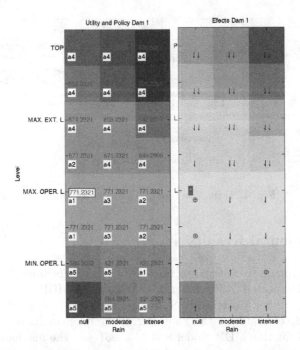

Fig. 5. (left) Value and utility functions . Dark colors represent low expected utility values and light colors represent high utility values. (right) Effects of the policy on the dam level at different rain conditions. Refer Table 3 for symbols interpretation (Color figure online).

a state with utility = 588.30 units, and in a third step it reaches the maximum utility value = 771.23 units.

In a second case, we initialized multiple dams at the conditions shown in Table 4, the algorithm is executed to check the optimization twenty executions.

Table 3. Policy effects on the dam level according to the rainfall condition (null, moderate or intense).

ID	Rain = Null	Rain = moderate	Rain = intense
A1	⊕	↑	↑↑
A2	↓↓	↓	⊕
A3	↓	⊕	↑
A4	↓↓↓	↓↓	↓
A5	↑	↑↑	↑↑↑
A6	↓	⊕	↑
A7	⊕	↑	↑↑
A8	↓↓	↓	⊕

Table 4. Initial states and expected utility values for a multiple dam system. The states variables are Level and Rain.

Dam	Level	Rain	Utility
1	MinOperL1	Null	427.68
2	MaxOperL2	Moderate	771.23
3	MinOperL2	Intense	621.23
4	MaxExtL2	Intense	542.20

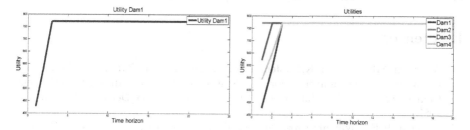

Fig. 6. Utility plot. (left) Utility for a single-dam system. (right) Utility for multiple dams (Color figure online)

As shown in Fig. 6 (right) the Dam1 (blue line), which started with a low level, reached the optimum value in 3 steps. The Dam2 (green line) started in a goal state (optimal value) and remains. The Dam3 (red line), which started with max extraordinary level , and it achieves the maximun utility in 2 state transitions. Finally, the Dam4 (light blue line) that was initialized with a high level got its optimal value in 3 steps.

6   Discussion and Future Work

In this paper, we showed a conceptual model of a real-world application of factored Markov Decision Processes to dam management. The idea was to demonstrate that it is possible to efficiently automate the construction of operation policies by modelling compactly the problem as a sequential decision problem that can be easily solved using stochastic dynamic programming. Using factored representations it is possible not only to represent the uncertainty of the rainfall behavior but also to deal with the curse of dimensionality and make hard problems more tractable. We provided an analysis of the resulting value and policy functions in a conceptual hydroelectric process and showed how a single-dam system or a multiple-dam system can easily achieve an optimal operation state.

Due that this is a demonstration of the feasibility to use the framework of factored MDPs to solve problems in a hydroelectric domain, and that several assumptions were made, there are still many challenges to face with this problem when it grows to a real-world application. One of this challenges has to do with how to optimize a multiple-dam system simultaneously without losing compactness in the representation. Other challenges suggest the use of reinforcement learning to approximate state transitions from historical data in a real system and consequently avoid the need of depending on a group of specialists to perform the task of building operation policies manually.

Acknowledgments. Authors wish to thank the Control, Electronics and Communication department and the Enabling Technologies division of the Electrical Research Institute-Mexico for the financial support to perform this research.

References

1. Andersen, S.K., Olesen, K.G., Jensen, F.V., Jensen, F.: HUGIN: a shell for building bayesian belief universes for expert systems. In: Proceeding Eleventh Joint Conference on Artificial Intelligence, IJCAI, pp. 1080–1085, Detroit, 20–25 August 1989
2. Bellman, R.E.: Dynamic Programming. Princeton U. Press, Princeton (1957)
3. Boutilier, C., Dean, T., Hanks, S.: Decision-theoretic planning: structural assumptions and computational leverage. J. AI Res. **11**, 1–94 (1999)
4. Darwiche, A., Goldszmidt, M.: Action networks: a framework for reasoning about actions and change under understanding. In: Proceedings of the Tenth Conference on Uncertainty in AI, UAI-1994, pp. 136–144, Seattle (1994)
5. Dean, T., Kanazawa, K.: A model for reasoning about persistence and causation. Comput. Intell. **5**, 142–150 (1989)
6. Lamond, B.F., Boukhtouta, A.: Water reservoir applications of Markov decision processes. In: Feinberg, E.A., Shwartz, A. (eds.) Handbook of Markov Decision Processes, Methods and Applications. Kluwer, US (2002)
7. Haddawy, P., Suwandy, M.: Decision-theoretic refinement planning using inheritance abstraction. In: Hammond, K. (ed.) Proceedings of the Second International Conference on Artificial Intelligence Planning Systems. AAAI Press, Menlo Park (1994)
8. Howard, R.A., Matheson, J.E.: Influence diagrams. In: Howard, R.A., Matheson, J.E. (eds.) Principles and Applications of Decision Analysis, Menlo Park (1984)
9. Loucks, D.P., van Beek, E.: Water resources systems planning and management: an introduction to methods, models and applications. In: Dynamic Programming. United Nations Educational, Scientific and Cultural Organization (UNESCO) (2005)
10. Veloso, M., Carbonel, J., Perez, A., Borrajo, D., Fink, E., Blythe, J.: Integrating planning and learning: the prodigy architecture. J. Exp. Theor. AI **1**, 81–120 (1995)
11. Majercik, S.M., Littman, M.L.: MAXPLAN: a new approach to probabilistic planning. In: Simmons, R., Smith, S. (eds.) Proceedings of the Fourth International Conference on Artificial Intelligence Planning Systems, pp. 86–93. AAAI Press, Menlo Park (1998)
12. Pearl, J.: Probabilistic reasoning in intelligent systems: networks of plausible inference. Morgan Kaufmann, San Francisco (1988)
13. Puterman, M.L.: Markov Decision Processes. Wiley, New York (1994)
14. Quinlan, J.R.: Induction of decision trees. Mach. Learn. **1**(1), 81–106 (1986)

Forecasting

Fishery Forecasting Based on Singular Spectrum Analysis Combined with Bivariate Regression

Lida Barba[1,2](✉) and Nibaldo Rodríguez[2]

[1] Engineering Faculty, Universidad Nacional de Chimborazo,
33730880 Riobamba, Ecuador
lbarba@unach.edu.ec
[2] School of Informatics Engineering, Pontificia Universidad Católica de Valparaíso,
2362807 Valparaíso, Chile

Abstract. The fishery of anchovy and sardine has a great importance in the economy of Chile; they are important resources used for internal consumption and for export. The forecasting based on historical time series is a fishery planning tool. In this paper is presented the forecasting of anchovy and sardine by means of the monthly catches in the Chilean northern coast ($18°S - 24°S$), during the period January 1976 to December 2007. The forecasting strategy is presented in two stages: preprocessing and prediction. In the first stage the Singular Spectrum Analysis (SSA) technique is applied to extract the components interannual and annual of the time series. In the second stage the Bivariate Regression (BVR) is implemented to predict the extracted components. The results evaluated with the efficiency metrics show a high prediction accuracy of the strategy based on SSA and BVR. Besides, the results are compared with a conventional nonlinear prediction based on an Autoregressive Neural Network (ANN) with Levenberg-Marquardt; it was demonstrated the improvement in the prediction accuracy by using the proposed strategy SSA-BVR with regard to the results obtained with the ANN.

1 Introduction

The Chilean continental shelf is rich in fishery resources, their properly exploitation maximizes the economy of coastal towns. Anchovies (Engraulis ringens) and Sardines (Sardinops sagax) have great economical importance in this country; these species are main food in the coastal and two important exportation resources.

Due to the significant fluctuations of the marine ecosystem, the stock of anchovy and sardine is in dependence of the environmental conditions. Considering the information of the Fishery National Service [1], it is observed that during the last decade the anchovy stock has grown up, while the sardine stock has been decreasing, it is advisable to keep track of the evolution of these species and it is essential the establishment of exploitation policies and control rules.

Forecasting based on historical time series is an important tool in fisheries planning. Autoregressive techniques have been evaluated to model the fishery behavior of different marine species as pacific sardines and anchovies [2–5].

© Springer International Publishing Switzerland 2015
O. Pichardo Lagunas et al. (Eds.): MICAI 2015, Part II, LNAI 9414, pp. 487–497, 2015.
DOI: 10.1007/978-3-319-27101-9_37

The fisheries time series have a complex nonlinear structure which involves the use of complex models with a big number of variables. An efficient alternative is the prediction based on the components extracted from the time series [6]. The Singular Spectrum Analysis (SSA) is associated with the publications of Broomhead and King [7], nowadays is a potent technique of data analysis; SSA does not require a priori knowledge about the number of periodicities and period values. Trend, seasonality, and noise are commonly extracted with SSA [8–14].

In this work is proposed the fishery stock prediction based on the components extraction by means of Singular Spectrum Analysis (SSA) combined with the linear method. SSA involves four steps, in the first step the window length is selected through the singular values energy information, it is used to embed the time series in a Hankel matrix. The Singular Value Decomposition, grouping and diagonal averaging are the next steps applied to extract the components of low and high frequency. The results are compared with a nonlinear conventional method based on an Autoregressive Neural Network with the Levenberg-Marquardt learning algorithm.

The paper is structured as follows. Section 2 describes the Components extraction based on Singular Spectrum Analysis. Section 3 presents the Prediction with the Bi-variate Regression. Section 4 describes the nonlinear prediction with a conventional Autoregressive Neural Network. Section 5 describes forecasting accuracy metrics. Section 6 presents the Results and Discussions. The conclusions are shown in Sect. 7.

2   Components Extraction with Singular Spectrum Analysis

The Singular Spectrum Analysis is described in four steps: embedding, decomposition, grouping and averaging [15].

2.1   Embedding

The embedding step maps the time series x of length N, to a sequence of multidimensional lagged vectors.

The window length L is an integer with values $1 < L < N$, the embedding creates $K = N - L + 1$ lagged vectors

$$H_i = (x_i, \ldots, x_{i+L-1})^T, \quad 1 \leq i \leq K \tag{1}$$

The L-lagged vectors are the rows of the trajectory matrix (Hankel matrix), which is represented with:

$$H = \begin{pmatrix} x_1 & x_2 & \cdots & x_K \\ x_2 & x_3 & \cdots x_{K+1} \\ \vdots & \vdots & \vdots & \vdots \\ x_L & x_{L+1} & \cdots & x_N \end{pmatrix}. \tag{2}$$

The elements $H_{i,j} = x_{i+j-1}$, and the matrix H has the same elements on the anti-diagonals.

The window length is significant in the forecasting model. In Sect. 5 will be presented the method to find the optimal value of L. The window length L is significant in the forecasting model, in this work, the optimal L is found through the computation of the singular values energy E as follows:

$$E_i = \frac{s_i^2}{\sum_{i=1}^{L} s_i^2} \tag{3}$$

where s_i is the i-th singular value, and L is initially computed with $L = N/2$. The new optimal L is visualized through the highest peak of energy, and the embedding step is executed again.

2.2 Singular Value Decomposition

The SVD of the trajectory matrix H has the form

$$H = \sum_{i=1}^{L} \sqrt{\lambda_i} U_i V_i^T, \tag{4}$$

where each λ_i is the ith eigenvalue of the matrix $S = HH^T$ arranged in decreasing order of magnitudes. $U_1, \ldots, U_L$ is the corresponding orthonormal system of eigenvectors of the matrix S.

Standard SVD terminology calls $\sqrt{\lambda_i}$ the ith singular value of the matrix H; U_i its ith left singular vector, and V_i its ith right singular vector. The collection $[\sqrt{\lambda_i} U_i V_i]$ is called ith eigentriple of H.

Elementary matrices can be represented with

$$H_i = \sqrt{\lambda_i} U_i V_i^T. \tag{5}$$

2.3 Grouping

The grouping step arranges the matrix terms H_i. Assume that $m = 2$, $I_1 = 1, \ldots, r$ and $I_2 = 1, \ldots, d$ for $r + d = L$. The time series will be separable by decomposition if there exist an indexes collection such that

$$Y_{I_1} = \sum_{i \in I_1} H_i, \tag{6a}$$

$$Y_{I_2} = \sum_{i \notin I_1} H_i. \tag{6b}$$

The purpose of the grouping step is to separate the time series additive components. From the set of indexes I_1 can be obtained the grouped matrices Y_{I_1} and Y_{I_2}. Therefore $Y_{I_2} = H - Y_{I_1}$.

The matrices Y_{I_1} and Y_{I_2} are trajectory matrices, then there exist series that can be called components, c_{I_1} and c_{I_2} such that $x = c_{I_1} + c_{I_2}$. The terms of each component are obtained in the next step.

2.4 Diagonal Averaging

This step is applied to transform the grouped matrices Y_{I_1} and Y_{I_2} into new series of length N.

Let Y be an $L \times K$ matrix with elements $y_{i,j}$, $1 \leq i \leq L, 1 \leq j \leq K$, with $L < K$, $N = L + K - 1$, and $k = i + j$.

Diagonal averaging transfers the elements of the matrix Y(Y_{I_1} and Y_{I_2} to the component by the equations

$$c_{i,j} = \begin{cases} \frac{1}{k-1} \sum_{m=1}^{k} y_{m,k-m}, & 2 \leq k \leq L, \\ \frac{1}{L} \sum_{m=1}^{L} y_{m,k-m}, & L < k \leq K+1, \\ \frac{1}{K+L-k+1} \sum_{m=k-K}^{L} y_{m,k-m}, & K+2 \leq k \leq K+L. \end{cases} \tag{7}$$

3 Prediction with Bi-Variate Regression

The predictions of the anchovy and sardine are obtained from the components extracted with SSA ($c_{i,j}$); which are labeled with annual(x_a) and interannual(x_{ia}). The prediction is computed with the addition of both predicted components with the equation:

$$\hat{x}(n+1) = \hat{x_a}(n+1) + \hat{x_{ia}}(n+1), \tag{8}$$

where n represents the time instant.

The annual component has influence of the interannual component, therefore x_{ia} is used as external input in the prediction of x_a. The prediction of the components is obtained with:

$$\hat{x_a}(n+1) = \sum_{i=0}^{m-1} \alpha_i x_{ia}(n-i) + \sum_{i=0}^{m-1} \beta_i x_a(n-i), \tag{9a}$$

$$\hat{x_{ia}}(n+1) = \sum_{i=0}^{m-1} \alpha_i x_{ia}(n-i), \tag{9b}$$

where m is the size of the time window (number of lagged values), α_i and β_i are the ith coefficients.

The coefficients estimation is based on the linear Least Square Method (LSM), by using the training sample, the components x_{ia} and x_a are represented with the linear relationship expressed in the equations

$$x_{ia} = \alpha Z_{ia}, \tag{10a}$$

$$x_a = \beta Z_a, \tag{10b}$$

where Z_{ia} is the regressor matrix of N_t rows and m columns, and α a vector of m rows and one column; while Z_a is the regressor matrix of N_t rows and $2m$ columns, and β a vector of $2m$ rows and one column. The coefficients are computed by using the Moore-Penrose pseudoinverse $Z_{ia}\dagger$, and $Z_a\dagger$ as follows

$$\alpha = Z_{ia}\dagger x_{ia}, \tag{11a}$$

$$\beta = Z_a\dagger x_a. \tag{11b}$$

4   Prediction with an Autoregressive Neural Network

The Autoregressive Neural Network has a common structure of a Multilayer Perceptron of three layers [16], the inputs are the lagged terms, which are contained in the regressor matrix Z, each row is a regressor vector z_i, at the hidden layer is applied the sigmoid transfer function, and at the output layer is obtained the predicted value. The ANN output is:

$$\hat{x}(n) = \sum_{j=1}^{Q} b_j h_j, \tag{12a}$$

$$h_j = \sum_{i=1}^{m} w_{ji} z_i(n), \tag{12b}$$

where $\hat{x}$ is the estimated value, n is the time instant, Q is the number of hidden nodes, b_j and w_{ji} are the linear and nonlinear weights of the ANN connections respectively, the sigmoid transfer function is computed with

$$f(x) = \frac{1}{1 + e^{-x}}. \tag{13}$$

The ANN is denoted with $ANN(m, Q, 1)$, with m inputs, Q hidden nodes, and 1 output.

The ANN weights b and w are updated with the application of the learning algorithm.

4.1   Levenberg-Marquardt Learning Algorithm

The weights of the ANN connections are updated with the Levenberg Marquardt algorithm. The scalar u is a parameter used in LM to determine the algorithm behavior, if u increases the value, the algorithm works as the steepest descent algorithm with low learning rate; whereas if u decreases the value until zero, the algorithm works as the Gauss-Newton method ([17]). The weights of the ANN connections are computed with:

$$\omega_{n+1} = \omega_n + \Delta(\omega_n), \tag{14a}$$

$$\Delta(\omega_n) = -[J^T(\omega_n) \times J(\omega_n) + u_n \times I)]^{-1} J^T(\omega_n) \times e(\omega_n), \tag{14b}$$

where ω is the weight vector composed by $(w_{ji}, \ldots, b_j)$, $\Delta(\omega_n)$ is the weight increment, J is the Jacobian matrix, J^T is transposed Jacobian matrix, I is the identity matrix, e is the error vector and n is the time instant.

The fitness function used here with LM is MSE (Mean Squared Error), the elements of the Jacobian matrix corresponds to the partial derivative of the fitness function regarding each weight, as follows

$$J(\omega_{j,i}) = \left[\frac{\partial e(\omega_{j,i})}{\partial \omega_{j,i}} \right], \tag{15}$$

where the order of the matrix (J) is $N \times k$; N is the sample size, and k is the total number of weights.

5   Forecasting Accuracy Metrics

The forecasting accuracy is evaluated with diverse criteria. The differences between the observed and predicted values are quantified by using forms more sensitive to significant over or underprediction, such as the modified Nash-Sutcliffe efficiency (E)[18], the Mean Absolute Percentage Error $(MAPE)$, and the Relative Percentage Error (RPE). Additionally is computed the Generalized Cross Validation (GCV) to calibrate the time window of the autoregressive models.

$$E = 1 - \frac{\sum_{i=1}^{N_v} |x_i - \hat{x}_i|}{\sum_{i=1}^{N_v} |x_i - \bar{x}|} \times 100, \tag{16}$$

$$MAPE = \left[\frac{1}{N_v} \sum_{i=1}^{N_v} |(x_i - \hat{x}_i)/x_i| \right] \times 100, \tag{17}$$

$$RPE = \left[\frac{(x_i - \hat{x}_i)}{x_i} \right] \times 100, \quad i = 1 \dots N_v, \tag{18}$$

$$GCV = \frac{RMSE}{(1 - P/N_v)^2}, \quad RMSE = \sqrt{\frac{1}{N_v} \sum_{i=1}^{N_v} (x_i - \hat{x}_i)^2} \tag{19}$$

where N_v is the validation data set size, x_i is the ith observed value, $\hat{x}_i$ is the ith forecasted value, and P is the length of the input regressor vector.

6   Results and Discussion

The results of the implementation of the proposed strategy is described in two stages: data preprocessing and prediction.

6.1   Data

The time series data analyzed in this work corresponds to the monthly fish catch of anchovy and sardine along the Chilean northern coast $(18°S - 24°S)$, from January 1976 to December 2007 obtained from SERNAPESCA [1]. Figure 1a shows the raw data in metric tons, from Figure is observed a complex nonlinear behavior. For the prediction this sample has been divided into two groups, training and validation; the training sample represents the 75% of the data, and consequently the validation sample represents the 25%. The sample contains some null values due to the fishery banning policy. In Fig. 1, the anchovy and sardine fisheries are presented from year 1976; the biomass growth was held between 1976 and 1986, later a declining trend is observed. The current status of the resource is diminished abundance, which is associated to adverse environmental conditions, the ecosystem of the northern of Chile is dominated by the anchovy; the anchovy stock has had an increasing growth in contrast to the sardine stock.

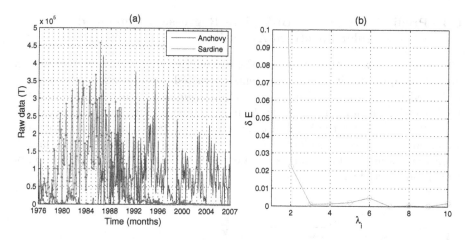

Fig. 1. (a) Anchovy and Sardine catches (b) Differential energy of eigenvalues

6.2 Components Extraction with Singular Spectrum Analysis

The components extraction from the time series was applied with the steps detailed in Sect. 2. The initial window length used was $L = N/2$; where N is the training sample size. The differential energy of the eigenvalues obtained with second step of SSA are plotted to find the highest energy concentration as shows Fig. 1b; the highest peak was used as the optimal window length, in this case $L = 6$. The preprocessing restarts with this optimal value. The components extracted from the Anchovy time series with SSA are shown in Fig. 2a; the components extracted from the Sardine time series with SSA are shown in Fig. 2b, from Figures is observed that the interannual component x_{ia}, shows the trend; while the annual component x_a shows the periodic behavior.

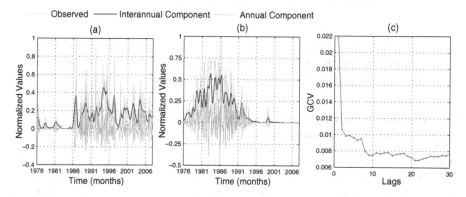

Fig. 2. (a) Anchovy: Observed data and Components Extracted (b) Sardine: Observed data and Components Extracted (c) Lagged values calibration

6.3   Prediction with the Bi-Variate Regression Combined with Singular Spectrum Analysis

The prediction with the Bi-variate Regression (which process was detailed in Sect. 3) is applied with the components extracted through SSA. The number of lagged values was found with the training sample of Anchovy by using the GCV metric, which is shown in Fig. 2c, in this case the same time window length $m = 21$ was used for the Sardine time series. The testing is executed with the validation sample, the results are presented in Figs. 3a and 4a, Tables 1 and 2; from Figures and residual values is observed high accuracy in the prediction of the anchovies and sardines stock.

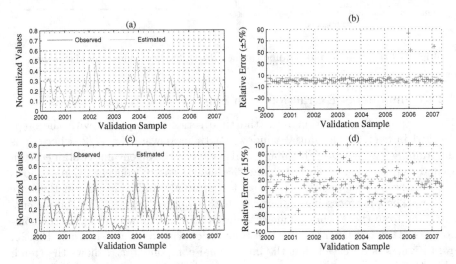

Fig. 3. Anchovy: (a) Prediction based on SSA-BVR (b) Relative Error (SSA-BVR) (c) Prediction based on ANN-LM (d) Relative Error (ANN-LM)

The Relative Percentage Error is presented in Figs. 3b and 4b; for the Anchovy, the 88.4 % of the points presents a lower RPE than ±5 %; for the Sardine, the 86.7 % of the points presents a lower RPE than ±15 %.

6.4   Prediction with the Autoregressive Neural Network Based on Levenberg-Marquardt

In this section the prediction is presented with the Autoregressive Neural Network based on Levenberg-Marquardt. The ANN structure was presented in Sect. 4. The number of hidden nodes is computed with $Q = log(N_t)$ (the formula normally used in our experiments), where N_t is the training sample size. The inputs are the lagged values, the time window length was found with the training sample through the computation of the GCV metric.

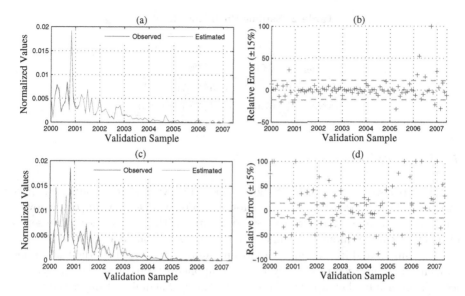

Fig. 4. Sardine: (a) Prediction based on SSA-BVR (b) Relative Error (SSA-BVR) (c) Prediction based on ANN-LM (d) Relative Error (ANN-LM)

The training process of the neural network was performed with 30 repetitions of 1000 epochs; each repetition took 5 seconds. The prediction through the best configuration with the validation sample is shown in Figs. 3c and 4c, Tables 1 and 2. From Figures and residuals values, lower accuracy was reached by using the ANN-LM model in the prediction of anchovies and sardines catches with regard to the model SSA-BVR.

The Relative Percentage Error is presented in Figs. 3d and 4d; in the prediction of Anchovies the 36.7 % of the points presents a lower RPE than ±15 %; in the prediction of Sardines, the 26.7 % of the points presents a lower RPE than ±15 %. Tables 1 and 2 present the evaluation of the Bi-variate Regresssion enhanced with SSA (SSA-BVR), and the conventional nonlinear model (ANN-LM). The best model is SSA-BVR with the lowest residuals values, the highest efficiency criteria, and the highest Relative Percentage Error.

Table 1. Anchovy Prediction Results

Models	MAPE (%)	E (%)	RPE (%)
SSA-BVR	4.3	98	88.4(±5 %)
ANN-LM	29.9	67.2	36.7(±15 %)

Table 2. Sardine Prediction Results

Models	MAPE (%)	E (%)	RPE (%)
SSA-BVR	7.8	94.5	86.7(±15%)
ANN-LM	67.6	55.8	26.7(±15%)

7   Conclusions

In this paper was presented the Singular Spectrum Analysis to enhance the performance of the Bi-variate Regression, for one-step ahead forecasting of anchovies and sardines fishing. The strategy was evaluated with the historical time series of monthly catches along the Chilean northern coast from year 1963 to 2007.

The annual and interannual components were extracted from the time series by using Singular Spectrum Analysis; the components keep the ecosystem dynamics. The interannual component is the low frequency signal and shows the trend; whereas the annual component is the high frequency signal and shows the periodic behavior.

The components were predicted with the proposed model SSA-BVR and an Autoregressive Neural Network with Levenberg-Marquardt. The model based on SSA shows high prediction accuracy of anchovies and sardines catches, with a Nash-Sutcliffe efficiency of 98% and 94.5% respectively. The gain in efficiency (E) of the model SSA-BVR over the ANN-LM model is of 45.8% for anchovy and of 69.3% for sardine.

Due to the promising results, this model will be evaluated with other time series related with fishery, and other diverse knowledge areas.

Acknowledgments. This work was supported in part by Grant CONICYT/ FONDE-CYT/Regular 1131105 and by the DI-Regular project of the Pontificia Universidad Católica de Valparaíso.

References

1. SERNAPESCA (2015). https://www.sernapesca.cl//
2. Stergiou, K., Christou, E., Petrakis, G.: Modelling and forecasting monthly sheries catches: comparison of regression, univariate and multivariate time series methods. Fish. Res. **29**(1), 55–95 (1997)
3. Gutiérrez-Estrada, J.C., Yánez, E., Pulido-Calvo, I., Silva, C., Plaza, F., Bórquez, C.: Pacific sardine (Sardinops sagax, Jenyns 1842) landings prediction. a neural network ecosystemic approach. Fish. Res. **100**(2), 116–125 (2009)
4. Yánez, E., Plaza, F., Gutiérrez-Estrada, J.C., Rodríguez, N., Barbieri, M., Pulido-Calvo, I., et al.: Anchovy (Engraulis ringens) and sardine (Sardinops sagax) abundance forecast of northern chile: a multivariate ecosystemic neural network approach. Prog. Oceanogr. **87**(14), 242–250 (2010)

5. Kim, J.Y., Jeong, H.C., Kim, H., Kang, S.: Forecasting the monthly abundance of anchovies in the South Sea of Korea using a univariate approach. Fish. Res. **161**, 293–302 (2015)
6. Rodríguez N., Cubillos C., Rubio, J.M.: Multi-step-ahead forecasting model for monthly anchovy catches based on wavelet analysis. Journal of Applied Mathematics. vol. 2014, Article ID 798464 (2014)
7. Broomhead, D., King, G.: Extracting qualitative dynamics from experimental data. Phys D: Nonlinear Phenom. **20**, 217–236 (1986)
8. Xiao, Y., Liu, J.J., Hu, Y., Wang, Y., Lai, K.K., Wang, S.: A neuro-fuzzy combination model based on singular spectrum analysis for air transport demand forecasting. J. Air Transp. Manag. **39**, 1–11 (2014)
9. Marques, C., Ferreira, J., Rocha, A., Castanheira, J., Melo-Gonalves, P., Vaz, N., et al.: Singular spectrum analysis and forecasting of hydrological time series. Physics and Chemistry of the Earth, Parts A/B/C. **31**(18), 1172–1179 (2006)
10. Hassani, H., Webster, A., Silva, E.S., Heravi, S.: Forecasting U.S. tourist arrivals using optimal singular spectrum analysis. Tourism Management. **46**, 322–335 (2015)
11. Abdollahzade, M., Miranian, A., Hassani, H., Iranmanesh, H.: A new hybrid enhanced local linear neuro-fuzzy model based on the optimized singular spectrum analysis and its application for nonlinear and chaotic time series forecasting. Information Sciences. **295**, 107–125 (2015)
12. Telesca, L., Lovallo, M., Shaban, A., Darwich, T., Amacha, N.: Singular spectrum analysis and Fisher-Shannon analysis of spring flow time series: An application to Anjar Spring, Lebanon. Physica A: Statistical Mechanics and its Applications. **392**(17), 3789–3797 (2013)
13. Chen, Q., van Dam, T., Sneeuw, N., Collilieux, X., Weigelt, M., Rebischung, P.: Singular spectrum analysis for modeling seasonal signals from GPS time series. Journal of Geodynamics. **72**, 25–35 (2013)
14. Viljoen, H., Nel, D.: Common singular spectrum analysis of several time series. Journal of Statistical Planning and Inference. **140**(1), 260–267 (2010)
15. Golyandina N, Nekrutkin V, Zhigljavsky AA.: Analysis of time series structure. Chapman & Hall/CRC. (2001)
16. Freeman, J.A., Skapura, D.M.: Neural Networks. Applications, and Programming Techniques. Addison-Wesley, Algorithms (1991)
17. Hagan M., Demuth H., Bealetitle M.: Neural Network Design. Hagan Publishing (2002)
18. Krause, P., Boyle, D.P.: Bäse F.: Comparison of different effciency criteria for hydrological model assessment. Advances in Geosciences. **5**, 89–97 (2005)

Artificial Hydrocarbon Networks
for Online Sales Prediction

Hiram Ponce[✉], Luis Miralles-Pechúan,
and María de Lourdes Martínez-Villaseñor

Universidad Panamericana Campus México,
Augusto Rodin 498, Col. Insurgentes-Mixcoac, México D.F., Mexico
{hponce, lmiralles, lmartine}@up.edu.mx

Abstract. Online retail sales have been growing worldwide in the last decade.
In order to cope with this high dynamicity and market share competition, online
retail sales prediction and online advertising have become very important to
answer questions of pricing decisions, advertising responsiveness, and product
demand. To make adequate investment in products and channels it is necessary
to have a model that relates certain features of the product with the number of
sales that will occur in the future. In this paper we describe a comparative
analysis of machine learning techniques against a novel supervised learning
technique called artificial hydrocarbon networks (AHN). This method is a new
type of machine learning that have proved to adapt very well to a wide spectrum
of problems of regression and classification. Thus, we use artificial hydrocarbon
networks for predicting the number of online sales, and then we compare their
performance with other ten well-known methods of machine learning regression, obtaining promising results.

Keywords: Prediction of online sales · Artificial organic networks · Artificial
hydrocarbon networks · Supervised regression · Sales forecasting

1 Introduction

Online retail sales have been growing worldwide in the last decade, and the trend is to
keep growing. Forrester Research Online Retail Forecasts 2013-2018 (US) report projected online retail sales to grow at an 11.1 % compound annual growth rate (CAGR) by
2018 in US [1]. Similar or more optimistic trends can be observed in other countries, for
example in China, Forrester experts forecast total online retail spending to grow at the
compound annual rate of nearly 20 % [2]. Asociación Mexicana de Internet (AMIPCI)
reported 42 % a growth of the total spending in e-commerce in Mexico from 2012 to
2013, and 34 % more from 2013 to 2014 [3].

"The internet has facilitated the creation of new markets characterized by large scale,
increased customization, rapid innovation and the collection and use of detailed consumer and market data" [4]. Internet markets and online sales channels have lower the
cost of creating and distributing product and services. Users acquire information about
the goods easily, and allow suppliers to collect and use their consuming preferences and
demands more rapidly. On the other hand, when choices of sales mechanisms, enabling

O. Pichardo Lagunas et al. (Eds.): MICAI 2015, Part II, LNAI 9414, pp. 498–508, 2015.
DOI: 10.1007/978-3-319-27101-9_38

devices and availability of information grow, competition between markets, product and service suppliers become ferocious. In order to cope with this high dynamicity and market share competition, enterprises have to adjust rapidly to the market, offer innovation constantly, and provide quality products and services. Online retail sales prediction and online advertising have become very important to answer questions of pricing decisions, advertising responsiveness, and product demand.

The aim of this work is to create a model to predict monthly online sales of a product with the best accuracy possible, based on a data set of consumer products. The data set contains information about the product features and advertisement campaign. In this paper we describe a comparative analysis of machine learning techniques against a novel supervised learning technique called artificial hydrocarbon networks (AHN). In literature, this method has been implemented for regression and classification problems [5, 6] because it can handle uncertain and imprecise information typically found in practice, e.g. sales prediction, offering excellent response in modeling [5], forecasting [5, 6], and other fields like control systems [5, 7] and signal processing [8]. In that sense, we aim to determine if artificial hydrocarbon networks are suitable for online sales prediction, providing a comparison between its performance and ten other well-known supervised learning methods.

The rest of the paper is organized as follows: in Sect. 2 we discuss the machine learning approaches for online retail sales prediction. We present our artificial hydrocarbon networks approach for online sales prediction in Sect. 3. We describe our experiments in Sect. 4, and discuss the results in Sect. 5. Finally, we conclude and outline our future work in Sect. 6.

2 Machine Learning Approaches for Online Retail Sales Prediction

A good sales forecast can be a decisive factor in the success of a business. Predict the exact number of sales can make an effective planning of all business processes. We can calculate the number of copies we make, we can make investments taking into account future benefits or we can predict the market value of the company [9].

For this reason, companies devote increasing resources to the construction of models using machine learning, and there are many people researching to make these models more accurate.

Some methods have been widely used in the past, as exponential smoothing and Autoregressive integrated moving average (ARIMA), have been surpassed. Increasingly sophisticated tools that take into account several factors are used. Since many products are subject to seasonality or associated with other variables such as temperature [9]. For example, to take into account the number of cars to be sold in one country would have to make an estimate of the economic situation, an estimate of whether the government will give aid to buy a car, a prediction of the price of gasoline, regardless of whether they will build high-speed railway lines and some other factors.

To make a good number of sales forecasts, in addition to good tools, experienced people able to find the most relevant factors in estimating sales are needed. These people often face very similar scenarios as the products lack an historical record, or databases are stored with irrelevant noise data that must be eliminated. Often databases do not have all values therefore have to reduce or to estimate the results. All models are exposed to some uncertainty as predicted values have variations due to unforeseeable external factors. A revolutionary invention of competition, a disaster at a nuclear plant or a natural disaster likes an earthquake, for example invalidates a forecast.

Game theory, simulation and statistical methods can be used to predict online sales [10]. Game theory methods study the behavior of buyers and other companies competing within a niche product. These models have as input relevant business factors.

Simulation methods are based on supervised machine learning regression models. These models can take into account seasonality as Bayesian model-based classification or Modular Time Series. There are models that do not take into account seasonality of the data as Recurrent Neural Networks or Mean-Reversion. These methods look for patterns or relationship to estimate the output from the inputs. Neural networks and support vector machines are also well-known machine learning techniques used for sales forecasting.

Statistical methods analyze the probability of an event or the repetition of a pattern to estimate future sales. These methods do not analyze the underlying behavior patterns. They are based on certain ranges of confidence interval. Stochastic models are occupied to model randomized processes that are a set of functions that model time series based on a random variable [10].

In this article we used simulation methods for our comparative analysis.

3   Artificial Hydrocarbon Networks Approach for Online Sales Prediction

This section introduces the artificial hydrocarbon networks learning algorithm in order to get an overview of the method employed in this work. In addition, it also describes how this algorithm can be used for online sales prediction.

3.1   Artificial Hydrocarbon Networks

Artificial organic networks (AON) technique is a class of supervised learning algorithms inspired on chemical organic compounds [5]. It aims to package information in modules called molecules (e.g. data patterns), and to organize them in levels of energy. The artificial organic networks technique defines heuristic mechanisms similar to chemical rules involved in natural organic compounds in order to get organized and optimized structures in terms of chemical energy [5, 6]. Some of the characteristics presented in artificial organic networks are [5]: modularity, inheritance, organization and structural stability.

A particularization of this technique is the artificial hydrocarbon networks (AHN) algorithm. It inherits all characteristics and mechanisms from AON and it is inspired on chemical hydrocarbon compounds. Artificial hydrocarbon networks clusters

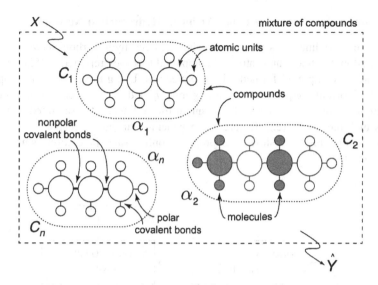

Fig. 1. Graph-model example of an artificial hydrocarbon networks.

information in molecules that only uses two different atomic units: hydrogen and carbon atoms that can be linked with at most one and four other atoms, respectively. In fact, these molecules can join together to form another type of structure so-called compounds, forming nonlinear relationships of clustered information [5, 8]. In a higher level, compounds can also be mixed them up forming a structure called mixture that is a linear combination of compounds. Currently, the artificial hydrocarbon networks algorithm is adequate for modeling issues, prediction, forecasting and classification [6]. An advantage of AHN is that it can deal with uncertain and imprecise data typically found in real applications [5–8].

Figure 1 shows a graph-model representation of artificial hydrocarbon networks. Mathematically, it can be explained as (1). For instance, artificial hydrocarbon networks receive a set of inputs X that is evaluated through n_i molecules that form the ith compound C_i using a set of coefficients H_i regarding to the hydrogen atoms of each compound in the whole structure. Then, artificial hydrocarbon networks compute a set of response outputs $\hat{Y}$ using a linear combination of all compounds weighted by the parameters α_i known as stoichiometric coefficients.

$$\hat{Y} = \sum_i \alpha_i C_i(X, H_i, n_i) \tag{1}$$

To this end, artificial hydrocarbon networks can be trained using the so-called simple AHN-algorithm reported in [5]. That algorithm is a supervised training method that finds the set of all hydrogen values H_i and stoichiometric coefficients α_i, given a training dataset of the form as $\langle X, Y \rangle$ representing multi-categorical inputs X and target outputs Y. Moreover, the simple-AHN algorithm minimizes a loss function such that $\hat{Y}$ approximates Y, using a learning rate coefficient $0 < \eta < 1$ [5].

3.2   Online Sales Prediction Using Artificial Hydrocarbon Networks

We propose an online sales prediction using artificial hydrocarbon networks. In this work, we adopt the linear and saturated compound topology reported in [5, 8] in which there is only a compound formed with n molecules. Using this particular compound, the AHN-algorithm requires the learning rate η and the number of molecules n occupied for training purposes. Thus, an artificial linear and saturated compound receives multiple inputs (e.g. features) and generates an output response (e.g. online sales prediction). Figure 2 shows our proposed online sales prediction using artificial hydrocarbon networks.

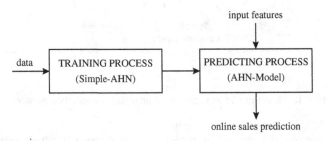

Fig. 2. Proposed online sales prediction using artificial hydrocarbon networks.

As noted in Fig. 2, the online sales data with previous features-target information is first used to train the AHN-model. The training process is computed with the simple-AHN algorithm [5] mentioned before. Once, the AHN-model is obtained it can be used to predict online sales given a set of input features and generating a proper output response.

4   Experiments

In order to compare our proposed online sales prediction model based on artificial hydrocarbon networks, first the proposed AHN-based online sales prediction model was trained and validated. Later on, other well-known learning methods were used to create other online sales prediction models, we presented ten with the best results: cubic-splines (CS), model-trees (MT), random forest (RF), linear regression (LR), quartile random forest (QRF), relaxed lasso (RL), Bayesian regularized neural networks (BN), support vector machines with radial basis function kernel (SVM), least angle regression (LAR), and independent component regression (ICR).

Finally, the AHN-based online sales prediction model was compared against the other ten models. Following, a description of the dataset is presented, then the methodologies for building AHN-based and other learning-based models are explained, and a comparative analysis is discussed lastly.

4.1 Dataset Description

Prediction models were trained and tested using a dataset downloaded from [11]. The data set represents information about consumer products: information about the product features and advertisement campaign. It has 558 attributes and 751 samples. The features, values and name of the fields are coded to maintain data privacy; given data is sensitive information for companies.

The dataset has twelve outputs representing the number of sales for twelve months ahead for a product. The rest of the attributes represent the model inputs. Of these entries, 513 have categorical values are represented by a number. Many are binary type and indicated by a "1" if the product has the feature and "0" otherwise. The other 33 entries correspond to qualitative values. There are two values that are particularly important: Date 1 is the number of days of the post-product launch campaign, and Date 2 is the number of days prior to the product launch campaign.

The dataset had some value NaN (Not a value) type. Some methods may not work with this type of variables so we applied a function that replaces all attribute values missing with the average value of the remaining values.

4.2 Feature Selection

There are two types of methods for feature selection. Filter methods calculate the importance of features without considering the model output; wrapper methods do consider the model output. Wrapper methods are much more laborious and slower as they have to generate several models to calculate the importance of the variables. In general, the filters are much faster but they have problems with the joint variables and give worse results. The wrapper is much slower, at risk of over fitting but give better results.

We applied the function nearZeroVar R that is a filter method of feature selection. The function detects nearZeroVar model those entries that have a unique value, that is, the variance is zero. It also detects those with very few unique values compared to total samples. Finally it detects those features for which the frequency of the most repeated value compared with the second more frequent value is to big. A threshold is set and the features above this threshold are rejected. This method has reduced the number of features from 546 to 163.

After applying the nearZeroVar function, we create a dataset for each of the twelve months. Each dataset contains the input features and one month. We ran the Recursive Feature Selection (RFE) [12] method for each of the twelve datasets, obtaining a new set of input features for each month. RFE method is of type wrapper, it creates several models to consider the best combination. This method generates very good results, and has a relatively fast construction time. On average, we reduced the number of input features in the twelve datasets from 163 to 87.5.

4.3 Methodology and Evaluation

For our online sales prediction comparative analysis, we used Caret Package from R Studio. The training sets were constructed with 70 % of each data set (525 samples) in order to generate the model. The remaining 30 % of the samples (226) were used to test the models.

Each method has several parameters that can be configured. In order to evaluate the models with the best configuration for each method, repeated cross-validation (Repeated CV) was used. Repeated CV created several partitions. Some of them are used for training and others for test. This method allows generating many models with different combination of parameters, obtaining more reliable results. For each of the methods, we applied five times cross-validation with ten partitions. Then we calculated the accuracy of the different configurations of each model as the mean of the fifty models generated. With the best configuration of each model, a new model was created using all the samples of the training set. Subsequently, we used the model to predict test samples.

Evaluation. To assess the accuracy of the model used root-mean squared error (RMSE) metric. This metric is the square root of the average difference between house of the samples and the predicted value for these samples. RMSE is commonly used for regression evaluation, because it is very suitable for measuring the error in numerical predictions for regression methods. The main difference between (mean squared error) MSE and RMSE is that RMSE gives more weight to larger errors.

The RMSE of a model prediction with respect to the estimated variable X_{model} is defined as:

$$RMSE = \sqrt{\frac{\sum_{i=1}^{n}\left(X_{obs,i} - X_{model,i}\right)^2}{n}} \tag{2}$$

where X_{obs} is observed values and X_{model} is modelled values at time/place i.

5 Results and Discussion

We randomly divide the dataset in two subsets: a training set of 525 samples and a testing set of 226 samples for all the experiments.

Then, we proposed 12 AHN-models, one per month predicted in given dataset. Each AHN-model for online sales prediction consisted on an artificial linear and saturated compound [5, 8] with a number of n molecules of the form as in (3); where, CH_k means a molecule of order k, and straight lines represent simple bonds or relationships. In addition, these 12 AHN-models were trained with the simple-AHN algorithm reported in [5] to find suitable values of H. Table 1 summarizes the number of molecules and the learning rate value for each AHN-model. These values were obtained using a cross-validation approach.

$$CH_3 - CH_2 - \cdots - CH_2 - CH_3 \quad \text{with} \quad 2 : CH_3, (n-2) : CH_2 \tag{3}$$

After training, the twelve AHN-models for online sales prediction were validated with the testing data set obtaining 5,828 RMSE in average. Table 2 shows this result and each of the RMSE values computed by each of the twelve AHN-models.

Table 1. Summary of parameters employed for training purposes in AHN-models for online sales prediction.

AHN-Model	Molecules (n)	Learning rate (η)
1	11	0.25
2	17	0.50
3	7	0.04
4	20	0.50
5	5	0.80
6	5	0.60
7	13	0.60
8	17	0.13
9	17	0.50
10	15	0.60
11	9	0.54
12	10	0.50

Table 2. Root-mean square error values obtained from the twelve AHN-models for online sales prediction. The average of these results is also presented.

AHN-Model	RMSE	AHN-Model	RMSE	AHN-Model	RMSE
1	29,641	5	4,258	9	1,608
2	13,046	6	2,689	10	1,274
3	8,603	7	1,833	11	848
4	3,868	8	1,214	12	1,057
		Average	5,828		

It can be seen from Table 2 that the first and second months were the most difficult ones for prediction using artificial hydrocarbon networks. In contrast, the eleventh month was the best accurate model found.

In order to compare the prediction results from artificial hydrocarbon networks, other ten supervised learning models were computed. Figure 3 shows the average RMSE values of each learning models in comparison with the AHN-model. This graph reported that the AHN-model (5,828 RMSE) with cubic-splines (5,870 RMSE), model-trees (5,995 RMSE), Bayesian regularized neural networks (6,323 RMSE) and random forest (6,439 RMSE) are the top five learning model for this online sales prediction case study. Contrasting, support vector machines, least angle regression and independent component regression were positioning at the last of the list with 8,803 RMSE, 8,988 RMSE and 9,310 RMSE, respectively. A complete summary of results is shown in Table 3.

Even though the difference between the RMSE of AHN and CS is small ($5870 - 5828 = 42$), it is very meaningful since the sales of this case study are in the order of thousands of US dollars. This means that, in average, the prediction of AHN is more accurate than predictions from the CS method.

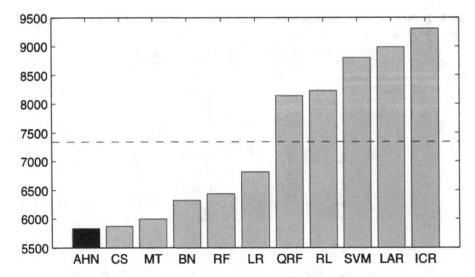

Fig. 3. Summary of results showing the RMSE value obtained with each of the supervised learning methods employed for comparison purposes. AHN reported 5,828 RMSE, cubic-splines (CS), model-trees (MT), Bayesian regularized neural networks (BN) and random forest (RF) are in the top five of the analysis. Independent component regression (ICR) reported 9,310 RMSE positioning at last. Dashed line shows the average value 7,340 RMSE of these results.

6 Conclusions and Future Work

In this paper we presented an online sales prediction using a novel supervised learning technique called artificial hydrocarbon networks. In fact, we compare and analyze the proposed learning model with other ten well-known supervised learning methods in terms of the root-mean squared error.

From the results of the comparative analysis, we conclude that the online sales prediction model based on artificial hydrocarbon networks had the best performance against the other methods. In particular, the proposed model obtained an average value of 5,828 RMSE while the second and third models, i.e. cubic-splines and model-trees, obtained 5,870 and 5,995, respectively. It is remarkable to say that support vector machines, one of the most the used supervised learning models, obtained high RMSE value (8,803) in this comparative analysis due to the fact that this method is better for classification than for regression purposes.

For future work, we are planning to increase the number of metric evaluations for a better comparison. In addition, we are analyzing more applications of this online sales prediction in order to increase the number of analysis tools for online retailing.

Table 3. Root-mean squared error values obtained by the eleven supervised learning models for online sales prediction. The average of these results is also presented. Bold numbers represent the minimum RMSE obtained by a learning model in that specific month.

Method	RMSE Average	1	2	3	4	5	6	7	8	9	10	11	12
AHN	5,828	29,641	13,046	8,603	3,868	4,258	2,689	1,833	**1,214**	1,608	1,274	**848**	1,057
CS	5,870	33,061	**11,608**	8,484	4,118	**3,405**	1,959	1,693	1,418	1,591	1,198	886	1,022
MT	5,995	32,414	12,157	8,401	4,158	4,184	2,352	1,839	1,428	1,742	1,340	870	1,060
BN	6,324	**29,358**	16,580	9,843	4,798	4,786	2,110	1,734	2,072	**1,291**	1,363	885	1,063
RF	6,439	36,310	15,055	**8,342**	**3,690**	4,363	**1,905**	**1,670**	1,332	1,737	**1,085**	869	**907**
LR	6,815	37,773	15,196	8,807	4,171	5,022	2,325	1,840	1,425	1,905	1,298	969	1,046
QRF	8,142	52,114	15,859	9,204	4,803	4,403	2,348	1,869	1,429	2,104	1,360	1,012	1,200
RL	8,228	48,787	19,179	9,444	4,699	5,702	2,422	1,827	1,386	1,903	1,274	1,040	1,077
SVM	8,803	54,395	20,172	8,956	5,405	5,452	2,434	1,908	1,464	1,998	1,286	1,034	1,127
LAR	8,988	54,557	22,676	9,071	5,777	4,955	2,325	1,801	1,422	1,912	1,289	976	1,090
ICR	9,310	55,593	23,851	9,229	5,669	5,602	2,353	1,935	1,603	2,223	1,425	1,054	1,178

References

1. Wu, S.: Forrester Research Online Retail Forecast, 2013 To 2018 (US), Q4 2014 Update, Forrester Forrester Research, Inc., Created January 26, 2015, Updated March 3, 2015, Consulted June 10, 2015 (2015). https://www.forrester.com/Forrester+Research+Online +Retail+Forecast+2013+To+2018+US+Q4+2014+Update/fulltext/-/E-res121011
2. Zeng, V. et al.: China Online Retail Forecast, 2014 to 2019, Forrester Forrester Research, Inc., Created February 4, 2015, Consulted June 10, 2015 (2015). https://www.forrester.com/ China+Online+Retail+Forecast+2014+To+2019/fulltext/-/E-res118544?al=0
3. Asociación Mexicana de Internet (AMIPCI): Estudio Comercio Electrónico en México 2015, Created June 24, 2015, Consulted June 25, 2015 (2015). https://amipci.org.mx/ estudios/comercio_electronico/Estudio_de_Comercio_Electronico_AMIPCI_2015_version_ publica.pdf
4. Levin, J.D.: The Economics of Internet Markets, NBER Working Paper No. 16852 March 2011 JEL No. C78, D4, D44, L10, L14, O33, Presented in Econometric Society World Congress in Shanghai, Consulted June 20, 2015 (2011). http://www.nber.org/papers/ w16852.pdf
5. Ponce, H., Ponce, P., Molina, A.: Artificial Organic Networks: Artificial Intelligence Based on Carbon Networks. Studies in Computational Intelligence, vol. 521. Springer, Switzerland (2014)
6. Ponce, H., Ponce, P.: Artificial organic networks. In: Proceedings of IEEE Conference on Electronics, Robotics, and Automotive Mechanics, pp. 29–34 (2011)
7. Molina, A., Ponce, H., Ponce, P., Tello, G., Ramirez, M.: Artificial hydrocarbon networks fuzzy inference systems for CNC machines position controller. Int. J. Adv. Manuf. Technol. 72(9–12), 1465–1479 (2014)
8. Ponce, H., Ponce, P., Molina, A.: Adaptive noise filtering based on artificial hydrocarbon networks: an application to audio signals. Expert Syst. Appl. 41(14), 6512–6523 (2014)
9. Beheshti-Kashi, S., Karimi, H.R., Thoben, K.D., Lütjen, M., Teucke, M.: A survey on retail sales forecasting and prediction in fashion markets. Syst. Sci. Control Eng. Open Access J. 3 (1), 154–161 (2015)
10. Haghi, H.V., Tafreshi, S.M.: An overview and verification of electricity price forecasting models. In: International Power Engineering Conference, IPEC 2007, pp. 724–729. IEEE, December 2007
11. Kaggle Inc.: Online Product Sales, Data files, Updated May 4th, 2012, Consulted June 20, 2015 (2012). https://www.kaggle.com/c/online-sales/data
12. Granitto, P.M., Furlanello, C., Biasioli, F., Gasperi, F.: Recursive feature elimination with random forest for PTR-MS analysis of agroindustrial products. Chemom. Intell. Lab. Syst. 83(2), 83–90 (2006)

Data-Driven Construction of Local Models for Short-Term Wind Speed Prediction

Joaquín Salas[✉]

Instituto Politécnico Nacional, Mexico City, Mexico
jsalasr@ipn.mx

Abstract. Currently, there is a growing interest in improving the methods applied to the prediction of wind speed. In this document, we propose to combine physically-based decision rules, inferred through a data-driven process, with local regression models. Specifically, quantitative and qualitative analysis of historical records lead us to define a regression structure with a decision tree at the top and local regression models at each leaf. Specifically, our results suggest that this encoding improves the predictions for wind speed for a number of regression schemes, including radial basis neural networks, binary regression trees, support vector regression, adaptive network-based fuzzy inference systems, and bagging trees. A reduction of about 14 % in the RMSE is shown for the latter.

1 Introduction

Currently, there is a growing interest in improving the methods applied to the prediction of wind speed, especially as energy production by means of wind turbines is becoming a valid alternative to fossil fuels [13]. Nonetheless, the subject has attracted wide interest in the past as an important element to assess weather conditions for general activities, such as the air propulsion of merchant ships [22] and enhancements to high-speed trains safety [25]. In our case, our interest is to improve the current one-hour wind speed forecasts to safely fly small Unmanned Aerial Vehicles (UAVs). Wind speed prediction models can be divided into numerical weather prediction [7], artificial intelligence [1] and statistical models. The former are used for predictions over days, weeks, or months ahead, while the latter are used for predictions that are seconds, minutes, or a few hours ahead. Since we are interested in short-term predictions, we focus our attention on the latter type of models.

Wind speed prediction is an important but elusive problem that has attracted considerable attention and has many different facets. To tackle it, researchers have been exploring methods including those based on Neural Networks [2], Support Vector Regression [14], Fuzzy Logic [9], k-nearest neighbors [27], chaotic phase space reconstruction [11], and fractal interpolation [26], with various degrees of success. To a large extent, the complexity of the problem lies in the difficulty to model the physical components involved, to take measurements unobtrusively and with enough resolution, and to compute reliable prediction models quickly enough.

© Springer International Publishing Switzerland 2015
O. Pichardo Lagunas et al. (Eds.): MICAI 2015, Part II, LNAI 9414, pp. 509–519, 2015.
DOI: 10.1007/978-3-319-27101-9_39

In this study, we break down the general prediction problem into local models; each local model defined in terms of temporal periods of cycles observed in historical records. The main contribution of this paper is to show that this data-driven interpretation of the physical model improves the prediction performance of several machine learning strategies. Depending on the applications, researchers have tried to optimize the prediction for the next few seconds [15] (*e.g.*, for wind turbine control), the next minute [17], the next ten minutes [8], or the next few hours (*e.g.*, for power system scheduling), or the next few days [3]. In our method, we calculate the cycles present in the historical measurements and apply this knowledge to further constrain the solution to the problem of predicting wind speed. Specifically, the quantitative and qualitative analysis of the records lead us to divide the data in periods, each one of them defining a regression model for that period. Our evidence suggests that for a several regression techniques including radial basis neural networks, binary regression trees, bagging trees, support vector regression, and adaptive network-based fuzzy inference systems, the encoding of this *prior* knowledge with the use of a decision tree results in improved wind speed predictions.

The rest of this document is organized as follows. In Sect. 2, we describe the wind speed data used in our research qualitatively and quantitatively. The latter serves us as the base upon which we construct the global decision tree structure. Then, in Sect. 3, we show how the incorporation of local models for wind prediction improves performance. In particular, we use the historical records, from January 1, 2007 to May 13, 2014, for *El Batán* Meteorological station (http:// tinyurl.com/elbatansmn) in Querétaro, México. Finally, we conclude and enumerate several possible directions of research.

2   Long-Term Observation of Wind Speed Data

Nowadays, it is possible to acquire considerable amounts of wind speed data. In our case, we asked the Mexican National Weather Service for historical records from *El Batán* meteorological station. *El Batán* dam is located at coordinates 20°29'54"N and 100°24'33"W, about 2 Km away from our UAV's test flight site[1], in the municipality of Corregidora in Querétaro. The data includes the period between January 1, 2007, and May 13, 2014. Measurements include: (1) wind gust direction; (2) wind direction; (3) relative humidity; (4) pressure; (5) cumulative rain; (6) sparse rain; (7) air temperature; (8) wind gust speed; (9) wind speed; and (10) battery voltage. In practice, measurements are recorded every hour with periods without observations that can sometimes last for months, without observations. Frequently, the reported measurements are zero for unusually long periods of time. Figure 1 provides a graphical representation of the observations included in this data set. In total, there are at most 44,031 measurements for each of the variables.

---

[1] Club de Aeromodelismo los Halcones.

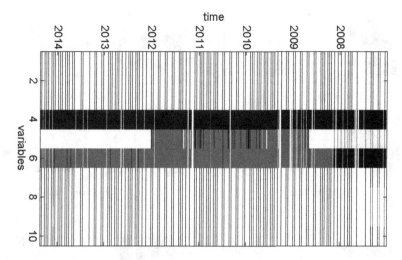

Fig. 1. Observations made at *El Batán* meteorological station from January 1, 2007, to May 13, 2014. The variables observed include: (1) wind gust direction; (2) wind direction; (3) relative humidity; (4) pressure; (5) cumulative rain; (6) sparse rain; (7) air temperature; (8) wind gust speed; (9) wind speed; and (10) battery voltage. In the figure, white means no data, black means data, and gray means zero.

2.1   Qualitative Analysis

Figure 2 illustrates the behavior for some of the observed variables for periods of days and years. There are some interesting features that are worth mentioning. For instance, when observed throughout the years, it seems clear that there are two prevailing wind gust directions 50° or 220°, with a larger variability around the former (Fig. 2 (a)). It is worth noting that by mid-2012 there is a shift in the measurements after a six-month period without observations. At that point, the meteorological station broke down and the direction sensors were not placed in their original positions. Correspondingly, the same prevailing directions can be observed in a 24 h period. The same directions can also be observed for wind direction (Fig. 2 (b)). However, the variability seems to be more spread out. The relative humidity has a seasonal behavior (Fig. 2 (c)) where it is dry in autumn and winter and more humid (above 30 %) during spring and summer. Throughout the day, the period between 10:00am and 3:00pm is dry. Then, after 3:00pm, the relative humidity starts to pick up and has a peak of about 35 % at around 5:00am. In Fig. 2(d) it can be appreciated that the rainy season starts in May and ends in September, with disproportionate peaks. Air temperature is illustrated in Fig. 2(e), it has a smooth and harmonic behavior during the observed period. However, there are some observations in the middle of 2013 that are off the charts. Clearly, the temperature is milder during the fall and winter and rises in the spring and summer, in synchrony with the relative humidity. Throughout the day, as expected, the temperature goes down during the nighttime, picks up as the sun rises and then goes down again after midday. Wind gust, illustrated

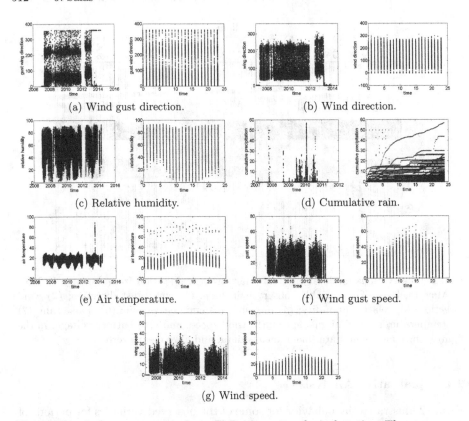

(a) Wind gust direction.

(b) Wind direction.

(c) Relative humidity.

(d) Cumulative rain.

(e) Air temperature.

(f) Wind gust speed.

(g) Wind speed.

Fig. 2. Historical measurements from *El Batán* meteorological station. They are organized by year and by time of day. Please, see text in Sect. 2 for a detailed description of the figure.

in Fig. 2(f), also has a slightly marked seasonal behavior; it has a wide range and daily peaks at around 3:00pm. Finally, in Fig. 2(g), we have wind speed, our variable of interest. It has a mild seasonal harmonic behavior as well. Normally, throughout the day, the wind speed stays below 20 km/h and may reach peaks slightly above 40 km/h between 10:00am and 3:00pm. The figures that lead to this analysis show us that there is an underlying physical model that dictates trends occurring at least during the day and throughout the year. We study this using frequency analysis in the next section.

2.2   Quantitative Analysis

In the context of harmonic phenomena, the classic tool for study is Fourier analysis [18]. The Fourier transform for a discrete signal c_k is given as [5]

$$F(f_j) = \frac{1}{n} \sum_{k=0}^{n-1} c_k \exp\left(-2\pi i f_j t_k\right), \tag{1}$$

where c_k corresponds to observations at equally spaced intervals t_k, for $k = 0, \ldots, n - 1$, $i^2 = -1$, and where f_j is the value of the frequency and it is given by

$$f_j = \frac{j}{t_{n-1} - t_0},$$ (2)

for $j = 0, \ldots, n - 1$. At its end, n corresponds to the number of observations during the period. In Fourier analysis one assumes that the signal represented by c_k repeats before and after the period described. The resulting function F is in general complex, although sometimes it is represented by both its magnitude and phase. The magnitude of F provides some indication about its energy content. In particular, it is very often used to unveil the main frequencies in the signal. On the other hand, the phase provides us with some temporal information about when the periodic behavior has peaks or valleys. This is important in our application as, for instance, it allow us to distinguish periodicity that peaks at a particular hour during the morning or the afternoon, or during particular months in the spring or in autumn. The square of the magnitude of the signal F, also known as the power spectrum, is given by [10]

$$P(f) = |F(f)|^2 = \frac{1}{n} \left\{ \left(\sum_{j=1}^{n} c_j \cos(2\pi f t_j) \right)^2 + \left(\sum_{j=1}^{n} c_j \sin(2\pi f t_j) \right)^2 \right\}.$$ (3)

For a finite set of frequencies, $P(f)$ is also known as the periodogram.

However, there is a fundamental technical difficulty in using the Fourier transform in our problem since, even though the signal is obtained at regular intervals most of the time, there are periods at which there is no signal. In the mid-1970s and early 1980s, the astronomers Lomb [16] and Scargle [21] were facing a similar problem. In their case, the observations for their work had to be stopped during the daytime or on rainy nights. Fundamentally, regular observation involves orthogonality between sines and cosines. This assumption does not hold when observations are missed or when the observations are not equally spaced. For these cases, Lomb and Scargle proposed an approximation for (3) by identifying the shift of phase for which the sines and cosines of a particular frequency are orthogonal. The expression, known as the Lomb-Scargle normalized periodogram, is defined as [19]

$$P(f_k) = \frac{1}{2\sigma^2} \left\{ \frac{\left(\sum_{j=1}^{n} c'_j \cos(2\pi f_k t'_j) \right)^2}{\sum_{j=1}^{n} \cos^2(2\pi f_k t'_j)} + \frac{\left(\sum_{j=1}^{n} c'_j \sin(2\pi f_k t'_j) \right)^2}{\sum_{j=1}^{n} \sin^2(2\pi f_k t'_j)} \right\},$$ (4)

where $t'_j = t_j - \tau$, $c'_j = c_j - \bar{c}$, and $\bar{c}$ and σ^2 are the mean and variance of the data, and are defined as

$$\bar{c} = \frac{1}{n} \sum_{j=1}^{n} c_j \text{ and } \sigma^2 = \frac{1}{n-1} \sum_{j=1}^{n} c'_j{}^2, \tag{5}$$

and τ, the phase shift that makes $P(f_k)$ independent of shifting all the t_j by any constant [19], is defined as

$$\tau(f_k) = \frac{1}{4\pi f_k} \arctan \left(\frac{\sum\limits_{j=1}^{n} \sin{(4\pi f_k t_j)}}{\sum\limits_{j=1}^{n} \cos{(4\pi f_k t_j)}} \right). \tag{6}$$

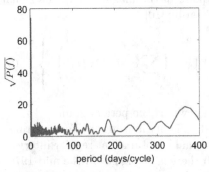

(a) Periodogram in a yearly scale.

(b) We zoom in on the Periodogram in (a) for the high frequencies.

Fig. 3. Wind speed Lomb-Scargle periodogram. For our data, the three largest peaks are located at 1.0, 365.9, and 0.5 days.

The Lomb-Scargle approximation for the wind speed data set is shown in Fig. 3. The three strongest signals are at 24 h ($P(1/24 \text{ hours}) = 74.4^2$), 365.9 days ($P(1/365.9 \text{ days}) = 18.2^2$), and 12 h ($P(1/12 \text{ hours}) = 17.5^2$). Nonetheless, to obtain information about when the peaks and valleys are reached, we need the phase. This can be obtained using an approximation to the discrete Fourier transform, which is given by [10]

$$F(f_k) = F_0(f_k) \sum_{j=0}^{n-1} \left\{ A(f_k)c_j \cos{\left[2\pi f_k t'_j\right]} + iB(f_k)c_j \sin{\left[2\pi f_k t'_j\right]} \right\}, \tag{7}$$

where the value of F_0 for f_k is given by

$$F_0(f_k) = \sqrt{\frac{n}{2}} \exp(-i2\pi f_k(t_f - \tau)), \tag{8}$$

and the coefficients for the harmonic functions are defined as

$$A(f_k) = \left(\sum_{j=1}^{n} \cos^2 \left(2\pi f_k t'_j \right) \right)^{-1/2}, \text{ and } B(f_k) = \left(\sum_{j=1}^{n} \sin^2 \left(2\pi f_k t'_j \right) \right)^{-1/2},$$

(9)

respectively and where $\tau = \tau(f_k)$. Finally, the sinusoid associated with frequency f_p is given by

$$y(t) = 2\sqrt{2} \frac{|F_p|}{N} \cos \left(2\pi f_p t + \phi \right),$$

(10)

where $\phi = Im(F_p)/Re(F_p)$ is the associated phase angle, $|F_p|$ is the magnitude of $F(f_p)$, and N is the number of frequencies resulting out of the Lomb-Scargle analysis.

The previous analysis makes clear the underlying physical model that operates on the wind speed observations. This model explains the fluctuations of the observations in a yearly and daily scale. This evidence will be used to develop a model for wind speed prediction in the next section.

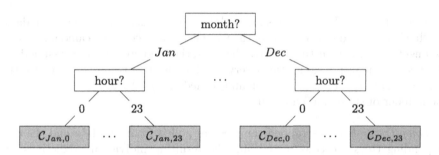

Fig. 4. Decision tree for wind speed prediction (using the notation in [20]). The frequency analysis performed in Sect. 2 suggests us to divide the observations by month of the year and later on by hour of the day. The leaves of the tree label the local regression model used, e.g., $C_{Dec,23}$ stands for the model of the 23th hour for all Decembers.

3   A Data-Driven Model

Here, we describe how we combine the prior information about frequency, that the analysis of historical records provides us, with local regression models. This idea is illustrated in the decision tree in Fig. 4. The quantitative analysis of the data leads us to naturally organize it by month and time of day. To construct the model, we learn for each hour of the day of a particular month of the year a local regression model C_{kj}, for $k \in \{Jan, \ldots, Dec\}$ and $j \in \{0, \ldots, 23\}$. During operation, the particular month of the year, for the particular hour of the day, defines which regression model is used. Nonetheless, we may not have enough data to construct this model. For instance, if we divide 44,031 measurements by 24 hours of one day, times 12 months in a year, the result is about

150 measurements, which may not be enough to construct a robust regression model. Therefore, we restrict ourselves to divide the observations by hour, which represents the strongest cycle detected in our analysis. For the experiments, 70 % of randomly chosen observations were used for training and 30 % of them for testing. The training and test phases were repeated 30 times. Let s_t be the wind speed for time t. The model used for either training and testing was $s_t = f(s_{t-1}, s_{t-2})$. Let $\hat{s}_t$ correspond to the prediction. The error measurement used was the Root Mean Square Error (RMSE). Several methods were used to construct C_{kj}; these included Radial Basis Neural Networks [6], Binary Regression and Bagging Trees [4], Support Vector Regression (SVR) [23], and Adaptive Network-based Fuzzy Inference Systems (ANFIS) [12].

Radial Basis Neural Networks. We used a radial basis network [6] for regression. These networks have two layers. In the first one, there is a radial basis function, which is typically modeled as a Gaussian distribution. In the second one, there is a linear function. We varied the spread of the radial basis function from 0.1 to 5 in intervals of 0.1 and finally settled at a value of 1.0, which gave us the best performance.

Binary Regression Trees. In this method, training finds rules to divide the data, which when applied at each level of the tree effectively reduce the amount of data to consider [4]. Then, at the leaves of the trees, the predicted value corresponds to the mean of the responses for the observed values used for training. We varied the minimum number of parents chosen and settled on 170. In addition, we explored the number of splits and chose 50.

Bagging Trees. B bootstrapped samples are polled from the data and the corresponding trees are constructed [4]. The resulting individual predictions are obtained by consensus. In our dataset, we tried different values of B given comparable results, finally settling on 20.

SVR. The goal is to find a function $f(x)$ which is at most ϵ deviation from the observations y_i of the training data while being as flat as possible [23]. We tried linear, polynomial, and radial basis functions. Interestingly, linear kernels gave the best results.

ANFIS. This method integrates neural networks and fuzzy logic [12]. It may be seen as a generalization of a regression tree. The Fuzzy system represents prior knowledge as a set of constraints reducing effectively the search space. Then, the neural network tunes the parameters. The neurons of an AFIS network can be either membership functions, rules, normalization factors, functions, or outputs. The inference corresponds to fuzzy IF-THEN rules.

The results are shown in Table 1. In it is interesting to note that all regression models provide a similar level of performance. In addition, it is worth pointing out that in all regression models there was a significant improvement in the wind speed prediction. Furthermore, the largest improvement occurred in the case of bagging trees, where we observed a 13.9 % reduction in RMSE. Recently, Troncoso *et al.* [24] presented a study where they compared favorably Classification and Regression Trees (CART) with other soft-computing alternatives, such as neural networks, support vector regression, multilinear regression, and Chi-squared Automatic Interaction Detection. It is noteworthy to observe that when we use the whole historical records our results do not distinguish a clear prime method. Although wind speed is a global concept, local factors including geography and climatology make it hard to compare absolute values. Nonetheless, our results do show a remarkable improvement for a variety of regression techniques, noticeable with a large degree of statistical certainty. In order to promote the comparison of results, we are making our database available upon request.

Table 1. Prediction performance. Several machine learning methods were applied to the wind speed data. Their performance, in terms of the RMSE, was assessed for the cases where the method was applied to the whole set, as it is usual, and when they were applied to a data-driven physically based subsets of the data, as we propose. In all cases, improvements were observed.

Method	Traditional		Stratified		Gain
	μ	σ	μ	σ	
Radial Basis Neural Networks	3.24	0.02	3.09	0.02	4.6 %
Binary Regression Trees	3.27	0.02	3.19	0.03	3.0 %
Bagging Trees	3.32	0.02	2.86	0.02	13.9 %
Support Vector Regression	3.27	0.03	3.06	0.03	6.4 %
Adaptive Network-based Fuzzy Inference Systems	3.23	0.03	3.04	0.02	5.9 %

4 Conclusion

Successful prediction systems make use of good abstractions of the reality as the foundation for satisfactory performance. Data-driven models have found their way in a myriad of applications. Yet, for wind speed prediction, the incorporation of physical rules has shown to be challenging. Based on the analysis of historical records, we have incorporated natural rules governing wind speed periodicity into the prediction models. For the regression schemes tested, which include radial basis neural networks, binary regression trees, bagging trees, support vector regression, and adaptive network-based fuzzy inference systems, the proposed approach produces better predictions. Furthermore, we have shown that for the case of bagging trees the performance has increased by about 14 %.

In the future, we are planning to extend our analysis to other meteorological stations and study the predictive limits for this problem. Overall, these results, and the methodology developed in this paper, may provide to be useful for the safe operation of light weight UAVs.

Acknowledgement. This work was partially supported by the FOMIX GDF-CONACYT under Grant No.189005, IPN-SIP under Grant No. 20150281. We thank Patricia Moreno for her comments to the document and the Facultad de Ingeniería at UAQ for providing a warm environment for the development of this work.

References

1. Ak, R., Fink, O., Zio, E.: Two machine learning approaches for short-term wind speed time-series prediction. IEEE Trans. Neural Networks Learn. Syst. **99**, 1–14 (2015)
2. Ata, R.: Artificial neural networks applications in wind energy systems: a review. Renew. Sustain. Energy Rev. **49**, 534–562 (2015)
3. Barbounis, T., Theocharis, J., Alexiadis, M., Dokopoulos, P.: Long-term wind speed and power forecasting using local recurrent neural network models. IEEE Trans. Energy Convers. **21**(1), 273–284 (2006)
4. Breiman, L., Friedman, J.H., Olshen, R.A., Stone, C.J.: Classification and Regression Trees. CRC Press (1984)
5. Brigham, O.: The Fast Fourier Transform and its Applications. Prentice Hall, Upper Saddle River (1988)
6. Broomhead, D., Lowe, D.: Radial basis functions, multi-variable functional interpolation and adaptive networks. Technical report, Defense Technical Information Center (1988)
7. Cassola, F., Burlando, M.: Wind speed and wind energy forecast through Kalman filtering of numerical weather prediction model output. Appl. Energy **99**, 154–166 (2012)
8. Chiang, C.T., Lu, W.L., Jhuang, H.A.: Extremely short-term wind speed prediction based on RSCMAC. In: Asian Control Conference, pp. 1–6 (2013)
9. Damousis, I., Alexiadis, M., Theocharis, J., Dokopoulos, P.: A fuzzy model for wind speed prediction and power generation in wind parks using spatial correlation. IEEE Trans. Energy Convers. **19**(2), 352–361 (2004)
10. Dilmaghani, S., Henry, I., Soonthornnonda, P., Christensen, E., Henry, R.: Harmonic analysis of environmental time series with missing data or irregular sample spacing. Environ. Sci. Technol. **41**(20), 7030–7038 (2007)
11. Gao, Y., Aoran, X., Zhao, Y., Liu, B., Zhang, L., Dong, L.: Ultra-short-term wind power prediction based on chaos phase space reconstruction and NWP. Int. J. Control Autom. **8**(5), 325–336 (2015)
12. Jang, J.S.R.: ANFIS: adaptive-network-based fuzzy inference system. IEEE Trans. Syst. Man Cybern. **23**(3), 665–685 (1993)
13. Jena, D., Rajendran, S.: A review of estimation of effective wind speed based control of wind turbines. Renew. Sustain. Energy Rev. **43**, 1046–1062 (2015)
14. Jiang, P., Qin, S., Wu, J., Sun, B.: Time series analysis and forecasting for wind speeds using support vector regression coupled with artificial intelligent algorithms. Mathematical Problems in Engineering, pp. 1–14 (2015)
15. Kani, P., Ardehali, M.: Very short-term wind speed prediction: a new artificial neural network-Markov chain model. Energy Convers. Manage. **52**(1), 738–745 (2011)
16. Lomb, N.: Least-squares frequency analysis of unequally spaced data. Astrophys. Space Sci. **39**(2), 447–462 (1976)
17. Nielsen, H.A., Madsen, H., Sørensen, P.: Ultra-short term wind speed forecasting. In: European Wind Energy Conference & Exhibition, pp. 1–6 (2004)

18. Papoulis, A.: The Fourier Integral and its Applications. McGraw-Hill, New York (1962)
19. William H Press. Numerical Recipes: The Art of Scientific Computing. Cambridge University Press, Cambridge (2007)
20. Russell, S., Norvig, P.: Artificial Intelligence: A Modern Approach. Prentice Hall (1995)
21. Scargle, J.: Studies in astronomical time series analysis. II-statistical aspects of spectral analysis of unevenly spaced data. Astrophys. J. **263**, 835–853 (1982)
22. Schenzle, P.: Standarised speed prediction for wind propelled mechant ships: possible technologies and potential performance. In: Symposium on Wind Propulsion of Commercial Ships, pp. 1–16 (1980)
23. Smola, A., Schölkopf, B.: A tutorial on support vector regression. Stat. Comput. **14**(3), 199–222 (2004)
24. Troncoso, A., Salcedo-Sanz, S., Casanova-Mateo, C., Riquelme, J., Prieto, L.: Local models-based regression trees for very short-term wind speed prediction. Renewable Energy **81**, 589–598 (2015)
25. Xiaodong, C., Xiaolei, C.: An algorithm for wind speed prediction for safety of high speed train based on expert system and neural network. Exp. Technol. Manag. **3**, 0–34 (2010)
26. Xiu, C., Wang, T., Tian, M., Li, Y., Cheng, Y.: Short-term prediction method of wind speed series based on fractal interpolation. Chaos, Solitons Fractals **68**, 89–97 (2014)
27. Yesilbudak, M., Sagiroglu, S., Colak, I.: A new approach to very short term wind speed prediction using k-nearest neighbor classification. Energy Convers. Manage. **69**, 77–86 (2013)

A Tool for Learning Dynamic Bayesian Networks for Forecasting

Pablo H. Ibargüengoytia[✉], Alberto Reyes, Inés Romero,
David Pech, Uriel A. García, and Mónica Borunda

Instituto de Investigaciones Eléctricas, Cuernavaca, Morelos, Mexico
{pibar,areyes,uriel.garcia,monica.borunda}@iie.org.mx
{senileon,davidpech_01}@hotmail.com

Abstract. Renewable energy is increasing its participation in power generation in many countries. In Mexico, the strategy is to generate 35 % of electricity from renewable sources by 2024. Currently only 18.3 % of the generated energy is obtained from renewable and clean sources. The integration of renewable energies in the energy market is a challenge due to their high variability, instability and uncertainty. Hence, energy forecast is the required service by the power generators to offer energy with certain degree of confidence. Dynamic Bayesian networks (DBNs) have proved to be an appropriate mechanism for uncertainty and time reasoning; however there is no basic tool that builds DBN using time series for a process. This paper describes the design, construction and tests for a DBNs learning tool. This tool has already been used to construct dynamic models for wind power forecast and in this paper it is used to describe the variation of the dam level caused by rainfall in a hydroelectric power plant.

1 Introduction

This paper deals with Forecast. Forecasting is the process of making statements about events which have not yet been observed. It is by nature, an uncertain process.

One approach to solve problems dealing with uncertainty is with Probabilistic Theory and Statistics. Indeed, by assigning potential events an uncertain probability of occurrence allows to quantify this uncertainty. Bayesian network (BN) is a probabilistic graphical model that models the causal relationships between a set of variables and their conditional dependencies via a directed acyclic graph, where the variables are represented by nodes and the causal dependencies between variables are the arcs connecting nodes. Moreover, Dynamic Bayesian Networks (DBNs) captures temporal dependencies by adding temporal arcs between variables, such that they model sequences of variables. In other words, DBN are directed graphical models of stochastic processes and are widely used in biology, medicine, image processing, data fusion, engineering, gaming, risk analysis and so on. In particular, in the engineering field they have become

© Springer International Publishing Switzerland 2015
O. Pichardo Lagunas et al. (Eds.): MICAI 2015, Part II, LNAI 9414, pp. 520–530, 2015.
DOI: 10.1007/978-3-319-27101-9_40

popular in prediction processes such as weather forecast, power generation prediction [9], failure prediction in power generation systems [7], etc.

This research group has been working on applications of Artificial Intelligence (AI) techniques to problems of the energy world [7–9]. We have utilized probabilistic graphical models, specifically Bayesian networks in the construction of models that represents industrial real problems that requires uncertainty management. Moreover, most of the real energy problems represent a dynamic behavior. As a consequence, an extension of Bayesian networks dealing with time was necessary.

There exist a number of software tools that allows representing and inferring over Dynamic Bayesian Models. However many of them do not support a variety of learning algorithms or do not include auxiliary tools for data processing. In some cases the user interfaces are not very friendly. For instance, the Bayes Net Toolbox (BNT) [1, 10] is an open-source Matlab package for directed graphical models. It supports many kinds of nodes (probability distributions) exact and approximate inference, parameter and structure learning, and static and dynamic models. However it does not count with a friendly user interface nor have auxiliary processing tools. GeNIe [2] is a development environment for building graphical decision-theoretic models. It implements Bayesian graph search, the PC [12] learning algorithm for static models, and different variations to represent the naïve Bayes model. In spite that it has a friendly-user interface, it does not include data preprocessing tools or machine learning algorithms for dynamic models. Elvira [5] does not support dynamic Bayesian learning however it does support a variety of algorithms for static Bayesian models. Perhaps the most complete and recent software tool for Bayesian modelling is Hugin Expert [3]. It allows representing and inferring dynamic Bayesian models and includes several learning algorithms to approximate models from data. It also has a friendly-user interface and many functions for data preprocessing. The weka package [6] is a powerful collection of data processing algorithms including static Bayesian networks learning modules. However, DBN are not included.

This paper describes an integrated machine learning-based software tool for constructing dynamic Bayesians models from data. The tool is called **RB-T**. Its main functions are dynamic Bayesian networks approximation using machine learning tools and configurable processing. The K2 [4] and PC [12] algorithms in **RB-T** are extracted from the Elvira and Hugin APIs to approximate dynamic models using static representation. The data processing functions are averaging, variable filtering, and an automated separation of training or testing data. The tool is tested in a case studio consisting in forecasting the level of a dam based on historic hydrometric data.

This paper is organized as follows. The next section introduces the theoretical base of the learning tool, namely, dynamic Bayesian networks (DBN). Next, Sect. 3 explains the design and construction of the software tool for learning DBN specialized in forecast. A block diagram is illustrated and the functions explained. Section 4 explains the case study conducted with the learning tool. This study concerns the forecast of dam level in hydroelectric power plants.

The DBN learned is depicted and the experiments for validation the dam level forecasting are included. This section also discusses the results of the experiments with emphasis in the DBN learning. Finally, Sect. 5 concludes the paper and directs the future work in this area.

2   Dynamic Bayesian Networks

Bayesian networks (BN) is the appropriate mechanism for representing knowledge and reasoning in applications that require uncertainty [11]. By definition, BN are directed acyclic graphs that provide a compact representation of a probability distribution, where nodes represent propositional variables and arcs probabilistic dependencies. For forecasting operations, the idea is to provide evidence in the nodes corresponding to related variables, and BN calculates a probabilistic forecast of a hypothesis variable. However, BN provides only a static view of the problem. A static BN works on an instant view of the application process. Forecast problems are generally dynamic, i.e., they deal with changes in the variables on time and events.

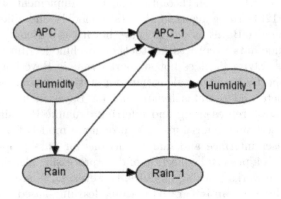

Fig. 1. Example of a transition model learned for the case study in forecasting.

Dynamic Bayesian Networks (DBN) [10] represent temporal process by replicating each variable for every time instant in the temporal range of interest, including dependency relations within and between temporal intervals (time is usually discretized according to fixed temporal intervals). In general, DBNs follow two basic assumptions:

Markovian process, so each variable depends only on variables from the previous and current time steps,
Stationary process, so the structure and parameters of the model remain the same for all time steps.

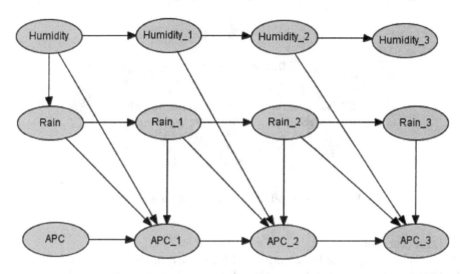

Fig. 2. An unrolled DBN for 3 time slices.

According to these assumptions, the dynamic Bayesian model considered in this project is formed basically by the two-slice temporal Bayes net which defines $P(X_t \mid X_{t-1})$ for all t in the process. This is called the transition model. In this model, there exist relations between variables in the same time slice and other relations between different time slices. For example, in the model of Fig. 1, *Humidity* and *Rain* are related at certain time t, and all variables maintain influence with these same variables at time $t + 1$ for all t. *APC_1* is probabilistically related with itself at previous time, with *Rain* and *Humidity* at previous time, and *Rain* at time $t + 1$.

The complete forecast model is obtained by *unrolling* the transition model in the number of time slices required for forecast. For example, if we define a daily time slice and we need three days in advance, then the DBN is unrolled to complete four slices (input slice and three more slices), as shown in Fig. 2.

An important decision is how to initialize the model. Since the initial time slice is formed by the same variables, and since we assume access to all the values, then the initial slice is only useful for entering the values of variables at time t. Thus, the propagation in the network produces a probability distribution of the forecasted value three days ahead (*APC_3*). This is an important parameter considered in this application, namely the forecast horizon (N). In the network shown in Fig. 2, $N = 3$.

3   A Software Tool for Learning DBN

This **RB-T** dynamic Bayesian networks learning tool has three applications that can be executed separately as shown in Fig. 3:

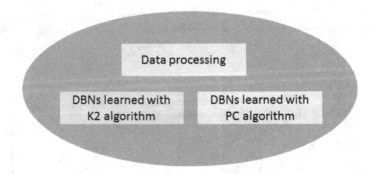

Fig. 3. A general block diagram of the system.

1. Data processing,
2. DBNs learning using PC algorithm [12] included in Hugin package [3]
3. DBNs learning using K2 algorithm [4] included in Elvira package [5].

A general block diagram of the system is shown in Fig. 3. First, the data processing module and next the option to learn the model using PC in Hugin, or K2 in Elvira.

The data processing module produces a specific file format from the original historical data file. It is able to execute four main functions:

Average, used to calculate the average when the time step required is longer than the original data. For example, if data values are every 10 min, and hourly information is required. This function establishes the time slice parameter used in forecasting.

Training and Testing, used when the original data set requires to be separated between data for training the model and data for testing. The parameter is percentage, e.g., 70 % for training and 30 % for testing.

Discretize, used when dealing with continuous value variables. In this version, DBN work only with discrete value variables. This function allows discretizing on equidistant intervals or manual setting of intervals.

Filter, used when only a specific part of the data set is required. For example, when data from daylight is required, filtering from the night data.

All these modules can be used when needed, independently, subject on the original data and the specific experiment needs, or altogether. Additionally, Fig. 3 shows two DBN learning modules. The first module utilizes the PC algorithm of the **Hugin** package. The second module utilizes the K2 algorithm of the **Elvira** package. They were designed for constructing different DBNs for testing them on different applications. Sometimes the PC algorithm is appropriate, while other times, algorithms like K2 or others may be the appropriate.

The main idea of **RB-T** learning tool is the integrated and automatic execution of the learning process, starting with the initial data file and ending with

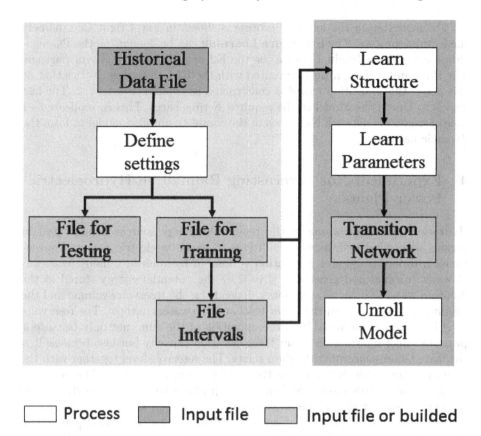

Process ▢   Input file ▣   Input file or builded ▣

Fig. 4. Procedure for the use of the DBN learning tool.

the dynamic model for forecasting. The procedure followed to achieve this learning process is shown in Fig. 4. Initially, an **Historical Data File** is required in text format separated by comma (.csv). It is assumed that the data registers are appropriate, i.e., a historical no gaps in time and obtained with calibrated instruments. Next, **Define Settings** includes the definition of the size of the time slice **T**, the time horizon as the number **N** of time slices ahead to forecast, and the percentage of the original file for testing and training. At this point, both files are defined: a file for training and a file for testing. Recall that these files are already accustomed, i.e., if the original time slice is shorter than **T**, then an average is calculated to obtain the new time slice. The next procedure is the discretization of the continuous variables. The learning tool maintains a default in the number and size of intervals for each variable. However, it allows changing the discretization of each variable. The learning process may finish here, producing a File for Testing (if a percentage assigned), a File for Training and a File Intervals.

The next step in the learning process is shown in Fig. 4 right side, namely the learning process. The **Structure Learning** can be done using the PC algorithm available in Hugin Package, or the K2 algorithm using Elvira package. The **Parameter Learning** is executed with the **EM** algorithm. Notice that at this point, the Transition model is constructed as explained in Sect. 2. The last step is to Unroll the Model to the required N time slices. This is, replicate t+1 slice of transition network N-2 times to the complete unrolled model to form the dynamic network.

4   Experiments for Forecasting Rainfall on Hydroelectric Power Plants

Hydroelectric energy is one of the renewable energy sources mostly used in regions with good hydropower conditions to generate electric power. Conventional hydroelectric power generation is done in hydroelectric dams by means of water turbines and generators driven by the potential energy stored in the dammed water. The generated power depends on the reservoirs volume and the height difference between the water level and the waters outflow. The reservoirs level is an important variable in the operation of the dam, not only because it provides direct information about the generation capacity but also because it is the main factor concerning the dam safety. The reservoir level together with the dam operating policies determine the way of draining the dam. Therefore the prediction of the reservoir level is a crucial problem to obtain a good and safe dam operation but also a complicated task.

The level of the reservoir is affected by different factors directly depending on the water cycle shown in Fig. 5. As it is shown clouds formation come mainly from condensation of sea water evaporation and evapotranspiration from ground, and depending on the atmospheric conditions eventually it will lead to rain, which is one of the important variables determining the reservoir level. On the other hand there is stored water in ice and snow uphill giving rise to a variable stream flow, which will also contribute to the variation of the water dam level. These conditions strongly depend on the meteorological and hydrological characteristics of the location which can be highly steady or highly variable. Moreover, there are some cases where there are interconnected dams and therefore each reservoir level depends on the others. In this case we will consider Grijalva river located in Chiapas, Mexico, with four dams: Angostura, Chicoasén, Malpaso and Peñitas, with a power generation capacity of 3.907 MW. The reservoir levels are discretized in 3 intervals: Minimum Operation Level (NAMinO), Maximum Operation level (NAMO) and Maximum Extraordinary Level (NAME) corresponding in Angostura to 380.0 msnm, 392.50 msnm and 395.0 msnm respectively (msnm stands for meters above sea level).

There are several methods to evaluate the reservoir level. Rainfall-runoff models are the most common based on physical-mathematical models and are classified depending on their methodology: statistical, empirical, conceptual and so on. However in this work we use a novel method based on Artificial Intelligence

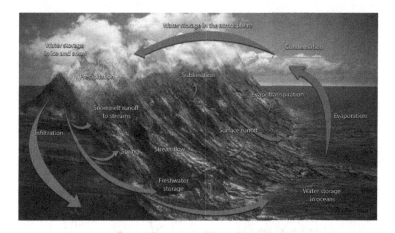

Fig. 5. The water cycle on earth.

techniques. We use our tool for learning DBN to predict the reservoir level. We build a DBN describing the transition probability between levels and with a huge historical measured database (rainfall, stream flow level and relative humidity) obtained from meteorological stations located in the 4 dams, the DBN learns with our tool and is able to predict the level of each reservoir.

Figure 6 shows the dynamic model learned for rain forecasting on the Angostura dam in Grijalva river. The historical data obtained consists in information from 4 hydrologic stations around the dam. Table 1 describes the variables utilized.

Table 1. Set of variables used to construct the model

ID	Description	Units
ACP	Inflow conduit	million cubic meters (Mm^3)
HR	Relative humidity	Percentage (%)
PP	Rainfall	millimeters (mm)
NR	Stream flow level	meters above sea level

The variable names included in Fig. 6 includes the measured variable, e.g., HR for relative humidity, plus a code for the hydrological station, e.g., $AngHR$, plus a script indicating the time stamp corresponding, e.g., $AngHR$-3.

It is worth mentioning that the forecasted variable is the inflow conduit or own contribution basin (ACP) which represents the total amount of water that falls over the basin. With this measurement in million cubic meters, there is a linear relation for calculating the dam level.

The model was learned using historical data from the hydrological stations from 2010 to 2014, and the validation tests uses data from the same stations in

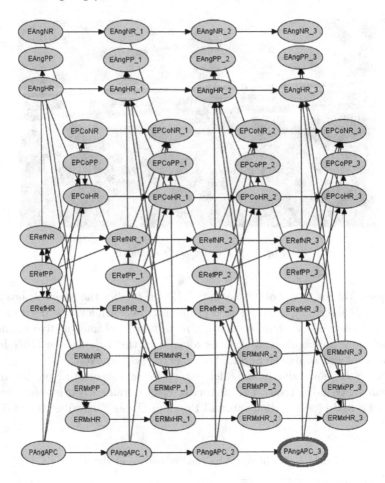

Fig. 6. Dynamic model learned using our tool for rain forecasting.

the beginning of 2015. The time stamp is per day, and the forecast corresponds to three days ahead. Figure 6 shows the resultant learned model. Notice that the model is formed by the variables *HR*, *PP*, *NR* and *APC* from 4 stations and 4 time slices. The forecasted variable is *PAngAPC_3* resulted in red, at the bottom right of Fig. 6.

The forecast process is conducted as follows. First, the current on–line information from all stations is loaded at the input nodes on the left side of Fig. 6. Next, the probability propagation is executed and a posterior probability distribution vector is calculated for *PAngAPC_3* node which is the 3 days ahead forecasted inflow conduit. Finally, a numerical value is calculated using the expected value:

$$PAngAPC\_3 = \sum_n PAngAPC\_3_i P_i$$

where $PAngAPC\_3_i$ is the central value of the interval i, and P_i is the corresponding probability of this interval.

Figure 7 shows a continuous graph with the daily value of the real measured inflow conduit (line with •) and the inflow conduit forecasted value (line with ×). The scale is indicated in the vertical axis in million cubic meters. The horizontal axis represents days. Even when the results look promising, there are some high errors in the forecasting as shown between days 100 and 120. This period corresponds to June to November 2014. The highest error corresponds to September 21–29 2014. These dates correspond to a hurricanes and tropical storms in this part of the country. The problem with the forecast model for meteorological phenomenon is that it requires longer periods of historical data to obtain closer models.

Nevertheless, this paper describes and evaluates the functions and performance of the **RB-T** learning tool for dynamic Bayesian networks.

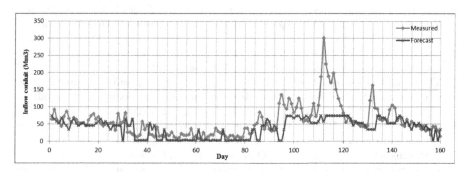

Fig. 7. Results obtained forecasting inflow conduit of the Angostura dam. The line with • represents the real measurement, and the line with × red represents the forecasted value.

5   Conclusions and Future Work

This paper has presented the construction of **RB-T**, a software tool that produces dynamic Bayesian networks that are utilized in forecasting. The forecasting task is specialized on the renewable energy domain. Some important variables to forecast are the wind speed (for wind power), solar radiation (for photovoltaic power), reservoir level (for hydroelectric power) and other energy applications like energy demand forecasting. In all these applications, the models are learned based on raw data that sometimes is noisy and with different time scales.

The **RB-T** software tool integrates the data conditioning, parameter setting and the learning of dynamical models specialized for forecast. **RB-T** utilizes learning algorithms included in the APIs of commercial packages like Hugin or Elvira. **RB-T** has been tested in this paper on the inflow conduit forecast that gives direct information to the reservoir level of Angostura dam, in the Grijalva river in Mexico. To learn the dynamic model, information of different hydrometric stations was recollected. The evaluation of the hydroelectric power forecasting, based on reservoir level forecasting is beyond the scope of this paper and it is straightforward. However, the results look promising for application in all hydroelectric power plants.

Future work is required in the use of this learning tool on different domains and incorporating additional data processing modules. For example, a specialized data cleaning and data discretization with different criteria is required.

References

1. Bayes net toolbox for matlab. Technical report, University of British Columbia, Canada (1997–2002)
2. Genie graphical network interface to smile software package to create decision theoretic models. Technical report, Pittsburgh University, USA (1998)
3. Andersen, S.K., Olesen, K.G., Jensen, F.V., Jensen, F.: Hugin: a shell for building Bayesian belief universes for expert systems. In: Proceedings of the Eleventh Joint Conference on Artificial Intelligence, IJCAI, 20–25 August 1989, Detroit, Michigan, USA, pp. 1080–1085 (1989)
4. Cooper, G.F., Herskovits, E.: A Bayesian method for the induction of probabilistic networks from data. Mach. Learn. 9(4), 309–348 (1992)
5. The Elvira Consortium: Elvira: An environment for creating and using probabilistic graphical models. In: Proceedings of the First European Workshop on Probabilistic graphical models (PGM 2002), pp. 1–11, Cuenca, Spain (2002)
6. Hall, M., Frank, E., Holmes, G., Pfahringer, B., Reutemann, P., Witten, I.H.: The WEKA data mining software: an update. SIGKDD Explor. 11(1), 10–18 (2009)
7. Ibargüengoytia, P.H., Reyes, A.: On-line diagnosis of a power generation process using probabilistic models. In: 16th International Conference on Intelligent Systems Application to Power Systems, ISAP 2011, Hersonissos, Crete Greece. IEEE PES (2011)
8. Ibargüengoytia, P.H., Reyes, A., Romero, I., Pech, D., García, U.: Evaluating probabilistic graphical models for forecasting. In: International Conference on Intelligent Systems Application to Power Systems, ISAP 2015, Porto, Portugal. IEEE PES (2015)
9. Ibargüengoytia, P.H., Reyes, A., Romero-Leon, I., Pech, D., García, U.A., Sucar, L.E., Morales, E.F.: Wind power forecasting using dynamic Bayesian models. In: Gelbukh, A., Espinoza, F.C., Galicia-Haro, S.N. (eds.) MICAI 2014, Part II. LNCS, vol. 8857, pp. 184–197. Springer, Heidelberg (2014)
10. Murphy, K.P.: Dynamic Bayesian networks: representation, inference and learning. Ph.D. thesis, University of California, Berkeley, CA, USA (2002)
11. Pearl, J.: Probabilistic Reasoning in Intelligent Systems: Networks of Plausible Inference. Morgan Kaufmann, San Francisco (1988)
12. Spirtes, P., Glymour, C., Sheines, R.: Causation, Prediction and Search. MIT Press, Cambridge (2000)

Intelligent Applications

More Accurate Inference of User Profiles in Online Social Networks

Raïssa Yapan Dougnon[1], Philippe Fournier-Viger[1(✉)], Jerry Chun-Wei Lin[2], and Roger Nkambou[3]

[1] Department of Computer Science, Université de Moncton, Moncton, Canada
{eyd2562,philippe.fournier-viger}@umoncton.ca
[2] School of Computer Science and Technology,
Harbin Institute of Technology Shenzhen Graduate School, Shenzhen, China
jerrylin@ieee.org
[3] Department of Computer Science, Université du Quebec à Montréal,
Montreal, Canada
nkambou.roger@uqam.ca

Abstract. Algorithms for social network user profiling suffer from one or more of the following limitations: (1) assuming that the full social graph is available for training, (2) not exploiting the rich information that is available in social networks such as group memberships and likes, (3) treating numeric attributes as nominal attributes, and (4) not assessing the certainty of its predictions. In this paper, we address these challenges by proposing an improved algorithm named PGPI+ (Partial Graph Profile Inference+). PGPI+ accurately infers user profiles under the constraint of a partial social graph using rich information about users (e.g. group memberships, views and likes), handles nominal and numeric attributes, and assesses the certainty of predictions. An experimental evaluation with more than 30,000 user profiles from the Facebook and Pokec social networks shows that PGPI+ predicts user profiles with considerably more accuracy and by accessing a smaller part of the social graph than five state-of-the-art algorithms.

Keywords: Social networks · Inference · User profiles · Partial graph

1 Introduction

Online social networks have become extremely popular. Various types of social networks are used such as friendship networks (e.g. Facebook), professional networks (e.g. ResearchGate) and interest-based networks (e.g. Flickr). An important problem for ad targeting on social networks is that users often disclose few information publicly [1,10]. To address this issue, an important sub-field of social network mining is now interested in developing algorithms to infer detailed user profiles using publicly disclosed information. Various approaches have been used to solve this problem such as relational Naïve Bayes classifiers [12], label propagation [9,11], majority voting [4], linear regression [10], Latent-Dirichlet Allocation [2] and community detection [13]. It was shown that these approaches can

© Springer International Publishing Switzerland 2015
O. Pichardo Lagunas et al. (Eds.): MICAI 2015, Part II, LNAI 9414, pp. 533–546, 2015.
DOI: 10.1007/978-3-319-27101-9_41

accurately predict hidden attributes of user profiles in many cases. However, all these approaches suffer from at least two of the following four limitations.

1. **Assuming a full social graph.** Many approaches assume that the full social graph is available for training (e.g. [9]). However, in real-life, it is generally unavailable or may be very costly to obtain or update [2,6]. A few approaches do not assume a full social graph such as majority-voting [4]. However, they do not let the user control the trade-off between the number of nodes accessed and prediction accuracy, which may lead to low accuracy.
2. **Not using rich information.** Several algorithms do not consider the rich information that is available on social networks. For example, several algorithms consider links between users and user attributes but do not consider other information such as group memberships, "likes" and "views" that are available on some social networks [1,4,9,11–13].
3. **Not handling numeric attributes.** Many approaches treat numeric attributes (e.g. age) as nominal attributes [1,4], which may decrease inference accuracy. Others are designed to handle numeric attributes but requires the full social graph, which is often unpractical [5,9,10,13].
4. **Not assessing certainty.** Few approaches assess the certainty of their predictions. But this information is essential to determine if a prediction is reliable and actions should be taken based on the prediction. For example, if there is a low certainty that a user profile attribute is correctly inferred, it may be better to not use this attribute for ad targeting, rather than showing an ad that is targeted to a different audience [3].

To address limitations 1 and 2, the PGPI algorithm (Partial Graph Profile Inference) was recently proposed [6]. PGPI lets the user select how many nodes of the social graph can be accessed to infer a user profile, and can use not only information about friendship links and profiles but also about group memberships, likes and views, when available. In this paper, we present an extended version of PGPI named PGPI+ to also address limitations 3 and 4. Contributions are threefold. First, we design a new procedure for predicting values of numeric attributes. Second, we introduce a mechanism to assess the certainty of predictions for both nominal and numeric attributes. Third, we introduce four optimizations that considerably improve the overall prediction accuracy of PGPI.

We report results from an extensive empirical evaluation against PGPI and four other state-of-the-art algorithms, for 30,000 user profiles from the Facebook and Pokec social networks. Results show that the proposed PGPI+ algorithm can provide a considerably higher accuracy for both numeric and nominal attributes while accessing a much smaller number of nodes from the social graph. Moreover, results show that the calculated certainty well assesses the reliability of predictions. Moreover, an interesting result is that profile attributes such as status (student/professor) and gender can be predicted with more than 95 % accuracy using PGPI+.

The rest of this paper is organized as follows. Sections 2, 3, 4, 5 and 6 respectively presents the related work, the problem definition, the proposed algorithm, the experimental evaluation and the conclusion.

2   Related Work

We review recent work on social network user profile inference. Davis Jr. et al. [4] inferred locations of Twitter users by performing a majority vote over the locations of directly connected users. A major limitation of this approach is that a single attribute is considered. Jurgens [9] predicted locations of Twitter/Foursquare users using a *label propagation* approach. However, it is an iterative algorithm that requires the full social graph since it propagates known labels to unlabeled nodes through links between nodes. Li et al. [11] proposed an iterative algorithm to deduce LinkedIn user profiles based on relation types. This algorithm also requires a large training set to discover relation types.

Mislove [13] applied community detection on more than 60k user profiles with friendship links, and then inferred user profiles based on similarity of members from the same community. Lindamood et al. [12] applied a Naïve Bayes classifier on 167k Facebook profiles with friendship links, and concluded that if links or attributes are erased, accuracy of the approach can greatly decrease. This study highlights the challenges of performing accurate predictions using few data. Recently, Blenn et al. [1] utilized bird flocking, association rule mining and statistical analysis to infer user profiles in a dataset of 3 millions Hyves.nl users. However, all these work assume that a large training set is available for training and they only use profile information and social links to perform predictions.

Chaabane et al. [2] inferred Facebook user profiles using Latent Dirichlet Allocation (LDA) and majority voting. The approach extracts a probabilistic model from music interests and additional information provided from Wikipedia. But it requires a large training set, which was difficult and time-consuming to obtain [2]. Kosinski et al. [10] also utilized information about user preferences to infer Facebook user profiles. Kosinski et al. applied Singular Value Decomposition to a huge matrix of users/likes and then used regression to perform prediction. A limitation of this work is that it does not utilize information about links between users and requires a very large training dataset.

He et al. [7] proposed an approach consisting of building a Bayesian network based on the full social graph to then predict user attribute values. The approach considers similarity between user profiles and links between users to perform predictions, and was applied to data collected from LiveJournal. Recently, Dong et al. [5] used graphical-models to predict the age and gender of users. Their study was performed with 1 billion phone and SMS data and 7M user profiles. Chaudhari [3] also used graphical models to infer user profiles. The approach has shown high accuracy on datasets of more than 1M users from the Twitter and Pokec social networks. A limitation of these approaches however, it that they assume a large training set for training. Furthermore, they only consider user attributes and links but not additional information such as likes, views and group membership.

Some of the above approaches infer numeric attributes, either by treating them as nominal attributes [1,2,4], or by using specific inference procedures. However, these latter require a large training set [5,9,10,13].

Besides, current approaches generally do not assess the certainty of predictions. But this information is essential to determine if a prediction is reliable, and actions should be taken based on this prediction. To our knowledge, only Chaudhari [3] provides this information. However, this approach is designed to use the full social graph.

3   Problem Definition

The problem of user profiling is commonly defined as follows [1,3,9,11–13].

Definition 1 (social graph). A *social graph* $\mathcal{G}$ is a quadruplet $\mathcal{G} = \{N, L, V, A\}$. N is the set of nodes in $\mathcal{G}$. $L \subseteq N \times N$ is a binary relation representing the links (edges) between nodes. Let be m attributes to describe users of the social network such that $V = \{V_1, V_2, ...V_m\}$ contains for each attribute i, the set of possible attribute values V_i. Finally, $A = \{A_1, A_2, ...A_m\}$ contains for each attribute i a relation assigning an attribute value to nodes, that is $A_i \subseteq N \times V_i$.

Example 1. Let be a social graph with three nodes $N = \{Tom, Amy, Lea\}$ and friendship links $L = \{(Tom, Lea), (Lea, Tom), (Lea, Amy), (Amy, Lea)\}$. Consider two attributes *gender* and *status*, respectively called attribute 1 and 2 to describe users. The set of possible attribute values for gender and status are respectively $V_1 = \{male, female\}$ and $V_2 = \{professor, student\}$. The relations assigning attributes values to nodes are $A_1 = \{(Tom, male), (Amy, female), (Lea, female)\}$ and $A_2 = \{(Tom, student), (Amy, student), (Lea, professor)\}$.

Definition 2 (Problem of inferring user profiles in a social graph). The problem of inferring the user profile of a node $n \in N$ in a social graph $\mathcal{G}$ is to guess the attribute values of n using the other information provided in $\mathcal{G}$.

The problem definition can be extended to consider additional information from social networks such as Facebook (views, likes and group memberships).

Definition 3 (extended social graph). An *extended social graph* $\mathcal{E}$ is a tuple $\mathcal{E} = \{N, L, V, A, G, NG, P, PG, LP, VP\}$ where N, L, V, A are defined as previously. G is a set of groups that a user can be a member of. The relation $NG \subseteq N \times G$ indicates the membership of users to groups. P is a set of publications such as pictures, texts, videos that are posted in groups. PG is a relation $PG \subseteq P \times G$, which associates a publication to the group(s) where it was posted. LP is a relation $LP \subseteq N \times P$ indicating publication(s) liked by each user (e.g. "likes" on Facebook). VP is a relation $VP \subseteq N \times P$ indicating publication(s) viewed by each user (e.g. "views" on Facebook), such that $LP \subseteq VP$.

Example 2. Let be two groups $G = \{book\_club, music\_lovers\}$ such that $NG = \{(Tom, book\_club), (Lea, book\_club), (Amy, music\_lovers)\}$. Let be two publications $P = \{picture1, picture2\}$ published in the groups $PG = \{(picture1, book\_club), (picture2, music\_lovers)\}$. The publications viewed by users are $VP = \{(Tom, picture1), (Lea, picture1), (Amy, picture2)\}$ while the publications liked by users are $LP = \{(Tom, picture1), (Amy, picture2)\}$.

Definition 4 (Problem of inferring user profiles in an extended social graph). The problem of inferring the user profile of a node $n \in N$ in an extended social graph $\mathcal{E}$ is to guess the attribute values of n using the information in $\mathcal{E}$.

But the above definitions assume that the full social graph may be used to perform predictions. The problem of inferring user profiles using a limited amount of information is defined as follows [6].

Definition 5 (Problem of inferring user profiles using a partial (extended) social graph). Let $maxFacts \in \mathbf{N}^+$ be a parameter set by the user. The problem of inferring the user profile of a node $n \in N$ using a partial (extended) social graph $\mathcal{E}$ is to accurately predict the attribute values of n by accessing no more than $maxFacts$ facts from the social graph. A *fact* is a node, group or publication from N, G or P (excluding n).

The above definition can be extended for numeric attributes. For those attributes, instead of aiming at predicting an exact attribute value, the goal is to predict a value that is as close as possible to the real value. Moreover, in this paper, we also extend the problem to consider the certainty of predictions. In this setting, a prediction algorithm must assign a *certainty value* in the [0,1] interval to each predicted value, such that a high certainty value indicates that a prediction is likely to be correct.

4   The Proposed PGPI+ Algorithm

We next present the proposed PGPI+ algorithm. Subsect. 4.1 briefly introduces PGPI. Then, Subsects. 4.2, 4.3 and 4.4 respectively present optimizations to improve its prediction accuracy and coverage, and how it is extended to handle numerical attributes and assess the certainty of predictions.

4.1   The PGPI Algorithm

The PGPI algorithm [6] is a lazy algorithm designed to perform predictions under the constraint of a partial social graph, where at most $maxFacts$ facts from the social graph can be accessed to make a prediction. PGPI (Fig. 1) takes as parameter a node n_i, an attribute k to be predicted, the $maxFacts$ parameter, a parameter named $maxDistance$, and an (extended) social graph $\mathcal{E}$. PGPI outputs a predicted value v for attribute k of node n_i. To predict the value of an attribute k, PGPI relies on a map M. This map stores pairs of the form

(v, f), where v is a possible value v for attribute k, and f is positive real number called the *weight* of v. PGPI automatically calculates the weights by applying two procedures named PGPI-G and PGPI-N. These latter respectively update weights by considering the (1) views, likes and group memberships of n_i, and (2) its friendship links. After applying these procedures, PGPI returns the value v associated to the highest weight in M as the prediction. In PGPI, half of the $maxFacts$ facts that can be used to make a prediction are used by PGPI-G and the other half by PGPI-N. If globally the $maxFacts$ limit is reached, PGPI does not perform a prediction. PGPI-N or PGPI-G can be deactivated. If PGPI-N is deactivated, only views, likes and group memberships are considered to make a prediction. If PGPI-G is deactivated, only friendship links are considered. In the following, we respectively refer to these versions of PGPI as PGPI-N and PGPI-G (and as PGPI-N+/PGPI-G+ for PGPI+).

PGPI-N works as follows. To predict an attribute value of a node n_i, it explores the neighborhood of n_i restricted by the parameter $maxDistance$ using a breadth-first search. It first initializes a queue Q and pushes n_i in the queue. Then, while Q is not empty and the number of accessed facts is less than $maxFacts$, the first node n_j in Q is popped. Then, $F_{i,j} = W_{i,j}/dist(n_i, n_j)$ is calculated. $W_{i,j} = C_{i,j}/C_i$, where $C_{i,j}$ is the number of attribute values common to n_i and n_j, and C_i is the number of known attribute values for node n_i. $dist(x, y)$ is the number of edges in the shortest path between n_i and n_j. Then, $F_{i,j}$ is added to the weight of the attribute value of n_j for attribute k, in map M. Then, if $dist(x, y) \leq maxDistance$, each unvisited node n_h linked to n_j is pushed in Q and marked as visited. PGPI-G is similar to PGPI-N. It is also a lazy algorithm. But it uses a majority voting approach to update weights based on group and publication information (views and likes). Due to space limitation, we do not describe it. The reader may refer to [6] for more details.

4.2   Optimizations to Improve Accuracy and Coverage

In PGPI+, we redefine the formula $F_{i,j}$ used by PGPI-N by adding three optimizations. The new formula is $F_{i,j} = W_{i,j} \times (T_{i,j} + 1)/newdist(n_i, n_j) \times R$. The first optimization is to add the term $T_{i,j} + 1$, where $T_{i,j}$ is the number of common friends between n_i and n_j, divided by the number of friends of n_i. This term is added to consider that two persons having common friends (forming a triad) are more likely to have similar attribute values. The constant 1 is used so that if n_i and n_j have no common friends, $F_{i,j}$ is not zero.

The second optimization is based on the observation that the term $dist(n_i, n_j)$ makes $F_{i,j}$ decrease too rapidly. Thus, nodes that are not immediate neighbors but were still close in the social graph had a negligible influence on their respective profile inference. To address this issue, $dist(n_i, n_j)$ is replaced by $newdist(n_i, n_j) = 3 - (0.2 \times dist(n_i, n_j))$, where it is assumed that $maxDistance < 15$. It was empirically found that this formula provides higher accuracy.

The third optimization is based on the observation that PGPI-G had too much influence on predictions compared to PGPI-N. To address this issue, we multiply the weights calculated using the formula $F_{i,j}$ by a new constant R. This

---

Algorithm 1. The PGPI algorithm

---

input : n_i: a node, k: the attribute to be predicted, $maxFacts$: a user-defined threshold, $\mathcal{E}$: an extended social graph

output: the predicted attribute value v

1 $M = \{(v, 0) | v \in V_k\}$;
2 // Apply PGPI-G
3 // ...
4 // Apply PGPI-N
5 Initialize a queue Q and add n_i to Q;
6 **while** Q is not empty and $|accessedFacts| < maxFacts$ **do**
7    $\quad$ $n_j = Q.pop()$;
8    $\quad$ $F_{i,j} \leftarrow W_{i,j}/dist(n_i, n_j)$;
9    $\quad$ Update (v, f) as $(v, f + F_{i,j})$ in M, where $(n_j, v) \in A_k$;
10   $\quad$ **if** $dist(n_i, n_j) \leq maxDistance$ **then for each** node $n_h \neq n_i$ such that $(n_h, n_j) \in L$ and n_h is unvisited, push n_h in Q and mark n_h as visited ;
11 **end**
12 **return** a value v such that $(v, z) \in M \wedge \nexists(v', z') \in M | z' > z$;

---

thus increases the influence of PGPI-N+ on the choice of predicted values. In our experiments, we have found that setting R to 10 provides the best accuracy.

Furthermore, a fourth optimization is integrated in the main procedure of PGPI+. It is based on the observation that PGPI does not make a prediction for up to 50 % of users when $maxFacts$ is set to a small value [6]. The reason is that PGPI does not make a prediction when it reaches the $maxFacts$ limit. However, it may have collected enough information to make an accurate prediction. In PGPI+, a prediction is always performed. This optimization was shown to greatly increase the number of predictions.

4.3 Extension to Handle Numerical Attributes

The PGPI algorithm is designed to handle nominal attributes. In PGPI+, we performed the following modifications to handle numeric attributes. First, we modified how the predicted value is chosen. Recall that the value predicted by PGPI for nominal attributes is the one having the highest weight in M (line 12). However, for numeric attribute, this approach provides poor accuracy because few users have exactly the same attribute value. For example, for the attribute "weight", few users may have the same weight, although they may have similar weights. To address this issue, PGPI+ calculates the predicted values for numeric attributes as the weighed sum of all values in M.

Second, we adapted the weighted sum so that it ignores outliers because if unusually large values are in M, the weighted sum provides inaccurate predictions. For example, if a young user has friendship links to a few 20 years old friends but also a link to his 90 years old grandmother, the prediction may be inaccurate. Our solution to this problem is to ignore values in M that have a weight more than one standard deviation away from the mean. In our experiment, it greatly improves prediction accuracy for numeric attributes.

Third, we change how $W_{i,j}$ is calculated. Recall that in PGPI, $W_{i,j} = C_{i,j}/C_i$, where $C_{i,j}$ is the number of attribute values common to n_i and n_j, and C_i is the number of known attribute values for node n_i. This definition does not work well for numeric attributes because numeric attributes rarely have the same value. To consider that numeric values may not be equal but still be close, $C_{i,j}$ is redefined as follows in PGPI+. The value $C_{i,j}$ is the number of values common to n_i and n_j for nominal attributes, plus a value $CN_{i,j,k}$ for each numeric attribute k. The value $CN_{i,j,k}$ is calculated as $(v_i - v_j)/\alpha_k$ if $(v_i - v_j) < \alpha_k$, and is otherwise 0, where α_k is a user-defined constant. Because $CN_{i,j,k}$ is a value in [0,1], numeric attributes may not have more influence than nominal attributes on $W_{i,j}$.

4.4   Extension to Evaluate the Certainty of Predictions

PGPI+ also extends PGPI with the capability of calculating a certainty value $CV(v)$ for each predicted value v. For numeric attributes, calculating the certainty value of a predicted value v requires to find a way to assess how "accurate" the weighted sum for calculating v is. Intuitively, we can expect it to be accurate if (1) the amount of information taken into account by the weighted sum is large, and (2) if values considered in the weighted sum are close to each other. These ideas are captured in our approach by using the relative standard error. Let $E_M = \{v_1, v_2, ...v_m\}$ be the set of values in the map M that were used to calculate the weighted sum. The amount of information used by the weighted sum is measured as the number of updates made by PGPI-N+/PGPI-G+ to the map M, denoted as *updates*. The relative standard error is defined as $RSE(v) = stdev(E_M)/(\sqrt{updates} \times avg(E_M))$. The RSE is a value in the [0,1] interval that assesses how close the average of the sample might be to the average of the population. Because we want a certainty value rather than an error value, we calculate the certainty value of v as $CV(v) = 1 - RSE(v)$. A drawback of the RSE is however that it is sensible to outliers. To address this issue, we ignore values that are more than one standard deviation away from the mean to when calculating $CV(v)$.

For nominal attributes, calculating the certainty value of a predicted value v is done differently. Our idea is to evaluate how likely the weight of value v in M is to be as large at it is, compared to other weights in M. To estimate this, we use a simulation-based approach where larger is defined in terms of standard deviations from the mean. Let $F_M = \{f_1, f_2, ...f_m\}$ be the weights of values in the map M, and $f_{M,v}$ be the weight of v in map M. We initialize a value $count = 0$ and perform 1,000 simulations. During the j-th simulation, we create a map B, and perform *updates* random updates to B. At the end of the j-th simulation, we increase the *count* variable by 1 if $(f_{B,v} - avg(F_B))/stdev(F_B) \geq (f_{M,v} - avg(F_M))/stdev(F_M)$. After the 1,000 simulations, the certainty value is calculated as $CV(v) = count/1000$, which gives a value in the [0,1] interval.

5   Experimental Evaluation

We compared the accuracy of the proposed PGPI+, PGPI-N+ and PGPI-G+ algorithms with the original PGPI, PGPI-N and PGPI-G algorithms and four additional state-of-the-art algorithms for predicting attribute values of nodes in a social network. The three first are Naïve Bayes classifiers [8]. Naïve Bayes (NB) infer user profiles strictly based on correlation between attribute values. Relational Naïve Bayes (RNB) consider the probability of having friends with specific attribute values. Collective Naïve Bayes (CNB) combines NB and RNB. To be able to compare NB, RNB and CNB with the proposed algorithms, we have adapted them to work with a partial graph. This is done by training them with $maxFacts$ users chosen randomly instead of the full social graph. The last algorithm is label propagation (LP) [9]. Because LP requires the full social graph, its results are only used as a baseline. Each algorithm was tuned with optimal parameter values.

Datasets. Two datasets are used. The first one is 11,247 user profiles collected from Facebook in 2005 [14]. Each user is described according to seven attributes: a student/faculty status flag, gender, major, second major/minor (if applicable), dorm/house, year, and high school, where year is a numerical attribute. The second dataset is 20,000 user profiles from the Pokec social network obtained at https://snap.stanford.edu/data/. It contains 17 attributes, including three numeric attributes: age, weight and height. Because both datasets do not contain information about groups, and this information is needed by PGPI-G and PGPI, synthetic data about groups was generated using the generator proposed in [6], using the same parameters. This latter generator is designed to generate group having characteristics similar to real-life groups.

Accuracy for nominal attributes w.r.t number of facts. We first ran all algorithms while varying the $maxFacts$ parameter to assess the influence of the number of accessed facts on accuracy for nominal attributes. The *accuracy* for nominal attributes is defined as the number of correctly predicted values, divided by the number of prediction opportunities. Figure 1 shows the overall results for the Facebook and Pokec datasets. Note that PGPI algorithms are not shown in these tables due to lack of space. It can be observed that PGPI+/PGPI-N+/PGPI-G+ provides the best results. For example, on Facebook, PGPI+ and PGPI-G+ provide the best results when 66 to 700 facts are accessed, and for less than 66 facts, PGPI-N+ provides the best results followed by PGPI+. No results are provided for PGPI-N+ for more than 306/6 facts on Facebook/Pokec because PGPI-N+ relies solely on links between nodes to perform predictions and the datasets do not contains enough links. It is also interesting to note that PGPI-N+ only uses real data (contrarily to PGPI+/PGPI-G+) and still performs better than all other algorithms. The algorithm providing the worst results is LP (not shown in the figure). LP provides an accuracy of 43.2 %/47.31 % on Facebook/Pokec. This is not good considering that LP uses the full social graph of more than 10,000 nodes. For the family of Naïve Bayes algorithms, NB has the best overall accuracy. It can be further observed that the accuracy of PGPI+

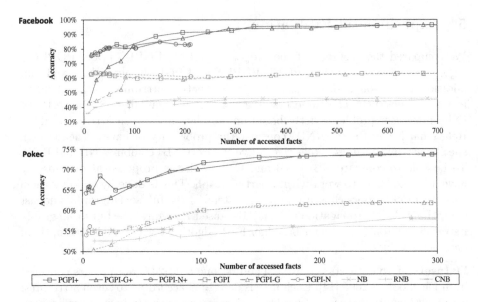

Fig. 1. Accuracy w.r.t. number of accessed facts for nominal attributes

algorithm is up to 34 % higher than PGPI, which shows that proposed optimizations have a major influence on accuracy.

Best results for each nominal attribute. We also analyzed accuracy for each nominal attribute separately. The best results in terms of accuracy for each attribute and algorithm for Facebook and Pokec are respectively shown in Tables 1 and 2. The last row of each table indicates the number of accessed facts to obtain these results. The best accuracy was in general achieved by PGPI+ algorithms for all attributes.

Table 1. Best accuracy results for nominal attributes on Facebook

Attribute	PGPI+	PGPI-N+	PGPI-G+	NB	RNB	CNB	LP
status	92.0 %	92.6 %	**93.0 %**	88.0 %	80.2 %	88.0 %	83.0 %
gender	**96.1 %**	84.7 %	95.8 %	51.1 %	57.7 %	47.3 %	50.4 %
major	**33.8 %**	30.4 %	32.8 %	16.6 %	15.0 %	9.0 %	16.7 %
minor	76.0 %	76.4 %	**76.6 %**	74.4 %	74.2 %	74.0 %	56.3 %
residence	**64.6 %**	62.4 %	64.4 %	55.6 %	55.0 %	54.8 %	49.1 %
school	7.4 %	**16.8 %**	7.0 %	10.6 %	9.8 %	10.6 %	10.1 %
$|facts|$	482	226	431	189	580	189	10K

Best results for each numeric attribute. We also compared the best accuracy of PGPI/PGPI+ algorithms for numeric attributes on Pokec/Facebook in

Table 2. Best accuracy results for nominal attributes on Pokec

Attribute	PGPI+	PGPI-N+	PGPI-G+	NB	RNB	CNB	LP
Gender	95.60 %	61.40 %	**95.77 %**	52.80 %	53.80 %	53.60 %	49.20 %
English	**76.35 %**	63.79 %	76.00 %	69.74 %	69.74 %	69.74 %	65.40 %
French	**87.46 %**	84.48 %	87.42 %	86.91 %	85.60 %	86.87 %	67.15 %
German	62.39 %	54.31 %	**62.85 %**	47.83 %	48.12 %	47.83 %	50.00 %
Italian	94.87 %	94.25 %	94.85 %	94.65 %	95.38 %	**95.41 %**	85.75 %
Spanish	**95.15 %**	94.54 %	95.14 %	94.38 %	95.08 %	94.29 %	80.52 %
Smoker	65.21 %	62.34 %	**65.42 %**	63.43 %	63.43 %	63.12 %	60.19 %
Drink	**71.65 %**	63.36 %	71.47 %	70.41 %	70.41 %	70.41 %	49.16 %
Marital status	**76.57 %**	70.86 %	76.40 %	76.11 %	76.02 %	76.07 %	69.92 %
Hip-hop	**86.51 %**	82.20 %	86.47 %	86.01 %	85.83 %	85.93 %	61.82 %
Rap	69.33 %	63.78 %	**69.52 %**	69.08 %	69.35 %	69.35 %	45.78 %
Rock	77.93 %	73.80 %	**78.09 %**	76.33 %	74.93 %	74.93 %	53.69 %
Disco	58.40 %	52.50 %	**58.56 %**	50.07 %	53.18 %	53.46 %	47.28 %
Metal	**86.19 %**	83.52 %	86.15 %	84.75 %	84.61 %	84.61 %	63.79 %
Region	18.60 %	10.20 %	**18.71 %**	6.20 %	6.20 %	6.20 %	10.00 %
$|facts|$	334	6	347	375	378	278	10k

terms of average error and standard deviation of predicted values from the real values. Results (Table 3) indicates that PGPI+ performs the best on overall. The other algorithms could not be compared for numeric attributes because they are designed for nominal attributes. We attempted to compare with the algorithm of Kosinski [10]. However, linear regression failed using a partial social graph for training.

Table 3. Average error and standard deviation for numerical attributes

Algorithm	Year	Age	Weight	Height
PGPI+	0.95 (0.85)	2.94 (4.55)	**9.83 (10.32)**	**7.70 (11.75)**
PGPI-N+	0.68 **(0.72)**	3.92 (4.56)	14.60 (12.56)	10.32 (12.55)
PGPI-G+	0.99 (0.89)	2.89 **(4.45)**	9.83 (10.37)	7.71 (11.76)
PGPI	0.46 (0.93)	2.55 (4.80)	11.67 (11.53)	8.75 (12.43)
PGPI-N	0.46 (0.87)	4.35 (5.11)	17.28 (15.61)	14.0 (36.52)
PGPI-G	**0.39** (0.93)	**2.20** (4.78)	10.75 (10.86)	8.35 (12.45)

Assessment of certainty values. We also assessed certainty values calculated by PGPI+. Figure 2 shows the best accuracy obtained for numerical attributes "year" and "age" for PGPI-N+. Each line represents the accuracy of predictions having at least a given certainty value. It can be seen, that a high certainty value

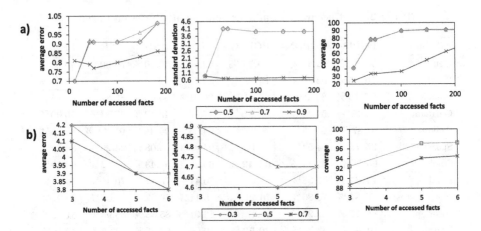

Fig. 2. Average error, standard deviation and coverage w.r.t. certainty for attributes (a) year and (b) age

generally means a low average error, standard deviation and coverage (percentage of predictions made), as expected. Results of PGPI+/PGPI-G+ are similar and not shown due to lack of space. For nominal attributes, the accuracy of predictions made by PGPI-N+/PGPI+/PGPI-G+ having a certainty no less than 0 and no less than 0.7 are respectively 59%/59%/61% and 91%/91%/93% on Facebook, which also shows that the proposed certainty assessment is a good indicator of accuracy.

Best results using the full social graph. We also compared the accuracy of the algorithms using the full social graph. The best accuracy obtained for each algorithm on the Facebook and Pokec datasets is shown in Table 4. It can be observed that the proposed PGPI+ algorithms provide an accuracy that is considerably higher than the accuracy of the compared algorithms, even when using the full social graph.

Table 4. Best accuracy for nominal attributes using the full social graph

Algorithm	Facebook	Pokec	Algorithm	Facebook	Pokec
PGPI+	**96.6**	73.8	PGPI-G	62.8	56.2
PGPI-N+	96.4	**73.9**	NB	48.67	57.48
PGPI-G+	84.9	65.9	RNB	50.11	56.37
PGPI	63.8	62.0	CNB	50.11	56.40
PGPI-N	63.8	62.1	LP	48.03	47.31

6   Conclusion

We proposed an improved algorithm named PGPI+ for user profiling in online social networks under the constraint of a partial social graph and using rich information. PGPI+ extends the PGPI algorithm with new optimizations to improve its prediction accuracy and coverage, to handle numerical attributes, and assess the certainty of predictions. An experimental evaluation with more than 30,000 user profiles from the Facebook and Pokec social networks shows that PGPI+ predicts user profiles with considerably more accuracy and by accessing a smaller part of the social graph than five state-of-the-art algorithms. Moreover, an interesting result is that profile attributes such as status (student/professor) and gender can be predicted with more than 95 % accuracy using PGPI+.

References

1. Blenn, N., Doerr, C., Shadravan, N., Van Mieghem, P.: How much do your friends know about you? Reconstructing private information from the friendship graph. In: Proceedings of the Fifth Workshop on Social Network Systems, pp. 1–6. ACM (2012)
2. Chaabane, A., Acs, G., Kaafar, M.A.: You are what you like! Information leakage through users interests. In: Proceedings of the 19th Annual Network and Distributed System Security Symposium. The Internet Society (2012)
3. Chaudhari, G., Avadhanula, V., Sarawagi, S.: A few good predictions: selective node labeling in a social network. In: Proceedings of the 7th ACM International Conference on Web Search and Data Mining, pp. 353–362. ACM (2014)
4. Davis Jr., C.A., et al.: Inferring the location of twitter messages based on user relationships. Trans. GIS 15(6), 735–751 (2011)
5. Dong, Y., Yang, Y., Tang, J., Yang, Y., Chawla, V.N.: Inferring user demographics and social strategies in mobile social networks. In: Proceedings of the 20th ACM International Conference on Knowledge Discovery and Data Mining, pp. 15–24. ACM (2014)
6. Dougnon, R.Y., Fournier-Viger, P., Nkambou, R.: Inferring user profiles in online social networks using a partial social graph. In: Barbosa, D., Milios, E. (eds.) Canadian AI 2015. LNCS(LNAI), vol. 9091, pp. 84–99. Springer, Heidelberg (2015)
7. He, J., Chu, W.W., Liu, Z.V.: Inferring privacy information from social networks. In: Mehrotra, S., Zeng, D.D., Chen, H., Thuraisingham, B., Wang, F.-Y. (eds.) ISI 2006. LNCS, vol. 3975, pp. 154–165. Springer, Heidelberg (2006)
8. Heatherly, R., Kantarcioglu, M., Thuraisingham, B.: Preventing private information inference attacks on social networks. IEEE Trans. Knowl. Data Eng. 25(8), 1849–1862 (2013)
9. Jurgens, D.: Thats what friends are for: inferring location in online social media platforms based on social relationships. In: Proceedings of the 7th International AAAI Conference on Weblogs and Social Media, pp 273–282. AAAI Press (2013)
10. Kosinski, M., Stillwell, D., Graepel, T.: Private traits and attributes are predictable from digital records of human behavior. Natl. Acad. Sci. 110(15), 5802–5805 (2013)
11. Li, R., Wang, C., Chang, K.C.C.: User profiling in an ego network: co-profiling attributes and relationships. In: Proceedings of the 23rd International Conference on World Wide Web, pp. 819–830. ACM (2014)

12. Lindamood, J., Heatherly, R., Kantarcioglu, M., Thuraisingham, B.: Inferring private information using social network data. In: Proceedings of the 18th International Conference on World Wide Web, pp. 1145–1146. ACM (2009)
13. Mislove, A., Viswanath, B., Gummadi, K.P., Druschel, P.: You are who you know: inferring user profiles in online social networks. In: Proceedings of the 3rd ACM International Conference on Web Search and Data Mining, pp. 251–260. ACM (2010)
14. Traud, A.L., Mucha, P.J., Porter, M.A.: Social structure of Facebook networks. Phys. A Stat. Mech. Appl. **391**(16), 4165–4180 (2012)

Credit Scoring Model for Payroll Issuers: A Real Case

José Fuentes-Cabrera[1] and Hugo Pérez-Vicente[2]([⊠])

[1] FES-Acatlán, National Autonomous University of Mexico, Av. Alcanfores, s/n, Col. Santa Cruz Acatlán, 53150 Naucalpan, State of Mexico, Mexico
[2] Center of Top Management in Engineering and Technology (CADIT), Anahuac University, Av. Universidad Anáhuac 46, Col. Lomas Anáhuac, 52786 Huixquilucan, State of Mexico, Mexico
hugo.perez@anahuac.mx

Abstract. In this paper we present the development of a credit score model for payroll issuers based on a credit scoring methodology. Typically, in the Mexican banking system, it is common to provide and administer payroll service for companies via third parties (outsourcing). This service allows employees to get payroll loans of which periodic payment is retained automatically by the creditor. However, if their relationship with the company is lost, the payment is omitted incresing the risk of default. Addressing the problem described, a statistical model was built to predict whether a payroll issuer will churn in the next six months, this allows the decision maker to determine the appropriate business retention actions in order to avoid future payment loan losses. Results showed that the developed model facilitates a practical interpretation based on scoring system and showed stability when it was implemented.

Keywords: Credit scoring · Logistic regression · Churn analysis · Data mining

1 Introduction

In the Mexican banking system, payroll loans are one of the most profitable businesses for credit issuers. This particular loan is given to those customers who receive their salary payment on a payroll account. The customer signs a contract giving permission to the bank to retain the corresponding amount (monthly, weekly, semimonthly, etc.) that pays for the credit. At this phase, the client's credit worthiness has been evaluated as well as his credit payment capacity (avoiding over-indebtedness), however, a potential risk can occur and may have a significant impact on the delinquency rates: churn of payroll issuers. If an issuer stops paying the payroll, every credit anchored to that issuer will default regardless of the clients credit quality.

The levels of financial education (good practices) in Mexico makes difficult to collect, even when the responsibility of paying is entirely on the customer side. If delinquency goes up, it will derive on several negative consequences, for example:

© Springer International Publishing Switzerland 2015
O. Pichardo Lagunas et al. (Eds.): MICAI 2015, Part II, LNAI 9414, pp. 547–559, 2015.
DOI: 10.1007/978-3-319-27101-9_42

- increase of regulatory credit reserves,
- increase of collections costs,
- deterioration of the relationship with the customers.

The aim of this paper is to provide an analytical tool that contribute to solve this specific problem. There are many reasons for a payroll issuer (company) to end its commercial relationship with a bank, some of them are listed below:

- bad service (operational issues) regarding payroll payments,
- company bankruptcy,
- asset migration to another institution.

On the one hand, the company relationship with the bank is managed by the wholesale banking, on the other hand, payroll loans are intended for individuals (retail banking). This difference in viewpoints creates a divergence of strategic purposes. Considering that this is an important problem to solve, we formulate two questions: (1) How can we to anticipate a possible churn of a payroll issuer? and (2) What actions should be triggered once the possible churn is detected?. To answer the first question, we will use the Credit Scoring Methodology to determine a stochastic model using issuer's transactional variables that allow us to infer whether an issuer will churn in the following months. For the second question, once the model is complete we will suggest a set of operative strategies to avoid churn risk and at the same time strengthen the bank's relationships with both customers and payroll issuers. The data used in this study was obtained from a real transactional data system from a Mexican bank.

The paper is organized as follows. We first present a brief literature review on credit scoring models. The next section provides the methodology for building the credit scoring models, results and business strategies. Finally, conclusions are presented and discussed.

2   Literature Review

2.1   Building Models

Analytical models are a statistical tool that provide scientific support to risk management in retail banking. As in Siddiqi [9], risk managers are challenged to produce solutions that do not only meet the criteria for creditworthiness but also keep the transactional costs low and lower the response time for applicants.

With the technological progress and the availability of analytical software solutions, additional to data processing tools via ETL (ExtractTransform-Load), the internal development of credit risk models grew in such a way that the inclusion of analytical techniques in decision making became more common. Classical analytical techniques to determine the risk regarding the credit of customers include logistic regression, discriminant analysis, neural networks and decision trees. Some other techniques compete as of late, seen in [3] where the use of new algorithms are proposed as in the support vector machines and least squares support vector machines.

Chen [4] mentions that alternative techniques have been used in order to improve the accuracy of classic modeling such as the difficulty to capture non-linear relationships/interactions among variables. Other efforts have focused on genetic algorithms which are more sophisticated models that attempt to improve the precision of existing models compared to artificial neural networks, logistic regression and decision trees [6].

Once the modeling technique is defined, it is possible to determine the advantages and disadvantages of this approach. Mester [5] proposed that building scoring models is faster, cheaper and more objective than "Expert" credit analysis. To assign a qualification dramatically reduces the time required to approve a credit line. Allen [2] states that the current process of loan approval averages 12 hours and a half when in the past it could take up to two weeks. This provides a substantial competitive advantage for institutions that depend on the quality of information of the acquired risk.

Additionally, scoring models do not represent a significant cost when compared to the size of the managed portfolios and also this cost is further reduced when the models are developed internally. Another underlying benefit is the intrinsic objectivity since these models are built on scientific methods, and techniques.

2.2   Credit Scoring Models

Credit scoring has as a concept many definitions in the scientific literature. We use the definition by [7] that consider it as the assessment of the risk associated to the lending to an organization or a consumer (an individual). Decision models and their underlying assumptions select for example, who will get the credit and also assess the risk associated with lending to that particular consumer. An introduction to this topic is presented in [11].

Typically, credit scoring is useful for banks and financial institutions. In fact, some reviews about these models and applications are shown in [1,7]. An important point argued in these works is that it is crucial to address the gap between academic and practical applications of credit scoring because most researchers lack real-world data sets. In that respect, we consider the main contribution in this work using a real case from a Mexican Bank in the context of payroll issuers. We think that currently credit scorecard practices are still popular in banking institutions.

As we mentioned in the literature review section, Logistic Regression models is one classic technique for credit scoring and so it is relevant to follow the model building process suggested in [10] as well as getting acquainted with the software used in that case. In addition, and for confidentiality reasons we omitted the identification of the data source and so, we only used these data for academic purposes.

3   Methodology

This section explains the process followed for constructing the credit scoring model. First, we had to build the database, then we proceeded to develop a data analysis: we ran a multicollineariaty analysis in order to select the variable involved in our study. Finally, we proceeded with the modelling exercise.

3.1   Data Description

The available data were collected in October 2014 as part of a transactional system from a Mexican bank and they consist of 19 tables, each one corresponding to a monthly summary for every issuer containing three variables:

- payroll amount (in US dollars),
- number of issued payroll payments, and
- number of distinct payroll payment dates.

Given the limitations of the available data regarding a timeline, we considered six months for observation as well as six months for performance. We organized 52 variables regarding observation for eight different time periods and then we overlapped each monthly anchor, in this way, we treated every single record as an input vector, thus, obtaining a simple random sample of 20,000 vectors in order to get the final representative dataset.

The variables dataset was obtained with upon the following algorithm:

```
%MACRO VAR;
  DATA VAR;
    SET FINAL2;
      ARRAY AM(6) M_1-M_6;
      ARRAY AN(6) N_1-N_6;
      ARRAY AF(6) F_1-F_6;
      %DO K=3 %TO 6;
        %MACRO MED(VARI);
        V_MED_&VARI._&K.=MEDIAN(OF &VARI._1-&VARI._&K.);
        %MEND;
        %MED(M);
        %MED(N);
        %MED(F);
        %MACRO AVG(VARI);
        V_AVG_&VARI._&K.=MEAN(OF &VARI._1-&VARI._&K.);
        %MEND;
        %AVG(M);
        %AVG(N);
        %AVG(F);
        %MACRO N_INC(VARI);
        V_INC_&VARI._&K.=0;
            DO I=1 TO &K.-1;
            IF A&VARI.(I+1)>A&VARI.(I) THEN V_INC_&VARI._&K.+1;
            END;
        %MEND;
        %N_INC(M);
```

```
%N_INC(N);
%N_INC(F);
%MACRO N_DEC(VARI);
V_DEC_&VARI._&K.=0;
    DO I=1 TO &K.-1;
    IF A&VARI.(I+1)<A&VARI.(I) THEN V_DEC_&VARI._&K.+1;
    END;
%MEND;
%N_DEC(M);
%N_DEC(N);
%N_DEC(F);
%MACRO RACHA(VARI);
V_RACHA_&VARI._&K.=0;
  AUX=0;
    DO I=1 TO &K.-1;
    IF A&VARI.(I+1)^=. AND A&VARI.(I)^=. THEN
    DO;
      AUX+1;
        V_RACHA_&VARI._&K.=MAX(V_RACHA_&VARI._&K.,AUX);
    END;
    ELSE
      AUX=0;
    END;
%MEND;
%RACHA(M);
%END;
DROP M_1-M_6 N_1-N_6 F_1-F_6 I AUX; RUN;
%MEND; %VAR;
PROC SURVEYSELECT DATA=VAR METHOD=SRS N=20000 OUT=VAR;RUN;
```

The macro takes the data table FINAL2 in order to obtain the final variables data table VAR. The FINAL2 data table contains the overlapped monthly anchors and it also includes the variables described below:

- M_1-M_6 payroll amount for last 6 months,
- N_1-N_6 number of issued payroll payments for last 6 months,
- F_1-F_6 number of distinct payroll payment dates,
- target variable.

Where "1" means current month and "6" means 5 months prior. All variables are measured at the interval level except the target variable which was measured at the nominal level. The sample data was partitioned at 70:30 that is 70 % for training and 30 % for validation sample.

In order to meet business requirements the target variable was defined as follows:

- Bad: an issuer that makes absolutely no payment within a month for all of its customers twice or more times in the performance period,
- Good: the complementary set.

The good/bad ratio has an 11 % of bad issuers. In Table 1 we show the description for the summarized variable where "n" goes from 3 to 6 months. After an exploratory data analysis, we note that no missing values were detected and the percentile revision was consistent with business behavior. Additionally, variables did fall within a normal distribution according to a Kolmogorov-Smirnov Test. Data mining softwares used were SAS Enterprise Guide 4.3 for data analysis and SAS Enterprise Miner 6.2 for modelling.

Table 1. List of variables in data set

Variable description	Variable name	Role
Issuer ID	ID	ID
Distinct monthly average payroll payment dates in the last n months	V_AVG_F_n	Input
Monthly payroll payment amount average in the last n months	V_AVG_M_n	Input
Average issued payroll payments in the last n months	V_AVG_N_n	Input
Number of decreases in monthly distinct payroll payment dates in the last n months	V_DEC_F_n	Input
Number of decreases in monthly payroll payment amount in the last n months	V_DEC_M_n	Input
Number of decreases in monthly issued payroll payment in the last n months	V_DEC_N_n	Input
Number of increases in monthly distinct payroll payment dates in the last n months	V_INC_F_n	Input
Number of increases in monthly payroll payment amount in the last n months	V_INC_M_n	Input
Number of increases in monthly issued payroll payment in the last n months	V_INC_N_n	Input
Median of distinct payroll payment dates in the last n months	V_MEC_F_n	Input
Median of payroll payment amount in the last n months	V_MED_M_n	Input
Median of monthly issued payroll payment in the last n months	V_MED_N_n	Input
Maximum consecutive payroll payment in the last n months	V_RACHA_M_n	Input

3.2 Multicollinearity Analysis

In order to minimize any possible multicollinearity among variables, we performed the SAS PROC VARCLUS procedure. As specified in [8] the VARCLUS procedure divides a set of numeric variables into disjoint or hierarchical clusters. This association is a linear combination of the variables in the cluster. In this way, 14 final input variables are obtained through the minimum $1 - R^2$ ratio selection within each cluster. We selected 14 clusters or variables (see Table 2) which represent each cluster that explains 90 % of the variance.

Table 2. Results after PROC VARCLUS procedure

Number of clusters	Total variation explained by clusters	Proportion of variation explained the clusters	Minimum proportion explained by a cluster	Maximum second eigenvalue in a cluster	Minimum R-squared for a variable	Maximum $1 - R^2$ ratio for a variable
1	15.358	0.295	0.295	10.152	0.001	1
2	25.075	0.482	0.377	6.598	0.010	0.995
3	28.461	0.547	0.482	6.586	0.124	0.919
4	31.384	0.604	0.486	6.586	0.124	0.919
5	34.195	0.658	0.582	6.586	0.286	0.817
6	36.268	0.698	0.620	6.586	0.286	0.817
7	42.839	0.824	0.653	2.138	0.588	0.534
8	44.181	0.850	0.770	2.138	0.669	0.438
9	44.921	0.864	0.805	2.138	0.707	0.444
10	45.298	0.871	0.819	2.138	0.724	0.444
11	45.693	0.879	0.820	2.138	0.724	0.444
12	46.048	0.886	0.827	2.138	0.785	0.444
13	46.524	0.895	0.846	2.138	0.785	0.369
14	**46.832**	**0.901**	**0.849**	**2.138**	**0.785**	**0.381**
15	48.969	0.942	0.866	0.438	0.785	0.381
16	49.208	0.946	0.875	0.438	0.785	0.381
17	49.587	0.954	0.878	0.310	0.844	0.381
18	49.816	0.958	0.878	0.310	0.844	0.369
19	50.125	0.964	0.878	0.239	0.844	0.369
20	50.356	0.968	0.879	0.232	0.853	0.363
21	50.574	0.973	0.918	0.164	0.918	0.233

3.3 Data Modelling

Before starting the modelling phase, a cluster analysis was performed but we did not find any interesting explanation in the business sense so we decided not to include these results in this paper. Initial steps for modelling process consist in to transform each input variable into its WOE (Weight Of Evidence) as presented in [9]. This step will organize the order of the variables according to its risk weight/factor facilitating the translation into scorecard for the final user to read. The scorecard points are easy to understand for business management teams in order to trigger better practices. The variable strength is given by its IV (Information Value). The rule of thumb for interpreting this number is provided in [9]. We suggest to choose the variables with IV greater or equal to 0.1, nevertheless, we decided to continue with the 14 variables because the use of overpredictive variables is subject to business understanding. The variable V_RACHA_M_5 is very important from a business perspective, and that is why the variable will be used in the present model. In Table 3 we show results for the process of transformation and also we show the Kolmogorov-Smirnov statistic or KS test that measures the distance between the distribution functions of the two distributions.

Table 3. Results for variable selection

Variable	Bins	KS	IV
V_DEC_F_5	4	10.486	0.064
V_DEC_F_3	2	14.861	0.089
V_INC_M_6	4	12.834	0.097
V_INC_M_3	3	10.793	0.101
V_AVG_F_4	5	14.448	0.107
V_INC_M_4	4	13.832	0.115
V_INC_F_3	2	16.134	0.116
V_INC_N_5	4	13.089	0.118
V_INC_N_3	3	11.826	0.127
V_INC_F_5	4	16.683	0.154
V_DEC_N_5	4	20.342	0.229
V_DEC_N_3	3	22.150	0.242
V_MED_N_4	8	23.821	0.256
V_RACHA_M_5	2	32.603	0.789

In credit scoring, we can apply a logistic regression model in order to perform the final scorecard transformation based on the estimated parameters for the model. Four different variable significance techniques were tested (Table 4). In addition, we calculated the main indexes that will be useful to choose an adequate model (see Table 4).

The Receiver Operating Characteristic (ROC) curves show that all models have a good predictive power. Indeed almost every single index is tied across to the models. However, the backward technique was chosen because of its parsimony (see Fig. 1).

Table 4. Values for indeces performance

Model	ROC	Gini index	KS index	Missclassification rate
None	0.75	0.51	0.39	0.10
Backward	0.75	0.51	0.39	0.10
Forward	0.75	0.50	0.39	0.10
Stepwise	0.75	0.50	0.39	0.10

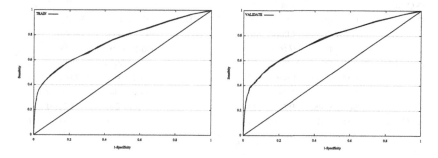

Fig. 1. ROC chart for training and validation sample.

3.4 Scorecard Transformation

Once obtained the model parameters for each input variable, we developed the process of scaling probability to get the scorecard points for each attribute. This scale is arbitrary and depends on each analyst's best fit for his/her own users. The credit scoring technique uses a odds base scaling. To do so, we calculated the factor and the offset. The factor is calculated according to the formula:

$$Factor = \frac{PDO}{\ln 2} \tag{1}$$

where PDO stands for Points to Double the Odds. For example, if we want that every 40 points the odds will double then the result factor is 57.70780164. The Offset is calculated with the following equation:

$$offset = score - factor * \ln(odds) \tag{2}$$

where $score$ represents the fix point by the reference odds. For example, in the case of the $odds$ of 4 at 600, we have:

$$offset = 600 - 57.70780164 * \ln(4) = 520 .$$

The final scorecards point transformation is given by the following formula:

$$points = (-WOE * \beta + \frac{\alpha}{n}) * factor + \frac{offset}{n} \tag{3}$$

Table 5. Scoring table

Variable	Rule	Points	Variable	Rule	Points
V_INC_F_3	001.$LOW - 0.0000$	22	V_DEC_N_3	001.$LOW - 0.0000$	14
	002.$0.0000 \leq HIGH$	14		002.$0.0000 \leq 1.0000$	19
V_INC_F_5	001.$LOW - 0.0000$	24		003.$1.0000 \leq HIGH$	22
	002.$0.0000 \leq 1.0000$	21	V_DEC_N_5	001.$LOW - 0.0000$	7
	003.$1.0000 \leq 2.0000$	14		002.$0.0000 \leq 1.0000$	14
	004.$2.0000 \leq HIGH$	4		003.$1.0000 \leq 2.0000$	20
V_INC_M_4	001.$LOW - 0.0000$	25		004.$2.0000 \leq HIGH$	24
	002.$0.0000 \leq 1.0000$	20	V_MED_N_4	001.$LOW - 12.0000$	-6
	003.$1.0000 \leq 2.0000$	15		002.$12.0000 \leq 24.0000$	13
	004.$2.0000 \leq HIGH$	7		003.$24.0000 \leq 40.5000$	17
V_INC_N_5	001.$LOW - 0.0000$	24		004.$40.5000 \leq 65.0000$	24
	002.$0.0000 \leq 1.0000$	22		005.$65.0000 \leq 109.0000$	25
	003.$1.0000 \leq 2.0000$	17		006.$109.0000 \leq 197.0000$	26
	004.$2.0000 \leq HIGH$	11		007.$197.0000 \leq 478.5000$	28
V_RACHA_M_5	001.$LOW - 3.0000$	-32		008.$478.5000 \leq HIGH$	31
	002.$3.0000 \leq HIGH$	28			

where α is the regression intercept, β is the variable coefficient in the regression equation and n is the number of characteristics (variables). Once the formula is applied, the final scorecard is obtained, see Table 5.

This scorecard allows an assignment of a risk qualification for each issuer.

3.5 Results

The final scale for the model was built with a PDO of 20, and the score goes from 20 to 200. The following figures show the score distribution, the cumulative distribution functions (good/bads), the odds ratio distribution and the separation rate for bads/goods issuers, respectively. See Figs. 2, 3 and 4.

Uniformity and consistency, smooth distribution, increasing rate event odds with exponential distribution and adequate separation of good and bad dis-tri-bu-tions is observed.

3.6 Business Strategy

Once the model was developed, the probabilistic selection of riskier issuers by decision makers becomes a straightforward process so it reduces the use of ma-te-ri-al and human resources for predicting the probability of churn, and consequently a low delinquency rate. Therefore, we answer the second question above (What actions should be triggered once the possible churn is detected?) with the following business actions to confront issuers churn risk:

- Implement preventive data collection strategies as well as financial education for the customers when issuer presents high churn probability (less than 50 points).

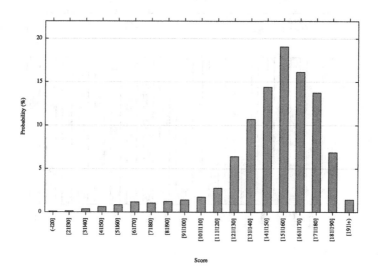

Fig. 2. Empirical distribution of scores of all clients.

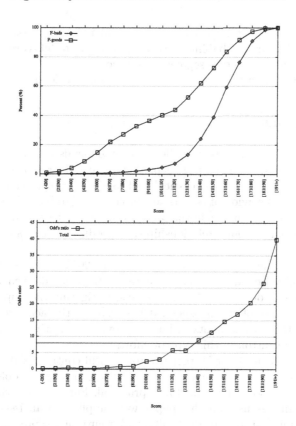

Fig. 3. Cumulative distribution functions and Odd's ratio distribution.

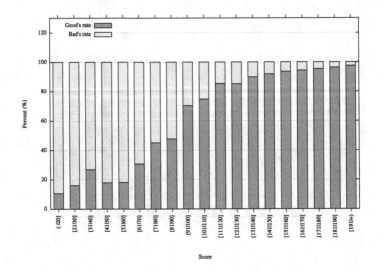

Fig. 4. Separation rate for bads/goods issuers.

- Make loyalty campaigns with the commercial network to issuers who have more than 0.5 churn probability (less than or equal to 90 score).
- Calculate technical reserves segmented by score.
- Block issuers of high risk (score less than 30) for new lending.

4   Conclusions

Predicting customer churn is a challenge that depends on many commercial, operational and market factors. The predictive model presented here allowed us to simulate those factors statistically through churn probability based on the transactional behavior of issuers available in a database. The results and conclusions are not exhaustive in the sense as to be able to understand a case by case review of each customer relationship that produces a high and unjustifiable cost.

The developed model was tested in December 2014. It has so far shown an adequate stability and discriminatory power. Strategies derived from it have brought benefits in dealing with credit losses, mitigating the impact of credits not returned because of churn issuers. It has also greatly facilitated monitoring the risk associated with accounts and it has provided objectivity gains by having a statistical tool control, in this type of efforts.

Although the definition of target variable is still controversial, we can argue that the proposed model is capable to solve these business problems. In fact, the validation was both theoretical and practical. Furthermore, the supervised modelling techniques used in this paper were applied to an issue that is not addressed in similar studies traditionally, and it currently represents a vital tool in the area of risk management.

The objectivity and simplicity of the model serves the purpose of the credit scoring practices focused on having only one number to interpret as a reliable indicator, which is easy to understand, related to the event probability under study and that considers and consolidates the available information in order to make an effective decision.

References

1. Abdou, A.H., Pointon, J.: Credit scoring, statistical techniques and evaluation criteria: a review of the literature. Intell. Syst. Acc. Finan. Manag. **18**, 59–88 (2011)
2. Allen, J.: A promise of approval in minutes, not hours. American Bankers (1995)
3. Baesens, A.: Benchmarking state-of-the-art classification algorithms for credit scoring. J. Oper. Res. **54**, 627–635 (2003)
4. Chen, I.F.: A two-stage green credit scoring model using nonparametric weighted feature extraction and multivariate adaptive regression splines. In: Advances in Industrial Engineering, Information and Water Resources. WIT Press, Great Britain (2013)
5. Mester, L.J.: What is the point of credit scoring? Business Review, Federal Reserve Bank (1997)
6. Ong, C.S., Huang, J.J., Tzeng, G.H.: Building credit scoring models using genetic programming. Expert Syst. Appl. **29**, 41–47 (2005)
7. Sadatrasoul, S.M., Gholamian, M.R., Siami, M., Hajimohammadi, Z.: Credit scoring in banks and financial institutions via data techniques: a literature review. J. AI Data Min. **1**, 119–129 (2013)
8. SAS Institute Inc.: SAS/STAT 9.3 User's Guide. SAS Institute Inc, Cary NC (2011)
9. Siddiqi, N.: Credit Risk Scorecards: Developing and Implementing Intelligent Credit Scoring. Wiley, USA (2005)
10. SAS Institute Inc.: Building Credit Scorecards using Credit Scoring for SAS Enterprise Miner. A SAS Best Practices Paper, pp. 1–23 (2009)
11. Thomas, L.C., Edelman, D.B., Crook, J.N.: Credit Scoring and Its Applications. Society for Industrial and Applied Mathematics, Philadelphia (2002)

Towards Autonomous Flight of Low-Cost MAVs by Using a Probabilistic Visual Odometry Approach

José Martínez-Carranza[1]([✉]), Esteban Omar Garcia[1], Hugo Jair Escalante[1], and Walterio Mayol-Cuevas[2]

[1] Instituto Nacional de Astrofísica, Óptica Y Electrónica, 72840 Puebla, Mexico
{carranza,eomargr,hugojair}@inaoep.mx
[2] University of Bristol, Bristol, UK
wmayol@cs.bris.ac.uk

Abstract. In this paper we present a methodology to localise and control low-budget Micro Aerial Vehicles (MAVs) in GPS-denied environments. The control law is based on a PD controller that controls height, orientation, roll and pitch in order to enable the MAV to fly autonomously towards a specific target. The core of our approach is the implementation of a fast probabilistic approach robust to erratic motion and capable of processing imagery data transmitted from the MAV to the Ground Control Station (GCS). The latter is due to the architecture of our low-budget MAVs which can not carry out any processing on board. However, images captured with the camera mounted on board the MAV can be transmitted via either wireless LAN or through analogue transmission to the GCS, where our fast probabilistic Visual Odometry system is used in order to rapidly obtain position estimates of the vehicle. Such estimates can be used accordingly to communicate back with the vehicle in order to submit control signals to drive its autonomous flight.

1 Introduction

Autonomous flight of MAVs has become focus of attention by many robotic research groups specialised in autonomous navigation [1–3]. In contrast to conventional terrestrial robotic platforms, aerial robots in the form of Unmanned Aerial Vehicles (UAVs) or Micro Aerial Vehicles (MAVs) imposes several challenges when it comes to control its dynamics, which maybe affected by strong perturbations such as wind currents, vibration of the motors, etc. But another challenge that we are particularly interested in this work is that of controlling the vehicle in environments where GPS signal is not accessible or not reliable, a common situation in indoor scenarios for the former, and when the vehicle flies through an urban canion, for the latter, where the GPS signal may be distorted due to the occlusion of signal reception provoked by metallic structures, buildings, trees, etc.

Similar to other research groups, our ultimate goal is that of achieving autonomous flight in GPS-denied environments. Typically, an autopilot system

© Springer International Publishing Switzerland 2015
O. Pichardo Lagunas et al. (Eds.): MICAI 2015, Part II, LNAI 9414, pp. 560–573, 2015.
DOI: 10.1007/978-3-319-27101-9_43

makes use of altitude, orientation and position (translation) of the vehicle in order to control it and take it to a desire waypoint in the air. But since GPS signal is assumed not accessible, then the vehicle's position information can not be observed directly. Even when the latter could be obtained by implementing dead-reckoning out of inertial measurements, such estimates would drift very quickly.

To address the lack of GPS signal, we estimate the 6D pose (translation and orientation) of the vehicle by processing visual data captured with an on-board monocular camera in a frame-to-frame fashion. For the latter, we propose to use a probabilistic visual odometry approach, which enables for fast simultaneous scene mapping and localisation of the 6D camera pose. Building a map of the scene mitigates, to some extend, drift in the estimation since a map that is continuously observed serves as a fixed reference. In this sense, visual odometry is by far better than dead-reckoning of inertial data. Even when error also accumulates in visual odometry, according to the literature, a probabilistic approach like ours has an accuracy of 1 % over the length of the trajectory, this is, we have an error of less than a meter in a 100 m trajectory [4, 5].

Another challenge we are interested in is that of working with low-budget UAVs or MAVs, which can not afford to lift extra payload or carry additional on-board computers to carry out intensive processing of the sensor data acquired during flight such as imagery data. Instead, inertial data and images have to be transmitted to the Ground Control Station (GCS) with the caveat that such data, and especially images, may arrive with delay. For this work, we have not tackled how to mitigate or avoid such delay, as we are more interested in assessing the effectiveness of our visual odometry approach robust to two main issues arising during the video reception: (i) received video gets frozen from time to time, thus, sudden changes in appearance of the observed scene may occur, which will lead to loss of tracking; (ii) delayed transmission plus fast manoeuvres or erratic motion induced by ground effect may also lead to loss of tracking since the received images may exhibit blur or distortion. For these reasons, we have also implemented a fast relocalisation mechanism based on fast and cheap-to-compare binary descriptors [6] that resumes tracking soon after the transmission becomes stable.

From the above, we present some examples of autonomous flight based on a PD controller[1] that uses position estimates obtained with our probabilistic visual odometry approach and without GPS signal. The obtained results indicate that our approach is effective an that we are on track in terms of developing a more sophisticated system to carry out a more complex autonomous flight in outdoor scenes. Thus, in order to present our work, this paper has been organised as follows: Sect. 1 presents the related work; Sect. 2 describes our probabilistic approach for 6D pose and map estimation; Sect. 4 described the MAV platforms used in this work; our experiments and results are described in Sect. 5; conclusions and future work are discussed in Sect. 6.

---

[1] We omitted the use of the integral controller as we found, empirically, that the proportional and derivative components were enough to our purposes.

2   Related Work

Vehicle localisation can be achieved by several approaches. In controlled environments, the most accurate technique is to use an external motion capture system [7,8]. Another approach is to use reference markers [1,9,10] and on-board cameras. Nevertheless, both methods are hard to implement on real situations because they need external components to be placed on systematic locations of the environment, so they are commonly used only for tests of control algorithms.

When the purpose is to navigate on real scenarios, GPS-independent aerial vehicles tend to use some sort of on-board sensors to discover their environment. Some approaches are based on scanning systems like Lidar [11,12], RGB-D sensors [13,14] or stereo cameras [4,12].

The more efficient technique in terms of weight and price is to use monocular vision. There are some useful approaches using a single on-board camera. The simplest algorithms use optic flow [15–17], which is useful to measure relative motion of the vehicle and might be used to discern between nearby and far away obstacles [18]. However, optic flow tends to accumulate error when used for long term trajectory estimation.

In most common not-controlled scenarios, features on images are a suitable to estimate position and locate 3D reference points. Some of such frameworks rely on the use of bundle-adjustment SLAM, such as PTAM [19]. PTAM has been used on quadcopters to perform simple tasks, like hovering on a reduced area [1, 2,20], but also in following some geometric paths indoors and outdoors [3]. A Recent technique called semi-direct monocular visual odometry [21] can also enable way-point-based autonomous navigation.

In this work, we aim to autonomously self-localise by only using monocular vision, which runs at high frame-rates. In addition to the mentioned approaches, the process is enhanced by making it more robust by fast visual re-localisation.

3   Probabilistic Visual Odometry

This section describes our probabilistic visual odometry system, which is based on the seminal work of [22]. Our framework is based on the EKF for monocular SLAM which is part of a family of stochastic solutions for monocular SLAM. A second branch is that of optimisation techniques, where bundle adjustment is the method that delivers the most accurate solution. Nevertheless, our choice is not based on the accuracy of the solutions, but in the ability of the EKF to initialise point features from the first frame of observation.

Optimisation methods, such as that of [19], use triangulation of image correspondences between two images in order to initialise a point feature given that the depth of the feature in a single view is unknown. However, triangulation requires an amount of parallax whose observation can lead to delayed initialisation or no initialisation at all if parallax is never observed. The latter could commonly arise in the case of a MAV flying forward or if the scene structure is too far w.r.t. the camera pose, in either case, observed features will not exhibit parallax.

In contrast, inverse-depth-like features will effectively cope with this problem, thus maintaining pose estimation whilst refining depth estimates, hence, it not surprising that optimisation-based methods use filtering approaches, similar to those based on the EKF, in order to firstly, initialise 3D points, and then insert converged points into the map to be optimised [23,24].

3.1 State Vector Definition

We begin by defining a joint state vector $\mathbf{x}$ as follows:

$$\mathbf{x} = \begin{bmatrix} \mathbf{x}_c^w, \mathbf{m}_1, \mathbf{m}_2, \ldots, \mathbf{m}_n \end{bmatrix}^\top \tag{1}$$

From above, $\mathbf{x}_c^w = [\mathbf{t}^w, \mathbf{e}^w]^\top$ corresponds to the 6D camera pose with a translation $\mathbf{t}^w$ and orientation component $\mathbf{e}^w$, with the latter expressed with the exponential map representation, note that w indicates that the components are defined w.r.t. the origin of the world. The vector also includes n map components where $\mathbf{m}_i$ corresponds to the i-th map component. A map component $\mathbf{m}_i$ can be of two types: a reference camera $\mathbf{m}_i = \mathbf{x}_{r_i}^w$ or an inverse depth value $\mathbf{m}_i = \rho_{ij}^c$, defined w.r.t. the reference camera $\mathbf{x}_{r_j}^w$, with $i = 1, \ldots, n, \, j = 1, \ldots, n$ and $i \neq j$.

As usual for EKF-based systems, the state vector $\mathbf{x}$ also involves the definition of a covariance matrix $\mathbf{P}_{\mathbf{xx}}$.

3.2 Dynamic Model

We use the *Constant velocity model*, as used by [22], to describe the motion of the camera in discrete time. The model includes linear and angular velocity representing the dynamics of the system up to the level of linear and angular accelerations (ν, Ω) affected by Gaussian noise. The model augments linear and angular velocity variables to the camera component as follows:

$$\mathbf{x}_c^w = \begin{bmatrix} \mathbf{t}^w, \mathbf{e}^w, \mathbf{v}^w, \omega^c \end{bmatrix}^\top \tag{2}$$

Thus, the dynamic model is defined as:

$$\mathbf{x}_{c_{k+1}}^w = \begin{bmatrix} \mathbf{t}_{k+1}^w \\ \mathbf{e}_{k+1}^w \\ \mathbf{v}_{k+1}^w \\ \omega_{k+1}^c \end{bmatrix} = \begin{bmatrix} \mathbf{t}_k^w + (\mathbf{v}_k^w + \nu)\Delta t \\ \mathbf{e}(\mathbf{q}(\mathbf{e}_k^w) \otimes \mathbf{q}((\omega_k^c + \Omega)\Delta t)) \\ \mathbf{v}_k^w + \nu \\ \omega_k^c + \Omega \end{bmatrix} \tag{3}$$

where $\mathbf{q}(\cdot)$ is the corresponding quaternion obtained from the exponential representation $\mathbf{e}_k^w$ and the angle-axis rotation vector $(\omega_k^c + \Omega)\Delta t$, $\otimes$ stands for quaternion multiplication, and the $\mathbf{e}(\cdot)$ indicates that the resulting quaternion from the multiplication is transformed back to the exponential map representation.

3.3 3D Point Initialisation

Let's assume that at a given time a 3D point has to be initialised. To this purpose, a first step is that of augmenting the state vector with a copy of the translation and orientation components of the current camera pose. Let's be $i = n+1$, where n is the current number of map components in the state vector, then $\mathbf{x}_{r_i}^w = [\mathbf{t}^w, \mathbf{e}^w]^\top$ is added to the state with the corresponding covariance propagation and augmentation of $\mathbf{P_{xx}}$.

As second step, a salient point with coordinates (u_d, v_d) on the image, chosen under some criteria, is used to construct the bearing ray $\mathbf{h}^c(u, v)$, where c indicates that such ray is defined w.r.t. the camera coordinate system. Note that we use the subscript d to indicate that the image position is obtained from a distorted image.[2], hence, the image position (u, v) corresponds to the undistorted image position. For the undistortion, we use the same radial distortion model used by [22]. Therefore, $\mathbf{h}^c$ corresponds to the bearing ray departing from the camera's optical centre and passing through the undistorted image position (u, v).

From the above, the state is augmented with a $i+1$-th component containing the inverse depth value of the 3D point defined by the bearing ray $\mathbf{h}^c(u, v)$, this is, $\mathbf{m}_{i+1} = \rho_{i+1,i}$, where $\rho_{i+1,i}$ is set as usual for the inverse depth parametrisation [24] at initialisation. Therefore, by assuming that $\mathbf{x}_{r_i}^w = [\mathbf{t}_i^w, \mathbf{e}_i^w]^\top$ and $\mathbf{m}_{i+1} = \rho_{i+1,i}$, a 3D point can be constructed as follows:

$$\mathbf{y}_{i+1}^w = \frac{1}{\rho_{i+1,i}} \mathbf{R}(\mathbf{q}(\mathbf{e}_i^w))\mathbf{h}^c(u, v) + \mathbf{t}_i^w \tag{4}$$

where $\mathbf{R}(\cdot)$ corresponds to the rotation matrix.

3.4 Measurement Model

As typically for visual slam systems, we use a pin-hole camera model in combination with perspective projection equations in order to define our measurement model. Therefore, given the current camera pose $\mathbf{x}_c^w$, a reference camera $\mathbf{x}_{r_i}^w$, an inverse depth value $\rho_{j,i}$, and in combination with Eq. 4, the measurement model for a 3D point corresponds to:

$$[\hat{u}_j, \hat{v}_j]^\top = \Pi(\mathbf{R}^c(\mathbf{y}_j^w - \mathbf{t}^w)) \tag{5}$$

where $\mathbf{R}^c = [\mathbf{R}(\mathbf{e}^w)]^\top$ and Π is the perspective projection model.

Due to space limitations we are not describing the corresponding Jacobians involved in the initialisation and measurement model, however, examples of similar calculations can be found in [24].

---

[2] Given that our goal in this work is that of achieving high frame rate, we avoid having to undistort the image, instead, we work directly on the distorted image, applying undistortion only when necessary.

3.5 Fast Recovery Against Loss of Tracking

During the mapping stage, each mapped visual feature is associated to a binary descriptor centred at the salient point where the visual feature was initialised. We use ORB descriptors [25] with length of 512 bits. These are organised by using a Locality-Sensitive-Hashing (LSH) technique [26], which enables us to store descriptors in hash tables at almost no cost and with no restriction to online increase of the database. The 3D world position of the salient point is available in the map and therefore can be attached to its binary descriptor. This means that whenever a binary descriptor is retrieved from any of the hash tables, we will have access to its 3D position as well.

Therefore, at relocalisation time, given a query image at some time step, salient points in the image are extracted using the FAST corner detector [27]. For each salient point $\mathbf{s}_i$ the corresponding ORB descriptor $\mathbf{b}_i$ is extracted. Each binary descriptor $\mathbf{b}_i$ is passed to the hash function, which simply takes subsets of bits from the binary number in order to access to the corresponding bins in the hash tables (where potential matches for $\mathbf{b}_i$ exist). A linear nearest neighbour search is performed with all the retrieved binary descriptors from the bins searching for the descriptor that minimizes the Hamming distance with $\mathbf{b}_i$.

Let $\mathbf{b}_{i_m}$ be the best match for $\mathbf{b}_i$ and let $\mathbf{p}_{i_m}$ be the 3D position of the best binary match $\mathbf{b}_{i_m}$. Then a set of 2D-3D pairs is augmented as follows: $\mathbf{C} = \mathbf{C} \cup \{(\mathbf{s}_i, \mathbf{p}_{i_m})\}$ and if $|\mathbf{C}| > c_{size}$ then it is passed to the pose estimation module, which is based on a three-point pose estimator plus RANSAC [6]. The relocalisation is considered successful if the pose estimator finds a minimum set of inliers in $\mathbf{C}$ such that these can be used to estimate a camera pose.

4 Low-Cost MAVs

Quadcopters are versatile vehicles that require a very small area to take-off and land and can hover on a specific spot. Compared to other aircraft, like helicopters, quadcopters have no complex mechanical parts and are much easier to build. Moreover, propelers are safer than helicopter's blades because they have less inertia. In this paper we focus in low-budget quadcopters (under 1,000 USD) that can carry a camera and transmit video to a ground station.

4.1 AR Drone

AR Drone, see Fig. 1a, is a quite popular quadcopter that costs no more than 400 USD and is ready to fly out of the box. The manufacturer has made the API available to make the development and research easier. The AR Drone can fly around 10 min carrying its protective hull, more if it is removed (not recommended for safety reasons). The video obtained from the on-board camera has a resolution of 640 × 480 pixels at 30 fps, it is encoded with H264 and then transmitted through WiFi to the ground station where it is processed.

For the communication with the AR Drone vehicle we used the cvdrone library [28], which enables roll, pitch, yaw and altitude control plus reading of the on-board camera images into a openCV image format.

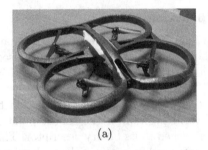
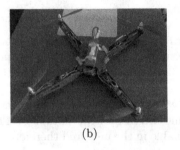

(a)   (b)

Fig. 1. Micro Aerial Vehicles used in this work: (a) commercial quadcopter AR Drone; (b) custom-built quadcopter.

4.2 Custom-Built Quadcopter

For some of the outdoor experiments we used a cheap custom-built quadcopter, see Fig. 1b, with total cost under 550 USD. Its frame is made of thin plywood with 680 mm of wheelbase diameter. It carries a GoPro Hero 2 camera with resolution of 720 × 480 and whose signal is in composite video. The video signal is sent through an analog video transmitter in 5.8 Ghz. On the ground station, the video signal is digitised using a USB video card EasyCap. The camera can be accessed using the openCV library, thus, camera frames can be allocated as openCV image objects. For this device we have not implemented the control (autopilot) yet, however, this is part of our future work.

5 Experiments

The next sections describe the experiments we carried out in order to assess our probabilistic visual odometry approach applied to imagery transmitted by our MAVs. The GCS receiving the imagery is a conventional computer with i5 quad-core processor running at 2.2 GHz and with 4 GB in RAM. Note that our visual odometry returns map and camera pose estimates up to a scale factor, however, when presenting our results, these estimates have been scaled appropriately.

5.1 Vision-Based Localisation of the AR Drone

The first step in this and the following experiments is that of flying the vehicle manually. After taking off and stable flight is achieved, driven by the pilot, and upon reception of the on-board camera images in the GCS, our visual odometry approach is kicked off, at the same time, the pilot flies the vehicle smoothly such that camera observations of the scene allow the visual odometry to build a 3D map of the scene. After a converged map has been created, the vehicle is flown following a rectangle-shape trajectory with the camera always facing forward. Thus, the goal in this experiment is to assess whether our approach can effectively estimate the vehicle's pose whilst traversing such path.

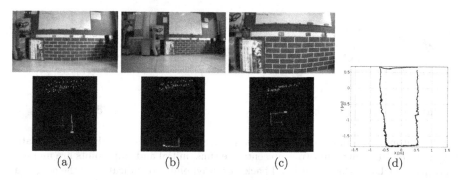

(a)   (b)   (c)   (d)

Fig. 2. Pose estimation of the AR Drone vehicle using our probabilistic visual odometry approach: first row in (a-c) show the camera view transmitted from the vehicle to the GCS where visual features are tracked (green circles) in real time, second row in (a-c) show a top view representation of the world where estimated 3D position of the visual features (green dots) is depicted as much as the estimated vehicle's position (turquoise rectangle with white trajectory); the full vehicle trajectory is shown in (d) (Color figure online).

Figure 2a–c correspond to snapshot examples of the flight where the vehicle is following the rectangle trajectory. Figure 2d corresponds to a top view plot of the total trajectory estimated by our approach. Note that the trajectory exhibits some irregularities and some deviation from the rectangle shape (see the third segment of the rectangle), however, this was in fact the trajectory that the vehicle followed since it was difficult for the pilot to follow a perfect rectangular shape. Nevertheless, the estimated trajectory indicates that our approach could effectively estimate the vehicle's pose from start to end.

5.2 Localisation and Control of the AR Drone

We carried out several runs where we used our visual odometry approach connected to a Proportional Derivative (PD) controller to command the vehicle to fly autonomously. For each one of these runs, as in the previous experiment, the pilot flew the vehicle in order to gain stability in the flight soon after which we started our visual odometry to build an initial map of the scene. After a map was built, the vehicle was moved accordingly in order to record forward and backward waypoints.

Soon after recording the way points, the *autonomous flight mode* was started. The goal of the controller in this mode is that of commanding the vehicle to perform a forward and backward flight using a cruise controller (PD controller) within the boundaries set by the waypoints. The controller also submit signals to control roll in order to keep the vehicle centred over the zero coordinate in the X-axis, this is, the X coordinate in the vehicle's translation vector should be close to zero. Other components of the control are the modules to maintain height hold and heading always facing forward.

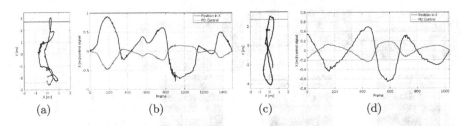

(a)   (b)   (c)   (d)

Fig. 3. Autonomous flight based on our approach: (a,c) top view of the vehicle's path driven by the PD control in two representative runs, initial and stop points are marked in green and red, and the forward and backward waypoints are indicated by the magenta and yellow lines respectively; (b,d) show the X estimated component in the position and the control signal calculated by the PD controller in order to bring the vehicle towards the zero value in the X-axis (Color figure online).

Figure 3 shows the results obtained during the autonomous flight. Figure 3a,c show a top view of the vehicle's position estimated in real time with our visual odometry approach. Note that such trajectory was produced while the vehicle was driven by our PD controller, which utilized the orientation and translation estimates from the visual odometry in order to calculate the control signal. Figure 3b,d show the X estimated coordinate together with the PD control signal. In this sense, the control signal behaves in opposite fashion to the behaviour exhibited by X, this is, if X gets away from the zero then the control signal reacts in opposite sign and with a proportional value to X aiming at driving the vehicle towards the zero.

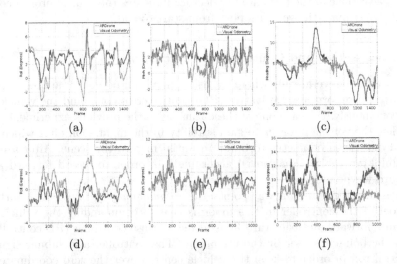

(a)   (b)   (c)

(d)   (e)   (f)

Fig. 4. Comparison of the vehicle's orientation estimates using our visual odometry appraoch (green) against those obtained with the AR Drone API using the cvdrone library (blue) (Color figure online).

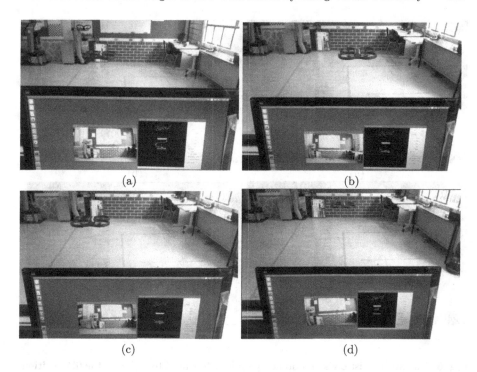

Fig. 5. Snapshots of a representative run with the order (a,b,c,d), the vehicle flies autonomously driven by the PD controller that uses our visual odometry approach to calculate the corresponding control signals.

Note that according to the figures mentioned above, the vehicle oscillates around the zero rather than following a straight line. However, this is a consequence of the delay reception of the images in the GCS. Nevertheless, the results indicate that our approach is effective in order to estimate the vehicle's position and that such estimates can be used by a PD controller to drive the vehicle autonomously. In fact, the total processing time of the system is shown in Table 1, in the first and second row for these runs. According to this, in average the system as a whole is running at more than 30 fps, whereas the visual odometry module only runs at around 40 fps. This clearly indicates that our approach runs in real time and that the delay in the transmission is the cause of the late response of the controller. Figure 5 shows snapshots of a run during the autonomous flight using our approach.

Furthermore, observe that in Table 1 we are reporting the number of frames where loss of tracking occurred due to either of the reasons mentioned before, however, our approach cope with this problem by effectively relocalising as soon as a next stable frame arrived. We should highlight that when a loss of tracking event occurs, the controller commands the vehicle to hover over the same point until tracking is resumed. Figure 4 shows the orientation estimates obtained with our visual odometry approach, for the runs described above, and compared

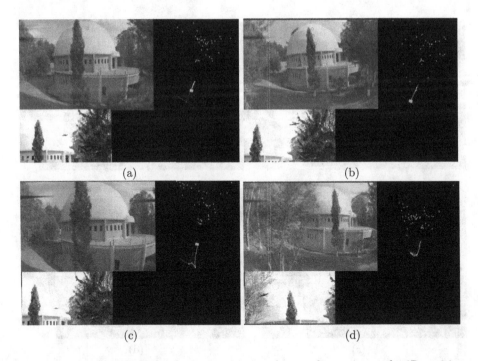

(a)   (b)

(c)   (d)

Fig. 6. Our probabilistic visual odometry approach is used to estimate the 6D position of our custom-built vehicle without requiring GPS or any other inertial sensor.

against those obtained through the AR Drone API (with cvdrone). Note that our estimation is comparable to that of the AR Drone.

Table 1. Average statistics obtained with our visual odometry approach for the different runs in the experiments.

Vehicle	Scene type	Image size	Total frames	Total FPS	Vis. Od. FPS	# Lost frames	# Tracked features	#Obs. features
AR Drone	Indoors	640 × 480	4688	39	42	238	40	30
AR Drone	Indoors	640 × 480	3687	36	37	9	31	20
Custom-built	Outdoors	720 × 480	6550	26	37	422	38	20

5.3 Outdoors Localisation

We finalise this work by presenting some preliminary results related to 6D pose estimation using our approach and obtained for our custom-built quadcopter fying outdoors. In this case, the vehicle was flown by our pilot in an outdoor scene, commanding the vehicle to fly backward/forward, left/right, to an altitude of about 20 m. Once in the air and with stable flight, our visual odometry was kicked off. Note that even when the observed scene structure is far from the vehicle (some 30 m away from the camera view point) our visual odometry still managed to initialise and map 3D points that can be used to localise the vehicle's position. Some snapshot examples of this run are shown in Fig. 6. Observe that, up to scale, our system manages to indicate that the vehicle is moving backwards, to the right and then forwards and to the left.

It's worth mentioning the our approach was robust to spinning propels appearing on the image and a little wobble effect (also called jello effect) due to rolling shutter CMOS sensor, which is common in cameras mounted on rotary-wing vehicles. Moreover, loss of tracking occurred when the vehicle observed some nearby trees with repetitive texture, but also due to the same reasons, as with the commercial vehicle, originated by the late transmission of the camera images to the GCS. However, the system resumed soon after the vehicle re-observed a known area with a stable flight. The third row in Table 1 shows the statistics corresponding to this run. Note that, in average, the estimation is also achieved in good real time, this is, between 25–30 fps.

Currently we are developing our own API to control the vehicle, therefore, from our current results, we are confident that we will be able to use our visual odometry approach in combination with a PD controller in order to carry out outdoors autonomous flight.

6 Conclusions

In this work we have presented a system that uses a probabilistic visual odometry approach for 6D pose estimation in real time (25–40 fps) of MAVs in indoor and outdoor scenes where GPS signal is assumed inaccessible. This estimation, however, does not run on-board the vehicles, instead, images are transmitted from the vehicles to a GCS where these are processed with our vision-based approach. In this sense, a main drawback in our implementation is that of not having a mechanism to mitigate the delayed reception of imagery data. Nevertheless, we still managed to couple our visual odometry approach with a PD controller in order to carry out indoor autonomous flight robust to loss of tracking due to erratic motion or problems with the video reception.

Our future work involves outdoors autonomous flight with our custom-built MAV by using our visual-based approach.

Acknowledgements. This work was funded by the Royal Society-Newton Advanced Fellowship with reference NA140454. We would like to thank David Carrillo López for his support on the experimental setup and video recording of this work.

References

1. Bloesch, M., Weiss, S., Scaramuzza, D., Siegwart, R.: Vision based MAV navigation in unknown and unstructured environments. In: ICRA (2010)

2. Achtelik, M.W., Achtelik, M.C., Chli, M., Chatzichristofis, S., Fraundorfer, F., Doth, K.-M., Kneip, L., Gurdan, D., Heng, L., Kosmatopoulos, E., Doitsidis, L., Lee, G.H., Lynen, S., Martinelli, A., Meier, L., Pollefeys, M., Renzaglia, A., Scaramuzza, D., Siegwart, R., Stumpf, J.C., Tanskanen, P., Troiani, C., Weiss, S.: sfly:swarm of micro flying robots. In: IROS (2012)

3. Engel, J., Sturm, J., Cremers, D.: Scale-aware navigation of a low-cost quadro-copter with a monocular camera. Robot. Auton. Syst. **62**, 1646–1656 (2014)

4. Martinez-Carranza, J., Calway, A., Mayol-Cuevas, W.: Enhancing 6d visual relo-calisation with depth cameras. In: IROS (2013)

5. Civera, J., Grasa, O.G., Davison, A.J., Montiel, J.M.M.: 1-point ransac for EKF-based structure from motion. In: IROS (2009)

6. Martinez-Carranza, J., Mayol-Cuevas, W.: Real-time continuous 6d relocalisation for depth cameras. In: MVIGRO workshop in conjunction with RSS (2013)

7. Mellinger, D., Kumar, V.: Minimum snap trajectory generation and control for quadrotors. In: ICRA, pp. 2520–2525. IEEE (2011)

8. Lupashin, S., Hehn, M., Mueller, M.W., Schoellig, A.P., Sherback, M., DAndrea, R.: A platform for aerial robotics research and demonstration: the flying machine arena. Mechatronics **24**(1), 41–54 (2014)

9. Nitschke, C.: Marker-based tracking with unmanned aerial vehicles. In: Robotics and Biomimetics (ROBIO) (2014)

10. Meier, L., Tanskanen, P., Fraundorfer, F., Pollefeys, M.: Pixhawk: a system for autonomous flight using onboard computer vision. In: ICRA (2011)

11. Grzonka, S., Grisetti, G., Burgard, W.: Towards a navigation system for autonomous indoor flying. In: ICRA (2009)

12. Achtelik, M., Bachrach, A., He, R., Prentice, S., Roy, N.: Stereo vision and laser odometry for autonomous helicopters in GPS-denied indoor environments. In: SPIE Defense, Security, and Sensing (2009)

13. Huang, A.S., Bachrach, A., Henry, P., Krainin, M., Maturana, D., Fox, D., Roy, N.: Visual odometry and mapping for autonomous flight using an RGB-D camera. In: International Symposium on Robotics Research (ISRR), pp. 1–16 (2011)

14. Bylow, E., Sturm, J., Kerl, C., Kahl, F., Cremers, D.: Real-time camera tracking and 3d reconstruction using signed distance functions. In: RSS 2013, vol. 9 (2013)

15. Schmid, K., Ruess, F., Suppa, M., Burschka, D.: State estimation for highly dynamic flying systems using key frame odometry with varying time delays. In: IROS 2012 (2012)

16. Grabe, V., Bülthoff, H.H., Giordano, P.R.: Robust optical-flow based self-motion estimation for a quadrotor UAV. In: IROS (2012)

17. Bristeau, P.-J., Callou, F., Vissiere, D., Petit, N., et al.: The navigation and control technology inside the AR. drone micro UAV. In: 18th IFAC (2011)

18. Zingg, S., Scaramuzza, D., Weiss, S., Siegwart, R.: Mav navigation through indoor corridors using optical flow. In: ICRA (2010)

19. Klein, G., Murray, D.: Parallel tracking and mapping for small ar workspaces. In: International Symposium on Mixed Augmented Reality (2007)

20. Kneip, L., Chli, M., Siegwart, R.: Robust real-time visual odometry with a single camera and an IMU. In: British Machine Vision Conference (2011)

21. Scaramuzza, D., Forster, C., Pizzoli, M.: Fast semi-direct monocular visual odom-etry. In: ICRA (2014)

22. Davison, A., Reid, I., Molton, N., Stasse, O.: Monoslam: real-time single camera slam. IEEE Trans. Pattern Anal. Mach. Intell. **29**, 1052–1067 (2007)

23. Eade, E., Drummond, T.: Scalable monocular slam. In: CVPR (2006)

24. Montiel, J., Civera, J., Davison, A.J.: Unified inverse depth parametrization for monocular slam. In: Proceedings of Robotics: Science and Systems (2006)
25. Rublee, E., Rabaud, V., Konolige, K., Bradski, G.: ORB: an efficient alternative to sift or surf. In: International Conference on Computer Vision (2011)
26. Gionis, A., Indyk, P., Motwani, R.: Similarity search in high dimensions via hashing. In: International Conference on Very Large Data Bases (1999)
27. Rosten, E., Drummond, T.W.: Machine learning for high-speed corner detection. In: Leonardis, A., Bischof, H., Pinz, A. (eds.) ECCV 2006, Part I. LNCS, vol. 3951, pp. 430–443. Springer, Heidelberg (2006)
28. cvdrone. https://www.openhub.net/p/cvdrone

Location and Activity Detection for Indoor Environments

Fernando Martínez Reyes$^{(\boxtimes)}$, Luis C. González Gurrola,
and Hector Valenzuela Estrada

Facultad de Ingeniería, Universidad Autónoma de Chihuahua, Chihuahua,
Chihuahua, Mexico
{fmartinez2004,gonzalezgurrola,undertolo}@gmail.com

Abstract. Location-based services require to process and infer knowledge based on the understanding of people daily activities. This information acquires relevance in cases when elder people live alone since it could be used to infer facts about his/her health. In this paper a platform for getting location and activity data for indoors is presented. Gathered information is processed, first, to locate people at room level and then to identify whether a person is sitting, standing, walking or even running. For classification purposes we used an artificial neural network, which report an accuracy as high as 97.75 %. A web page, which complements the platform, is made available for those persons who want to know about the rate of visits to the rooms and the rate of, for instance, walking exercise. In our next version we would like to extend the identification of activity by detecting the way the inhabitant interacts with artifacts.

1 Introduction

Pervasive technology is continually moving to our homes. Computing devices are at our fingertips and being used to support every day activities. Responsive and intelligent homes are expected to host objects and artifacts that are aware of user needs and desires. Such intelligent environments must get knowledge and understanding of how the dweller uses spaces and what kind of activity is being done. Location and activity information are valuable keys to offer computational services that, for instance, could help elders live alone and reasonable safe. The level of activity the person accomplishes could be an indicator of his/her healthiness.

The recognition of location and activity indoors are of great interest for the academic community but surprisingly often studied separately. In this work it is reported the integration of a technology platform for the collection of these pieces of information, and the processing and identification of the homes rooms use as well as if the person is sitting, standing or if s/he is walking.

The rest of the work is organized as follows. Section 2 reviews work aiming with the identification of location and work that motivates our interest for the recognition of the activity elders do indoors. Section 3 describes the implementation of the technology platform that help with the identification and recognition

© Springer International Publishing Switzerland 2015
O. Pichardo Lagunas et al. (Eds.): MICAI 2015, Part II, LNAI 9414, pp. 574–582, 2015.
DOI: 10.1007/978-3-319-27101-9_44

of location and activity. Section 4 documents the current system performance and the experiments done. Section 5 offers conclusions and future work.

2   Related Work

The identification of objects or individuals is a major growth area in the field of wireless technologies and has become an essential part of systems that provide location-based services. Smart home networks would integrate devices, resources and services to support the current user needs. Given the myriad of activities that take place in the home, however, it is important to design adaptive services that take into account the users dynamic situations [1]. The identification of the current users environment depends on the quality of the information it is possible to gather from indoors location technology. Furthermore, what pervasive technology could help us to know, understand and infer the kind of activity the inhabitant is doing. The most common of location systems uses WiFi, Bluetooth, ultrasound or RF communication based devices. Indoor location-aware services were firstly proposed for museums where the proximity of a person with a piece of art was used to deliver content that enhanced the users experience as illustrated in [2]. WiFi based location systems are also of interest because of the internet penetration in todays homes. A work that implements a WiFi location system to support indoor navigation is presented in [3]. In spite of that the navigation system is used for a robot it could be extended for tracking and supporting blind people in the home. Most of these technologies can be provided by today-smartphones and in conjunction with technologies can be found in the home, e.g. access points, robust location services can be implemented. In [4] for instance, the fusion of the WiFi, accelerometer and compass smartphone sensors give support to an indoor positioning system. The Bluetooth wireless technology was originally designed as a solution for short-range communication, however, given the availability of BT sensors in most of to date mobile technologies it is possible the design of complete location and navigation systems [5]. Tracking systems based on the BT technology make use of the signal strength measurements. In [6] the Received Signal Strength Indicator (RSSI) value of the Bluetooth protocol is used to get a correlation to the distance between the sender and the receiver. Euclidean distance is calculated and used to determine the sender location.

The other piece of information highly relevant for indoor smart environments is the identification of the human being activity. In the home context, especially for people with special needs, activity recognition systems can help to assist with the inference and prediction of potential accidents the inhabitant can face. For instance, an activity detection system can identify whether an adult fell and how long the person has been lying on the floor [7]. From the elders interaction with artifacts or appliances it can be possible to help users with, for instance, the home energy consumption or to remind them of whether appliances have been left on [8]. Ubiquicom [9] is a technology company that produces solutions for Real Time location for indoor and outdoor prevention and monitoring in the field of workplace safety using Bluetooth WiFi RFID, sensors: Tilt, triaxal accelerometer.

3   Implementation

This section presents the implementation of the systems facilities that support the location and detection of activity. We describe the integration of the technological platform, the collection and the processing of data, and the high level application that allows for the monitoring of the homes spaces usage as well as for the identification of a persons activity, in particular, if the person is sitting, walking or standing. Figure 1 shows the general architecture for the proposed system being the two main components the location system and the activity detection system.

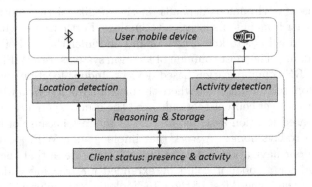

Fig. 1. Platform for the monitoring of location and activity for indoors.

3.1   Location Detection

The kitchen, the living and the study rooms were tagged with Bluetooth-enabled devices that support the service that identifies the presence of a person within the rooms. For the kitchen and the living rooms two Raspberry PI computers are used. In the studio room a desktop computer is used. In this computer, in addition to the service of presences location, there is running the detection of activity service and the web service, which is covered later in this section. The tag, i.e. the mobile device carried by the user, is a Samsung Galaxy Pro smart phone. All of the Bluetooth nodes (Raspberry PI, desktop computer and mobile phone) are manually registered in the location server. The presence of a person within a room is decided upon the magnitude of the Received Signal Strength Indicator (RSSI) signal strength. To determine if the mobile device is in the field of view of any of the presences detection nodes the RSSI signal is compared against a threshold (-15 in this case). The threshold was empirically calculated after the mobile phone was located at different places around the house. Figure 2 shows how RSSI events are processed to establish the connection status of a TAG, i.e. users location. A sample of 254 RSSI values is read from the mobile TAG, and its arithmetic mean obtained. If this average value is less than the threshold the TAG is considered as NO connected, or a TAG present event is registered by the presence server if the other way around.

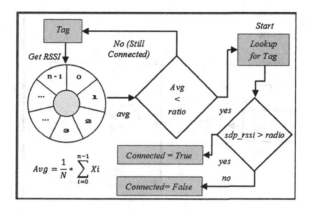

Fig. 2. RSSI data processing for the definition of a connected state of a TAG.

3.2 Activity Detection

The users mobile device is used to collect the readings that are later sent to the main server to be processed. Acceleration data is processed by means of two classification phases, each phase uses an artificial neural network for the classification task, see Fig. 3. The input to the first classifier is a sample of 420 feature vector values (1). A 50 % overlapping window is applied for consecutive acceleration events, also a smooth filter is applied to the samples. The characteristic function defined for the classifier consists of the statistical features of the axis magnitudes and the orientation angle value:

$$featureVector = [avg(mag), var(mag), std(mag), max(mag),$$
$$min(mag), sma, ae, avg(angle), var(angle), std(angle)] \tag{1}$$

Where, mag is the resultant magnitude of axis vectors, angle corresponds to the Euler angle between x-axis and y-axis, sma is the signal magnitude area and ae is the average energy.

The output from the first classifier consists of events identifying three types of classes: static, dynamic and transition. The next classifier has the task of filtering these classes and defining the events for the states of sitting and standing (static), walking and running (dynamic), and sitting-standing and standing-sitting (transition). The definition of each of these events is accomplished by using three neural networks, as shown in Fig. 3. For the first two classifiers, static and dynamic, the characteristic vector is given by:

$$featureVector = [ar1, ar2, ..., ar15, sma, avg(angle)] \tag{2}$$

Where, $ar1, ..., arn$ are autoregressive coefficients, sma is the signal magnitude area or the sum of the area under the module, angle is the tilt angle calculate using atan2(x,y).

Because transitional events are different from the static and dynamic ones, the third classifier must seek for changes on both the acceleration of any of

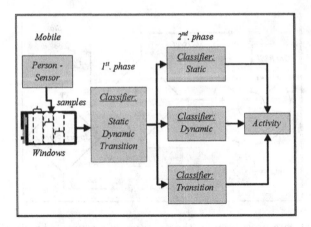

Fig. 3. System architecture showing where the classifiers (Artificial Neural Networks) were located.

the axis and the accelerometers orientation. The characteristic vector for this classifier is given by:

$$featureVector = [corrxy, corrxz, corryz, SEx, SEy, SEz, avg(mag), \tag{3}$$
$$max(mag), min(mag), std(mag)]$$

Where, corrxyz corresponds to the correlation coefficient between two acceleration axes, and SExyz represents the spectral entropy for acceleration data [10], mag is the resultant magnitude of axis vectors given by accelerometer.

A Multilayer Perceptron (MLP) neural network was implemented for the classification of activity. All of the four neural networks, one for the first classification phase and three for the second classification phase, were similarly configured: a hidden layer of 10 neurons, a learning factor of 0.1, a momentum of 0.9, a sigmoid activation function, goal set at 0.001 and a softmax function for the output layer. The main difference between the MLPs is regarding the input layer. The number of inputs depends on the features exposed by each of the characteristic vectors.

3.3 Web Interface

There is a web interface available for the monitoring of the activities occurring in the home, see Fig. 4. For instance, relatives would like to get informed of the level of physical activity adults accomplish during the day or if they have visited the kitchen which may suggest the person food intake. The web interface runs in the presence server and updates every 3 s.

4 Results

The implemented system identifies the location of a person within one of the homes spaces, and is able to determine if the person is sitting, standing or

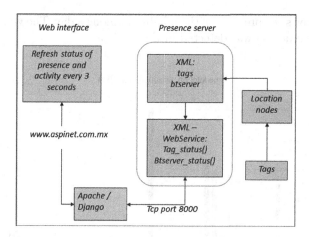

Fig. 4. The web interface refreshes the location and activity information every 3 s. This information is retrieved from the presence server which hosts a SQLite database.

walking. The technology was installed in a detached house, and tested for five weeks. The inhabitant was a person who works from 8 am to 6 pm. In the morning the person does some tasks in preparation to go to work between 6:30 am and 7:40 time when the inhabitant leaves home. The inhabitant is back at 2.30 pm for lunch and leaves home again at 4:00 pm. The person is back from work at 7 pm. Bedtime is said occurs between 9:30 to 10:00 pm.

Using the web interface, described later in this section, one can retrieve information and observe the activity happening within the home. For instance, the Fig. 5 shows the total time the tagged rooms have been in use for the weeks (x axis); being the kitchen the most visited space.

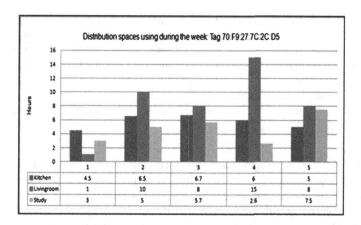

Fig. 5. The user's presence in each of the tagged rooms during the 5 weeks.

Figure 6 shows the presence of the inhabitant along a day. The y-axis indicates the minutes the person was detected in the kitchen.

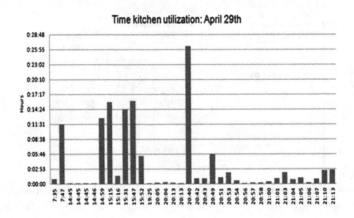

Fig. 6. Distribution of the time the kitchen was used in one day.

Regarding the neural network classifiers four experiments were conducted to validate their performance. Each of the experiments consisted on the collection and the processing of acceleration data. Different auto regressive coefficients were tested for the classifier of static and dynamic classes. For this classifier, we also worked with different filtering values and applied an LDA (Linear Discriminant Analysis). The confusion matrix that was obtained for this classifier is shown in Table 1.

Table 1. Confusion matrix for the activity classifier.

Classifier	LDA AR=10 Filter=19	LDA AR=20 Filter=19	LDA AR=10 Filter=19	LDA AR=20 Filter=19	LDA AR=10 Filter=2
Type (1 phase)	93.5	97.5	95.5	97.25	97.75
Dynamic (2 phase)	93.25	95.5	95.5	90.25	95.5
Static (2 phase)	94	95	93.73	94.5	94.5
Transitive (2 phase)	92.5	92.5	92.5	73.25	93.25
Average	**93.3**	**95.187**	**94.3**	**88.81**	**95.25**

Finally, Fig. 7 presents the web interface that allows for the monitoring of activity and rooms space usage. The left top section indicates the users detected in the house. The left bottom information indicates whether the monitoring system is activated. A button is provided to start or stop this service. The bar menu available on the top of the web interface is available for the management of the system for instance to register a new mobile phone with the system. The particular interest here is that it is by means of this interface that reports such

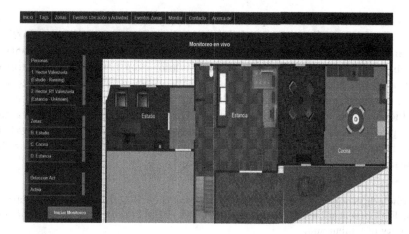

Fig. 7. The web interface that the inhabitant's relatives can use to monitor what activity the person is doing and in what room s/he is in.

as the one presented in Fig. 5 can be generated. For example, it is possible to review the rate of presence or the level of activity an individual is performing within the home.

5 Conclusions

This paper reports a technology platform for the location and the identification of four types of activity within the home, system that could help monitor the activity of an elder living alone. The technology used for the location service is based on Raspberry PI embedded computers. The location nodes communicate with the users mobile phone via Bluetooth, and use the RSSI strength of signal to determine whether the user is in a particular room. On the other hand, the users activity is identified from the acceleration data reported by the mobile phone the inhabitant worn. Four neural networks were used to process acceleration data to finally determine if the person was sitting, standing, walking or even running. After five weeks the system was running we observed an overall good performance. Both the location and the activities identification services seemed to provide adequate information to support a platform for the monitoring of a person living alone. Insights from the experiments done, however, indicate new opportunities for improving resources and facilities currently offered by the monitoring platform. First, the location services lacks information that could indicate what particular space within the room is being used by the inhabitant. For example, it would be interesting to get some understanding of the reasons for the person to spend much of his/her time in front of the TV set and what kinds of TV programs are of interest.

The activity detection system can detect if the person is sitting, standing, walking or running. The cell phone of the person is the means by which activity data is collected. The data is processed by applying four neural networks classifiers. The final configuration of the classifier has a quite competitive (95.25 %) performance. With the combination of the two systems, location and activity, it may be possible to monitor the person lifestyle or even better to have information that could offer a hint of the inhabitant well-being. The activity detection system, however, can be improved if the identification of other types of activities is included. For instance, we plan to extent this work to monitor the interaction of the person with artifacts, e.g. cooker, fridge, and microwave, among others. With the collection of a richest contextual data it would be possible to predict potentially risky activities the elder would face.

Acknowledgement. We would also like to thank the PROMEP for funding Platform for the Experimentation with Mobile Technologies (PEMT) project, at the Autonomous University of Chihuahua.

References

1. Cheng, B.C., Chen, H., Tseng, R.Y.: Context-aware gateway for ubiquitous sip-based services in smart homes. In: 2006 International Conference on Hybrid Information Technology, ICHIT 2006, vol. 2, pp. 374–381 (2006)
2. Tesoriero, R., Gallud, J., Lozano, M., Penichet, V.: Using active and passive RFID technology to support indoor location-aware systems. In: IEEE Consumer Electronics Society, pp. 578–583 (2008)
3. Biswas, J., Veloso, M.: Wifi localization and navigation for autonomous indoor mobile robots. In: IEEE International Conference on Robotics and Automation (ICRA) (2010)
4. Gallagher, T., Wise, W., Li, B., A.G.: Indoor positioning system based on sensor fusion for the blind and visually impaired. In: International Conference on Indoor Positioning and Indoor Navigation (2012)
5. Anastasi, G., Bandelloni, R., Conti, M., Delmastro, F.: Experimenting an indoor bluetooth-based positioning service. In: 2003 Proceedings 23rd International Conference onDistributed Computing Systems Workshops (2003)
6. Opoku, K.S.: An indoor tracking system based on bluetooth technology (2012). asXiv preprint 1209.3053
7. McKenna, S., Charif, H.N.: Summarising contextual activity and detecting unusual inactivity in a supportive home environment. Pattern Anal. Appl. **7**, 386–401 (2004)
8. Berenguer, M., Giordani, M., Giraud-By, F., Noury, N.: Automatic detection of activities of daily living from detecting and classifying electrical events on the residential power line. In: 2008 10th International Conference on e-health Networking, Applications and Services, HealthCom. (2008)
9. www.ubiquicom.it (2012)

Short-Term Motion Tracking Using Inexpensive Sensors

Filip Matzner[(✉)] and Roman Barták

Faculty of Mathematics and Physics, Charles University in Prague,
Malostranské náměstí 25, 118 00 Praha 1, Czech Republic
floop@floop.cz, bartak@ktiml.mff.cuni.cz

Abstract. Current consumer electronics is equipped with various sensors, among which accelerometer, gyroscope, and magnetometer represent typical examples. In this paper, we study the possibility of using these low-cost sensors for 3D motion and orientation tracking. In particular, we thoroughly describe a simple dead-reckoning algorithm for sensor data fusion which produces a 3D path of the device in real time. More importantly, we propose a method of automated stabilization every time the device stands still, which corrects the bias caused by sensor inaccuracies. This method extends the time when motion tracking is reliable. We evaluate the proposed pipeline in a variety of experiments using two common smartphones.

Keywords: Motion tracking · Sensor fusion · Signal processing · Inertial navigation · Visualization · Dead-reckoning · Smartphones

1 Introduction

Precise motion tracking is very important in robotics for navigation, however, it can also be exploited in many other areas such as mapping of surrounding environment or taking panoramatic snapshots using smartphones. The question that we ask in this paper is whether low-cost sensors included, for instance, in common smartphones and "toy robots" such as AR.Drone could be used for this purpose. The goal is to design a method for short-term tracking of device movement and orientation using only its on-board sensors – accelerometer, gyroscope, and magnetometer.

The approaches to motion tracking can be divided into two basic categories. The first one is to ignore the behaviour of the device (i.e., the way it moves) and to trust the data received from the sensors. Those are called *non-model methods*. The second one is to create a model of the device behaviour and to trust more the data in accordance with the model than the data contrary to the model. Those are called *model methods*. Model methods are particullary useful for objects with limited means of movement, such as cars and airplanes. For instance, when an airplane is flying forwards, it is highly unprobable that it stops in place and starts moving backwards even if the sensors claim so.

© Springer International Publishing Switzerland 2015
O. Pichardo Lagunas et al. (Eds.): MICAI 2015, Part II, LNAI 9414, pp. 583–601, 2015.
DOI: 10.1007/978-3-319-27101-9_45

Probably the most profound example of the model method is the Kalman filter [7] and its variants. It is a probabilistic method, which plays a key role in the inertial navigation of airplanes, vehicles, and in signal processing in general. It operates on sensor data containing noise and inaccuracies and produces a statistically optimal estimate of variables such as velocity, position, and orientation. With suitable parameters, even multiple contradicting sensors or measurements can improve the overall filter accuracy, therefore it is best used with additional sensors such as odometry [3], strategically placed RFID tags [16], rolling-shutter cameras [11], GPS [5], and ultrasound rangefinders [22]. The Kalman filter itself is well covered in [19,20], however, understanding of this paper does not require its deeper knowledge. Other examples of probabilistic model methods include unscented and extended Kalman filters, particle filters [12], and multi-model techniques [21]. Nonetheless, there also exist non-probabilistic model methods, such as human indoor navigation based on walking style utilizing fuzzy logic [10].

As we want to track the motion of smartphones, which can be moved in all directions and arbitrarily rotated, no reasonably strong model seems to be available. Therefore we decided to implement a straightforward non-model dead-reckoning method based on simple physics and linear algebra. To eliminate some kinds of inaccuracies, such as sensor drift, we propose a novel stabilization routine based on the fact that gravity and magnetic field keep pointing the same direction no matter the orientation and position of the device.

Our work might resemble the work by Neto *et al.* [14], which uses accelerometer, gyroscope, and magnetometer to track the position of a human hand during a common pick-and-place task. To eliminate the accelerometer inaccuracies, Neto *et al.* use the accelerometer data only when there is a significant motion and suspend the process when the hand stands still. We have improved the method by using the standstill moments to not only suspend the process but also to correct the supposed orientation of the device. Similar methods exist [4,6,16], however, they seem to exploit the fact that the object of interest moves on a horizontal plane whereas our approach is applicable to any 3D motion.

In Sect. 2, we briefly present the sensor technology and its problems. In Sect. 3, we thoroughly describe the sensor fusion procedure, first as a theoretical model and second as an outline of a practical implementation. In Sect. 4, we explain the proposed stabilization method in a step-by-step manner. In Sect. 5, all the presented techniques are evaluated in a variety of experiments using two common smartphones. Finally, in Sect. 6, our results are summarized.

2   Background on Sensors

The most widely used technology of smartphone sensors is called micro-electro-mechanical systems (usually denoted as MEMS). The size of these sensors is in the order of micrometers ($10^{-6}\,m$) and the previously mentioned triple of an accelerometer, a gyroscope, and a magnetometer might be manufactured on a single chip called inertial measurement unit (IMU). The low-cost alternatives of such chips mounted in smartphones are able to produce up to hundreds of readings per second.

The minimal requirements for smartphone sensors are low because they are almost exclusively used for detecting the orientation of the device and not its position. The orientation is afterwards used in games, mobile applications supporting both landscape and portrait view etc.

2.1 Noise and Bias

The sensors are affected by various sources of noise and bias. A thorough discussion of the sources of accelerometer noise and evaluation of the corresponding filters can be found in work by Khosla *et al.* [8]. The authors collected data from a flying rocket and during off-line data processing, they applied various filters to estimate the impact of individual noise natures. Conclusions are, that most significant sources of noise include bias (i.e., permanent misalignment of the sensor) and improper mounting. Unfortunately, the non-linearity and influence of the temperature on the accelerometer accuracy is not discussed.

It should be noted that there are contradicting opinions on whether smoothing of the accelerometer signal by, for example, Butterworth filter improves the tracking accuracy or not. In works by Baranski *et al.* [2] and Gusenbauer *et al.* [5], both focused on pedestrian navigation, the filter shows promising results. On the other hand, Khosla *et al.* [8], focused on localization of a rocket, demonstrated all but a neglegible impact of the filter on the overall accuracy.

Similar discussion of the various natures of gyroscope noise can be found in [1,3,17]. All the referred works agree on the fact that the gyroscope drift and accuracy is a strong function of temperature. Shiau *et al.* [17] use artificial neural networks to learn and compensate the temperature effect. Chung *et al.* [3], use analytical methods to estimate the non-linearity and temperature effects by higher order polynomials. Both achieve significant improvement over non-compensated data.

The magnetometer appears to be the least reliable sensor of all the three. When the sensor is moving close to, for instance, a Wi-Fi receiver, a mobile phone, or a large metal object, the magnetic field is significantly unstable. This interference can be at least partially eliminated by proper shielding or filtering [1,4].

We are focused on short-term tracking only, therefore we have not dealt with most of the mentioned problems. It was, however, neccessary to calibrate the magnetometer right before experimentation using the procedure provided by its manufacturer[1].

3 Sensor Fusion

In this section, we describe the process of fusing the sensor data to get the position of the device. The sequence of positions with their corresponding timestamps will specify the device movement path.

---

[1] In our case, the Android OS requires launching an application that uses the magnetometer and rotating the device in the "figure 8 pattern".

Before we begin, we have to define two coordinate systems we will be working with. The world frame of reference (world FoR) represents a fixed coordinate system the device was in at the very beginning of the process. The device frame of reference (device FoR), on the other side, is fixed to the device and rotates with it during its motion. Comparison of the two systems is depicted in Fig. 1. The data produced by the sensors are always relative to the device FoR, because the sensors are mounted to the smartphone case. Additionally, we will assume that at the beginning the device was standing still, i.e., the only force measured by the accelerometer in time 0 was gravity.

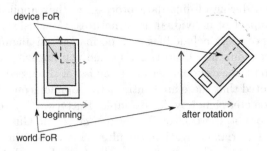

Fig. 1. World and device frames of reference.

The data produced by the sensors will be defined as follows:

- **Accelerometer data**, $acc(t) : \mathbb{R} \to \mathbb{R}^3$ specifies the acceleration vector in ms^{-2} in time t including the gravity force. Additionally, $acc(0)$ denotes gravity only.
- **Gyroscope data**, $gyro(t) : \mathbb{R} \to \mathbb{R}^3$ specifies the rotation rates (i.e., angular speeds) in $rad\ s^{-1}$ around the three coordinate axes x, y, and z in time t.
- **Magnetometer data**, $mag(t) : \mathbb{R} \to \mathbb{R}^3$ specifies the magnetic field strength in μT along the three coordinate axes in time t.

Throughout the paper, we use integration on vector functions. The result of such operation is again a vector function where the integration is performed piecewise as shown in Formula 1.

$$f : \mathbb{R} \to \mathbb{R}^3$$
$$f(x) = \langle f_1(x), f_2(x), f_3(x) \rangle$$
$$\int f(x)\mathrm{d}x = \langle \int f_1(x)\mathrm{d}x, \int f_2(x)\mathrm{d}x, \int f_3(x)\mathrm{d}x \rangle \qquad (1)$$

3.1 Theoretical Model

We will begin with the simplest possible model, where the device is not rotating during its motion and the sensors are perfectly accurate and provide continuous data. Because the orientation of the device does not change, the device FoR will have the same orientation as the world FoR during the entire motion. Therefore, we can process the sensor data as if they were relative to the world FoR.

Let us remind some basic physics. Velocity is defined as derivative of position with respect to time (Formula 2) and acceleration is defined as derivative of velocity with respect to time (Formula 3).

$$\text{linacc} : \mathbb{R} \to \mathbb{R}^3 \text{ acceleration in time } t \text{ without gravity}$$

$$\text{vel} : \mathbb{R} \to \mathbb{R}^3 \text{ velocity in time } t$$

$$\text{pos} : \mathbb{R} \to \mathbb{R}^3 \text{ position in time } t$$

$$\text{vel}(t) = \frac{\partial \text{pos}(t)}{\partial t} \tag{2}$$

$$\text{linacc}(t) = \frac{\partial \text{vel}(t)}{\partial t} \tag{3}$$

However, in our case, the only known variable is the acceleration, thus we will use the definition the other way around. That is, the velocity is the integral of acceleration (Formula 4) and the position is the integral of velocity (Formula 5).

$$\text{vel}(t) = \int_0^t \text{linacc}(u)\mathrm{d}u \tag{4}$$

$$\text{pos}(t) = \int_0^t \text{vel}(u)\mathrm{d}u \tag{5}$$

Note that the accelerometer sensor also measures gravity which has to be removed before the sensor data can be used in the formulas above. We have assumed that the device stands still at the beginning, thus the gravity can be denoted as acc(0). By putting velocity Formula 4 and position Formula 5 together and subtracting the gravity from the accelerometer data (Formula 6) we can express the position of the device using only the data from the accelerometer (Formula 7).

$$\text{linacc}(t) = \text{acc}(t) - \text{acc}(0) \tag{6}$$

$$\text{pos}(t) = \int_0^t \int_0^t (\text{acc}(u) - \text{acc}(0))\,\mathrm{d}^2 u \tag{7}$$

Unfortunately, once we take the rotation of the device into account, the device FoR will rotate with the device, thus accelerometer data from different times will be relative to different coordinate systems. Therefore, the data have to be converted to the world FoR and only after the conversion we can integrate the transformed data the same way we have done in Formula 7. To be able to calculate this conversion, we need to know the orientation of the device.

Orientation. Before we define our representation of the orientation, we have to define a 3D rotation matrix [13]. The 3D rotation matrix is used to represent and perform arbitrary rotation in 3D space. If we have a rotation matrix $A \in \mathbb{R}^{3 \times 3}$ and we want to apply the rotation it represents to a vector $u \in \mathbb{R}^3$, we can simply pre-multiply the vector by the matrix, i.e., Au. The construction of such matrix is, however, a little bit more difficult.

To make the construction easier, we will introduce a known Formula 8 for the rotation matrix representing rotation around an arbitrary axis through an arbitrary angle [13]. For our purposes a slightly simplified version where the axis is a unit vector is sufficient. This formula hardly has an intuitive explanation. However, the procedure that derives it is not that difficult and is clearly explained in [13].

$$R : \mathbb{R}^3 \times \mathbb{R} \to \mathbb{R}^{3 \times 3}$$

$$v \in \mathbb{R}^3 \text{ where } v = <a, b, c> \text{ and } \sqrt{a^2 + b^2 + c^2} = 1$$

$R(v, \theta)$ is a rotation matrix through the angle θ around the unit vector v

$$R(\langle a, b, c \rangle, \theta) = \begin{pmatrix} a^2 + (1 - a^2)\cos(\theta) & ab(1 - \cos(\theta)) - c\sin(\theta) & ac(1 - \cos(\theta)) + b\sin(\theta) \\ ab(1 - \cos(\theta)) + c\sin(\theta) & b^2 + (1 - b^2)\cos(\theta) & bc(1 - \cos(\theta)) - a\sin(\theta) \\ ac(1 - \cos(\theta)) - b\sin(\theta) & bc(1 - \cos(\theta)) + a\sin(\theta) & c^2 + (1 - c^2)\cos(\theta) \end{pmatrix}$$

$$(8)$$

Now, we can define the orientation of the device as the rotation matrix representing the rotation of the device FoR relative to the world FoR (i.e., relative to the initial orientation). The rest of this section describes how to construct such a matrix using the gyroscope data.

It might be tempting to integrate the raw gyroscope data (i.e., angular speeds) the same way we have integrated the accelerometer as shown in Formula 9.

$$\int_0^t \text{gyro}(u)\mathrm{d}u = ? \tag{9}$$

The result of such integration are three rotation angles around the axes x, y and z representing the rotation of the device from the beginning of the process. Unfortunately, those three angles just by themselves do not provide sufficient information to reproduce the orientation of the device. Even the fact, that rotation composition is not commutative in the 3D space (as depicted in Fig. 2), might give us multiple orientations corresponding to the same three rotation angles. Therefore the result of such integration is effectively useless.

We will solve this problem by sampling the gyroscope data into time intervals, whose duration is getting to zero. We may presume that during each such a short time interval the rotation speed was constant. This presumption allows us to construct rotation matrices representing the rotation of the device during each of these intervals. Finally, we can simply multiply all those matrices to create a matrix representing the rotation from the beginning to the time t as depicted in Fig. 3. This composed matrix will be the orientation matrix.

Let us describe the construction of the orientation matrix in detail. At first, we need the rotation angles representing rotation during a time interval (t_1, t_2). We can calculate these angles by integrating the gyroscope data and we will

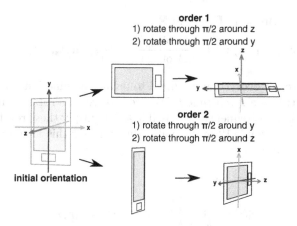

Fig. 2. Counterexample for rotation commutativity in 3D

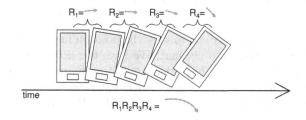

Fig. 3. Rotation sampling

denote this vector of rotation angles by the function $\Delta\mathrm{rot}_{\mathrm{ang}}(t_1, t_2)$ defined in Formula 10.

$$\Delta\mathrm{rot}_{\mathrm{ang}} : \mathbb{R} \times \mathbb{R} \to \mathbb{R}^3$$

$$\Delta\mathrm{rot}_{\mathrm{ang}}(t_1, t_2) := \int_{t_1}^{t_2} \mathrm{gyro}(t)\mathrm{d}t \qquad (10)$$

To convert this vector to a rotation matrix, we will use Formula 8. However, what angle and what axis should we use? Presuming a short time interval, the rotation speed might be considered to be constant. Therefore, the rotation around the coordinate axes x, y and z by the angles α, β and γ is the very same as the rotation around the vector $v =< \alpha, \beta, \gamma >$ through the angle $||v||$. Additionally, Formula 8 assumes a unit vector, thus we have to normalize the vector v to a unit vector. It can be achieved by dividing it by its own size, i.e., $v_{norm} = \frac{v}{||v||}$. Using these observations and substituting the $\Delta\mathrm{rot}_{\mathrm{ang}}(t_1, t_2)$ to the rotation matrix Formula 8, we can convert the function $\Delta\mathrm{rot}_{\mathrm{ang}}(t_1, t_2)$ returning a vector to a function $\Delta\mathrm{rot}_{\mathrm{mat}}(t_1, t_2)$ returning a matrix. This conversion is defined in Formula 11.

$$\Delta\text{rot}_{\text{mat}} : \mathbb{R} \times \mathbb{R} \to \mathbb{R}^{3\times3}$$

$$\Delta\text{rot}_{\text{mat}}(t_1, t_2) := R\left(\frac{\Delta\text{rot}_{\text{ang}}(t_1, t_2)}{||\Delta\text{rot}_{\text{ang}}(t_1, t_2)||}, ||\Delta\text{rot}_{\text{ang}}(t_1, t_2)||\right) \tag{11}$$

Now we have got everything required to define the function that returns the orientation matrix in a given time t. We need to create a rotation matrix out of the gyroscope data as frequently as possible and multiply these rotation matrices up to the time t. Formula 12 mathematically expresses this idea and defines the orientation function.

$$\text{ori} : \mathbb{R} \to \mathbb{R}^{3\times3}$$

$$\text{ori}(t) := \lim_{h\to0} \prod_{i=1}^{\lfloor t/h \rfloor} \Delta\text{rot}_{\text{mat}}((i-1)h, ih) \tag{12}$$

where h is the duration between two subsequent samples.

The Final Formula. Now we can modify the position function from Formula 7 so it takes the orientation into account. We have the accelerometer data relative to the device FoR and we have the orientation matrix of the device FoR. The only thing we have to do is to pre-multiply the accelerometer data by the orientation matrix to convert them to the world FoR. Formula 13 defines this modified version of the position function.

$$\text{pos} : \mathbb{R} \to \mathbb{R}^3$$

$$\text{pos}(t) := \int_0^t \int_0^t (\text{ori}(u)\text{acc}(u) - \text{acc}(0)) \, \mathrm{d}^2u \tag{13}$$

3.2   Practical Approach

The theoretical model can be implemented in a straightforward way or utilized in other algorithms for sensor fusion, such as the previously mentioned Kalman Filter.

The straightforward approach is based on Formula 13 and can be implemented as follows. We will process the gyroscope data and the accelerometer data separately. For each gyroscope reading, we integrate the data, convert them to a rotation matrix, and update the current orientation matrix. For each accelerometer reading, we multiply the data by the current orientation matrix (i.e., we convert the data to the world FoR), remove the gravity, and double integrate the result to calculate the position of the device. This implementation is fast enough to run as an online process without the need for high processing power.

The discrete integration itself might be implemented, for instance, as summation of values or the values can be approximated by a function whose integral can be easily calculated. We, however, recommend using the trapezoidal integration rule [9], as it improves the results significantly [8] and is very easy to implement. The trapezoidal integration is similar to the standard Euler's integration method which approximates a function by rectangles, however, the remaining space between the rectangle and the function is further approximated by a triangle, as depicted in Fig. 4.

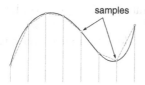

Fig. 4. Trapezoidal integration rule

4 Automated Stabilization

Even though gyroscope data are usually very accurate, the integration introduces drift, partially because of noise and partially because of insufficient sampling rate. Why is it such a problem? Because if the device orientation is just a few degrees off, Earth's gravity is removed from a wrong direction. If it creates a false acceleration of, for example, $0.1\,\mathrm{ms}^{-2}$ then after ten seconds it pulls the device $10\,\mathrm{m}$ off (calculation in Formula 14).

$$\int_0^{10} \int_0^{10} 0.1\mathrm{d}^2t = 10 \tag{14}$$

Fortunately, the Earth's gravity and magnetic field point a constant direction no matter the orientation and position of the device. We will use this property whenever the device is at rest[2], to adjust the orientation by comparing gravity and magnetic field vectors measured at the beginning with the current values of accelerometer and magnetometer.

4.1 Stillness Detection

The device is at rest, when it does not rotate and the only force measured by the accelerometer is gravity. To detect such a moment, we will utilize the high sensitivity of the gyroscope and implement something called an *angular rate energy detector* [18]. The implementation is as follows. Whenever squared magnitudes of the gyroscope data stay below a specified threshold α during a specified time window of length W, we will consider the device to be still (Formula 15). The selection of the threshold and the size of the time window

---

[2] The technique of updating the stored values when the device is at rest is usually called zero-velocity update [18].

depends on the quality of the sensor and various other aspects, such as whether the device lays on a table or is held in a shaking hand.

$$\text{still}(t) \Leftrightarrow \frac{1}{W} \int_{t}^{t+W} \|\text{gyro}(u)\|^2 du < \alpha \tag{15}$$

In theory, this technique would detect stillness, for instance, while moving in a straight line at a constant speed. In practice, however, it is very difficult to move the device in a way the gyroscope data would seem still. For a thorough discussion on various stillness detectors please refer to [18].

4.2 Zero Velocity

Even when we stop the motion and the device is at rest, the drift could cause that acceleration is not integrated to zero. It can be a serious problem because the integrated acceleration represents velocity and thus the algorithm behaves as if the device was moving even though it rests in place as depicted in Fig. 5. Therefore, it is very important to set the supposed velocity to zero whenever the device stands still.

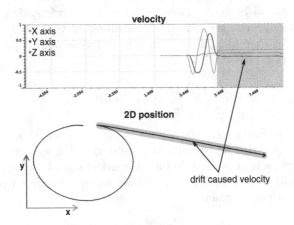

Fig. 5. Device is moved in a shape of a circle and then put to rest. The integrated false velocity keeps dragging the supposed position off.

4.3 Gravity Fix

When the device is still, the current acceleration vector in the world FoR should match the gravity vector measured at the beginning. If not, we will adjust the stored orientation to make it true as seen in Fig. 6.

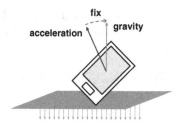

Fig. 6. Matching the acceleration to the gravity vector

Let's assume that the device is standing still and we have the following data:

- $gra \in \mathbb{R}^3$ is the gravity measured at the beginning.
- $acc \in \mathbb{R}^3$ is the vector currently measured by the accelerometer, including gravity. Since the device is still, it is nothing but the gravity in the device FoR.
- $ori \in \mathbb{R}^{3\times3}$ is the current orientation matrix.

Then we can fix the orientation drift in two steps:

1. Create a rotation matrix $fix \in \mathbb{R}^{3\times3}$ that rotates the vector $ori \cdot acc$ (i.e., acceleration in the world FoR) to match the vector gra (i.e., acceleration at the beginning). Formula 16 expresses this idea mathematically.

$$fix \cdot ori \cdot acc = gra \tag{16}$$

But how does a matrix that rotates a vector $a \in \mathbb{R}^3$ to match a vector $b \in \mathbb{R}^3$ look like? We will use the definition of the rotation matrix around an arbitrary unit vector through an arbitrary angle (Formula 8), but we need to find the vector to rotate around and the angle to rotate through. A very simple way of finding both is to use a known Formula 17 for cross product of two vectors [9]. Visual representation of the formula is depicted in Fig. 7.

$$a, b \in \mathbb{R}^3$$
$$\theta \text{ is the angle between } a \text{ and } b$$
$$n \text{ is a unit vector perpendicular to the plane}$$
$$\text{generated by } a \text{ and } b$$
$$a \times b = \|a\|\|b\|n\sin\theta \tag{17}$$

Having the definition of the cross product, it is not difficult to calculate the vector and the angle to be substituted into the definition of the rotation matrix (8). The result is a matrix that rotates a vector a to match a vector b, as shown in Formula 18.

$$R_{match}(a,b) := R\left(\frac{a \times b}{\|a \times b\|}, \arcsin\left(\frac{\|a \times b\|}{\|a\|\|b\|}\right)\right) \tag{18}$$

Having Formula 18, we can simply substitute appropriate vectors $ori \cdot acc$ and gra for the a and b to define the matrix fix mentioned in Formula 16. The result is shown in Formula 19.

$$fix := R_{match}(ori \cdot acc, gra) \qquad (19)$$

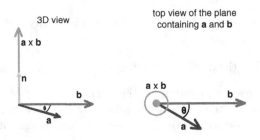

Fig. 7. Cross product visual representation

2. Pre-multiply the orientation matrix by the fix.

It should be mentioned that the magnitude of the Earth's gravity ($\approx 9.81 \text{ms}^{-2}$) should never be considered to be a constant, since the accelerometer sensitivity varies with the sensor orientation relative to the measured force. For instance, the devices evaluated in our experiment exhibited 1 - 1.5 ms^{-2} difference in the Earth's gravity measurement when the device is simply turned over.

4.4   Magnetic Field Fix

Even when the orientation of the device is fixed using the gravity vector, it still remains ambiguous as demonstrated in Fig. 8. To eliminate this ambiguity, we will use the magnetometer sensor. It might be tempting to repeat the same steps as we have done with the gravity fix, but this time with the magnetic field. Such an approach, however, could break the previous gravity fix and alter the orientation matrix in a way that the accelerometer data in the world FoR would not perfectly match the gravity measured at the beginning. In such a case, the gravity would again be removed from a wrong direction and that, as we have previously calculated, is a serious flaw. Therefore, after this process of fixing the orientation by magnetic field, we still require the acceleration vector in the world FoR to point the very same direction as the gravity.

The only way of adjusting the orientation matrix with the persistency of the accelerometer vector in the world FoR, is to perform the rotation around the accelerometer vector itself. To have the fix as accurate as possible at the same time, we will choose the rotation angle minimizing the distance between the current magnetic field vector in the world FoR and the magnetic field vector

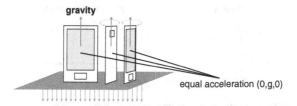

Fig. 8. The device measures the same acceleration in multiple orientations

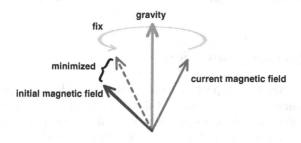

Fig. 9. Rotating around the gravity vector so that the initial and current magnetic vectors are as close as possible

measured at the beginning. The idea is depicted in Fig. 9, where the accelerometer vector in the world FoR is denoted as gravity as they are equal, thanks to the previously described gravity fix.

Such a fixing matrix can by constructed using just the tools we already have. Let's assume that the device is standing still, we have already fixed the orientation using gravity, and we have the following data:

- $mag_b \in \mathbb{R}^3$ is the magnetic field measured at the beginning.
- $mag_c \in \mathbb{R}^3$ is the vector currently measured by the magnetometer.
- $gra \in \mathbb{R}^3$ is the gravity measured at the beginning and the accelerometer vector in the world FoR at the same time.
- $ori \in \mathbb{R}^{3 \times 3}$ is the current orientation matrix.

The steps to fix the orientation are as follows:

1. Project the mag_b and mag_c vectors in the world FoR to the plane perpendicular to the gravity vector[3]. Denote the results as $pmag_b$ and $pmag_c$. It is equal to viewing the situation from such position that the gravity vector points right towards us, as demonstrated in Fig. 10.
2. Create a rotation matrix fix that rotates the vector $pmag_c$ to the vector $pmag_b$. We can observe that the rotation matrix has to represent a rotation around the gravity vector.
3. Pre-multiply the orientation by the fix.

---

[3] We can achieve the projetion by creating a rotation matrix that rotates the gravity vector to the z axis, then rotate the mag_b and $ori \cdot mag_c$ vectors using this matrix, set their z coordinate to zero and rotate them back.

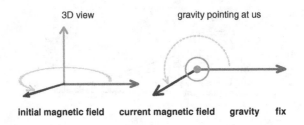

initial magnetic field   current magnetic field   gravity   fix

Fig. 10. The vectors from Fig. 9 after projection to the plane perpendicular to the gravity

5   Experimental Evaluation

We have implemented a computer software, which provides a user-friendly interface for processing and visualization of data produced by accelerometer, gyroscope, and magnetometer sensors (a screenshot is depicted in Fig. 11). The fusion method is based on the straightforward algorithm from the section Practical Approach and enhanced by the automated stabilization. We will perform a series of experiments with this software to demonstrate the properties of the algorithm.

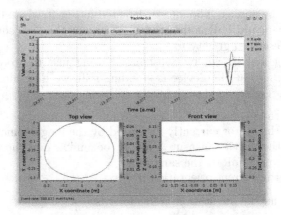

Fig. 11. TrackMe GUI screenshot

The situation will always be visualized from two angles, as demonstrated in Fig. 12. The top view observes the device from the direction of the z axis and the front view observes the device from the direction of the y axis. The color of each tracepoint will denote the distance from the viewer, with red being the closest and purple being the furthest. The entire spectrum is depicted in Fig. 13.

The first experiment will be performed on two different smartphones - Huawei Honor U8660 and Samsung Galaxy S III. We have chosen these particular devices

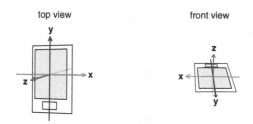

Fig. 12. Two views of a smartphone on a table

Fig. 13. Distance spectrum

for their significant difference in price and performance. Table 1 gives a comparison of sensor reading rates for both smartphones.

During the first experiment, the device will lay on a table and we will move it in the shape of a circle. The result is depicted in Fig. 14. The movement took less than three seconds and the result is surprisingly accurate. Especially for the Galaxy phone, the shape is smooth from both views. The Honor phone suffers from lower sensor reading rate and the motion path slightly drifts. From now on, we will perform the experiments with the Galaxy phone only.

Let us prolong the motion duration and draw the same circle three times in a row. The result drawn in Fig. 15a demonstrates that with longer motion the shape can no more be recognized because of the gyroscope drift and consequent false acceleration. The first circle is clearly visible but even the next one is off by a diameter. The reason is, that we have not given the stabilization system a chance to fix the drift and the result would actually be the same even if the stabilization would not be implemented at all.

To see the benefits of the automatic stabilization, we will insert a small pause (cca. one second) after each circle. During this pause, the software detects stillness and updates the orientation matrix. Figure 15b shows the same three circles with two pauses in between. The motion took twelve seconds and the Galaxy phone, again, draws a smooth and accurate picture. It has all the circles clearly visible and the starting position is almost the same as the ending position.

Table 1. Number of readings per second

	Samsung Galaxy S III	Huawei Honor U8660
Accelerometer	105	52
Gyroscope	206	61
Magnetometer	102	95
sum	**413**	**208**

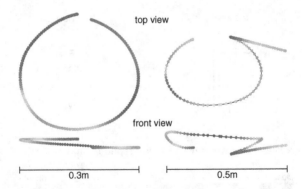

Fig. 14. Circle shape - 30 cm in diameter - Galaxy S III (left) and Huawei Honor (right)

To compare this result to the case where the stabilization system is turned off, we have performed the same experiment once again, but we have disabled all the corrections introduced in the section Automatic Stabilization. The drawing is demonstrated in Fig. 15c. Not surprisingly, the results are even worse than in the experiment without pauses (as shown in Fig. 15a), because the double integration of false acceleration introduces a drift whose strength rises quadratically with time. The last circle was drawn after twelve seconds of motion and ended up as nothing but a little curve in a fast nonexistent movement.

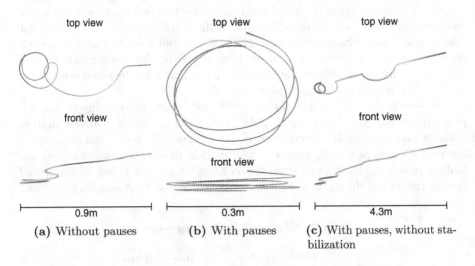

(a) Without pauses   (b) With pauses   (c) With pauses, without stabilization

Fig. 15. Three circles in a row with Samsung Galaxy S III

The last motion will be a walk. The author will hold the phone in his hand, will watch its display and will walk forward (i.e., in the direction of the y axis)

through a seven metres long horizontal path. The result is depicted in Fig. 16a. The phone suffers from a strong gyroscope drift and the path is far from reality.

We will perform the same trick as with the circles and insert a small pause after each two steps. The result is depicted in Fig. 16b. The result has significantly improved, thanks to the stabilization system, and even individual steps leave a trace. Figure 16c shows the real path for comparison.

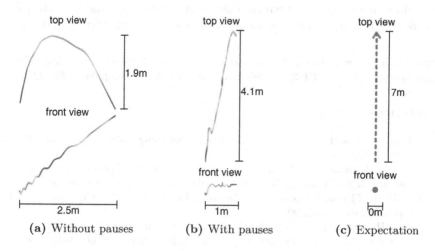

(a) Without pauses   (b) With pauses   (c) Expectation

Fig. 16. Walk - 7 m long - Samsung Galaxy S III

6 Conclusion and Future Work

In this paper, we presented a simple dead-reckoning method for tracking device movement and orientation using accelerometer, gyroscope, and magnetometer. A crucial role in our system plays a novel algorithm for correction of the supposed orientation whenever the device is at rest. We have evaluated the proposed methods in various experiments using two common smartphones.

We deliberately used a non-model method of tracking, which does not assume any knowledge about expected movement of the device. Exploiting some information about expected movements, for example using a Kalman filter, would undoubtedly be the way to further improve accuracy. Even without such information, minor improvements might be achieved by analyzing and eliminating sensor specific noise prior to the data fusion as discussed in Sect. 2.1.

Despite presence of the mentioned inertial sensors in modern electronics, these low-cost sensors are usually not accurate enough to be used for motion tracking. In this paper, we demonstrated that with some sensor data fusion we could track 3D motion with reasonable error for a couple of seconds, which might be useful for, e.g., gesture recognition. The proposed stabilization method can further extend this time, however, it requires the device to stop every few seconds. This requirement might be fulfilled, for instance, with shoe mounted systems such as [15,16,22], where the stabilization algorithm could be reliably executed when the shoe touches the ground. The open question is whether similar stabilization can be implemented without the necessity to stop the device.

In spite of the fact that the inertial sensors do not provide sufficient tracking information by themselves, they can be very useful when fused with additional sensors. For instance, excelent results are demonstrated in the work by Mingyang Li *et al.* [11], where data from smartphone rolling-shutter camera were fused with data from inertial measurement unit using the extended Kalman filter. The authors were able to retain high accuracy even after ten minutes of walking.

Acknowledgements. Research was partially supported by the Czech Science Foundation under the project P103-15-19877S and by SVV under the project 260 224.

References

1. Abbott, H., Powell, D.: Land-vehicle navigation using GPS. Proc. IEEE **87**(1), 145–162 (1999)
2. Barański, P., Bujacz, M., Strumillo, P.: Dead reckoning navigation: supplementing pedestrian GPS with an accelerometer-based pedometer and an electronic compass. In: Society of Photo-Optical Instrumentation Engineers (SPIE) Conference Series, vol. 7502, p. 16, June 2009
3. Chung, H., Ojeda, L., Borenstein, J.: Accurate mobile robot dead-reckoning with a precision-calibrated fiber-optic gyroscope. IEEE Trans. Robot. Autom. **17**(1), 80–84 (2001)
4. Fang, L., Antsaklis, P., Montestruque, L., McMickell, M., Lemmon, M., Sun, Y., Fang, H., Koutroulis, I., Haenggi, M., Xie, M., Xie, X.: Design of a wireless assisted pedestrian dead reckoning system - the NavMote experience. IEEE Trans. Instrum. Meas. **54**(6), 2342–2358 (2005)
5. Gusenbauer, D., Isert, C., Krosche, J.: Self-contained indoor positioning on off-the-shelf mobile devices. In: International Conference on Indoor Positioning and Indoor Navigation (IPIN), pp. 1–9, September 2010
6. Jimenez, A., Seco, F., Prieto, J., Guevara, J.: Indoor pedestrian navigation using an INS/EKF framework for yaw drift reduction and a foot-mounted IMU. In: 7th Workshop on Positioning Navigation and Communication (WPNC), pp. 135–143, March 2010
7. Kalman, R.E.: A new approach to linear filtering and prediction problems. Trans. ASME-J. Basic Eng. **82**(Series D), 35–45 (1960)
8. Khosla, P., Khanna, R., Sood, S.: Quantification and mitigation of errors in the inertial measurements of distance. MAPAN **30**(1), 49–57 (2015). http://dx.doi.org/10.1007/s12647-014-0115-z
9. Kreyszig, E.: Advanced Engineering Mathematics, 8th edn. Wiley, New York (1999)
10. Lee, S.W., Mase, K.: Activity and location recognition using wearable sensors. IEEE Pervasive Comput. **1**(3), 24–32 (2002)
11. Li, M., Kim, B.H., Mourikis, A.: Real-time motion tracking on a cellphone using inertial sensing and a rolling-shutter camera. In: IEEE International Conference on Robotics and Automation (ICRA), pp. 4712–4719, May 2013
12. Liu, M., Wang, H., Guo, Q., Jiang, X.: Research on particle filter based geomagnetic aided inertial navigation algorithm. In: 3rd International Symposium on Systems and Control in Aeronautics and Astronautics (ISSCAA), pp. 1023–1026, June 2010

13. Murray, G.: Rotation about an arbitrary axis in 3 dimensions (2013). http://inside. mines.edu/fs_home/gmurray/ArbitraryAxisRotation/ArbitraryAxisRotation.pdf. Accessed 24 September 2014

14. Neto, P., Norberto Pires, J., Moreira, A.: 3-D position estimation from inertial sensing: minimizing the error from the process of double integration of accelerations. In: 39th Annual Conference of the IEEE Industrial Electronics Society (IECON), pp. 4026–4031, November 2013

15. Ojeda, L., Borenstein, J.: Personal dead-reckoning system for GPS-denied environments. In: IEEE International Workshop on Safety, Security and Rescue Robotics (SSRR), pp. 1–6, September 2007

16. Ruiz, A., Granja, F., Honorato, P.J., Rosas, J.: Accurate pedestrian indoor navigation by tightly coupling foot-mounted IMU and RFID measurements. IEEE Trans. Instrum. Meas. **61**(1), 178–189 (2012)

17. Shiau, J.K., Huang, C.X., Chang, M.Y., et al.: Noise characteristics of MEMS gyros null drift and temperature compensation. Appl. Sci. Eng **15**(3), 239–246 (2012)

18. Skog, I., Handel, P., Nilsson, J.O., Rantakokko, J.: Zero-velocity detection - an algorithm evaluation. IEEE Trans. Biomed. Eng. **57**(11), 2657–2666 (2010)

19. Stuart, R., Norvig, P.: Artificial Intelligence: A Modern Approach, 3rd edn. Prentice Hall, New York (2010)

20. Thrun, S., Burgard, W., Fox, D.: Probabilistic Robotics (Intelligent Robotics and Autonomous Agents). The MIT Press, Cambridge (2005)

21. Toledo-Moreo, R., Zamora-Izquierdo, M., Gomez-Skarmeta, A.: IMM-EKF based road vehicle navigation with low cost GPS/INS. In: IEEE International Conference on Multisensor Fusion and Integration for Intelligent Systems, pp. 433–438, September 2006

22. Weenk, D., Roetenberg, D., van Beijnum, B., Hermens, H., Veltink, P.: Ambulatory estimation of relative foot positions by fusing ultrasound and inertial sensor data. IEEE Trans. Neural Syst. Rehabil. Eng. **23**(5), 817–826 (2015)

Conditional Colored Petri Net for Modelling an Automated GDM System

Joselito Medina-Marín[1], Virgilio López-Morales[2]([⊠]), and Oleksandr Karelin[1]

[1] Centro de Investigación Avanzada En Ingeniería Industrial,
Univ. Aut. Edo. Hidalgo, Carr. Pachuca Tulancingo Km. 4.5,
42184 Mineral Reforma, HGO, Mexico
[2] Centro de Investigación En Tecnologías de Información Y Sistemas,
Univ. Aut. Edo. Hidalgo, Carr. Pachuca Tulancingo Km. 4.5,
42184 Mineral Reforma, HGO, Mexico
virgilio@uaeh.edu.mx

Abstract. When a house/building is able to perceive the environmental conditions and regulate or control a priori internal/external parameters accordingly, we said that it has an intelligent behavior. A Smart House/Building (SH) is a home-like environment which is able to perceive the environmental conditions, administrative state and users' inputs in order to regulate, control or perform various tasks for achieving desired levels of comfort. Consequently a SH requires a distributed set of sensors, actuators and experts' knowledge bases which should be specialized for specific tasks or problems domains. In this framework a Group Decision Making (GDM) system becomes paramount to choose the best decision among the different experts' knowledge bases in order to supervise or control the security, administrative variables and users' components. In this paper a Conditional Colored Petri Net (CCPN) is shown to be an useful technique to model and validate concurrency and distribution among the different experts and components of our whole system. A CCPN is jointly used with a group decision making (GDM) system to solve possible nondeterminism and ambiguity in the real time control environment of a SH when two or more experts might have different advice/conclusions for a particular combination of events. In this paper a set of experts' knowledge bases are modelled and validated trough CCPN working with a GDM system. A physical example for SH supervision illustrates our approach.

Keywords: Group decision making · Petri nets · Supervision · Concurrency

1 Introduction

Home Automation, Smart Home, Intelligent House/Buildings or simply Domotics are the various labels of a trend line: An automated environment to perform several routine human tasks in an interconnected, intelligent and controlled setting.

© Springer International Publishing Switzerland 2015
O. Pichardo Lagunas et al. (Eds.): MICAI 2015, Part II, LNAI 9414, pp. 602–616, 2015.
DOI: 10.1007/978-3-319-27101-9_46

A Smart Home (SH) can be though as a home-like environment provided with advances services for its users. Technological developments made possible the idea of an intelligent space where devices and appliances can be enhanced with sensors to gather information about SH conditions, and in some cases, an action can be done independently of human intervention Cf. [3,13,15].

There exist a wide range of sensors and actuators applied in intelligent environments for providing support to disabled users (e.g. wheelchairs, rehabilitation robotics, specialized interfaces, etc.) or visually/hearing impaired subjects (e.g. tactile screens, teletype machines, etc.); for monitoring the lifestyle of inhabitants (e.g. physiological signs, heart rate, temperature, blood pressure, etc.); for delivering therapy (e.g. drugs delivery, hormone delivery, tremor suppression, etc.); or for being comfortable in the SH (e.g. intelligent households devices - dishwasher machine, refrigerator; smart objects - mailboxes, mirrors; smart leisure equipment - TV, home cinema programs; intelligent environmental control equipments - windows and doors) [2].

There are three major development axes of SH applications [5]:

1. Services provided by automated systems to human interaction and training the system via advance pattern recognition techniques for recognizing their actions, behaviours and health conditions,
2. Multi media captured within the smart homes with storing and retrieving services at different levels,
3. Surveillance and security services to analyze information and to protect the home and/or the resident from natural and anthropogenic hazards. In this area a special type of SH can help the occupant to reduce energy consumption by monitoring and controlling the devices and rescheduling their operating time according to the energy demand and supply.

Actually, according to what is to be automated and supervised, several expert knowledge bases on different domains need to be managed. When a set of experts in several areas (for instance surveillance security, energy cost efficiency, degraded system control, comfort, etc.) are concerned about solving a given problem in SH, various advice can be synthesized from a set of experts. Furthermore, different or completely opposed conclusions could be drawn from similar events involving various criteria and alternatives when a set of requirements are fulfilled. In this framework a Group Decision Making (GDM) system becomes paramount to choose the best decision among the different experts' knowledge bases in order to supervise or control the security, administrative, variables and users' components.

Then GDM is an important tool for evaluating and decision making. A well known method called the Analytic Hierarchy Process (AHP) provides an useful framework to drive GDM techniques via pairwise comparison matrices or Multiplicative Preference Relation (MPR). A MPR is called a subjective judgement matrix, adopted to express decision maker(s) preferences and is composed of judgements between any two criteria components which are declared within a crisp rank, called Saaty's scale $(1/9, 1/8, \cdots, 1/2, 1,2, \cdots, 8, 9)$.

On the other hand, a useful tool to model the set of experts' knowledge expressed in the form of If - Then rules, is a Colored Petri Net (CPN) [6,7] which can also integrate in our framework an interaction protocol among the different experts and various models from their knowledge bases.

In this work, we are proposing a framework based on a PN extension, called Conditional Colored Petri Net (CCPN) [8,9], which includes interaction protocols, knowledge bases, system model, and ambiguities or conflicts resolution. This framework allows the knowledge-based system taking advantage of the PN matrix representation and different analysis tools provided by PN theory. Furthermore, the proposed framework is able to model, simulate, analyze, verify and execute a rule set even in a real environment. All these tasks are carried out in the same framework, and it is not needed a different one for each functionality.

The paper is organized as follows: In Sect. 2 a GDM system is briefly described and the main architecture of our proposal is shown. In Sect. 3 the basis of the CCPN is introduced. In Sect. 3 is introduced the methodology to model and validate the production rules and their interaction with the GDM and CCPN. In Sect. 5 a study case is addressed to illustrate our approach. Finally, in Sect. 6 concluding remarks are stated and perspectives of the future work are given.

2   Group Decision Making and Smart Homes

In order to reach a certain level of consensus and inter operability among different systems (programs, electronics or humans) on the data or knowledge level, an ontology provides basic domain vocabulary to different messages and systems and their relationship among them.

In this case a high level of complexity can be obtained and the understanding of the ontologies and consequently of the coded messages are useful to elaborate the reasoning component that fulfill the objective and targets of the analyzed system. Thus, the whole system could be more complex to deal with their physical and logical structure in a real time framework.

Group Decision Making in this context has mainly two advantages: Synergy and sharing of information. Synergy is the idea that the whole is greater than the sum of its parts. When a group makes a decision collectively, its judgment can be keener than that of any of its members. Through discussion, questioning, and collaboration, group members can identify more complete and robust solutions and recommendations.

Group decisions take into account a broader scope of information since each group member may contribute unique information and expertise which in our case is managed with the knowledge bases. Sharing information can increase understanding, clarify issues, and facilitate movement toward a collective decision based on a GDM system [1].

Many managerial decisions involve consideration of more than one single criterion. Despite the development of GDM, decision support systems (DSS), and group decision support systems (GDSS) that are aimed at helping decision makers address these complex decisions, there is inadequate success in supporting GDM. Problems hindering the success of these systems may be due to their undue complexity, over-reliance on quantitative modelling, and failure to accommodate the dynamic learning needs of the people who use them [10].

In Group Decision Making (GDM), a problem resolution involves the aggregation of individual preferences into a single collective preference [18]. After the aggregation of the preferences, some prioritization methods such as Eigenvalue-based Methods (EM) [16,17], and the Row Geometric Mean Method (RGMM) [4]; are utilized to derive a priority vector to synthesize an ordered collective judgment matrix.

The aim of an automated GDM is to analyze and provide a system based on some models and numerical algorithms to make the best decision. Thus, once expert decision makers have proposed a set of MPRs considering different scenarios and their respective conclusions and or actions, a reliable priority vector characterizing the best decision among the experts[1] can be generated by the system. In this manner, decision making system could give a reliable decision to be implemented in a SH based on certain levels of consistency and group consensus. This can be done despite the inherent uncertainty and imprecision while accomplishing some a priori decision targets, rules and advice given by the current framework.

Since a drawback of a SH is the low level of standardization of the inter-connectivity among household appliances and consumer electronics, a system aiming to the management and regulation of a completely integrated SH, must have different manners for reaching various goals among those appliances and electronics as inter communication, control strategies, multi platform, etc.

Many reasons and technical problems are at the core of these goals: physical layer integration sharing the same platform and parameters is not actually agreed; and at the network layer, several component (routers) are necessary to provide the appropriate addressing and routing over the interconnected ecosystem for the shared information. Finally, there exists various problems also at the application level or the data semantics which range from the heterogeneity until the inter-operability among the relational data in databases which enable ontology reasoning and over digitized information.

In order to have a suitable integration of the different components, control strategies, and autonomy of the whole system, the scheme proposed is depicted in Fig. 1.

In order to reduce the energy consumption in the Smart House and at the same time to follow the instructions of the Customer, we propose a system based on extensive knowledge bases for storing all information needed to achieve the goals of energy efficiency and user comfort. The various different knowledge bases of our system are modelled and represented by CCPN considering at the same time the requested inter-connectivity to the outside world by means of the system based in JAVA which is a multi platform programming language.

The current paper is mainly focused on the description of the extensive knowledge bases, their representation trough the CCPN and the interaction with the

---

[1] i.e. a vector where individual consistency and group consensus respectively have been achieved.

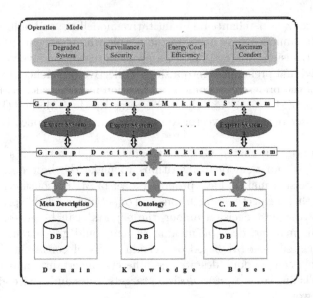

Fig. 1. System scheme.

GDM system. Thus, for further details about a GDM system where the best decision among a set of weighted experts is taken, please refer to [11].

When a conflict is found in the CCPN model among the different conclusions, this information is sent to the GDM system along with a priority vector (experts' weights). The GDM system takes this information (rules and experts involved, operation mode and experts' priority vector) to solve for the best group decision to be taken. This resolution is then sent back to the CCPN system which is then able to break up the deadlock (conflict) and continue to work. Furthermore, the rules priority is updated in a dynamic manner via the set of experts' bases in the GDM system.

3   Modelling and Implementing a CCPN

To define the reactive behavior in a SH, it is feasible to apply Event-Condition-Action rules (ECA rules), commonly used in rule's development of Active Data Base Systems (ADBS).

3.1   Active Databases

An ADBS is an extension of a *passive* DataBase System (DBS) with the capability to specify a reactive behavior. The essential part in an ADBS is the reactive rule definition, where the rule developer specifies how the ADBS will react to the occurrence of events in the DBS.

Currently, ECA rule model is used to define reactive rules and its general representation follows:

on *event*
if *condition*
then *action*

where *event* describes the happening in a specific moment to which the rule must be able to respond. The rule *condition* examines the context of the DB when the event happens. Finally, *action* describes a task that will be carried out if the corresponding *event* has taken place and the evaluation of the *condition* part is true.

An *event* could be a DB operation, i.e. insert or update instructions; a clock event; or external events, i.e. sensors monitoring temperature and sending data to the DB.

Furthermore, an event could be *primitive* or *composite*. A primitive event occurs when only one of the possible events takes place. On the other hand, a composite event is composed of a combination of primitive and/or composite events. Most useful composite events are *disjunction, conjunction, sequence, simultaneous, negation, first, last, history,* and *any* [14].

3.2 Petri Nets Preliminaries

A Petri Net (PN) is a graphical and mathematical modelling tool applied in different areas for modelling Discrete Event Systems (DES). Graphically, a PN is a directed and bipartite graph, which has two types of nodes named places and transitions. Directed arcs connect nodes of different types, either from transitions to places or from places to transitions. Places are represented by circles and transitions are denoted by rectangles.

In order to model the dynamic behavior of systems, a PN includes tokens, i.e., small dots drawn inside places, which are used to indicate event occurrences, or system components availability. Token distribution in the PN is known as *marking*, and it represents the state of the modelled system.

Formally, a PN can be defined as a tuple of 5 elements: a finite set of places P, a finite set of transitions T, a set of arcs F connecting places to transitions an viceversa, a weight function W, and the initial marking M_0 [12].

System behaviors can be modelled with the movement of tokens in the PN (token game animation), indicating the changes of system trough the time. The token game animation is performed according to the following firing rule:

1. A transition t is enabled if every input place of t has at least $w(p,t)$ tokens. $w(p,t)$ is the weight value for the arc connecting place p to transition t.
2. Depending on the modelled system, an enabled transition may be fired or not.
3. When an enabled transition t is fired, $w(p_i, t)$ tokens are deleted from input place p_i and $w(t, p_j)$ tokens are added to output place p_j.

3.3 Rule Representation Through CCPN

In order to describe rules based on GDM, a PN extension named CCPN model [8,9], is applied. The CCPN model was introduced as an alternative to define ECA rules in ADB environments, and it is able to store events, conditions and actions of ECA rules.

3.4   ECA Rule Elements in CCPN Model

CCPN model inherits the attributes and firing rule of PNs. Moreover, CPN concepts are also taken into account in CCPN model, such as data type definition, color (values) assignment to tokens, and data type assignment to places.

An ECA rule is composed of an *event* that enables it, and it could be fired depending on the evaluation of the conditional part. Primitive events are represented by an unique input place p_i, and if the primitive event occurs, then a token is placed in p_i denoting the event's happening.

On the other hand, composite events has their own representation as a CCPN structure [9]. Every constituent event is denoted as an input place connected to a special transition called *composite transition* and it is drawn as a double bar. This type of event occurs when its constituent events happen according to the composite event description. When each constituent event happens, a token is situated inside the corresponding place, and depending on the composite event description, it will happen or not. Every token stores a set of values (colors) about the event, such as the occurrence time (timestamp), record information, modified value, etc.

In order to trigger an ECA rule, a condition is evaluated. In CCPN model, the conditional part is defined as part of a transition. Then, by triggering an ECA rule in a CCPN model when the evaluated condition is true, a special type of transition is used. Rule transitions are drawn as rectangles in the PN graph, see Fig. 2.

The third element of the ECA rule is the action part. This element is executed once the *event* occurs and the conditional part is fulfilled. *Action* can modify the DB state and is represented in the CCPN model as an output place from the rule transition.

A CCPN is defined as follows [8]:

Definition 1. *A Conditional Colored Petri Net (CCPN) is a 11-tuple:*

$$CCPN = \{\Sigma, P, T, F, N, C, Con, Act, D, \tau, I\}$$

where:
Σ is a finite set of data type, called colors.
P, T and F are the same as traditional PNs.
$N : F \rightarrow P \times T \cup T \times P$ is a node function.
$C : P \rightarrow 2^{\Sigma}$ is a color function.
Con is a function that evaluates the conditional part.
Act is a function that executes the action part of the ECA rule.
D is a time interval function, used in composite events that includes time periods or intervals.

$\tau : M(p) \to R^+$ *is a timestamp function.*
$I : P \to C(p)$ *is a function for initializing tokens in the CCPN model.*

4   GDM Rules Modeled by CCPN

Traditionally GDM rules are modeled as *Condition-Action* (CA) rules instead of ECA rules. Thus, in order to represent GDM rules as a CCPN structure, first we need to apply the ECA rule model to GDM rules. The CA rule model lacks of the event part, and most of time its conditional part contains the event that enables the rule, considered as a condition to trigger it. Thus, we can separate the conditional part of a CA rule into events and conditions, and be able to define the three elements of an ECA rule. For instance, the rule:

```
if rain_sensor, then close_windows & close_domes
```

contains only the conditional and the action part. The condition *if rain_sensor* can be divided in two parts: first, the rain sensor is detecting the rain, thus it can be considered as an event that changes the state of the environment. Secondly, the value of the sensor changes from a *false* value into a *true* value, which can be defined as the conditional part. Now, we are able to define an ECA rule with its three elements as follows:

```
ON UPDATE_RainSensor_value, IF update.value = true, THEN UPDATE
WindowStatus set status = 'close'  & UPDATE DomeStatus set status
= 'close';
```

The CCPN of the previous rule is shown in Fig. 2.

A similar strategy can be applied to convert a GDM rule set into ECA rules, and after that, in a CCPN structure.

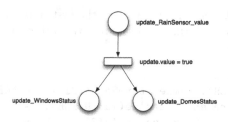

Fig. 2. A GDM rule denoted as a CCPN model.

5   CCPN Methodology for GDM Systems

In order to validate the feasibility of our proposal, to discover and solve non-determinism and ambiguity in a set of group knowledge rules, we apply this methodology to a set of GDM rules obtained from the consensus (agreement) of several experts from different SH supervision areas, such as Energy Saving, Comfort and Security.

5.1   Excerpt of a GDM Rules Set

In order to provide support to inhabitants of a SH and based on the environment temperature, SH security and lighting, seven rules of our GDM Rules Set are figured out on the CCPN structure. The rule set contains the following rules:

R1: if rain_sensor then close_windows & close_domes

R2: if temperature_sensor > 40 & temperature_sensor < ext_temperature_sensor & expert_mode = 'energy saving' then open_windows & open_domes

R3: if temperature_sensor > 40 & expert_mode = 'comfort' then open_windows & open_domes

R4: if temperature_sensor < 15 & air_conditioner_status = 'on' then air_conditioner_status = 'off'

R5: if ~presence then electronic_lock_status = 'on'

R6: if ~presence & lighting_sensor then lighting_status = 'off'

R7: if presence & ~lighting_sensor then lighting_status = 'on'

These rules are originally defined as CA rules, and transformed into ECA rules in the next section.

5.2   ECA Rule Definition

To transform the CA rules into ECA rules, the first step is to identify the event and condition for each CA rule, and separate them to create the corresponding ECA rules as follows.

```
// Table definition
Expert(mode INTEGER); TemperatureSensorR1(id INTEGER, value
FLOAT); TemperatureSensorOutside(id INTEGER, value FLOAT);
PresenceSensor(id INTEGER, value INTEGER); RainSensor(id INTEGER,
value INTEGER); WindowState(id INTEGER, status INTEGER);
DomeState(id INTEGER, status INTEGER); AirConditionerState(id
INTEGER, status INTEGER); ElectronicBolt(id INTEGER, status
INTEGER); LuminositySensor(id INTEGER, status INTEGER);
CommonLight(id INTEGER, status INTEGER);

// Event definition
e0: UPDATE_TemperatureSensorR1_value; e1: UPDATE_RainSensor_value;
e2: UPDATE_PresenceSensor_value; e3:
UPDATE_LuminositySensor_status;
```

```
// Rules definition
Rule 1: ON UPDATE_RainSensor_value, IF update.value = 1, THEN
UPDATE WindowState set value=0 & UPDATE DomeState set status=0;

Rule 2: ON UPDATE_TemperatureSensorR1_value, IF update.value > 40
& update.value < TemperatureSensorOutside.value & Expert.mode =
'Energy saving', THEN UPDATE WindowState set status = 'Open' &
UPDATE DomeState set status = 'Open';

Rule 3: ON UPDATE_TemperatureSensorR1_value, IF update.value > 40
& Expert.mode = 'Comfort', THEN UPDATE AirConditionerState set
status = 'On';

Rule 4: ON UPDATE_TemperatureSensorR1_value, IF update.value < 15
& AirConditionerState = 'On', THEN UPDATE AirConditionerState set
status = 'Off';

Rule 5: ON not(e2), IF PresenceSensor.value = 'Off', THEN UPDATE
ElectronicBolt set status = 'Close';

Rule 6: ON and(not(e2):e3), IF PresenceSensor.value='Off' &
LuminositySensor.value='On', THEN UPDATE CommonLight set
status='Off';

Rule 7: ON and(e2:not(e3)), IF PresenceSensor.value='On' &
LuminositySensor.value='Off', THEN UPDATE CommonLight set
status='On';
```

5.3 CCPN Rule Set

The ECA rule set is now transformed into a CCPN structure (Fig. 3). The relationship among ECA rules and CCPN elements is described in Table 1, where transitions denoted as rectangles $(t_2, t_3, t_4, t_5, t_{12}, t_{14}, t_{15})$ to represent ECA rules; transitions are drawn as bars (t_1, t_6, t_8, t_{10}) and transitions are depicted with a double-line for indicating composite events $(t_7, t_9, t_{11}, t_{13})$.

Places are divided into four categories. $i)$ Places drawn with a single line represent primitive events $(p_1, p_5, p_6, p_7, p_8, p_9, p_{11}, p_{20}, p_{22})$; $ii)$ Places denoted by a double solid line circumference correspond to *negation* composite events (p_{14}, p_{15}); $iii)$ Places depicted as a double circumference, with its inner circumference as a dashed one, indicate event replicas utilized in different rules or to be considered in a composite event $(p_2, p_3, p_4, p_{10}, p_{12}, p_{16}, p_{17}, p_{18})$; and places drawn as a dashed circumferences (p_{19}, p_{21}) represent the rest of composite events.

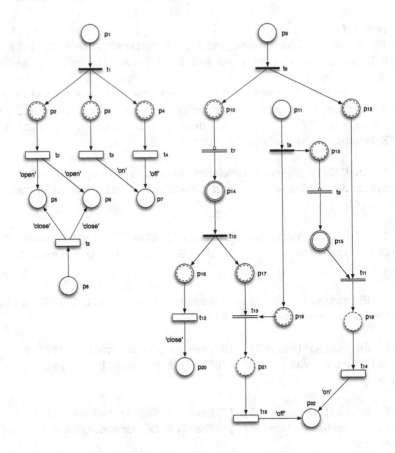

Fig. 3. CCPN model for an excerpt of a GDM rule set.

5.4   CCPN Matrix Representation

A CCPN model with m transitions and n places can also be represented as an $m \times n$ matrix.

In the CCPN model of Fig. 3, the representation of Rule 1 to Rule 4 includes places $p_1, p_2, \ldots p_8$ and transitions $t_1, t_2, \ldots, t_5$. Thus, the incidence matrix corresponding to this part of the CCPN model and representing Rule 1 to Rule 4 is shown in Eq. (1).

$$
A = \begin{array}{c} \\ t_1 \\ t_2 \\ t_3 \\ t_4 \\ t_5 \end{array}
\begin{array}{c} p_1\ p_2\ p_3\ p_4\ p_5\ p_6\ p_7\ p_8 \\
\left[\begin{array}{rrrrrrrr}
-1 & 1 & 1 & 1 & 0 & 0 & 0 & 0 \\
0 & -1 & 0 & 0 & 1 & 1 & 0 & 0 \\
0 & 0 & -1 & 0 & 0 & 0 & 1 & 0 \\
0 & 0 & 0 & -1 & 0 & 0 & 1 & 0 \\
0 & 0 & 0 & 0 & 1 & 1 & 0 & -1
\end{array} \right]
\end{array}
\tag{1}
$$

Table 1. Places and transitions meaning.

Place	Description	Transition	Description
p_1	UPDATE_TemperatureSensorR1_value	t_1	Copy of p_1
p_2	Copy of p_1	t_2	Condition of rule 2
p_3	Copy of p_1	t_3	Condition of rule 3
p_4	Copy of p_1	t_4	Condition of rule 4
p_5	UPDATE_WindowState_status	t_5	Condition of rule 1
p_6	UPDATE_DomeState_status	t_6	Copy of p_9
p_7	UPDATE_AirConditionerState_status	t_7	Composite event Neg
p_8	UPDATE_RainSensor_value	t_8	Copy of p_{11}
p_9	UPDATE_PresenceSensor_value	t_9	Composite event Neg
p_{10}	Copy of p_9	t_{10}	Copy of p_{14}
p_{11}	UPDATE_LuminositySensor_status	t_{11}	Composite event And
p_{12}	Copy of p_9	t_{12}	Condition of rule 5
p_{13}	Copy of p_{11}	t_{13}	Composite event And
p_{14}	Composite event Neg	t_{14}	Condition of rule 7
p_{15}	Composite event Neg	t_{15}	Condition of rule 6
p_{16}	Copy of p_{14}		
p_{17}	Copy of p_{14}		
p_{18}	Copy of p_{11}		
p_{19}	Composite event And		
p_{20}	UPDATE_ElectronicBolt_status		
p_{21}	Composite event And		
p_{22}	UPDATE_CommonLight_status		

The incidence matrix can be utilized to detect inconsistencies in a ECA rule set[2]. From Fig. 3, we note that input arcs for places p_5, p_6, p_7, and p_{22} are in conflict, since all of them have opposite action commands. Analytically, the identification of this kind of conflicts can be done by applying the next algorithm to the incidence matrix.

Algorithm 1: CCPN Conflict Detection and Resolution

Step 1: Identify the places having two or more input arcs.
$P_x = \{p|p \in P, |{}^\bullet p| > 1.\}$
In this case: $P_x = \{p_5, p_6, p_7, p_{22}\}$

Step 2: For each place in P_x, detect the places having the same action for every input action command, and remove them from P_x.
$P_y = \{p|p \in P, Action_i(p) = Action_j(p)\}$, $P_x = P_x - P_y$
In this case: $P_y = \emptyset$, $P_x = \{p_5, p_6, p_7, p_{22}\} - \emptyset = \{p_5, p_6, p_7, p_{22}\}$

---
[2] represented in a CCPN scheme.

Step 3: For each place p_j in P_x, analyze if its input arcs have the same origin, i.e. if in the incidence matrix previous places to p_j can be located. For each positive integer value located in column j, search for negative integer values in their corresponding row. Then, for each negative value located, search for positive integer values in their corresponding column.

Step 4: If there are no more either positive or negative values in the same column or row, respectively, stop.

Step 5: If there is at least one place belonging to different paths, it means that one rule produces the same action with different values through different paths. Nondeterminism and ambiguity is detected. Go to Step 7.

Step 6: If the analyzed place p_j is not the same at the different paths, it means that the sources for p_j come from different places. Nondeterminism and ambiguity is nonexistent. Go to Step 7.

In our example, places p_5, p_6, p_7, and $p_{22} \in P_x$, however not all of them have the same origin. Input arcs for p_5 and p_6 come from different initial places. Thus, they can be deleted from P_x. In Eq. (2) the paths found for the place p_5 are shown. The first one contains places $\{p_2, p_1\}$, and the second one contains the place $\{p_8\}$. $\{p_2, p_1\} \cap \{p_8\} = \emptyset$, thus p_5 can be removed from P_x. The same procedure is applied for removing p_6.

$$
A = \begin{array}{c} \\ t_1 \\ t_2 \\ t_3 \\ t_4 \\ t_5 \end{array}
\begin{array}{c} p_1\ \ p_2\ \ p_3\ \ p_4\ \ (p_5)\ \ p_6\ \ p_7\ \ p_8 \\
\left[\begin{array}{cccccccc}
-1 & 1 & 1 & 1 & 0 & 0 & 0 & 0 \\
0 & -1 & 0 & 0 & 1 & 1 & 0 & 0 \\
0 & 0 & -1 & 0 & 0 & 0 & 1 & 0 \\
0 & 0 & 0 & -1 & 0 & 0 & 1 & 0 \\
0 & 0 & 0 & 0 & 1 & 1 & 0 & -1
\end{array} \right]
\end{array}
$$

$$(2)$$

Step 7: Identify if the composite event *Negation* is contained in any rule.

For this example, $p_{22} \in P_x$ has the same initial places (p_9 and p_{11}), and both input arcs come from composite event *Conjunction*, however, both conjunctions include the composite event *Negation*, then it never will occur that p_{22} receive two tokens at the same time, and it can be removed from P_x.

Step 8: If $P_x \neq \emptyset$, there is at least one place having the same origin place and coming from different paths. The expert who has the highest priority takes the decision about the rule that will be fired. At this moment, the GDM system receives the information and support the decision-making process. After that, the CCPN system triggers only the rule(s) chosen by the GDM system.

Step 9: End.

In this example, $P_x = \{p_7\}$, and Eq. (3) shows how p_7 is reached from different paths but starting at the same initial place p_1.

$$A = \begin{array}{c} \\ t_1 \\ t_2 \\ t_3 \\ t_4 \\ t_5 \end{array} \begin{array}{c} \begin{array}{cccccccc} p_1 & p_2 & p_3 & p_4 & p_5 & p_6 & \boxed{p_7} & p_8 \end{array} \\ \left[\begin{array}{cccccccc} -1 & 1 & 1 & 1 & 0 & 0 & 0 & 0 \\ 0 & -1 & 0 & 0 & 1 & 1 & 0 & 0 \\ 0 & 0 & -1 & 0 & 0 & 0 & 1 & 0 \\ 0 & 0 & 0 & -1 & 0 & 0 & 1 & 0 \\ 0 & 0 & 0 & 0 & 1 & 1 & 0 & -1 \end{array} \right] \end{array}$$

$$(3)$$

6 Concluding Remarks and Future Work

An extended PN model, called Conditional Colored Petri Net, CCPN) has been applied to represent rules in SH, which are denoted as ECA rules. The CCPN is able to detect changes or events in the environment, and if enabled rules are true, then they execute their action part via their actuators in the SH. Furthermore, the CCPN works together with GDM system to solve possible nondeterminism and ambiguity in the rule set definition. Furthermore, the rules set defined for smart environments can be modelled, analyzed, simulated, verified and executed in the same framework based on CCPN.

In order to show the feasibility of our approach, an excerpt of seven CA rules are presented and converted into ECA rules, and then depicted as a CCPN structure. The CCPN incidence matrix was used to detect those rules that could produce ambiguity in the rule set, and the GDM system sets the execution priority to the rules in conflict.

As a future work, the CCPN model will be enhanced with fuzzy logic theory, in order to model uncertainty in the SH behavior. On the other hand, new analysis tools and algorithms based on PN theory can be included in the proposed framework to carry out a more complete study in SH rules.

Acknowledgments. This work was financially supported by the "Consejo Nacional de Ciencia y Tecnología - CONACYT-Mexico" within the Project Grant CB-2014-01-236818. The authors would like also to express their gratitude to the anonymous reviewers for their very useful comments.

References

1. A Boundless Concept Version 7: Advantages and Disadvantages of Group Decision Making. Boundless Management (2015). https://www.boundless.com/management/textbooks/boundless-management-textbook/decision-making-10/managing-group-decision-making-81/advantages-and-disadvantages-of-group-decision-making-388-5156/
2. Chana, M., Esteve, D., Escriba, C., Campo, E.: A review of smart homespresent state and future challenges. Comput. Methods Progr. Biomed. **91**, 55–81 (2008)
3. Cook, D.J., Augusto, J.C., Jakkula, V.R.: Ambient intelligence: applications in society and opportunities for AI. Pervasive Mob. Comput. **5**, 277–298 (2009)
4. Crawford, G., Williams, C.: A note on the analysis of subjective judgement matrices. J. Math. Psychol. **29**, 387–405 (1985)

5. De Silva, L.C., Morikawab, C., Petraa, I.M.: State of the art of smart homes. Eng. Appl. Artif. Intell. **25**(7), 1313–1322 (2012)
6. Jensen, K.: Coloured Petri Nets. Basic Concepts, Analysis Methods and Practical Use. Basic Concepts, vol. 1. Springer, Berlin (1992)
7. Jensen, K.: Coloured Petri Nets. Basic Concepts, Analysis Methods and Practical Use. Analysis Methods, vol. 2. Springer, Berlin (1994)
8. Li, X., Medina, J., Chapa, S.V.: Applying petri nets in active database systems. IEEE Trans. Syst. Man, Cybern. Part C: Appl. Rev. **37**(4), 482–493 (2007)
9. Li, X., Medina, J., Chavarría, L.: Composite event specification in active database systems: a petri nets approach. In: Proceedings of the Fifth Workshop and Tutorial on Practical Use of Coloured Petri Nets and the CPN Tools, pp. 8–11 (2004)
10. Limayem, M., Chelbi, A.: Improving multicriteria group decision making with automated decision guidance. In: Proceedings of the Systems, Man, and Cybernetics. Computational Cybernetics and Simulation, vol. 2, pp. 1890–1895, October 1997
11. López-Morales, V., Medina-Marín, J.: Methods and Algorithms for an Automated Group Decision-Making System. Technical report from Instituto de Ciencias Básicas e Ingenierías, UAEH, ICBI (2015)
12. Murata, T.: Petri nets: properties, analysis and applications. Proc. IEEE **77**(4), 541–580 (1989)
13. Nugent, C., Augusto, J.C.: Proceedings of the 4th International Conference on Smart Homes and Health Telematic (ICOST 2006), Belfast, UK. Assistive Technology Research, vol. 19, June 2006
14. Paton, N.W., Díaz, O.: Active database systems. ACM Comput. Surv. **31**(1), 63–103 (1999)
15. de Ruyter, B.E.A.: Ambient intelligence: visualizing the future. In: Proceedings of the Working Conference on Advanced Visual Interfaces (2004)
16. Saaty, T.: The Analytic Hierarchy Process. McGraw-Hill, New York (1980)
17. Saaty, T.: Decision-making with the ahp: why is the principal eigenvector necessary. Eur. J. Oper. Res. **145**, 85–91 (2003)
18. Wu, Z., Xu, J.: A consistency and consensus based decision support model for group decision making with multiplicative preference relations. Decis. Support Syst. **52**(3), 757–767 (2012)

Author Index

Printed in the United States
By Bookmasters